Dr. YOUNGSAM KIM'S
CLINICAL NOTES

Easy Simple Safe Efficient Minimally Invasive & Atraumatic *Gangnam Style* Extraction of Third Molars

AUTHOR

Youngsam Kim DDS, MS, PhD

CO-AUTHORS

Jae-wook Lee
Min-gyo Seo
Jonathan Jong-hwan Lim
Dae-yong Kim
Young-hoon Pyun

SUPERVISION

Seung-O Ko

TRANSLATORS

Jong Wook Hur
GiTae Kwon
Jong Yoon
Scott J-S Park
Ryan Dongchan Seo
Min Ji Kwon
Addie Yoojung Chang
YouRee Lim
Edward Jh Lee
Leandro Choe
Joung Lee

EASY, SIMPLE, SAFE, EFFICIENT,
MINIMALLY INVASIVE & ATRAUMATIC *Gangnam Style*
EXTRACTION OF THIRD MOLARS

1st Publication : 2018-11-10
2nd Publication : 2019-5-20
3rd Publication : 2019-12-20
4th Publication : 2022-05-15
5th Publication : 2024-07-20

Author : Youngsam Kim
Editor : Su-in Han
Text Designer : Ji-won Shin
Cover Designer : Jae-wook Kim
Illustrator : Hak-yeoung Yu

Permissions may be sought at Koonja's rights department:
Tel: (82)-31-943-1888
Fax: (82)-31-955-9545
www.koonja.co.kr

Printed in South Korea
First Edition, © 2019 Koonja publishing, Inc.
ISBN 979-11-5955-380-6

USD 220.00

Easy Simple Safe Efficient
Minimally Invasive & Atraumatic
Extraction of Third Molars GANGNAM STYLE

AUTHOR

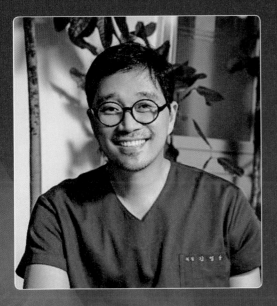

Youngsam Kim DDS, MS, PhD

Jeonju Highschool
Chonbuk National University School of Dentistry
Chonbuk National University Masters Degree
Chonbuk National University PhD
University of Toronto Faculty of Dentistry Periodontics-Implant CE
UCLA School of Dentistry Periodontics Preceptorship

Current

Principal Dentist at Gangnam Dental Clinic
Associate professor at Jeonbuk National University School of Dentistry
Associate professor at Yonsei University College of Dentistry
Associate professor at Pusan National University School of Dentistry
Faculty member of Ostem(Hiossen) Implant Korea
Head director of Dentis Implant continuing education
Director of Gangnam Academy of Wisdom tooth Extraction (GAWE)
Director of Gangnam Academy of Dental Implantology (GADI)
UCLA School of Dentistry Oral Maxillofacial Surgery Preceptor

Contact

⊚ youngsamkimdds
f youngsamkimdds
▶ youngsamkimdds

CO-AUTHORS

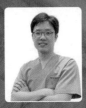

Jae-wook Lee
Oral Maxillofacial Surgeon
Kyoung Hee University School
of Dentistry,
Kyoung Hee University School
of Dentistry,
Department of Oral
Maxillofacial Surgery

Min-gyo Seo
Oral Maxillofacial Surgeon
Chonbuk National University
School of Dentistry,
Chonbuk National University
School of Dentistry,
Department of Oral
Maxillofacial Surgery

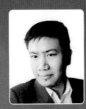

Jonathan Jong-hwan Lim
Oral Maxillofacial Surgeon
Seoul National University School of
Dentistry
Samsung Medical Centre Oral
Maxillofacial Surgery

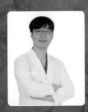

Dae-yong Kim
Kyungpook National University,
School of Dentistry
Faculty member of GAWE,
GADI,
Dentis Implant

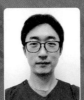

Young-hoon Pyun
Oral Maxillofacial Surgeon
Chosun University Dental
College
Inha University School of
Dentistry,
Department of Oral
Maxillofacial Surgery

Supervision
Seung-O Ko

Oral Maxillofacial Surgeon
Professor at Chonbuk National University
Department of Oral Maxillofacial Surgery

TRANSLATORS

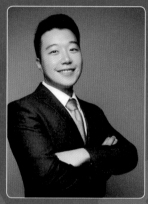

Dr. Jong Wook Hur
BOH DSc, GD Dent.

🇦🇺 **Griffith University School of Dentistry**

🇦🇺 **New South Wales, Australia**

Chapter 1   Chapter 2

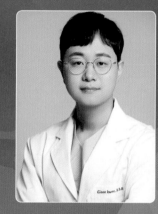

Dr. GiTae Kwon DDS

🇺🇸 **New York University College of Dentistry**

🇺🇸 **Connecticut, USA**

Chapter 3

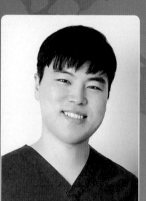

Dr. Jong Yoon DDS

🇺🇸 **University of California, San Francisco**

🇺🇸 **Washington, USA**

Chapter 4

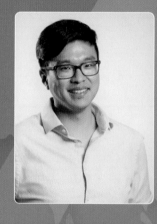

Dr. Scott J-S Park BDSc

🇦🇺 **University of Queensland**

🇦🇺 **Canberra, ACT, Australia**

Chapter 5

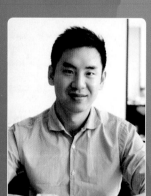

Dr. Ryan Dongchan Seo
BDSc

🇦🇺 **University of Queensland**

🇦🇺 **Brisbane, Australia**

Chapter 5-1

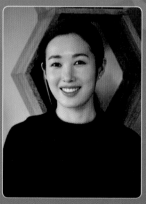

Dr. Min Ji Kwon BDSc

🇦🇺 **University of Queensland**

🇦🇺 **Griffith, NSW, Australia**

Chapter 5-2

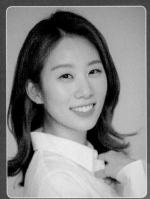

Dr. Addie Yoojung Chang
DMD

🏳️ **Tufts University School of Dental Medicine**

🏳️ **Seattle, Washington, USA**

Chapter 6

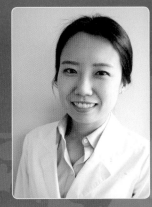

Dr. YouRee Lim DDS

🇨🇦 **University of Toronto**

🇨🇦 **Toronto, ON, Canada**

Chapter 7

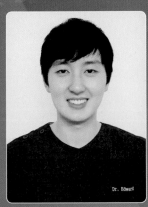

Dr. Edward Jh Lee
Bdent. Mdent. MSc. FICOI. DICOI.

🇦🇺 **La Trobe University**

🇩🇪 **Goethe-University Frankfurt**

🇦🇺 **Melbourne, Australia**

Chapter 8

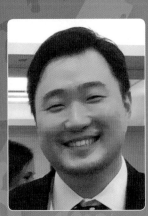

Dr. Leandro Choe DMD

🏳️ **Tufts University School of Dental Medicine**

🏳️ **Los Angeles, CA, USA**

Chapter 9

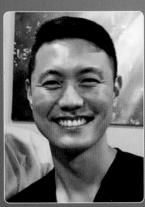

Dr. Joung Lee DMD

🏳️ **Nova Southeastern University**

🏳️ **San Antonio, TX, USA**

Chapter 10

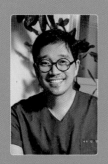

Youngsam Kim

Principal Dentist
at Gangnam Dental Clinic
in Korea

Foreword by Author

Hello, my name is Youngsam Kim, a dentist who loves to do wisdom teeth extractions.

Let me briefly explain how I have first become recognised as a leader of the field in South Korea, which was long before I was invited to lecture all around the world. When I opened my own practice in 2002, even the most surgically challenging third molar extraction surgery had a government enforced fee-schedule of approximately 30-40USD per tooth. It is merely 1/100th of the cost of a dental implant at the time. This is because basic dental care is a publicly funded health service in South Korea. Once a treatment is categorised to be a part of 'essential public care', it is illegal for dentists to charge any more than the fee schedule outlined by the government. The 'low fee, high risk' factor drove most dentists away from third molar extractions to focus more on higher production procedures. I saw this as an opportunity and started extracting third molars that the others refused to operate on. Eventually, as much as half of my day consisted of third molar extractions. On average, I was extracting up to 20 wisdom teeth a day and as many as 3-400 a month on a busy month. According to Korean government records, I was top of the nation in the number of wisdom teeth extracted over past 17 years.

I've become better and faster as I've extracted more and more wisdom teeth. My passion for wisdom teeth surgery continued to grow and finally, several years ago, I started writing columns and giving lectures on third molar extractions. As implants grew quite popular in South Korea, there was this newly stirred up interest in third molar extractions as well, which, in turn, made me quite famous as an expert in the field. Interestingly, since providing third molar extractions are much better compensated in other countries, my book and courses received even more attention and demand abroad. So with gratitude, here I am translating my book into English.

In South Korea, where implants are already quite popular, more than 80% of dentists place their own implants these days. In other countries, the proportion may be less, but I believe that it will eventually reach the comparable level, and this will naturally increase the demand for dentists around the world to perform extractions themselves including third molars. I have noticed that most dentists who extract third molars routinely tend to think that they are quite good at what they do, perhaps because at the end of the day, the teeth are all out and the patients all survive. This may explain the overall lack of resources and platforms available for dentists to learn and improve on this particular topic. In my opinion, however, successful third molar extractions or any other extractions should involve more than just the physical removal of teeth. They should also be performed in a way that is as atraumatic and minimally invasive as possible, so that the patient's post-operative discomfort is minimized. This book outlines the techniques and skills I have developed throughout my career to achieve the goals of "Easy, Simple, Safe, and Efficient" while also being atraumatic and minimally invasive. I strongly believe that these principles will also allow you to perform all surgical procedures more efficiently and predictably.

I debated until the very last moment whether I should publish this book…

As you read this book, you may find some typos and words that do not flow well. Even after the translation process was completed, I kept asking myself if I should take more time before publishing this book. Whenever I reviewed, there were always some new things I noticed that could be improved, and this made me wish my English had been better.

However, since it's very hard and rare to find textbooks that are specifically on third molar extractions, I have been told by many dentists around the world have been waiting for my book to be translated into English. It was so humbling to hear that some even purchased my Korean prints to read using Google Translator, which as we all know is far from perfect and often misrepresents the message. For such passionate dentists and colleagues, I decided to publish it as soon as possible without further ado. My hope is that even if translation isn't perfect, the book will still be meaningful as the very first English version and will be far better than just Google Translate.

Therefore, I apologize in advance if you find some loose ends in this book. I hope I can publish the second version with all those tied up, along with some revisions and improvements based on the feedback from you readers in the future.

CONTENTS

03
CHAPTER

Wisdom Tooth Coronectomy

04
CHAPTER

Anesthesia, Incision, Surgical Flap Design, Suture for highlighted all other Wisdom Tooth Extraction

CONTENTS

CONTENTS

CONTENTS

08
CHAPTER

Horizontally Impacted
Wisdom Tooth

09
CHAPTER

Upper Third Molar

CONTENTS

10
CHAPTER

Common Problems
related to Extractions of
Third Molars

APPENDIX

CHAPTER

Issues with Third Molars

How to navigate through this book ★★★

I want to be someone who is good at teaching how to perform third molar extractions well, not someone who is good at extracting wisdom teeth.

I have been lecturing on wisdom tooth surgery for ten years, and it has been more than five years since I became one of the first dentists in Korea who launched a dental education institute dedicated for wisdom tooth surgery. The reason I am sharing this information as an author is because I genuinely hope that you can improve your surgical competency by following my advice in the book. I think my guide can still be helpful for already competent dentists in oral surgery because you can still incorporate my useful tips into your usual surgical routine. However, if you are just starting wisdom tooth extractions in your practice, reading through this book just once will not all of a sudden turn you into a proficient operator. I would strongly encourage you to get involved in a long-term wisdom tooth study club (accredited by your state/country jurisdiction) at least once a month. For most inexperienced dentists, it may be difficult to gain the surgical skills necessary to remove wisdom teeth right away. I encourage you to attend hands-on seminars to hone your surgical skills whilst treating your patients. Repetition is required to improve your surgical skills.

I would like you to take this same approach when reading this book. Although it may only take a few days to finish the entire book, beginners may not find this book very helpful the first time through. Therefore, I would strongly encourage you to follow my guide below.

I've separated this book into three sections by the number of stars. Start by first lightly skimming through sections with three-stars (★★★) which is indicated on top of the page. I would not recommend the readers to read the book too thoroughly from the beginning to the end because some parts are repeated numerous times. It may sound confusing, but it may be beneficial to skim through the content of each chapter and then to go back to the beginning. Then, start with simple extractions in your practice followed by reading the sections with two-stars (★★). You may skip the part with one-star (★) in the beginning. Once you find joy in wisdom tooth surgeries and develop more interest, you can go back to this section later. It would not be too late to go back to the one-star (★) section then if you are in the process of learning my surgical technique and incorporating it into your routine. I hope you find the book easy to read because the textbook has numerous illustrations throughout the book. Please think of me as a helpful educator rather than a dentist who is merely good at wisdom teeth extractions. I encourage you to follow my guidance above.

Because this book is an amalgamated version of numerous PowerPoint presentation of my wisdom tooth surgery lectures (usually 12 hrs in duration or longer over 2 days), terminology and literary style may be different throughout the book. All details are from previously created PowerPoint files that I have been working on for a long time. There could be overlapping or repeated information throughout the book. Some lectures were presented from the beginning to the end in continuation whereas some were presented by focusing only on specific subjects. Therefore, I hope you understand the reason behind some repeated information in the book. Nonetheless, several pieces of information are purposely reemphasized for their importance. I ask that you please have an open mind as you are reading my book.

If this is your first time reading this book, read through ★★★ sections first.

Before you read further!

I decided to write in the most basic Korean/English language as possible

A lot of dentists from overseas showed interest in my lectures when I uploaded them to the internet. There were particularly strong interests from Korean dentists residing in North America and Australia. However, many of these Koreans dentists immigrated when they werein their teenage years. Therefore, they are not familiar with Korean dental words such as the crown, mesial, distal, or coronal, etc. To complicate matters even more, most Korean dental terminologies stem from old language that is not commonly used in casual conversations. I received lots of questions about dental are not familiar with so I tried to use the most basic Korean words in my book wherever I can. Just as I had done so for my Korean prints, I attempted to do the same in my English version for ease of reading and understanding so that even if English is not your first language, it would be easier to read and understand my messages. As I mentioned before, the content of the book is from my previous PowerPoint lecture presentations I made a long time ago and thus there is some inconsistency in certain terminology used throughout the book. I feel embarrassed for not having the most stylistically written book, but some people would prefer a book that is informal and easy to read. I ask that you please focus on my intentions and messages rather than the style of the way it is written and translated.

There aren't enough photos

Not even a single image in the book is altered or edited although the quality of the printed copies become less than ideal when compared to the digital images. I was tempted to enhance the images to make them more palatable, but I wanted to document everything as factual as possible to maintain the integrity of the book.

It was not easy to document photos before or during surgery since my clinic is an incredibly fast-paced private practice and not an academic institution. I got into a habit of piecing together the separated crown and roots like a puzzle on top of the surgical apron for photos after discharging my patients. My schedule is quite busy and I rarely have the time to take quality photos. Sometimes I asked my clinic staff to piece the sectioned teeth together for photographs, but many were unusable for presentation because they were incorrectly put together.

In my clinic, after having wisdom teeth removed from one side, patients return to have wisdom teeth removed from the opposite side. You can often predict how the other side will pan out by examining the previous post-operation photos. I usually do not take any pictures of extracted wisdom tooth which did not require tooth sectioning. However, this information would also be useful because I can predict to some degree that I would not need to section the opposite side either.

I had been planning to write a wisdom tooth surgery book for the past 4~5 years, but I could not put together satisfactory contents because I only had post-operative images after the extractions. I tried to collect more before and during surgery images while writing this book. This process was more challenging than I had anticipated. I hope you can understand why I could not document more images in the book for the reasons stated above. Most pictures taken during surgery are from patients who are my relatives, clinic staff, and their family and friends. Thorough documentation still proved difficult even if knew the patients well and had their consent for photography because often my staff were too busy to take multiple progress photographs for during surgeries due to the busy clinic schedule. To overcome this problem, I decided to launch my wisdom tooth surgery hands-on courses. I could document more efficiently during my live surgeries and take necessary images and videos. This way I could include these valuable data in my book.

Dr. Youngsam Kim's ESSE Dental Philosophy ★★★

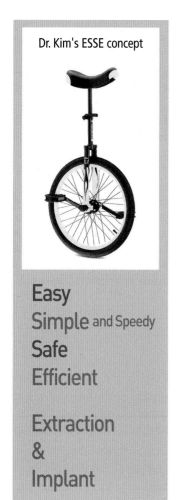

Dr. Kim's ESSE concept

Easy
Simple and Speedy
Safe
Efficient

Extraction
&
Implant

ESSE Extraction of Third Molar

My philosophy of wisdom tooth extraction could be described as ESSE (Easy, Simple, Safe, and Efficient). People who watch my extraction surgery frequently say the same thing. Rather than praising my surgical ability, they say that I make the procedure look easy. If I extract one or two teeth easily, it can be seen as a coincidence, but after watching my surgeries for a while, they say all of my treatments appear effortless. All wisdom teeth are extracted by implementing the same principles with similar surgical technique. You will get to know how I could do them effortlessly once you read this book till the end.

I added the word "safe" in my philosophy because if the surgery is not performed safely, regardless of how quickly and effortlessly, it cannot be a practice builder. The dentist must compensate the patient for any injuries and this carries tremendous psychological stress and fear associated with any major surgical complication that can arise. Lastly, The reason I emphasized "Efficient" especially in my Korean version of this book is because the hard fee schedule for extractions set by the Korean national dental insurance is very low. When I first opened my practice, all senior dentists told me the same thing--instead of performing wisdom tooth surgeries, I should just rest or exercise because wisdom tooth extractions have a little return on investment. In South Korea, the unfortunate reality is that dentists must reduce as much overhead as reasonable to make any profit in performing extractions without sacrificing the quality of care, which is challenging. Although the cost of extraction is low and unproductive it was a blessing in disguise because I was able to perform numerous extractions as much as I wanted, which I enjoy a lot.

Now, let's learn about wisdom tooth surgery by following the principles of ESSE. Some dentists want to include "Speedy" in the abbreviation, but if the surgery is easy and simple, it is difficult not to be speedy. Therefore, I found the word to be redundant but decided to keep it in a smaller font right next to "Simple" simply because there happens to be enough space for this word in the box.

We're not trying to learn to ride a unicycle

Every dentist's ability and skills are all different. A dentist's physique, physical strengths, athletic ability, and spatial awareness are entirely different from another. Some may learn to ride a unicycle within a few hours whereas others may never be able to ride it even with extensive training.

Therefore, I wrote this book like I'm teaching how to ride a bicycle. Most people can learn how to ride it with some practice. I'm sure some still will not be able to ride it well but most learn to ride it well with practice. Before starting our lessons together, not only is it important to recognize one's current skill level but it is also essential to be aware of how much you can improve as a dentist.

Let's analyze your ability. I think spatial awareness is the most crucial ability in wisdom tooth surgeries. Having adequate physical strength also helps immensely.

In this book, I would like to believe that I explained how to ride a bicycle, that most people can learn eventually with enough practice and trial and error.

Now, let's get on a bicycle and go on this ride together.

Let's purchase these instruments before you proceed further ★★★

Please invest in the following instruments before you read this book. I recommend Hu-Friedy 222 forceps for mandibular and Hu-Friedy 10S forceps for the maxillary wisdom teeth. It is not necessary to buy these forceps if you are currently satisfied with what you are already using. But I would highly recommend these forceps if you do not have a favorite one. The next instrument I highly recommend is Hu-Friedy EL3C elevator. It would be pointless to continue reading this book without this instrument. This instrument is a must buy, and I cannot emphasize this enough. It is inexpensive, and I have been recommending this elevator at my seminars for a long time. I have not received any negative feedback about this instrument, yet. Trust me and purchase this elevator. Even if you are working at an office that is not your own, buy this elevator at your own expense, and you will not regret it.

In the picture below are the periosteal elevator (Hu-Friedy P9) and surgical currette (Hu-Friedy CM11). Any similar instruments would be fine. However, the periosteal elevator should be designed with a knife-like edge in one end to reflect a clean flap; and the surgical currette should not be too large (approximately 2.5 mm in diameter). The downside of such a smaller currette is that it can break and therefore I would encourage beginners to use a reliable brand such as Hu-Friedy. And as I will mention later in the book, I recommend purchasing long shank surgical round burs. I use KOMET #4 and #6 surgical round bur.

I get asked by vendors to recommend other brands as well, but I cannot suggest or recommend any products I am not familiar with...I will let you decide what you want to use and what works in your hands.

These recommended brands are analogous to Benz, BMW, etc., which are internationally well recognized. You will be able to purchase them through your local dental suppliers easily. If you do not have a dental supplier, you can contact the suppliers below. These suppliers know my instruments. They even sell the instruments in a package. You may get a good deal through them.

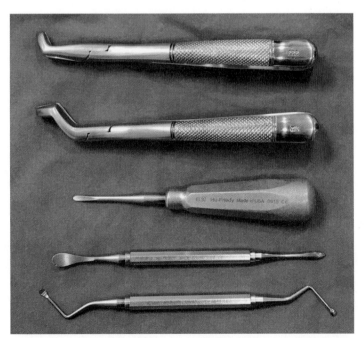
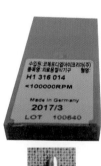
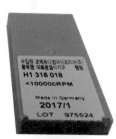
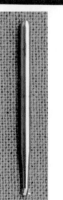
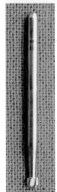

In the Korean version, several companies that I purchased my instruments from were introduced but in the English version, the information was edited out because it may be irrelevant based on where you practice. However, in this book, most of the burs are from Komet, and instruments are from Hu-Friedy.

Follow my extraction technique by reading this book ★

Since I am very interested in the topic of wisdom tooth surgeries, I enjoy meeting and discussing with other well-seasoned dentists who share common interests. One thing is clear -each dentist has his or her own technique- and believes that his or her methods are the because it has worked well so far. Most seemed as though they do not need to learn additional skills because they are very content with their current methods. Moreover, some even claim to be the best at wisdom tooth surgeries where they practice. Admittedly, I used to have the same mindset before, but after discussing with numerous experienced dentists, I became more humble and changed my attitude. Nowadays, I think that "there are plenty of dentists who can extract wisdom teeth better than II can, and I should always try to improve further.", "I am not the best at wisdom tooth extractions. Moreover, my techniques may be only suitable for me." This is how I think now.

The reason I am sharing this with the readers is that I would like to say that you do not have to follow all of my methods. Instead, develop a style that works best for you after studying my techniques and methods. This book may be more beneficial for dentists who are familiar with wisdom tooth surgeries already because you can enhance your routine by incorporating my tips to what already works well in your hands. But if you are a beginner, I encourage you to follow my technique step by step. Not only do I extract lots of teeth, I also educate other dentists-I've become familiar with what areas many beginners need the most help.

Analysing Dr. Youngsam Kim's wisdom tooth extraction by numbers ★

I was just a mediocre dentist when I first opened my dental clinic. Ironically, I saw great potential in wisdom tooth surgeries from the very beginning because it was not a popular procedure performed by other successful dentists. For this reason, I had many wisdom tooth surgery patients from the get-go. Before hiring an oral maxillofacial surgeon, between 2002 and 2004, I extracted a few hundred wisdom teeth every month. My record at the time was performing 27 extractions (including extractions for orthodontic treatments) in one day. I broke the record in February of 2016, extracting 32 wisdom teeth in one day, while spending half of my schedule on check up and recall exams. I personally administered local anesthetic and sutured all my patients.

After hiring an oral maxillofacial surgeon in 2004 spring, approximately 100 wisdom teeth were extracted on a regular basis for the last ten years. This information was based on the data from the national dental insurance program. However, there could be much more that were not in-

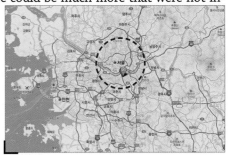

cluded in the data because, in Gangnam, there are many foreigners from other countries who do not subscribe to the national dental insurance. Moreover, in the past, I also removed wisdom teeth for orthodontic treatments, which were not covered by the national dental insurance. But now almost all patients requiring extraction for most treatments (including orthodontics) are covered by national dental insurance.

Ever since I opened Gangnam Leon Dental Clinic, more than 400 wisdom teeth were extracted per month. In 2017, with the help of one additional dentist, more than 5000 wisdom teeth extractions were expected.

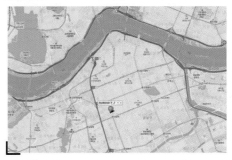

If you are interested in the number of wisdom tooth extractions you are performing, you can request this information from the insurance database. You may realize that the numbers are significantly lower than what you had imagined. When I checked my monthly statistics, I was surprised to see that I had extracted only about half of what I actually felt like I had extracted. The readers of this book may feel the same way. Check the national dental insurance statistics if you want to compare your wisdom tooth surgery numbers from other dentists.

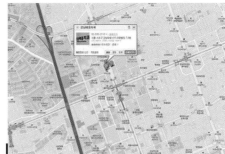

These are close up maps showing Gangnam Leon Dental Clinic and Gangnam station. The Gangnam district has heavy foot traffic because of the metro station and various bus routes to Seoul (capital city of South Korea) and Gyeonggi Do. Although the rent is extremely high, I cannot leave Gangnam because of my long time, loyal patients. If I were to open a clinic again, I don't think I would open in Gangnam again...

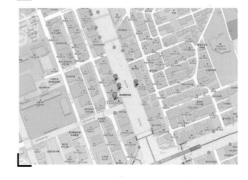

Analysing the number of wisdom tooth extractions in South Korea

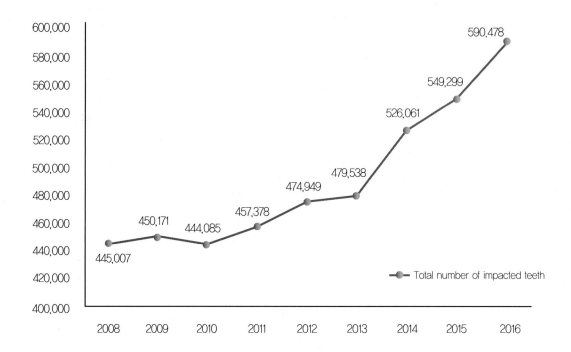

How many wisdom teeth do South Korean dentists extract? The graph above shows the number of impacted wisdom teeth extractions performed by South Korean dentists in the last few years. The most recent data shows 590,478 extractions in 2016. There were 17,000 dental clinics at the time which means it would be logical to assume that a typical dental clinic extracted 34.7 wisdom teeth yearly and 2.89 monthly. A typical dental clinic removed 4-5 wisdom teeth per month even if we include uncomplicated wisdom tooth extractions.

As mentioned earlier, not all wisdom teeth are billed as impacted extractions because many are also classified as uncomplicated extractions. Including University dental hospitals and advanced medical facilities, I think the total number of wisdom tooth extracted nationally is approximately 80,000~90,000 per year.

From the graph, it is surprising to see the opposite trend of declining younger population vs. rise in the reported number of impacted wisdom extraction cases. However, as I often mention this in my dental insurance seminars, many South Korean dentists study the dental insurance codes and therefore correctly bill impacted wisdom tooth extractions. In the past, some complicated impacted extractions were mistakenly invoiced as uncomplicated extractions. Consequently, now I assume there is a significant increase in the ratio of impacted wisdom tooth extraction numbers than the ratio of the total number of tooth extractions.

Wisdom tooth extraction cost in South Korea ★★★

In South Korea, all wisdom tooth extraction procedures are covered by the national dental insurance. Therefore for whatever reason, a dentist cannot charge a patient for any procedures which are not subscribed by the national dental insurance.

It is illegal to charge fees for additional procedures on top of routine extraction fees. For example, a dentist cannot bill an additional procedure such as IV/GA sedation or any other treatment that can help patients feel more comfortable along with extraction.

Let's discuss a scenario together.

A typical uncomplicated wisdom tooth extraction costs 7,360 won (approx. USD $7). The total cost becomes 30,000 won (approx. $30) even after including local anesthetic and x-rays. The cost is very low when compared to other countries. In other developed nations, an average extraction costs approximately USD $100~$500. When compared to other OECD (The Organisation for Efficient Co-operation and Development) countries, the cost of extraction in Korea can be considered extremely low.

The most expensive wisdom tooth extraction procedure is as follows:

The most costly tooth extraction procedure in South Korea is an impacted wisdom tooth which is positioned ⅔ in the bone. It can be analyzed from the radiograph, and the cost is approximately 59,750 won (approx. USD $59). After including medical tax, panoramic x-ray, periapical x-ray, and local anesthetic, the final cost is around 110,000 won (approx. USD $110). How does the most complicated wisdom tooth procedure fee compare with other nations? From my research, even in the country with the cheapest dental fee schedule charges over USD $500. In the United States, where we have the closest ties typically charges between USD $1,000~5,000.

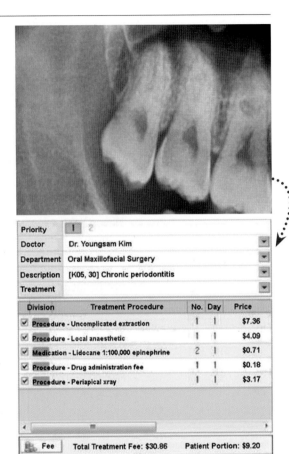

Priority	1 2			
Doctor	Dr. Youngsam Kim			
Department	Oral Maxillofacial Surgery			
Description	[K05, 30] Chronic periodontitis			
Treatment				

Division	Treatment Procedure	No.	Day	Price
☑ Procedure - Uncomplicated extraction		1	1	$7.36
☑ Procedure - Local anaesthetic		1	1	$4.09
☑ Medication - Lidocane 1:100,000 epinephrine		2	1	$0.71
☑ Procedure - Drug administration fee		1	1	$0.18
☑ Procedure - Periapical xray		1	1	$3.17

Fee	Total Treatment Fee: $30.86	Patient Portion: $9.20

The cost of uncomplicated wisdom tooth extraction in South Korea. This is the cost breakdown of uncomplicated forcep extraction including x-ray and local anesthetic.

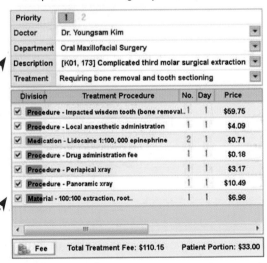

Priority	1 2			
Doctor	Dr. Youngsam Kim			
Department	Oral Maxillofacial Surgery			
Description	[K01, 173] Complicated third molar surgical extraction			
Treatment	Requiring bone removal and tooth sectioning			

Division	Treatment Procedure	No.	Day	Price
☑ Procedure - Impacted wisdom tooth (bone removal..		1	1	$59.75
☑ Procedure - Local anaesthetic administration		1	1	$4.09
☑ Medication - Lidocaine 1:100, 000 epinephrine		2	1	$0.71
☑ Procedure - Drug administration fee		1	1	$0.18
☑ Procedure - Periapical xray		1	1	$3.17
☑ Procedure - Panoramic xray		1	1	$10.49
☑ Material - 100:100 extraction, root..		1	1	$6.98

Fee	Total Treatment Fee: $110.15	Patient Portion: $33.00

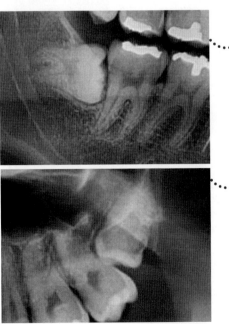

The most expensive tooth extraction procedure in South Korea is an impacted wisdom tooth which is ⅔ in the bone and procedurally involves bone removal and tooth sectioning. The fee here includes local anesthetic and x-ray. Usually, a dentist is limited to charging CBCT and periodontal treatment (i.e., scaling) along with the extraction.

★★

I included the x-ray and local anesthetic fees in the final cost. However, the price in other countries mentioned previously do that even include these fees in the final cost. Some countries charge x-rays and local anesthetic administration separately just like South Korea. I have also heard some countries that have separate fees for suturing, post-operative instruction, and post-operative care such as giving gauze after extraction. In South Korea, these services are all included in the extraction fee.

Moreover, dentists in some countries may charge patients more than double the cost of treatment by combining surgery with deeper forms of sedation so that patient can undergo surgery without anxiety.

Nevertheless, I extract wisdom teeth because I love doing the procedure. Although it can be challenging at times, my dental practice is doing well. I encourage you to study the correct wisdom tooth extraction codes set by your national dental insurance. Learn to remove wisdom teeth if you are a young dentist wanting to open a dental practice. It may be hard on the body, and it may not be lucrative, but you will not go out of business. Moreover, you will gradually improve your surgical skills without even realizing.

Many people think I am the first person who lectured and wrote a book that teaches about national dental insurance. To learn more about correct dental insurance billing, I sent a lot of wisdom tooth extraction claims to the national dental insurance. I can comfortably say that I removed many wisdom teeth in the process.

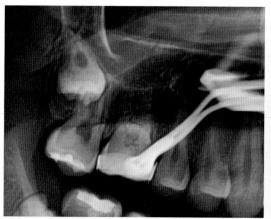 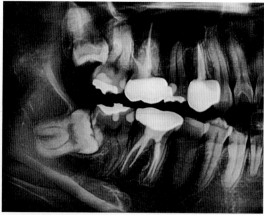

━━ Above x-rays are examples of challenging complicated impacted wisdom tooth cases where one cannot claim additional procedure codes to the national dental insurance. I believe the cost of more challenging wisdom tooth extraction should be increased and there should be an additional classification for more difficult extractions.

To make up for the cheaper cost of wisdom tooth surgery, some dentists are charging additional fees and billing procedures that includes hemostatic agents and PRP (protein-rich-plasma). These additional fees billed on top of wisdom tooth surgery are considered illegal in South Korea.

I think I would have been a very successful dentist enjoying my life only doing wisdom teeth extraction if I were a dentist in the United States or another country.

Why have wisdom tooth extraction seminars become so popular now?

The direct answer is…

It is difficult as a dentist to shy away from oral surgery now that implants have become the standard of care. I have been lecturing numerous topics in dentistry for a long time, but I have noticed a rise in popularity of wisdom tooth extraction seminars. Could this be the cause of challenging economic situation driving dentists to perform unlucrative procedures? Not long ago, I lectured to Korean dentists practicing in the United States and Canada. As soon as this book got published, I used the contents of the book to lecture in Australia as well. Even dentists in developed countries are showing a keen interest in wisdom tooth surgery.

Why is this happening? This is because of the popularization of implants.

Previously, many general dentists did not perform oral surgery in South Korea. This was probably more evident in developed countries because specialized dental procedures are routinely referred out to the specialists. However, as implants became a more common treatment, many general dentists began placing implants. On average, I think implant surgery is more straightforward than some challenging extractions.

It is a common knowledge that surgical placement of an implant is one of the most crucial aspects of implant treatment. Oral maxillofacial surgeons or periodontists who place implants usually refer to prosthodontists to restore the implant. Due to this reason, they may feel as though they are at a loss when they refer the cases out to prosthodontists. Some oral surgeons and periodontists are restoring implants after realizing that they are well capable of restoring implants on their own. Meanwhile, prosthodontists are also placing more implants. Some general dentists in the middle are thinking they are better than prosthodontists at placing implants and even better than periodontists at restoring implants. I think many general dentists are placing implants and restoring crowns for this reason. Moreover, with the spread of computer-guided implants, many general dentists are gaining confidence at performing full mouth implant cases.

Another reason for the popularity of wisdom tooth surgery is due to declining cost of implants globally.

I think a dentist can attract more patients by performing wisdom tooth surgery. I have many patients requesting second molar implants since I do lots of wisdom tooth extractions. Most of these cases are done at the same time. Moreover, the trend towards immediate implant placement after extraction is increasing. From this perspective, it is illogical to refer out patients to another dentist only for extraction if a dentist is capable of placing implants in his or her clinic. Dental students tell me that more general practitioners are doing extractions and therefore it makes sense that more dentists are showing interest in wisdom tooth seminars. At my seminars, even dentists over sixty years old who were not interested in oral surgery before tell me that they are now learning implants because it is becoming the norm and implants are covered by national dental insurance. Some older dentists tell me that they are learning even if they will practice for only 5 or 10 years because they fear of being labeled out-of-date.

Wisdom tooth extraction is not just about extracting the problematic tooth. It can be considered a start of comprehensive dental treatment. Many aspects of oral surgery such as raising a flap, implant placement, and bone grafting will become more natural if you become proficient at wisdom tooth surgery. I want to emphasize that I am not encouraging you to remove all wisdom teeth, but instead <do not to give up on all wisdom teeth>. Once you start wisdom tooth cases that are easier and master the safe method of extraction, you will be able to gain more confidence in other aspects of oral surgery such as implants.

Gangnam Academy of Wisdom tooth Extraction ★

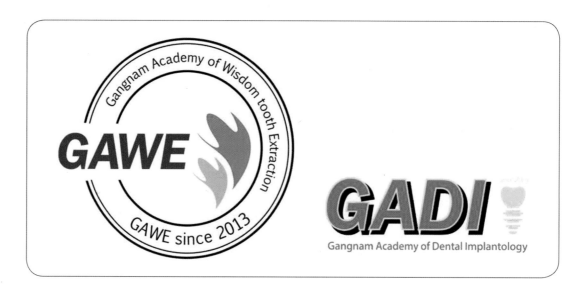

▶ YouTube^{KR}

Gangnam Academy of Wisdom tooth Extraction

I have learned so much by teaching and sharing knowledge with other dentists. An educator, Edgar Dale once said: "teaching is learning." I modified his motto to "The best way to learn is to teach." I would not be as competent as now at oral surgery if I did not teach wisdom tooth surgery. Likewise, if I did not decide to write this book, I would not have documented and organized so many cases. I love teaching wisdom tooth surgery because I can learn at the same time.

The picture above is the logo of my Gangnam Academy of Wisdom tooth Extraction. Although I lectured wisdom tooth surgery for a long time, I started advertising and teaching for a fee since 2013. This is why it says "since 2013" in the logo. I did not have a logo before, but some dentists wanted the certificate of attendance, so I decided to make one. I pondered about the word that goes in front of "Academy of Wisdom Tooth Extraction" and considered "Korea", "Daehan" or "Seoul" but selected "Gangnam". Gangnam is a place where I practiced for 16 years, and it has become a popular place internationally. The image next to it is a logo of GADI (Gangnam Academy of Dental Implantology). I also do implant seminars because, in Korea, there are many dentists showing keen interest in both wisdom tooth and implant surgeries. I would like to acknowledge Dr. Jong Hwan Lim for helping me with the English names of my Academy.

I hope the logos and the book become more widespread in the dental community.

Dr. Youngsam Kim's YouTube channel

I do not have an official website, but I manage my YouTube channel. Please join me if you are interested.

▶ YouTube^{KR}

Dr. Youngsam Kim's You-Tube channel

Introduction and Chapter 01 translated by

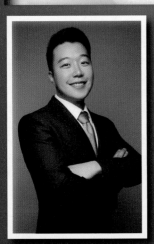

Dr. Jong Wook Hur BOH DSc, GD Dent.

Griffith University School of Dentistry
New South Wales, Australia

I am a general dentist from Australia who graduated from Griffith University dental school in 2015. It is an honour to be part of the translating team for the second edition of this fantastic book. I first met Dr. Kim when I attended his wisdom teeth seminar in 2018. His lecture really resonated with me and since then, I've attended all of Dr Kim's lecture series including the Mexican Live Surgery course. I even have the privilege of simultaneously interpreting his wisdom teeth surgery lectures in Australia. If you haven't done so already, I highly recommend that you attend his lecture series on wisdom teeth extractions and on implant surgery.

01
Tooth notation ★★★

Dentists learn tooth numbering systems as soon as they enter into dental school. However, some dentists in the United States were unfamiliar with the numbering system that I referenced in my book and lectures. Therefore, I decided to include this section to help all dentists familiarize with the tooth notation used throughout the book.

A	B	C	D	E	F	G	H	I	J		1	2	3	4	5	6	7	8	9	10	11	12	13	14	15	16
T	S	R	Q	P	O	N	M	L	K		32	31	30	29	28	27	26	25	24	23	22	21	20	19	18	17

Beginning from the most upper right tooth in the maxilla, deciduous teeth are written in capital alphabet letters and permanent teeth are written in increasing numbers in a clockwise direction in "Universal Notation". As far as I know, the United States may be the only country using this tooth classification system despite its name. It is likely to be named this way because it is the first notation to include numbers to identify tooth. There has been some modification to this system over time. There are usually two factors that are required to make a change in formal designation or unit system.

An effective national education system is required to reduce a large gap between a small number of educated elites vs. the average population. Another critical factor is a strong willingness to make a change at a national level. I believe the United States is still using the Universal Notation and Customary units possibly due to these factors which are difficult to change.

However, all orthodontists use FDI notation to classify teeth. I believe this is because symmetry is crucial in orthodontics. Perhaps, it could be because orthodontic specialty was recently formally established by "the father of American orthodontics", Dr. Edward Angle in the 1900s and thus this specialty became very well established in the United States.

E	D	C	B	A	A	B	C	D	E		8	7	6	5	4	3	2	1	1	2	3	4	5	6	7	8
E	D	C	B	A	A	B	C	D	E		8	7	6	5	4	3	2	1	1	2	3	4	5	6	7	8

FDI World Dental Federation notation is a dental notation system that is used internationally. This system is used globally including Canada and Mexico, which are geographically close to the United States.

This book uses the FDI notation to identify teeth. It is important to note that all teeth notated as 8 are third molars, and 7 are second molars. In Korea, dentists prefer to remove third molars from one side and wait for healing before removing the opposite side instead of removing all four third molars at once. This could be attributed to how the national dental insurance works in South Korea. I prefer to remove third molars from one side at a time to lessen patient discomfort, and I favor right side third molar extraction over the left side. The last four digits of my cell phone are 1848 for this reason. I am currently on sabbatical at UCLA with my family after accepting a preceptor position at UCLA department of oral maxillofacial surgery. Ironically, the current address of my residence is 2838. Perhaps a higher being is encouraging me to favor the left side third molar extractions from now on. Let's remember that 18, 48, 28, and 38 are third molars.

Primary Teeth										Permanent Teeth															
Upper Right								Upper Left		Upper Right														Upper Left	
55	54	53	52	51	61	62	63	64	65	18	17	16	15	14	13	12	11	21	22	23	24	25	26	27	28
85	84	83	82	81	71	72	73	74	75	48	47	46	45	44	43	42	41	31	32	33	34	35	36	37	38
Upper Right								Lower Left		Upper Right														Lower Left	

02
This book is written to help readers remove wisdom teeth that are... ★★★

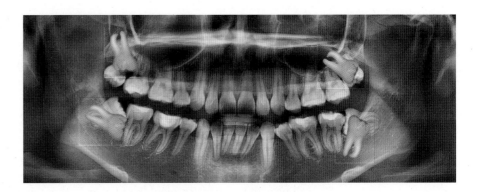

This book is intended to help readers extract third molar impactions like the ones shown in the panoramic x-ray. The main objective is to remove teeth safely, efficiently, and quickly. I encourage dentists to start with less complicated to more challenging impactions.

Gaining surgical skills is necessary, but most importantly, dentists should concentrate on doing surgery safely to avoid complications. Safety is the most crucial aspect of third molar surgery.

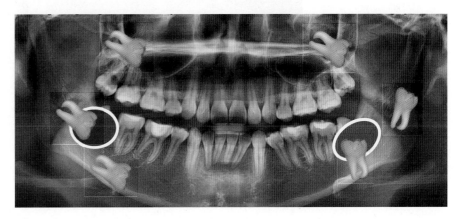

Consider referring patients to university oral maxillofacial surgery department for severely impacted third molars as shown in the panoramic x-ray above. Also, consider referral if the patient is severely medically compromised or has a large cyst. It would be very challenging to accomplish safe, easy, and fast extraction under these difficult circumstances. Most importantly, the teeth should be taken out as atraumatically as possible. This will lead to less postoperative discomfort. In South Korea, some experienced oral maxillofacial surgeons elect not to extract very difficult impactions. The low cost may be a factor as national dental insurance scheme does not provide sufficient remuneration for time taken to perform such extractions and cyst removal procedures. I think it is essential to consider the patients' medical history and check for conditions such as diabetes, hypertension, or other compromised systemic conditions. A dentist must be able to make a clinical decision on when it will be beneficial for the patient to be referred to an OMFS, so that the surgery may be carried out in a safer environment where appropriately trained personnel and equipment for emergencies are readily available. Many oral surgery residents and oral maxillofacial surgeons reference basic oral surgery techniques from my book and seminars due to the popularity of my surgical style. I suggest you stop reading the book right here if you thought you were going to learn how to extract extremely challenging cases such as the ones shown in the second panoramic x-ray. I wanted to include extremely challenging surgeries that I performed in my book but decided against it because the intention of the book is not to showcase my skills. In fact, it was more challenging to leave some of those cases out but I thought the readers wouldn't appreciate the book as much if my intention was to brag about my skills.

03
Can you respect treatments like this? ★★

Crown on the second molar without extraction of the third

I often come across cases where patients present to my surgery for wisdom teeth extractions and the second molars haven't received the best possible treatment or the restorative margins are defective. In some cases I don't know how to break the bad news to the patients. Sometimes I wonder why the previous dentist hasn't extracted the wisdom teeth especially if the case doesn't even seem to be very challenging. In some cases the 7s'were treated when the patients were very young but most of the time I find such treatments were done in their adulthood. The patients claim that they were either informed that the wisdom teeth extraction was optional rather than compulsory or in worst case scenario weren't even informed about the wisdom teeth. If your life calling is to be a dentist, wouldn't you agree that wisdom teeth extraction in these cases are compulsory rather than optional?

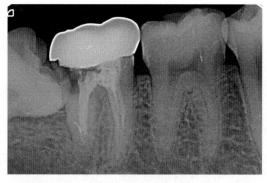

As a result of leaving the wisdom tooth behind, severe secondary carious lesion developed on the distal of second molar.

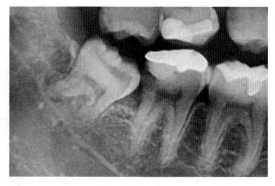

Again, due to the wisdom tooth being left behind, the second molar ended up with defective distal margin which resulted in large recurrent carious lesion.

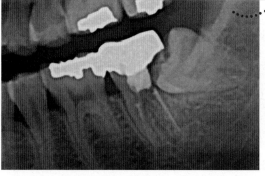

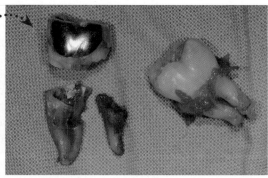

Another case where the patient lost both 7 and the 8 due to not extracting the 8 prior to treatment of 7. For cases like this, even if you are a general dentist who doesn't do extraction of wisdom teeth, I recommend you refer the patient to another clinician who does, to incorporate wisdom teeth extraction to your treatment plan. When I get referrals from other dentists for an extraction of wisdom teeth for cases like this, I always commend very highly of the referring dentist to the patient because the dentist is fulfilling his/her duty of care.

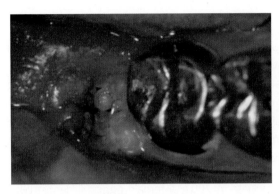
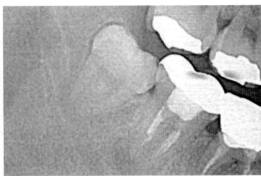

This is a case of severe gingival inflammation from treating second molar without removal of the third. It makes the extraction more challenging as the gold crown on the second molar can dislodge in the process. Usually a wisdom tooth like this will be easily extracted using only an elevator if the gold crown wasn't present. However, in this particular case I sectioned the mesial portion to take extra precaution and remove the mesial undercut.

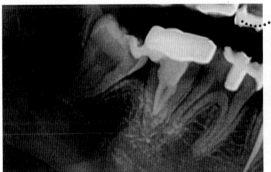
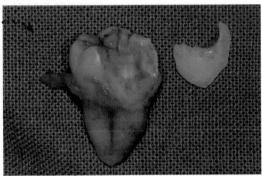

It's a similar case to the one mentioned above. Again, mesial portion of the 8's crown inferior to the distal of 7 was removed first for safer extraction of the 8. This is done routinely if there is a crown or an onlay to prevent them from dislodging. Of course, we get consents from the patient that they acknowledge the crown/onlay can dislodge in the process of extraction. The most important lesson here is to avoid this situation by removing the wisdom tooth prior to the treatment of second molars.

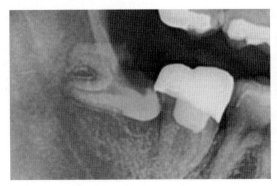
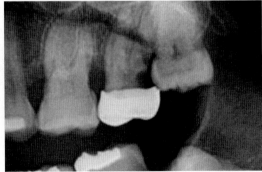

Again, 7s were treated without extraction of 8s. Both cannot be deemed ideal as it significantly reduces marginal fitting accuracy for any restorative work done on distal of 7s.

Wait!

Practice wisdom teeth extraction to increase proficiency of other oral surgery procedures

 ★★★

When I first opened up my private clinic, it wasn't easy to replicate what I learnt from flap surgery course or implant seminars. However, as I got into doing more wisdom teeth extractions, essential oral surgery skills such as incisions, sutures, detaching periosteum etc were unavoidable. As I repeatedly performed wisdom teeth extraction I noticed huge improvements in my implant and periodontal surgery skills. When you become more comfortable with wisdom teeth which is as far as you can get in the mouth, you will notice even implants on 7s which some clinicians find challenging, to be easily approachable.

Back when I was an associate in 2001, a female principal dentist with 12 years of experience forecasted implants to be the future of dentistry. She then started practicing suturing after every extraction case even if it was a simple extraction from the maxilla. Her theory was that one must master suturing techniques in order to perform successful implant surgeries. I think it was her influence that got me working hard on wisdom teeth extractions as part of implant surgery training.

I share this story with every young inexperienced dentist I meet. I recommend wisdom teeth extraction as a starting point to improve their surgical skills. Many dentists still avoid doing wisdom teeth extractions so its easier to choose cases if they wish. I advise them to put their focus on becoming proficient in different types of incisions, raising full thickness flaps, bone removal and suturing. As you continue to educate yourself with wisdom teeth surgeries, other implants or periodontal surgeries in more accessible part of the mouth will start to feel easier and you will start to perform better.

Wait!

Why do many dentists claim they are the best at wisdom teeth extractions?

 ★★

I rarely come across dentists who claim that they are the best at crown preparations or root canal treatments. Even some of the best clinicians are modest and never say that they are the best. Some dentists say they are best at implant surgery to their patients but i rarely see them making the same claim to other dentists. Why? I think it's because extractions don't leave any evidence behind. No one knows what the process of extraction was like and how difficult it was other than the operators. This lack of evidence has increased number of dentists who claims they are the best at it. I've seen some colleagues of mine in Korea whom I couldn't agree with their claims of being top 10 wisdom teeth surgeon in the country. I am not saying all of these people are liars. What I am trying to say is you can make claims like that too with some proper education and training!

04

Confidence in wisdom teeth surgery: A pre-requisite for a successful dental practice

Benefits of being proficient in wisdom teeth surgery

- Walk-in or one off patients are retained within the practice

- Easy clientele builder

- Easy to claim from National Health Care or other health insurance patients have.

- Patient believes you are proficient in other dental procedures too. (Which is truth over time as wisdom teeth surgery improves your other clinical skills)

- You become especially proficient in periodontal and implant surgeries

- When I first opened my practice I only did wisdom teeth to find my feet. But now they are big part of my billings.

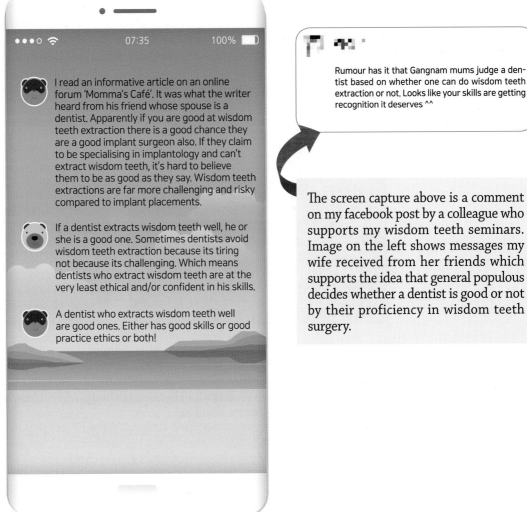

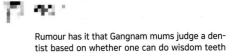

The screen capture above is a comment on my facebook post by a colleague who supports my wisdom teeth seminars. Image on the left shows messages my wife received from her friends which supports the idea that general populous decides whether a dentist is good or not by their proficiency in wisdom teeth surgery.

05
Gain trust from patients by being good at wisdom teeth extractions

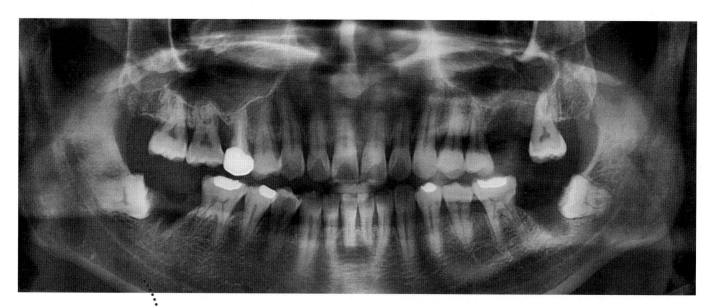

Initially, the patient presented with 26,37 and 47 already extracted from another dental practice. The patient decided to visit our clinic as the previous dentist said they don't do wisdom teeth extractions. Since visiting our practice, the patient advised that he/she lost trust in the previous dentist and wanted to continue the implant treatment at our practice. Since it was the patient's decision to visit our surgery rather than being referred by another colleague, we provided the patient with the necessary treatments as per patient's request.

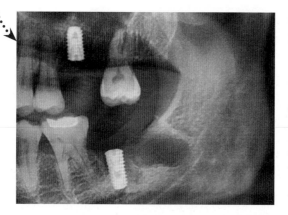
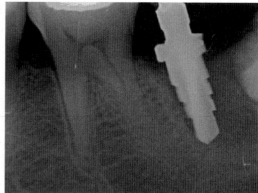

This is a radiograph following 38 extraction and implant placement. To prevent excessive bleeding, I performed 26 sinus lift and implant placement prior to 37 implant placement and 38 extraction. On a side note, you can see that I prefer to use the osteotomy burs over implant guide pins to take mid-surgery PA xrays for checking pathways. A lot of my seminar attendees find this tip helpful during my implant seminars.

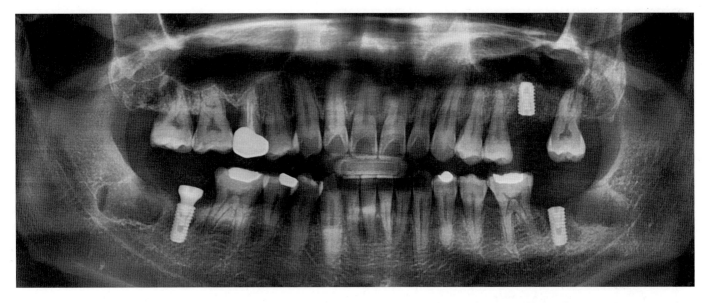

A month later, patient returned for #48 extraction and #47 implant placement. We aimed to preserve the alveolar bone surrounding the crown of #48 as much as possible to ensure primary stability of #47. Crown of #48 was decoronated prior to extraction as per my usual impacted wisdom tooth extraction routine. In these cases the operator needs to decide whether to do the implant or extraction first. I personally place implant prior to extraction if alveolar bone distal to the implant is sound.

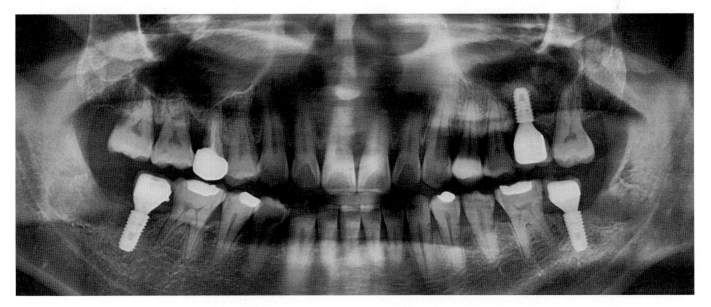

1 month follow up after restoration of the implants. Patient was very satisfied with the outcome and all implants and crowns are still fully healthy and functional after a few years.

06
Wisdom teeth = Unconditional trust for the dentist ★

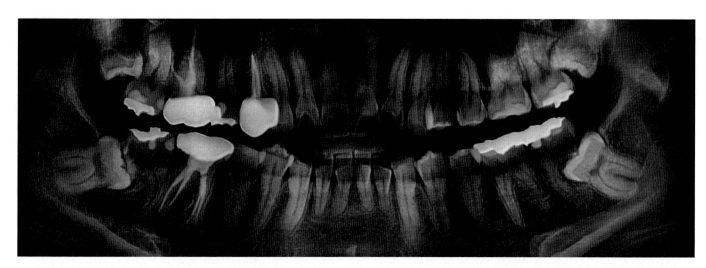

The patient was advised to have both #37,38 extracted at another dental clinic, but patient decided to visit our surgery after some online research. The patient had both teeth removed in a single visit.

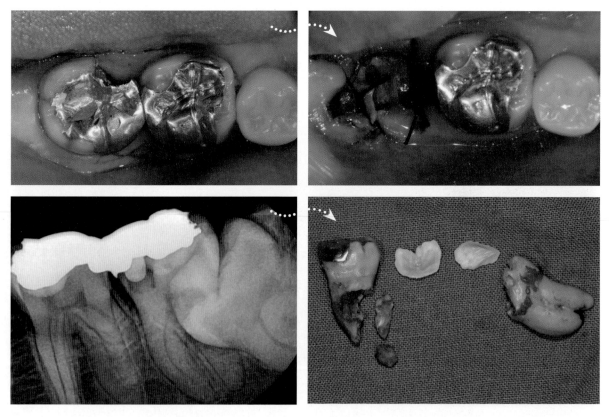

Teeth were extracted without any incision and collagen plug (Terplug M size from Olympus Terumo(Japan)) was placed within the socket prior to suturing to aid the healing process.

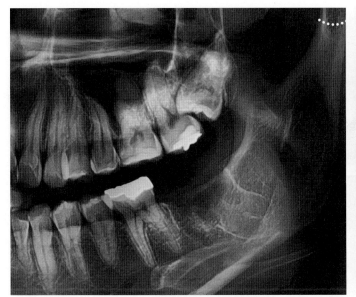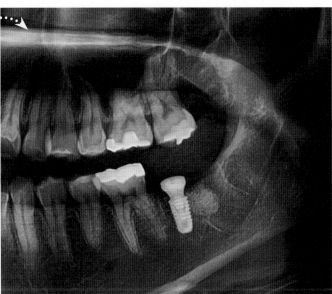

2 months later, patient returned for #37 implant placement and #28 extraction. There was insufficient bone formation on the distal of #37 so little bit of xenograft material (Cerabone 0.25g) was placed despite having sufficient primary stability. No membrane was placed as my philosophy is "Perfectly cut and detached periosteum is the best membrane."

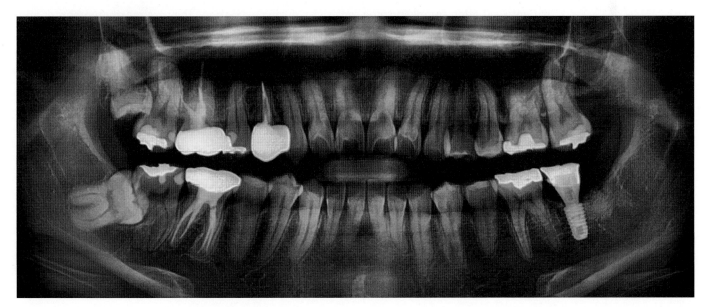

2 months later, implant crown was delivered. In this appointment patient requested the remaining #48 to be extracted.

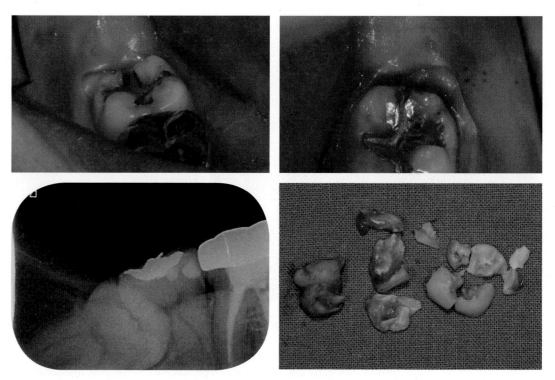

Small portion of #48 was supragingival and tooth was removed with caution. For 2-3 days immediately following extraction, patient complained of minor numbness and pain on premolar region. However, all the symptoms disappeared in approximately 2 weeks. We will cover this topic later in the book but if IAN canal and the root of the wisdom tooth is in contact with each other, patients will often complain some sensitivity during extraction. They are mostly temporary and will recover from it immediately.

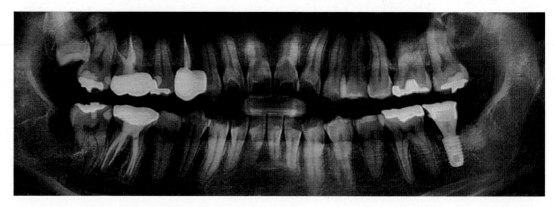

1 month Post Operative OPG following #48 extraction.

07

Wisdom tooth extraction site from another clinic still in pain ★

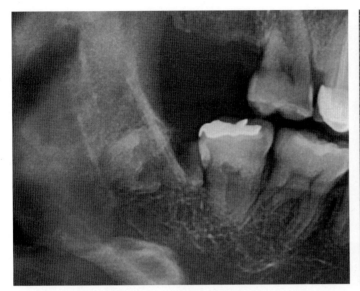 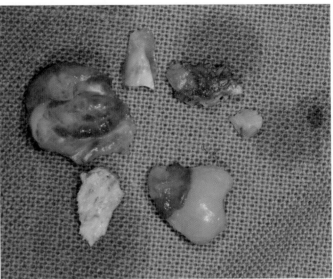

Patient presented with chief complaints of pain in area where wisdom tooth was extracted by a dentist in another practice. Radiograph showed retained root of significant size and patient agreed to have it removed.

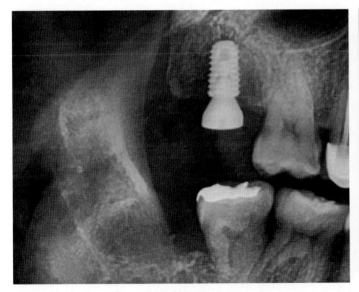 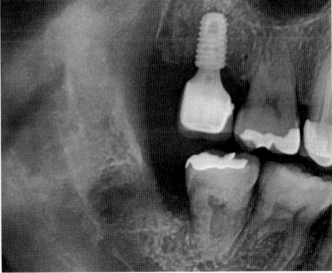

This was a female patient in her late 20s preparing to study abroad in the US. She wanted all her dental treatment done prior to departure and requested an implant on #17. As I mentioned many times earlier, competency in wisdom tooth extraction gains unconditional trust from patients. This patient left for study in the US after the implant surgery but had her entire family visit our practice for their dental care.

08
Continued treatment for patients whose initial chief complaint was wisdom teeth

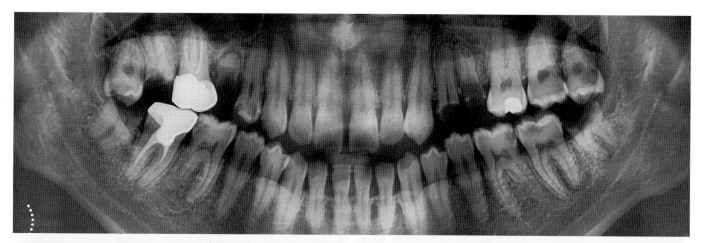

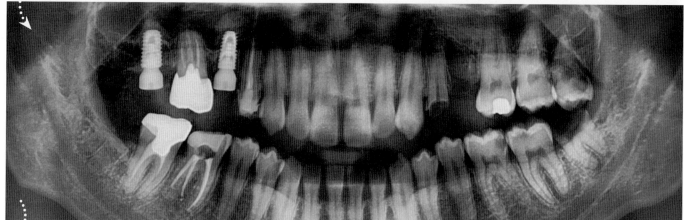

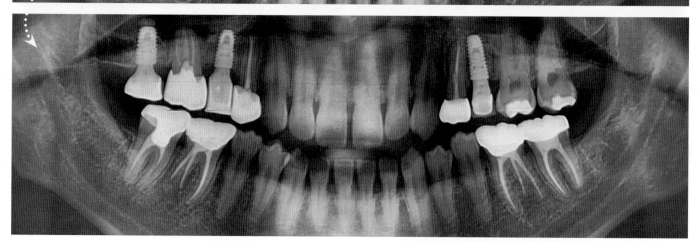

The patient presented with tooth ache from wisdom teeth. Just like some of the other teeth, wisdom teeth were carious. We extracted the wisdom teeth first then explained the needs for treatment in other teeth and completed them. I see many cases where the patients first visit my practice for wisdom teeth issues and end up staying for all other treatments and even routine hygiene appointments thereafter. A result of trust built up from the initial wisdom teeth extractions.

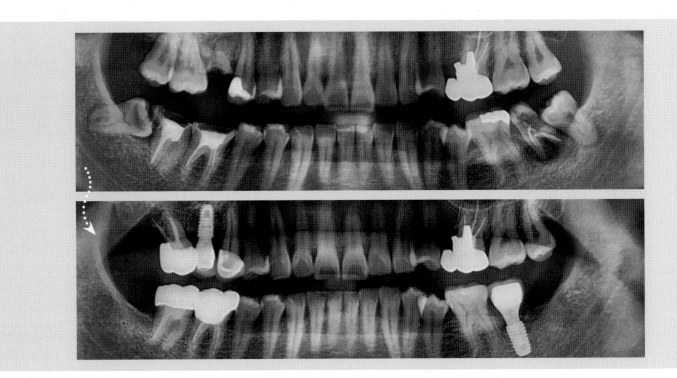

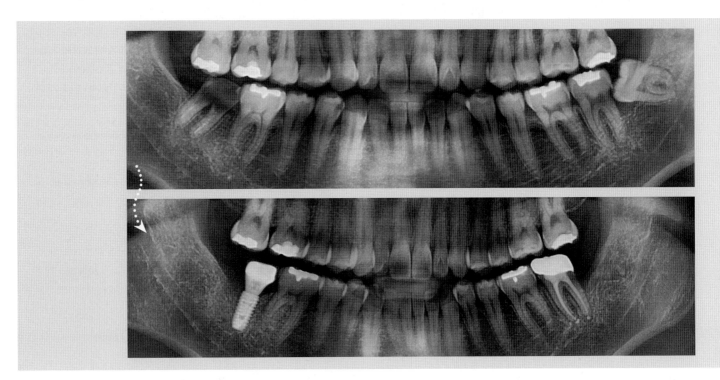

All the cases above are patients who initially visited my practice for wisdom teeth. Not everyone needs complex treatment following extraction of wisdom teeth. In a lot of cases, wisdom teeth extraction can be very easy and allows you to work on all quadrants of the mouth. If you are a young dentist just starting up a practice, try and become more proficient at wisdom teeth extractions first. It will make other treatments feel easier for you.

Wait!

Focus on avoiding one disaster that makes you sad rather than
the 99 successes that makes you happy

Why do some dentists avoid wisdom tooth extraction?

There has to be a reason why some dentists dislike wisdom teeth extractions. Any dentist should be able to extract wisdom teeth with some practice. But over time, more and more dentist avoid third molar extractions all together. Why? Most likely because they got traumatised a few times. What could cause such trauma?

- Patients complain about post operative complications (Bleeding and pain)
- Took too long or gave up half way.
- Nerve damage, altered sensations
- Pain on adjacent teeth following extraction
- Pain on TMJ following extraction.

To be proficient in wisdom teeth extraction is not just about the speed. It's more about how much you've avoided the above-mentioned complaints.

I've extracted lots of wisdom teeth over an extended period of time but I still love doing them as I rarely face any post-operative complications mentioned above. First and second complications from the list will improve over time and practice. Of course, you have to train yourself in minimal incision and bone removal. In particular, for the second one, when you are more experienced you will learn when and how to finish off the extraction with intentional coronectomy. You will also notice the third one to improve over time. It really isn't easy to damage IAN while extracting wisdom teeth as they are quite obvious on the radiograph. Lingual nerve is a bigger problem as no one can accurately know where exactly the lingual nerve travels. We will discuss this in the later chapters of the book.

I take pride in the fact that I NEVER had a patient with nerve damage. I will share how it was achievable in this book.

Patients complaining of TMJ pain during and after extractions will become more infrequent as you learn proper use of forceps and become quicker and better at extractions. This will reduce the mouth opening duration for the patients which prevents such complications.

Last and one of the biggest reasons for beginner dentists to give up on wisdom teeth extraction is actually due to patients complaining of toothache from adjacent second molar. Unlike other complications there isn't a whole lot we can do about this and is a cause of huge mental stress for dentists.

Lets learn about how to reduce such complications in the coming chapters of this book.

Interpretation of Panoramic Radiographs for Third Molars

Chapter 02 translated by

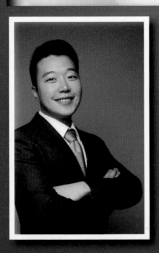

Dr. Jong Wook Hur BOH DSc, GD Dent.

Griffith University School of Dentistry
New South Wales, Australia

I am a general dentist from Australia who graduated from Griffith University dental school in 2015. It is an honour to be part of the translating team for the second edition of this fantastic book. I first met Dr. Kim when I attended his wisdom teeth seminar in 2018. His lecture really resonated with me and since then, I've attended all of Dr Kim's lecture series including the Mexican Live Surgery course. I even have the privilege of simultaneously interpreting his wisdom teeth surgery lectures in Australia. If you haven't done so already, I highly recommend that you attend his lecture series on wisdom teeth extractions and on implant surgery.

01
Why this chapter was written

For a long time, I have had interactions with younger dental practitioners while giving third molar extraction seminars. To my surprise I've noticed that a lot of dentists weren't proficient in interpreting panoramic x-rays. We have all spent a lot of time and effort studying them in our dental schools and it was reinforced to us time and time again over multiple disciplines of dentistry including Oral Maxillofacial surgery. So why do the dentists still struggle to interpret the panoramic radiographs when it comes to third molar surgeries?

I think it's because we just memorise what is written in the books without full understanding of the topic. It will be very difficult to retain the knowledge we gained for the sake of passing written exams without adequate exposure to clinical experience while in dental schools.

So this one time, I decided to give a brief run down of a few critical points when it comes to interpretation of OPGs prior to my wisdom teeth seminar. The attendees absolutely loved it because it let them replenish their knowledge on OPG through my explanation just when they needed it. Things they've learned and forgotten and things that they've forgotten that they've learned.

Multiple attendees complimented me saying "is he a genius?" after the lecture that day. With the confidence boost from the seminar, I did the same again on the next seminar. The reaction was as good as the first. With the overwhelming excitement, I've given the segment proper name of "Interpretation of Panoramic Images" and expanded my lecture slides from 5~6 pages Power-Point presentation to 80 pages and allocated more time for it in the next lecture series. However, it was not as well received as before.

I was very disappointed but it got me questioning why. A conclusion I reached was that it's probably because the lecture felt like dental school all over again with lengthy and overwhelming amount of slides. This experience made me consider many things as I was preparing this book. In the end I decided to trim away unnecessary details and only mention the critical core points. As much as I liked the sound of being called a "Genius", I did add a lot more details compared to my first few lectures because I figured listening to a seminar and reading a book are different when it comes to content delivery.

Interpretation of panoramic radiograph is a very important factor in third molar extraction surgery. I urge you to read this chapter very thoroughly to gain good understanding of it. If you need, go back to your old textbooks from dental school and refresh your knowledge.

02
Interpretation of third molar and IAN Canal relationship ★★★

If you look at existing radiology textbooks regarding interpretation of relationship between IAN and the third molar, most of them mentions Deflection, Narrowing, Bifid and Blurred Dark band of roots, Interruption, Constriction, Diversion of IANC. Most of the time these books are written by radiology specialists whose capability to read and interpret radiographs are far superior compared to myself. Personally, I would like to see more dental radiology specialists to actively engage in clinical dentistry and beyond. When I was running a large dental practice with a few other partners, I even hired a dental radiology specialist as an associate dentist despite all my partners being against the idea. So without any intention to disregard their expertise, I would like to briefly discuss what I think is more clinically relevant to interpret especially when it comes to third molar extractions.

I have a habit of taking photos of every third molar after extraction when it involves sectioning of crown and/or roots and it helped a lot when it came to comparing what it looked like on OPG versus what it actually looked like in the mouth. You can already find numerous texts explaining the relationship between third molar and IANC with quick Google search. However, there are too many exceptions in actual clinical cases and therefore some of the descriptions lack effectiveness. In this chapter, I will discuss what I deem most clinically relevant (dark band around the roots, diversion of IAN canal) by comparing the OPGs and post-extraction tooth photos. Below is a review of already well-known common IAN canal to 3rd molar root relationship patterns.

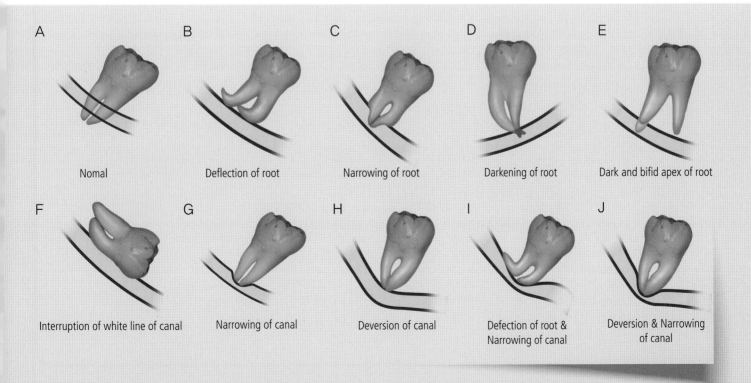

A — Nomal

B — Deflection of root

C — Narrowing of root

D — Darkening of root

E — Dark and bifid apex of root

F — Interruption of white line of canal

G — Narrowing of canal

H — Deversion of canal

I — Defection of root & Narrowing of canal

J — Deversion & Narrowing of canal

Make sure your re-visit this chapter later!

When I was first organising the chapters, I wanted this chapter and the next (Crown sectioning) to be part of the appendix at the end of the book. But as I've mentioned before, over the years that I've been delivering wisdom teeth seminars, I've found out that most dentist forget about what they've learned in dental school and only retain knowledge they got from practicing clinical dentistry. Which is why I think my seminar attendees praised me to be a genius when I added OPG interpretation and crown sectioning at the end of my seminars. Because quite often you think you know everything but in actual fact you have forgotten about a lot of things.

I decided to pull these 2 chapters forward because I think that the most important thing in 3rd molar extraction isn't about methodology of how you perform the extraction. Rather, I thought they were

1. Case Selection
2. Handling complications
3. Dealing with incomplete tooth removal.

As I said, main purpose of this chapter is to compare the OPG and the actual orientation of the 3rd molars intraorally. So don't worry about the methodology of sectioning in this chapter yet as it will be discussed in copious detail in the following chapters.

However, I do strongly recommend that you re-visit this chapter and the next (the coronectomy chapter) once you finished reading through the extraction technique chapters. It will help solidify your knowledge on most important aspects of wisdom teeth surgery; case selection, identifying and managing high risk situations.

03
Is the Inferior Alveolar Nerve Canal a soft tissue? ★

Is IAN Canal soft tissue? No. It isn't. As the name suggests, it is a nerve canal which allows passage of a nerve and is a hard tissue. It varies from person to person as does the bone density and anatomy. Therefore, when roots of the dentition meet the canal, it can be in many different shape and form.

Roots of mandibular third molar starts forming around mid to late teens and completes around early 20s when the roots come in contact with the IAN Canal. As seen on the diagram below, roots will encounter the IAN canals of varying density. From pipes (canals) as hard as a metal pipe to as soft as a Styrofoam tube. Aside from the influence of cortical bone or other surrounding tissues, formation of root apex will heavily rely on the density and hardness of the canal the roots meet during development.

1. They are exclusive and doesn't influence one another.
2. The pipe is as hard as metal which will cause the roots to bend
3. The pipe is like plastic and bends due to developmental force of the roots.
4. The pipe is like Styrofoam and gets constricted as the roots develop.

Of course, there are other factors coming into play, but I always take the type of IAN canal I am dealing with into consideration. If an IAN canal is hard, it will be less affected by the amount of pressure I apply to it. Conversely, if the IAN is not surrounded by any hard tissue at all, nerve damage would not occur, with slight pressure or movement, as the nerve itself would be bendable.

In addition, the speed and force at which the roots forms is as relevant as the strength of the roots itself. In my experience, extraction is harder if the tooth and/or roots are very weak. Much like how it's much easier to remove a live, healthy tree root from the ground compared to dead and rotten ones.

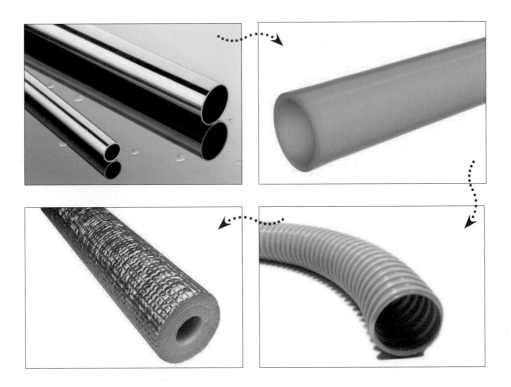

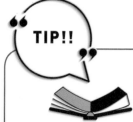

TIP!!

Analysis of CT scans on the relationship between wisdom teeth and the IANC ★★

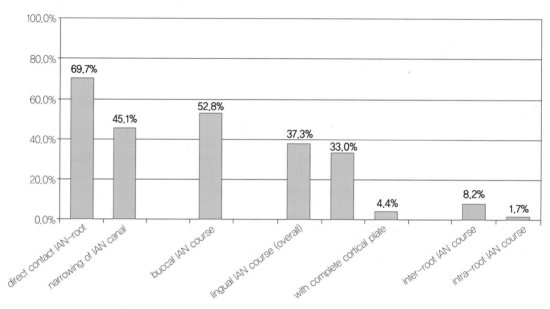

Anatomy of impacted lower third molars evaluated by computerized tomography:
is there and indication for 3-dimensional imaging?(Oral Surg Oral Med Oral Pathol Oral Radiol Endod 2011:111:547-550)

I prefer to discuss my experience in the of clinical notes in this book. But I thought journal articles are a great way to approach anatomy. So here are some literature reviews.

According to the research above, IAN and the root is in direct contact with each other in 69.4% of the cases and constricts the canal in 45%. IANC travels lingually 37.3% and buccally 52.8% of the time which is 1.42 times more prevalent. But this result is odd for us as a Korean dentist. Why? I think it's because in Korea, we are only permitted to take CBCT under national health care if the roots and the IANC overlaps on the OPG. Perhaps due to the lack of available space on lingual side of the jaw, if IANC travels lingual to the root of the tooth we see more of the alarming overlaps. Also probably because x-ray of the OPG originates bucco-inferiorly. So in the cases where CBCT is available, most IANC travels lingually,contrary to the statistical data from the research above. Personally, I do own a CBCT machine but I select my cases very carefully and only take it in cases where I believe the IANC and the root(s) of the mandibular third molar are severely involved with each other. Surely, when we take selective CBCTs like that, we find more IANC to be travelling lingually.

TIP!!

Analysis of CT scan on the relationship between the wisdom tooth and the IANC ★

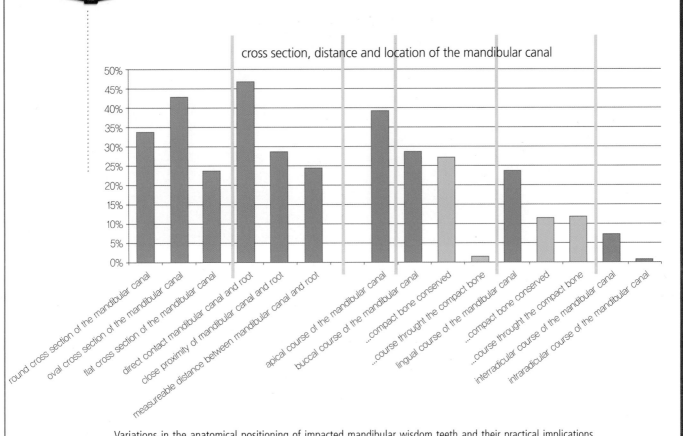

cross section, distance and location of the mandibular canal

Variations in the anatomical positioning of impacted mandibular wisdom teeth and their practical implications
(SWISS DENTAL JOURNAL 124: 520–529 (2014))

Above is a study from Switzerland in 2014 regarding the relationship between mandibular third molar and the IANC. I didn't want to create any misunderstanding so I won't add any extra comment on it. Only use this as a point of reference. I recommend you to search for the journal and have a read yourself. But I believe there is significant racial variation so please take that into consideration as well. Just to briefly explain the graph, in this study, 29.0% of the IANC travelled buccally which is more than the 23.8% that travelled lingually. However, this particular study has a separate category for inferiorly travelling IANC so if you only consider ratio of buccal to lingual, you could say that the result from this study (Buccal is 1.22 times more prevalent) is similar to the previous study (Buccal is 1.42 times more prevalent). On the contrary, the previous study describes 'constriction of IANC' in 45% of the cases where as this one describes it as 'Flat Cross Section' in 23.6% of the cases. If you would like to find out more about this, please look this journal up and have a read.

04
A direct comparison: IANC and Third Molar vs Bow string and Arrow ★★★

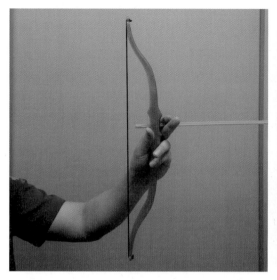 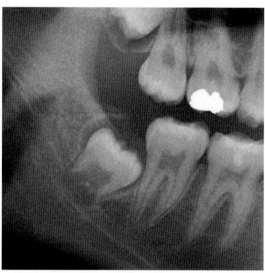

Let's say the IANC is the bow string and the dentition is the arrow. The IANC has elasticity to allow itself to bend much like the bow string. So what would happen if developing roots comes in contact with the nerve canal?

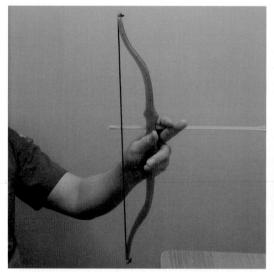 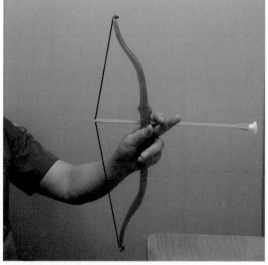

The left photo is when the root and IANC didn't meet each other and the right one is when root comes in contact with the nerve canal causing it to bend. Of course, in the latter, if the nerve canal is as hard as a metal pipe or the developing root is soft and cannot exert a lot of force on the canal, the arrow might bend when it meets the bowstring. Any of the above may appear mixed together to the lesser extent. Obviously, there are more factors to consider; age of the patient may lead to ankylosis of the root to the IANC or the lingual cortical wall. But these factors are very hard to tell on the OPG. What I deem noteworthy from my personal clinical experience is when the IANC gets constricted or bent because the canal external wall is weak and fragile. This is because ultimately, IAN damage will always be accompanied by IAN canal wall damage.

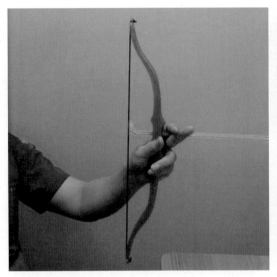
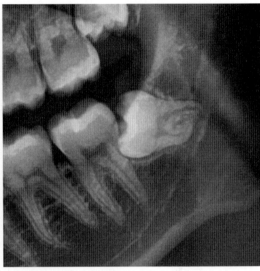

You can see that the arrow has been bent as it encountered the bowstring. Perhaps the bowstring is as hard as a metal pipe? Maybe we can extract this third molar without being too concerned about damaging the IAN. On the OPG you can see that the mesial root has bent upwards as it encountered the IAN canal.

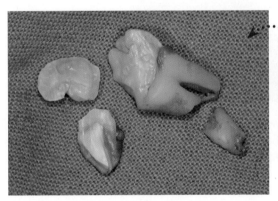
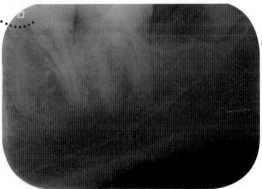

The mesial root has fractured during extraction. The remaining root is evident on the PA x-ray. I've removed the remaining root knowing that the nerve is safely protected within a hard IAN canal. However, perhaps it is a waste of your time and effort to try and remove root tips like this regardless of how skillful you are. I will explain the statement above in the next chapter (Coronectomy) in more depth but it is often wise to leave root tips like this one.

05
Can roots really bend when it meets the IAN Canal? ★

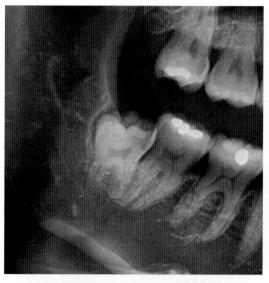
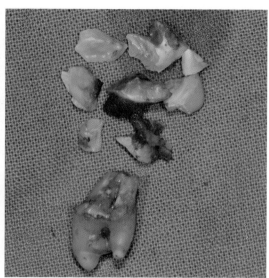
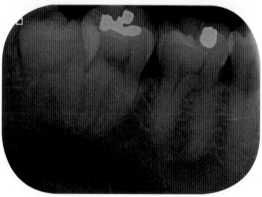

You can see blurring of distal root on the OPG but PA also suggests the ML root to have a little curve at the tip. If you look closely you can see that there are 3 roots. As you can see from the photo of the extracted tooth, the MB root has formed normally, the ML root has been bent as it encountered the IAN canal. We will discuss blurring and darkening of the root on the radiograph in much more detail later in this chapter. Anyhow, when I tackle a case like this, I think the IAN canal must be hard enough to change the direction of a root entirely. But when I sectioned the crown of the tooth and applied force with an elevator, portion of the tooth would chip off. So either cortication around the canal is very strong or the tooth is very weak and fragile.

ALWAYS REMEMBER. Weak tooth = difficult extraction.

06
Superimposition on the OPG ★★★

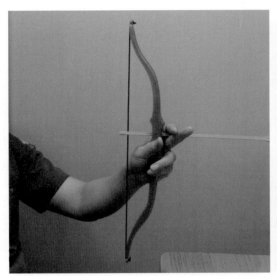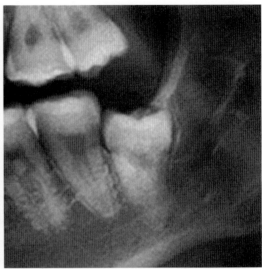

This is when the root and the nerve canal are does not meet or interfere with one another. The root will develop as per norm and the nerve canal remains unaffected.

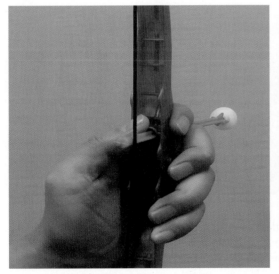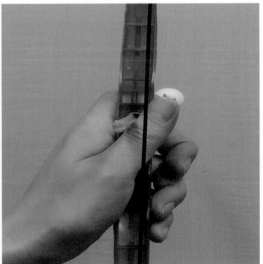

However, the proximity of the IANC and the roots may change our approach. As the left photo above shows, if the root and the nerve canal are in contact, they may have influenced each other. Either the nerve canal would've been pushed outwards or if the canal was strong like a metal pipe it would've caused deformation of the root. Let's take a look one by one.

07
Appears to be superimposed on the OPG but actually not ★★

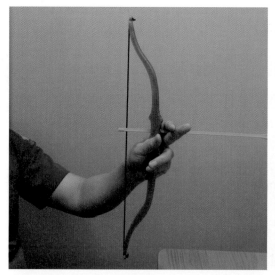 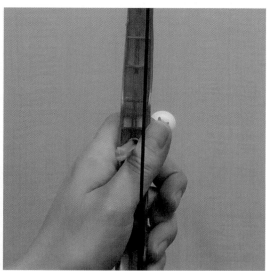

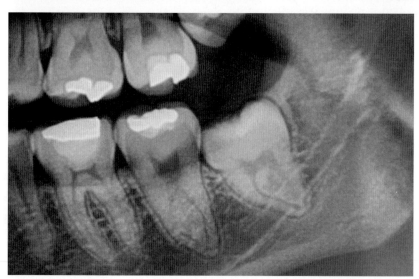

If the root of the third molar and the IAN canal is completely separate and exclusive, it may seem overlap on the OPG but you do not notice any anomaly on the OPG. All the structure are shown on OPG with continuous line. Since I strive to minimise bone removal with my third molar extractions, I ignore the IAN canal unless root tip fracture happens.

★★

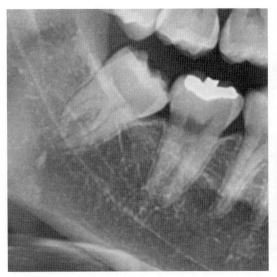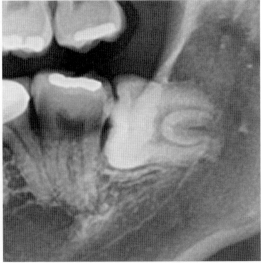

Again, in the radiograph above, the third molar and the nerve canal seems to overlap. However, we can't observe any anomaly on the formation of the roots and continuation of the nerve canal and the roots. This means that nerve canal and the roots of the third molar are completely exclusive to one another. If you take a CBCT of cases like this, you will see that the IANC is travelling bucco-inferiorly, far from the actual root.

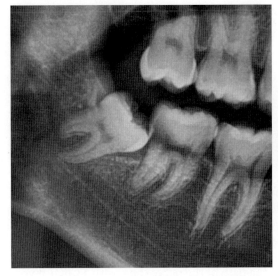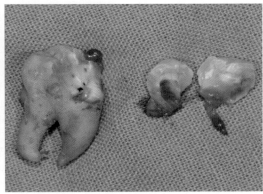

Again, the roots and the IANC seems to be overlapping but there are no anomalies on the radiograph, proceeded with extraction as per normal.

08
Third molar extraction : Appears superimposed on the OPG but without ★★★
complications

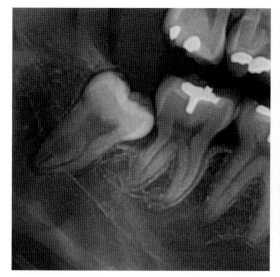 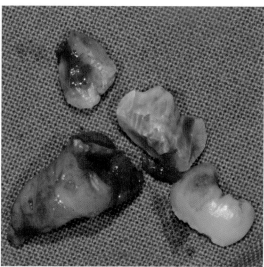

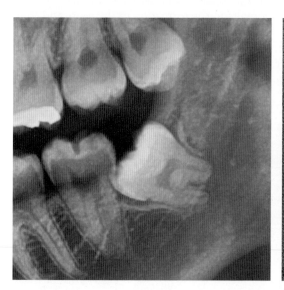 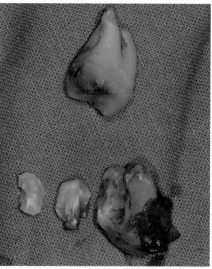

I've extracted the third molar which appeared superimposed on the OPG but with no apparent complication. As evident from the photo of the extracted dentition, no anomaly is noted from the root and you may proceed as per your normal extraction protocol without being concerned about the IANC. However, caution is necessary if there is a root fracture and you are required to do a lot of bone removal. In my experience, the IANC travels buccally in most cases like this. However, double check the path of the nerve canal with a CBCT if you have one handy.

09
The dark band: Superimposed on OPG and root and the IANC is ★★★ in contact with each other

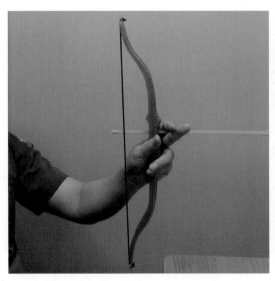 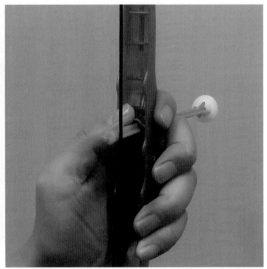

Although the root of the third molar is not heavily involved with the IANC, if the two are in contact with each other, then it may appear as radiographic distortion. The most common one being the dark band where the root suddenly darkens on the radiograph.

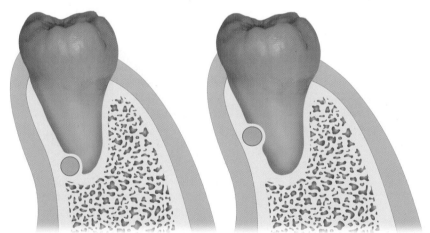

As seen on the diagram on the left, the root has deformed as it encountered the IANC. Obviously, you want to take precaution as the root is touching the IANC but formation of the dark band instead of distortion of the IANC means that the nerve canal is the metal pipe type we discussed earlier. I tend to proceed with extraction without much concern for the IANC but it is important to tell your patients to let you know when they feel nerve sensitivity during elevation, as this means you are applying pressure to the nerve. On a similar note, if a root tip fractures, it's quite often better to leave them alone instead of trying to fish them out and potentially cause nerve damage.

10
Typical dark band ★★★

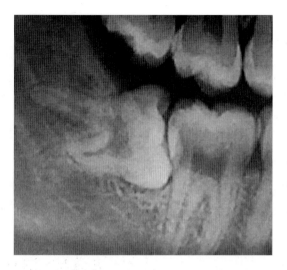

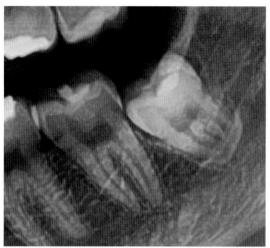

Dark band is obvious in the middle of the mesial root and root appears very clearly for the distal root. This can mean that the mesial root splits in two half way down but it's very difficult to know that. Considering the IANC travels without any obstruction it is more likely that the IANC is very hard and rigid.

Typical dark band formation in the middle of both roots. You may proceed with your normal extraction protocol but if patient complains of nerve pain half way through the extraction despite having sufficient anaesthesia, I recommend considering intentional coronectomy.

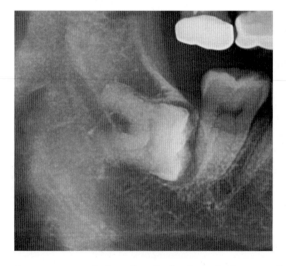

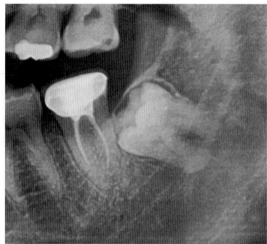

Same patient, left and right both with distinct dark band around the roots. From my experience, this type of radiographic presentation was usually a sign of a very strong nerve canal.

11

Case Study: Comparison of left and right where both sides appear to have ★★ root to IANC superimposition

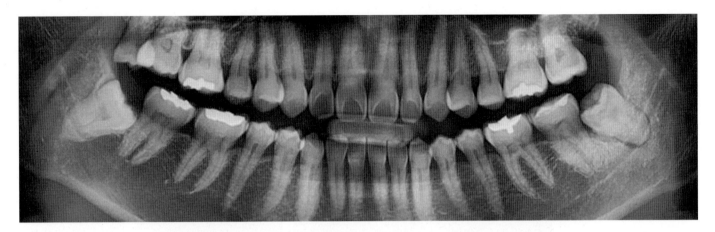

Female patient in her late 40's was referred to my practice for pericorinitis of 38. Dark band is clear around the #48 on the OPG but although the #38 has dark shadow around the dentition, there is no anomaly where the root and IANC is superimposed. It was a lot clearer on the monitor than on the printed x-ray above.

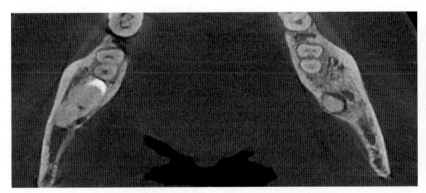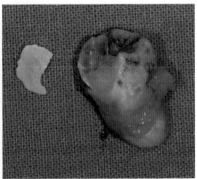

If you compare the cross-section of the left and right, IANC is travelling lingually and is in close contact with the #48. Whereas on the left the IANC is travelling buccally and is completely separate from the #38. Radiolucency is much larger around the #38 on the OPG but the dark band is a lot more distinctive in #48. I think the #38 would look a lot more normal if it wasn't for the bone resorption around the tooth. This case was referred to me by a professor in a dental school as he wasn't comfortable with extracting these third molars from his older sister. The cross section x-ray seems like a slice from a head and neck CT scan which the professor recommended her to bring to the appointment. I briefly discussed the differential diagnosis but the patient just requested extraction. Oddly, she just said thank you and left the practice without settling the account after the extraction. When my staff tried to stop her, she just said "Don't worry I will get post-op care from my brother". From time to time, when my colleague or their family visits, I don't charge them out of courtesy, but I was left a little dumbfounded when she took it for granted like that

12
Case Study 1: Extraction of third molars with the dark band ★★★

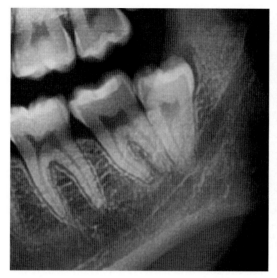 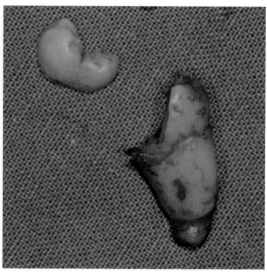

I took the photo of the extracted tooth from the buccal side where you can clearly see the passage of the IANC.

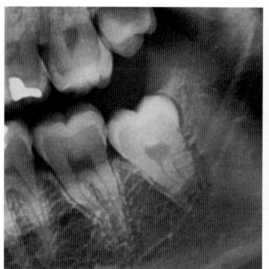 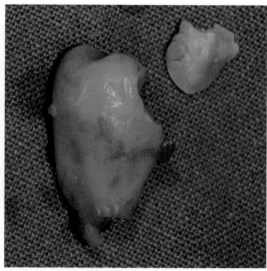

The tooth photo was taken from the lingual side of the tooth. You can observe the root malformation due to the developing root interacting with the IANC. For the first case, I sectioned off the distal part of the crown before elevating. Mesial portion of the crown was sectioned prior to elevation for the second case. Again, details of sectioning are discussed later in the book so let's remain focused on the shape of the roots for now. Neither patient complained of pain or sensitivity for the extractions. Perhaps the IAN canals were the metal pipe type for both?

Case Study 2: Extraction of third molars with the dark band ★★

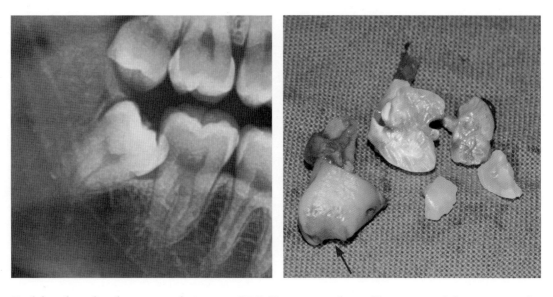

Dark band on distal root was obvious on OPG. You can see the malformation of the root near the apex of the distal root on the buccal side.

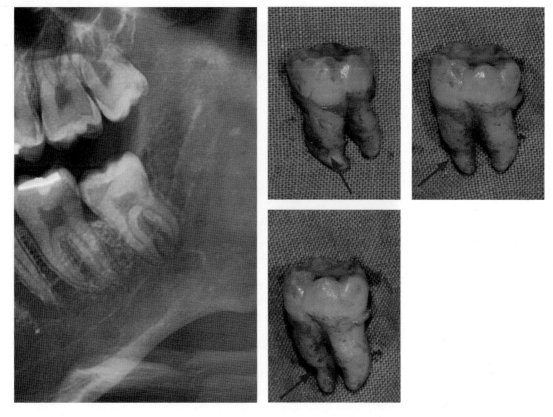

This is a rare case where the nerve canal is in contact with buccal aspect of the mesial root as it travels through. Even for cases like this, I tend not to raise a flap and extract the tooth only using an elevator as per usual.

Case Study 3: Extraction of third molars with the dark band ★★

Same patient left and right

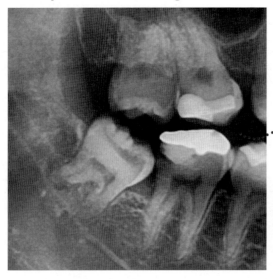

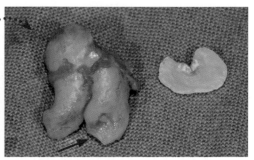

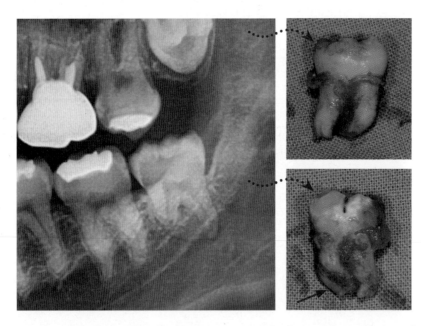

On the OPG the root of the #48 seems severely distorted. Looking at the tooth outside the jaw you can see the apex has been bent and pressed after meeting the IANC. You can observe the mesial root of the #38 to be darker and more blurred compared to the distal root. Even after extraction tooth shows no anomaly from buccal view, but from lingual aspect you can confirm where the developing root has encountered the IAN canal.

Seeing as both left and right third molar roots were affected in their development as they came to contact with the IAN canals, we can assume that the nerve canal would be as hard as a metal pipe.

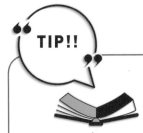

Another form of the "Dark Band" ★★

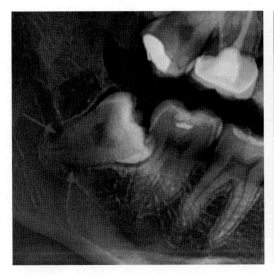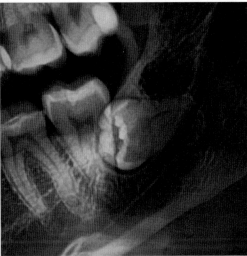

Again, both sides of the same patient. Dark band is evident but you also notice that the dark band extends beyond the root of the tooth.

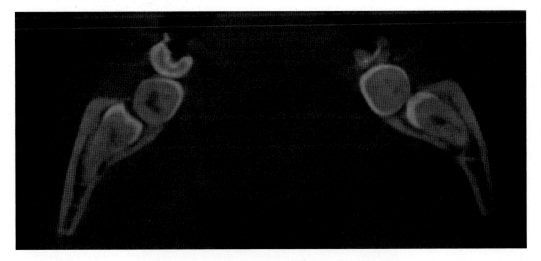

For cases like these, it's mostly because the growing root has pushed the IANC into the lingual cortical plate causing the nerve canal to travel within the lingual cortical plate. The nerve canal doesn't have a steep 90degree bend when its pressured by the roots. Rather, it bends and gets pushed like a bowstring. Hence there is a gradated resorption of lingual cortical plate before and after the nerve canal is completely embedded in the cortical plate which creates the radiolucency pattern as shown in the OPG above.

Wait!

Warning** Case Study 1: When the IANC travels between ★★ the roots

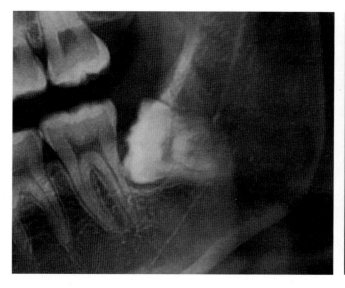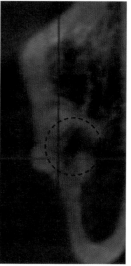

There was a blurring of the distal root on the OPG above. Something didn't quite sit right with me so I decided to take a CBCT. Turns out, there were 4 roots and the IANC was right in the middle of the roots. The blurring isn't exactly same as the dark band but I think the fundamental reason behind it is the same. When you see blurring of the roots, be very cautious in removing the roots.

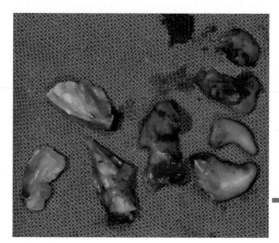

The tooth had 4 roots and distal roots on the top of the photo seems to have either C-shape or two root canals. Clearly the IANC travels in between the root.

My ego made me extract the tooth but I think if you are a less experienced GP you must consider intentional coronectomy. You have to be very conscious about the patient's reactions such as pain or sensitivity to the movement of the tooth you make.

Wait!

Case Study 2: When the IANC travels between the roots

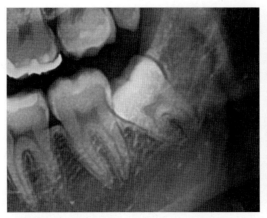
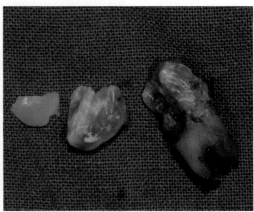

The roots and the nerve canal are appearing superimposed. The roots have maintained its shape in growth but you can observe that the IANC has lost its continuity. This doesn't always mean that the IANC is traveling in between the roots but it certainly warrants a further investigation. The photo on the right shows the mesial view of the tooth. There will be detailed description of sectioning methods later in the book so we won't discuss it here. You can observe that the IANC had travelled through the furcation of the roots as seen in the CBCT below.

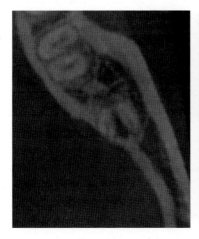
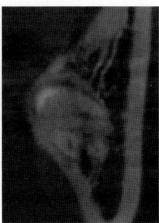
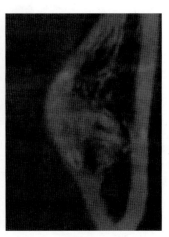

The cross-sectional slice on the far left shows the IAN canal to be located in between the roots. Again, its paramount that you observe the patient's reaction to pressure during extraction. Even on the 2 coronal slices, you can observe the IANC before and after it enters the furcation of the roots. During the extraction procedure the patient constantly complained of nerve sensitivity; the extent of which, was carefully checked and monitored. All up it took myself about 2 minutes to complete the extraction with no report of nerve damage post-extraction.

13
When in doubt, perform an Intentional Coronectomy ★★★

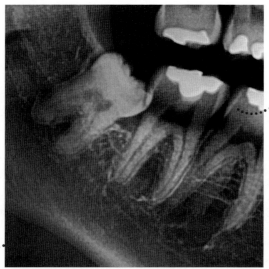

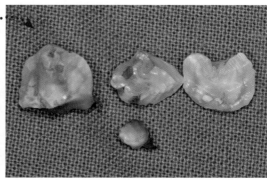

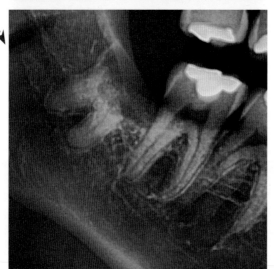

If there is distinctive dark band which could pose difficulty in extraction, don't waste your time attempting to fully extract, instead start with the intention to perform a coronectomy. The OPG below was taken a week after the procedure during the suture removal visit. After a 1-year follow-up, the patient is not bothered by the remaining root at all. He lives very far away so he couldn't physically visit our surgery. Instead, we've spoke on the phone to see if he had any concerns.

Attention!

MORE EXCEPTIONS THAN YOU THINK!

Yes, the dark band is a sign that the nerve canal and the roots are in close proximity. However, absence of dark band doesn't necessarily mean that they are apart. There are cases where the two are in close contact even when you see no evidence of it on the OPG.

In addition, there are many other variables that can arise from the relationship between the IANC and the lingual cortical wall as the IAN canal travels lingually to the roots for most cases where the dark band is observable.

14
When the pressure of developing roots cause IANC diversion ★★★

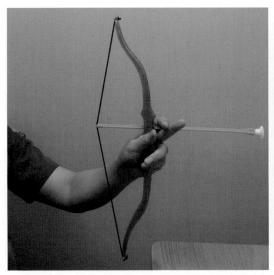
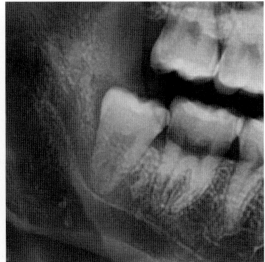

The roots have come in contact with the IANC in the process of its development and dsiplaced the nerve canal out of its way. You can see the alteration of the path of the IANC as if an arrow is pushing the bow string back. If you notice such features on the OPG, there is a high chance that the IANC is located directly inferior to the apex of the roots so you must not apply too much force in the event of root-tip fracture.

Another very important point to remember here is that at least when the encounter of the developing root and the IAN canal happened, the canal was not as strong as a metal pipe. Rather, it would've been a plastic pipe or weaker. It is the weakness of the bone tissue surrounding the IAN which allows the force of root development to be able to displace the nerve as seen on the OPG. You must take the weakness of the IAN canal into consideration when you are performing extraction in a case such as this one. Always ask the patient to express any pain during the procedure and be very careful if you must remove a fractured root tip.

★★

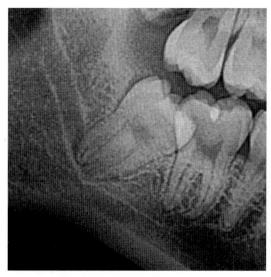 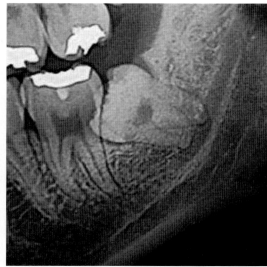

Left and right of the same patient. We can easily assume that when the root was forming the nerve canal was very elastic.

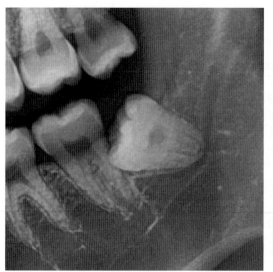 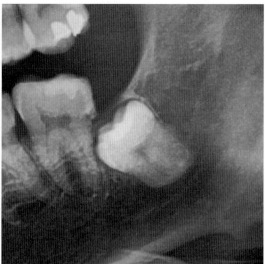

The case above on the left shows that the displacement of the IANC is very limited to where the root apex is, as opposed to the entire canal being pushed away as like a bowstring. This is a very common presentation. The case on the right shows a bent root upon encountering the IANC but the root shape is very clear without any blurring all the way down to the apex. However, not only was the nerve canal displaced but it was also constricted. We can infer that either the force of root formation was very strong or the nerve canal was weak at the time of root development. Therefore, these are the cases I would be most cautious about.

15
Extraction of mandibular third molars with distinctive signs of IANC diversion ★★★

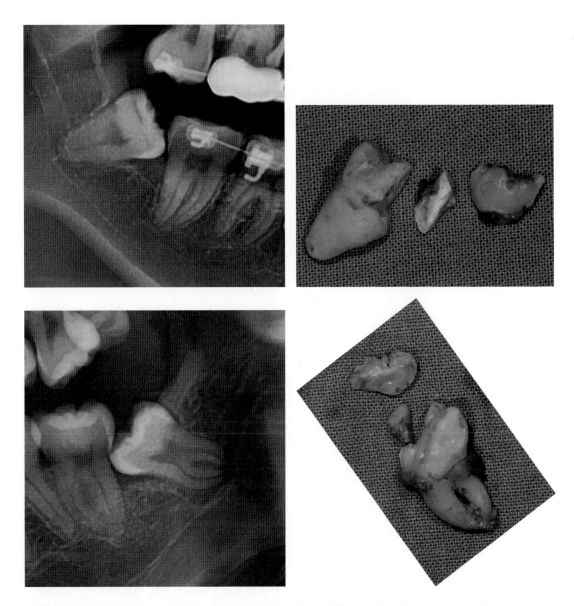

With the cases above, the nerve canals were displaced like a pulled bow string with no signs of anomaly on the root morphology. For the case of the #38 above, there were no symptoms of nerve damage following extraction even though part of the interseptal bone was extracted with the tooth. However, it wouldn't be a bad choice to consider coronectomy from the beginning instead of taking an unnecessary risk.

16
Dark band & Diversion ★★★

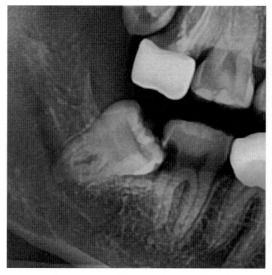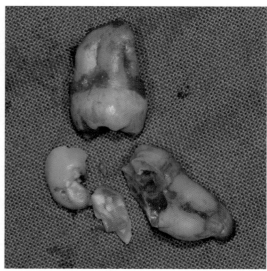

The photo was taken to show lingual aspect of the extracted third molar. You can clearly observe where the IANC was in contact with the root near the apex.

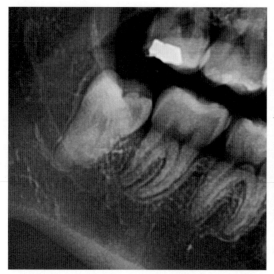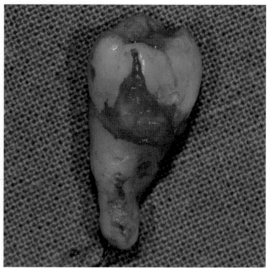

Although it's not as prominent, you can still observe mild dark band from IANC bending. You do NOT have to worry about the IANC too much during extraction. Proceed as you would normally with ~5 mm gingival incision and an elevator.

17
Case Study 1: Constricted and Diverted IAN Canal ★★★

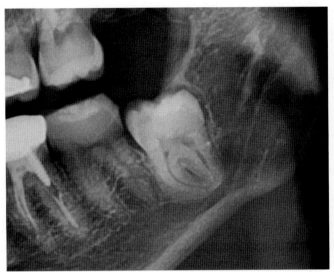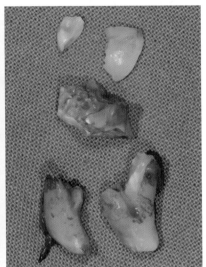

Above case shows IAN canal to be constricted AND diverted. You can observe that the formation of root had applied enough force on the IAN canal to be pushed all the way down to the cortical bone of the inferior border of the mandible. Again, this is my personal opinion but, the IAN canal is a pipe-like hard tissue of varying hardness. If it was strong enough, the root would be deformed or bent as it encountered the canal. However, if the canal was displaced and thinned out then it may mean that the external wall of the canal wasn't hard at all. This doesn't change the methodology of the third molar extraction though. For the case above, I did consider stopping after coronectomy but decided to proceed with root sectioning. As I mentioned earlier, I always ask the patient to express any nerve sensation (sharp pain, electric tingling etc.) during extraction. Extra caution is mandatory for cases like this.

Generally speaking, it is said that the lower border of the inferior alveolar canal is a little bit harder and the top border is a little softer. In that sense, when you look at constrictions on panoramic radiographs, we can infer that the inferior border of the canal space is hard cortical bone and the superior border is relatively softer bone. As the tooth root developed, the softer superior border flexed while the harder inferior border held firm. Therefore, when you notice a constriction effect on the radiograph, you must be extra careful not to exert too much apical force when removing root tips – to avoid crushing and damaging the nerve with root tips when the nerve is resting on a hard surface with no flexibility below to soften the pressure.

18
Case Study 2: Constricted and Diverted IAN Canal ★★

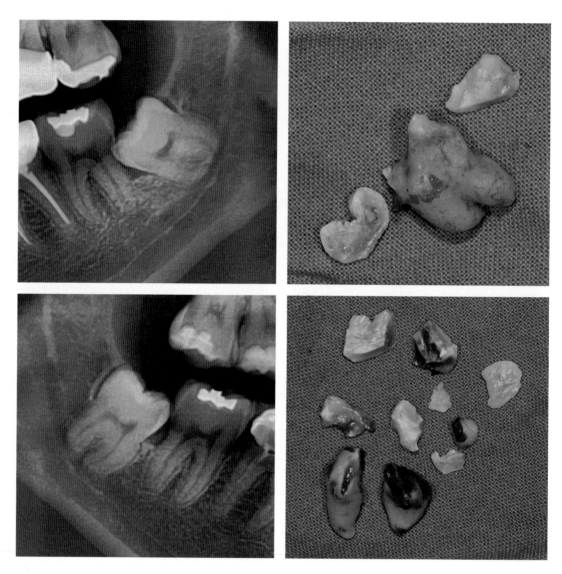

This is a case of 35y.o female who lived in Germany for a long time. She returned home in Korea and couldn't find a dental practice where she could get her third molars extracted until she visited my surgery. She had the #38 extracted first, waited a month and got the #48 extracted. Above are the OPG and post-extraction photos. My policy is usually 'same-day consult and extraction' as I rarely get OPGs in advance to do surgery planning. #38 was extracted on her first visit and it was a very simple 5-minute extraction.

★★

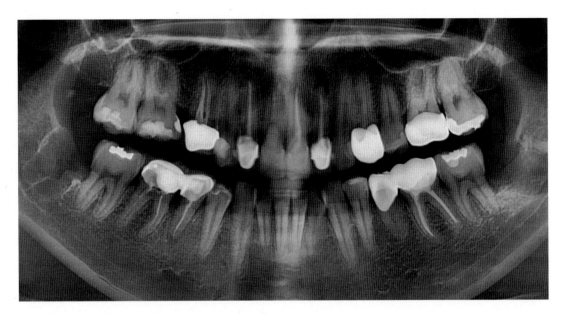

Although the #48 was approached with the same method as the #38, the procedure panned out a little differently. I will discuss the extraction methods later in the book, but usually with impacted third molar cases I tend to remove the mesial portion of the tooth first rather than removing the buccal bone. However, with this particular case, angulation of the handpiece forced the sectioned lingual portion to be much larger than I would've liked. As I applied force on the distobuccal part of the tooth to elevate the tooth, remaining crown of the third molar fractured off. In the end, the cervical portion of the crown and the roots were extracted separately in about 20minutes.

The next day as the patient returned to dress the wound, she reported sensory changes so we've taken another OPG (shown above). The OPG was unremarkable and the issue was resolved eventually. However, we can observe a clear, white densely corticated lamina dura which explains why the extraction was challenging.

In conclusion, the constricted and diverted IAN canal could be the result of the canal not being surrounded by hard cortical casing. Therefore, we should be very cautious to NOT apply excessive force onto the roots in the process of extraction and should consider refraining from fractured root removal at times.

19
Treatment Notes for the patent above ★

This was taken directly from the treatment notes of the patient

Nov.12   #48 extraction (#38 was extracted 21st. September 2015)

Nov.14   Post-op dressing visit. Patient reported swelling on the right side and mild numbness as if the anaesthetic hasn't worn off. Advised that it may be temporary, watch and wait.

Nov.16   Post-op care call by reception staff.

Patient: My sensory changes hasn't improved at all since Saturday. Dr. Kim mentioned taking steroids if the issue persists. Should I start taking them now or should I wait till Thursday?

Staff: I will double check with Dr Kim and call you back.

Nov.18   Return phone call

Staff: I checked with Dr Kim and he says there's no need for steroid and also said your senses will return to normal soon. Don't worry too much! We will also double check when you come for your suture removal visit

Nov.18   Phone call to change appointment time.

Staff: Hi Ms Lee, Dr Kim wants to attend to you personally and we wanted to change appointment time. Any chance we can see you on Friday or today even?

Patient: I can't do today but I can do Friday morning. There is still mild numbness on the right-hand side. I will come in Friday 10 am. Can I bring my child for a check-up then too?

Nov. 20   Suture removal appointment

Patient: Everything is still the same as when you first anaesthetised it.

Me: Don't worry, your senses will come back to normal. We will continue to monitor.

Dec. 07   Patient called the surgery. (A Happy call!)

02:09 PM Patient: Numbness improved a little bit. I know you said it can take a while to recover so I am happy to continue monitoring. I am honestly not sure if I've gotten used to it or if things have improved.

After the 1-month follow-up, I contacted the patient personally

It's always my policy to make the care calls myself when there are active complaints or issues with the treatment. It reduces stress for my staff and I also learned through experience that it is usually a lot quicker for myself to resolve this personally.

Dec. 17   Contacted patient on personal messenger

Me: Hi Mrs Lee! It's Dr Youngsam Kim from Gangnam Leon Dental. How are you feeling now?

Patient: Hello Doctor. Thank you for getting in touch personally. To be completely honest, the numbness is still there. However, I don't think it's because of your lack of skill at all. I just had an odd-looking tooth. A lot of dental clinics have refused to extract my tooth. Thank you for your concerns, I will wait a little longer as you've said. Have a nice day.

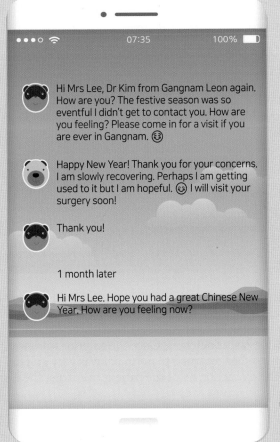

To the left is messages exchanged after another month have passed. She reported signs of improvement. I've sent her a message again after another month have passed but the number 1 next to the message indicating she hasn't read my message yet hadn't disappeared for a long time. Rare occasion where I was happy that I didn't get a reply back from a lady.

However, there was a problem after a month.

This is a conversation between me and my patient, talking about the healing process. Last message was not read by the patient.

Problem was that the patient has asked for aesthetic work on the anteriors.

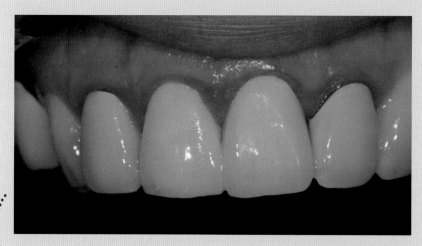

She said she never used to care too much about aesthetics of her upper anteriors but living in Korea made her conscious about her smile and asked me to improve her smile for her. When we were providing quote for her treatment, she casually mentioned that the extraction site is still a little uncomfortable 😊 Of course, I've given her some extra discount for the treatment.

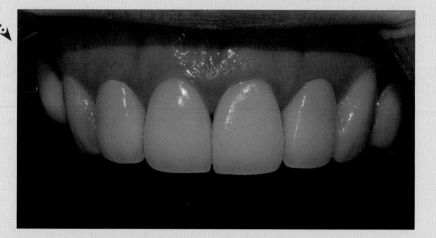

She had mild chronic gingivitis, but through continuous oral hygiene reinforcement and education she now has health gums and a healthy smile. Thanks to the prosthetic work I could maintain a trusting relationship with a patient who could've been my only nerve injury patient. She is very satisfied with the aesthetic outcome. Once the anterior work was complete, she also advised us that the extraction site has returned to normal. I was very grateful to hear that. Again, being proficient at third molar extraction helps the patient to entrust the dentist very easily.

Inflammation around the Third Molars ★★★

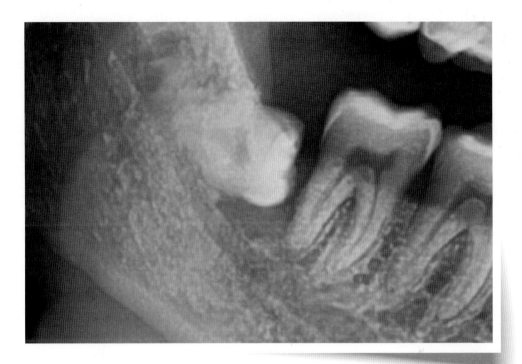

Normally dentists think that the dentition affected by periodontitis are easy to extract. True if we are talking about normal molars where the periodontitis had progressed deep down into the root. But inflammation around the third molars are a little different. Unlike usual presentation of periodontitis, excessive periodontal tissue around the crown of the third molars act as deep pockets and inflammation often presents itself as form of pericoronitis. This could apply pressure to the tooth much like a cyst could, which can result in movement of the roots. Let's take a look at how such chronic inflammation could affect the difficulty of extractions and how its presented on the radiographs.

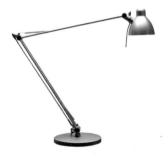

01
Case Study 1: Chronic inflammation may alter the location of the third molars

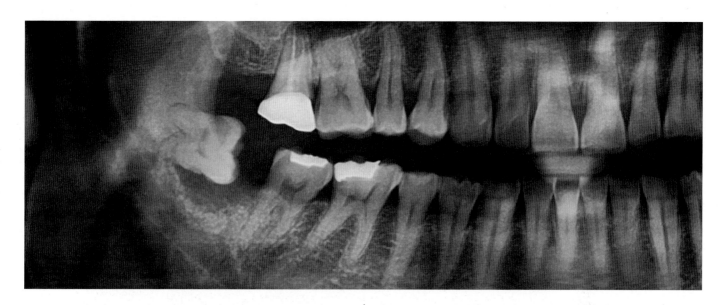

You can observe the disto-superior displacement of the #48 due to the severe pericorinitis. It's similar to how a cyst around the roots would displace a tooth. Regardless of the source being an inflammation or a cyst, the pressure from the local soft tissue swelling displaces the tooth towards the direction of its roots. Same principles as an orthodontic intrusion. For such cases, the roots are embedded deeper into the alveolar bone leading to narrowing of the PDL space or sometimes even ankylosis. Consequently, this can lead to increased difficulty of extraction.

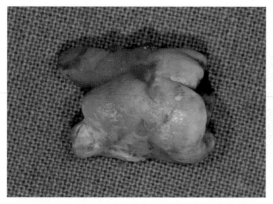 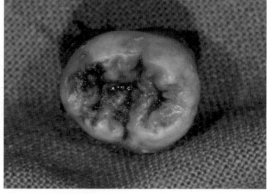

This particular case didn't require any sectioning despite the tooth being horizontally impacted. In most cases you will discover food, calculus and inflammatory tissue surrounding the crown of the tooth. Instead of being ankylosed, this tooth had severe periodontitis and therefore the extraction was as simple as extracting any other periodontally affected dentition.

02
Case Study 2: Pericorinitis pushed horizontally impacted third molar backwards ★★★

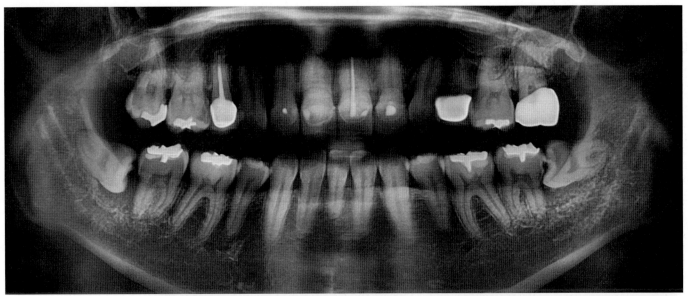

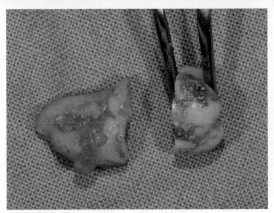
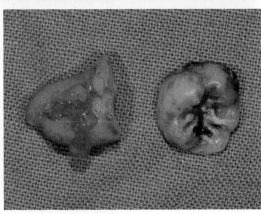

Severe inflammation is evident on both #38 and #48 on the OPG and you can clearly see a lot of calculus remaining on the teeth. That is after removing a lot of it during the extraction procedure. A point to note for cases like these is that the inflammation makes the sectioning (and removal of sectioned pieces) safer and easier. Even if the coronal portion of the dentition is very close to the IANC, you can easily fracture the sectioned pieces to remove them without drilling too deep. The space between the 47 and 48 will allow for easy removal of the pieces. It's even easier when there is plenty of space between the crown of the tooth and the IAN canal. With a long shank round bur, you will and should feel a 'drop' similar to that of entering the pulp during extirpation. This ensures that you are sectioning right down to the inferior border of the crown. This particular case was relatively simple due to the tooth being pushed superiorly. However, this won't always be the case. As I mentioned earlier, pressure from inflammation may cause the tooth to be ankylosed.

03
Case Study 3: Narrowing of PDL space due to the third molar being pushed back ★★★

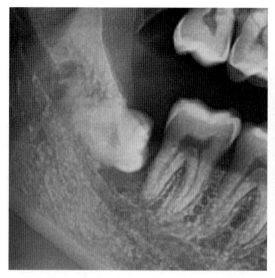

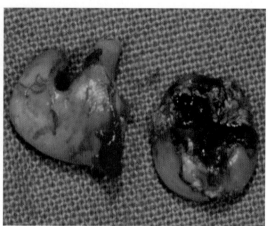

It's very challenging to insert the elevator into the PDL space if the root had been pushed further into the alveolar bone. As you can see in the photo (Distal Crown Cutting- To be discussed in horizontal impaction chapter) I've created a little trench across the distal surface of the root to engage the elevator and delivered the tooth. You can tell how severe the inflammation was by looking at the removed crown.

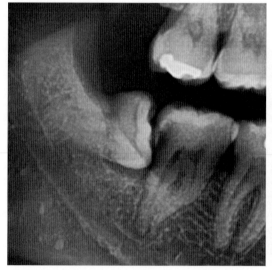

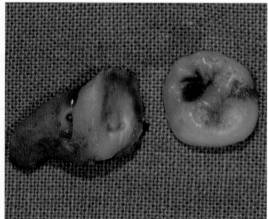

Same principle and technique as above. I created a little trench, engaged the elevator and moved it in a 'rowing motion' to extract and deliver the tooth.

04
Case Study 4: Cases with increased difficulty ★★

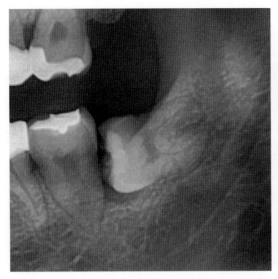 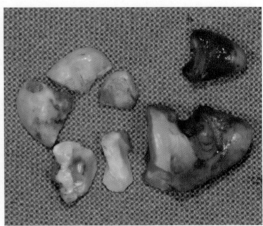

Although the chronic inflammation had made the sectioning of the crown easier, the tooth was positioned too inferiorly and the roots were intentionally sectioned in multiple segments before removal. It is very challenging to estimate the difficulty on the radiograph. You can approach every case in a similar fashion for any horizontally impacted third molar but be prepared to section the roots if you encounter difficulty in removing the remaining roots. We will further this discussion in later chapter; "Horizontally Impacted Third Molar"

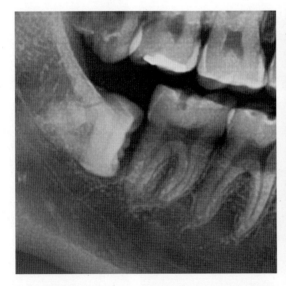 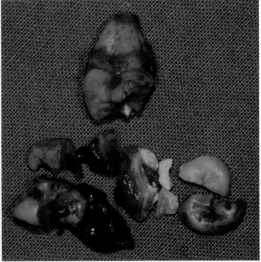

Severe ankylosis made the case above very challenging. In addition, you may think that the abundance of inflammatory tissue would make the crown removal easier, but the crown was positioned very inferiorly and in a close proximity with the IANC. You can observe that the tooth itself was rotated with severe curvature on the mesial root. The roots had to be sectioned for safe removal of the tooth.

05
Case Study 5: Age increases likelihood of ankylosis ★★

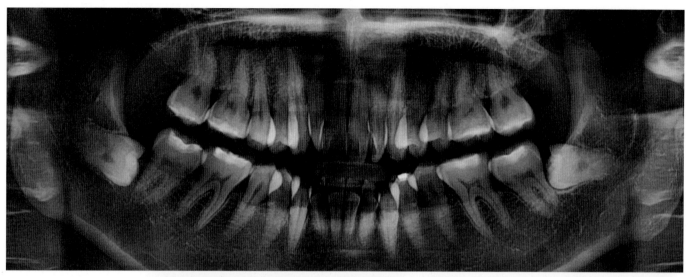

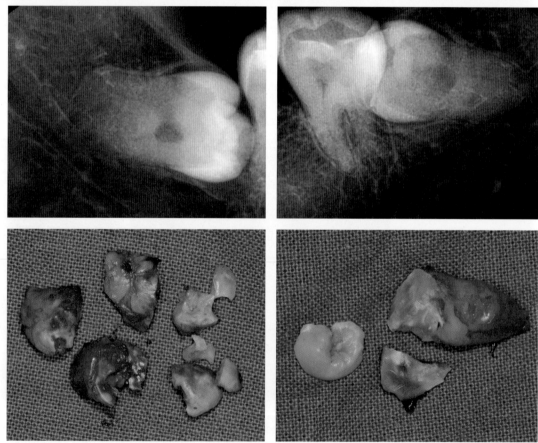

Not every extraction is easy. The crown was positioned inferiorly, pericorinitis would've been applying constant force towards the alveolar bone for a while. Chance of ankylosis is very high. Especially if you follow my methods of conserving buccal bone and extracting the third molar by only using an elevator. There simply isn't enough PDL space to engage the elevator. The patient was a 44 years old female and the #48 in particular posed a lot of challenge.

06
Case Study 6: Longest extraction in 2015 ★

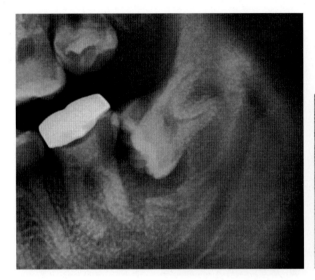
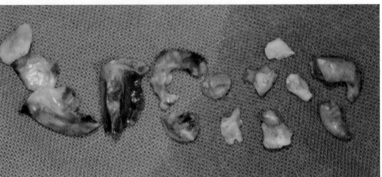

Severe pericorinitis pushed the roots superiorly and caused ankylosis. In addition the roots were severely curved. The patient's younger brother brought the patient to my surgery after getting his third molar removed by me. Among thousands of third molars I extracted in 2015, this was by far the toughest one. Almost took me 40 minutes to extract this one.

The reason I am emphasising how difficult this case was, is because it doesn't look particularly challenging on the radiograph. Many factors can contribute to varying difficulty of third molar extractions. Even with my years of experience, I rarely encountered cases I thought would be very challenging that were actually difficult. Rather, cases like the one shown above where you'd think it will be a routine and easy extraction, quite often end up being unexpectedly challenging.

STOP!

Why you must read this book at least twice

Because I have too many cases, I rarely have to discuss the same case repeatedly. But the case shown above really left a strong impression on me and you will see this case again in the later chapter; Extraction of horizontally impacted Third Molars. If you are wondering how I've extracted this tooth, please read on. Once you've finished reading the whole book and come back to this part, you will have far better understanding of what had happened here.

07
Case Study 7: Root ankylosis ★★★

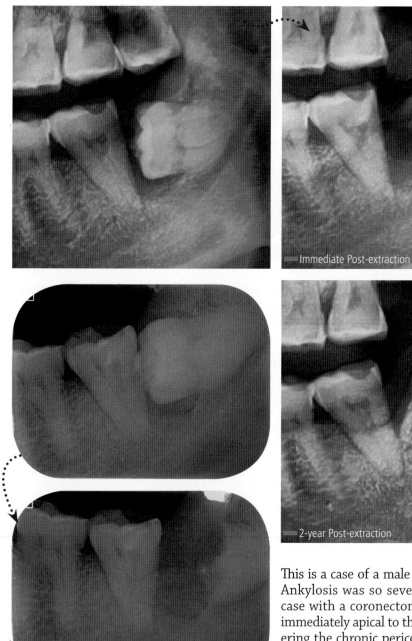

Immediate Post-extraction

2-year Post-extraction

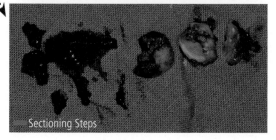

Sectioning Steps

This is a case of a male patient in his mid-50s. Ankylosis was so severe, I had to finish the case with a coronectomy. The IAN canal was immediately apical to the root apex and considering the chronic pericorinitis which would've pressured the tooth further apically, there was heightened possibility that the roots were fused to the external wall of the IAN canal. Patient was asymptomatic and happy after the 2 years follow-up and the OPG was taken 2 years and 10days after the extraction. The roots have shown no movement and I suspect it to be due to the ankylosis.

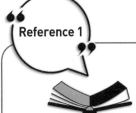

Case Study 8: Distobuccal Bone Resorption from pericorinitis ★★

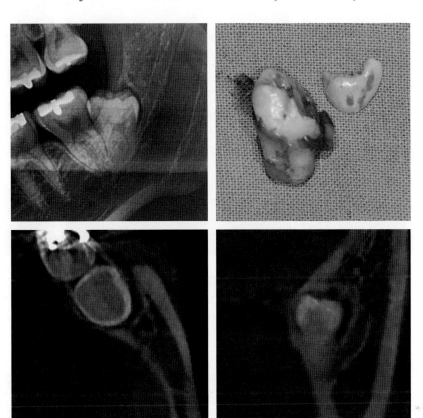

Chronic pericorinitis on a distally and vertically impacted third molar can result in severe bone resorption of the area. It also pushes the root mesiobuccally or further inferiorly. The difference between such cases and other vertically impacted cases in general may not be great, but the PDL space is a variable that is hard to predict. As it could either be very tight from further impaction or very wide from periodontitis. If space between buccal cortical bone and the tooth is very wide, then the Hu-Friedy EL3C (3 mm diameter) might be too narrow to be engaged. It will rotate pointlessly without engagement. These are the cases where the broader EL5C (5 mm diameter) or a pair of forceps becomes useful. We will discuss this further in the Vertically Impacted Third Molar chapter.

STOP!

Root Ankylosis is actually very rare

In actual fact, root ankylosis is very rare. We should not assume that the roots are ankylosed just because the patient is old and the dentition was non-functional for a long time encased in the alveolar bone. However, partial ankylosis may happen to small, limited parts of the roots in these cases. Moreover, in some of the case studies, I've used the word ankylosed for the cases where the PDL space was diminished to an extreme just to help you understand what it feels like.

08
Case Study 9: Pericorinitis and surrounding bone resorption

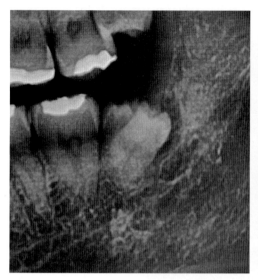
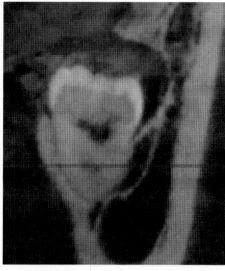
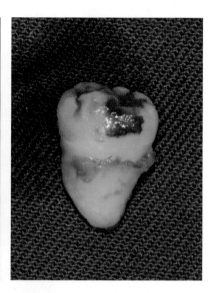

30 years old female patient. Bone loss is evident even on the OPG. Cross section on the CBCT shows abnormality around the crown of the dentition. When you extract a tooth like this, its very common to find a lot of calculus on the tooth. Any bigger radiolucency than what is shown, I might have considered biopsy to rule out cyst.

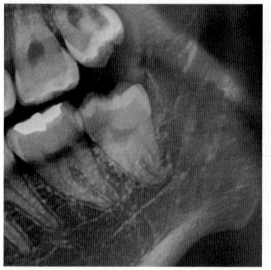
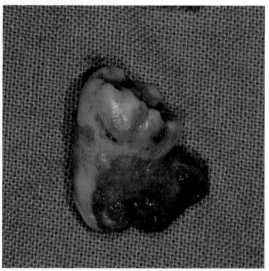

24 years old female patient who wanted extraction due to severe pericorinitis. Sometimes you will see inflammatory soft tissue attached to the extracted tooth which resembles a cyst. It's important to remember to provide adequate curettage and saline irrigation following the extraction to remove any detached calculus and debris from the extraction.

Third Molar Roots and Lingual Cortical Bone ★★★

Youngsam's sign

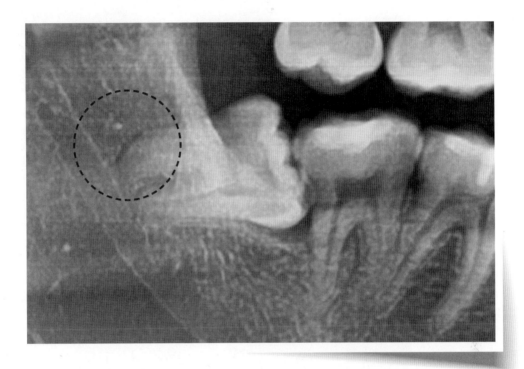

I dared to name this particular radiographic phenomenon which seemed to increase the difficulty of the third molar extraction, a 'Youngsam's Sign'. We will discuss the details in the following pages but I would like to ask you a small favour ahead of this. If you find this helpful on your extraction journey, please call this phenomenon a 'Youngsam's sign' too. It is my aspiration to have it named after myself.

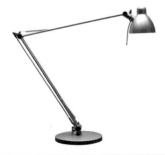

01
Youngsam's Sign Case 1: Case from "Inflammation around the Third ★★★ Molars"page

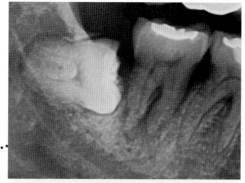

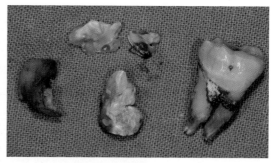

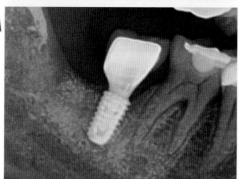

We've seen this radiograph earlier in this chapter. Male patient, 50 years of age. Let's take a look at the photos of extracted teeth first. It seems like extraction of the #48 would be very easy once the #47 has been extracted, but you can see evidence of struggle from the sectioned #48.

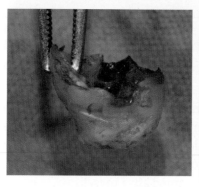

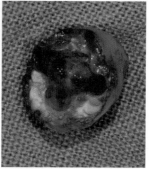

You can see that the root was sectioned multiple times in multiple direction. Until the apical third of the root was removed, all the other parts were fractured and suctioned up. Why was this third molar which seems so simple and easy, a challenge?

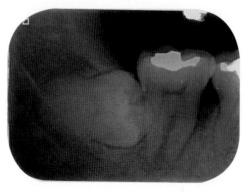

You can see the widening of the PDL space from the PA X-ray to the left. It's even more prominent from the OPG above. You can see that the strip of dark radiolucency is surrounding the root and it comes up beyond the middle third of the root. We are going to call this 'Youngsam's Sign' from now on. I know it probably doesn't roll off the tongue very easily but you will see Youngsam's sign discussed not only in this chapter but throughout the entire book.

02
Why did this root fracture? ★★★

Why do you think the root has fractured in the case below? Neither does it have severe curvature on the root nor can I find any other obvious predisposing factors for a root fracture. Once you study Youngsam's Sign from this chapter, it will be more obvious to you. As discussed earlier, there are many factors that can affect the difficulty of a third molar extraction. However, I consider Youngsam's sign to be one of the most important factors. I am yet to come across any other text to discuss this so I would like you to take this away from the book and consider Youngsam's sign in your everyday clinical practice.

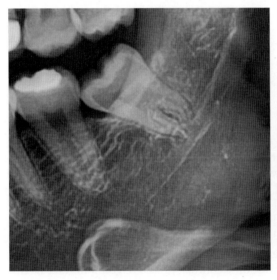 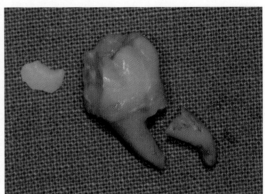

You can see Youngsam's Sign on the apex of #38's distal root on the OPG above. Distal root had fractured during the extraction and the photos were taken after removal of distal root separately. Why do you think the distal root fracture? No severe curvature there, also seems like the mesial root had fractured a little at the tip too.

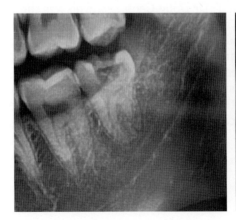 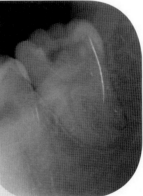 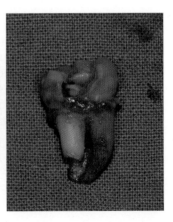

Again, Youngsam's sign around the distal root of the #38. It is more distinctive from the PA radiograph. Sometimes an OPG taken at a different time may show Youngsam's sign to a different extent too. The photo to the far right was taken from the lingual aspect. You can see that the distal root was fractured during extraction.

03
What is this dark radiolucency surrounding the root which indicates ★★★ widened PDL space?

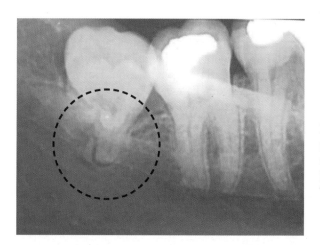

I run the third molar extraction seminars on a regular basis with multiple lecturers and one of the videos shown by another lecturer (Dr Minkyo Seo) had the radiograph to the left. It was about how he removed the fractured meisal root and you can see a typical Youngsam's sign from the radiograph.

So why was the root tip fractured? This is where we consider why Youngsam's Sign appears on the radiograph. It is when the root tip(s) are embedded in the lingual cortical bone. I haven't heard any other third molar extraction gurus discuss this and even the dental radiologists were either unaware or had a vague response such as 'I think I've heard of it somewhere'. I discuss this in my seminars a lot but there was no defined name for this radiographic appearance. You may see it being described as 'dark sign around the apex', 'thickening', burn out etc but because all those descriptions are used elsewhere as well and does not describe this phenomenon exclusively. Therefore, to save you some confusion, we are going to refer to this as 'Youngsam's sign' from now on in this book.

I think this radiographic appearance deserves its own name because it significantly increases the difficulty of the extraction procedure and frequently causes root fracture. Remember bi-cortical implant theory all those years ago when the implants first started? It's similar to that. Recently, I lectured in a seminar hosted by 'Osstem Implant Korea' on 'Reading Panoramic Radiographs for Safe Third Molar Extraction'. Dr Dong-Geun Lee, who was the vice-president at the time, informed me that his cadaver research from a while back showed about 30% of the mandibular third molar to have part of their roots intruded into the lingual cortical bone. Even in one of the journals we looked at earlier in this chapter; "Variations in the anatomical positioning of impacted mandibular wisdom teeth and their practical implications"[SWISS DENTAL JOURNAL 124: 520–529 (2014)] shows similar statistics. 31.4% of the mandibular third molar roots were intruding into the lingual cortical bone and as anyone can predict, only 4.3% of the roots were intruding into the buccal cortical bone.

04
Wait! Only lingual cortical bone? ★

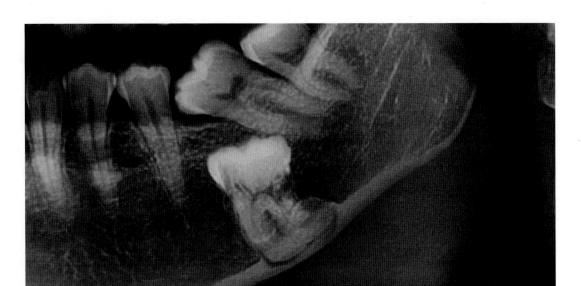

You can see that the root has bent from encountering cortical bone of inferior border of mandible. Radiolucency around the roots that are similar to the ones we've seen on Youngsam's sign discussion are also visible. So every time you see a similar radiographic appearance, it's safe to assume that it's due to the roots that have intruded into cortical bone (buccal or lingual). Obviously, you need to adapt your sound clinical judgement to distinguish Youngsam's Sign from different causes of similar radiolucency, under developed root apex or periapical periodontitis from irreversible pulpitis to name a few.

Anyway, when you see Youngsam's sign on the OPG, please bear in mind that there is a good chance that the extraction is going to be challenging and/or the root tip may fracture. In addition, the risk of fractured root tip being lodged into the sublingual space is also higher as you only have thin layer of cortical bone underneath that root tip. I have had cases where I had my finger on the lingual bone while trying to remove the root tip and I could feel the movement of the fractured root underneath the soft tissue. If you are still a novice, please refrain from trying to remove this root tip. Always remember that it is more important NOT to create one case that makes you sad than to have 100 cases that makes you happy. If you have removed the coronal part of the tooth successfully, leave the remaining root tip behind. We will discuss this further in the next chapter; The Intentional coronectomy.

Statistically speaking, I want to say Youngsam's sign has positive predictive value higher than 99%. But the probability of false negative is also quite high. In other words, absence of Youngsam's sign does NOT necessarily indicate that the root tips aren't intruding into the cortical plate. Just to make matters more complicated, different OPGs of the same patient may present the same tooth differently but always remember that many research papers has shown that 30% of the mandibular third molar roots were involved in the lingual cortical bone. Sometimes when you see the roots being involved with the buccal cortical bone on the CBCT, you can easily tell because the PDL space appears to have widened to a greater extent. But on the OPGs, the intrusion into the buccal cortical bone is less obvious when compared to Youngsam's signs you see on the cases where the roots have intruded into the lingual cortical bone.

05
Youngsam's Sign ★

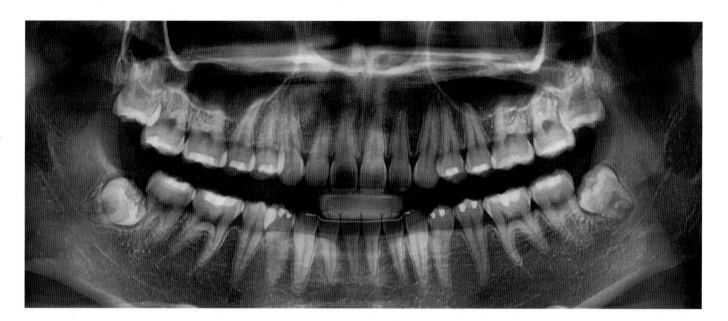

Female patient in her mid-20s. Root seems to have completed. We decided to take a CBCT because the angulation towards the lingual side tends to increase the difficulty of the extraction.

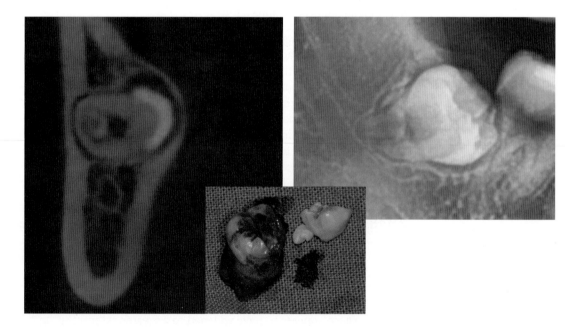

CBCT shows lingually inclined dentition with its apex intruding into the buccal cortical bone. Widened PDL space is also visible. Again, if the apex is positioned buccally, PDL space widening will be more obvious in a CBCT than on an OPG.

06
So what does Youngsam's Sign mean? ★★★

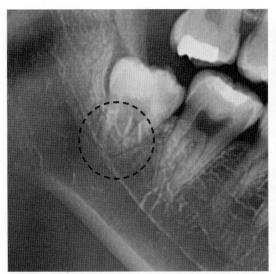 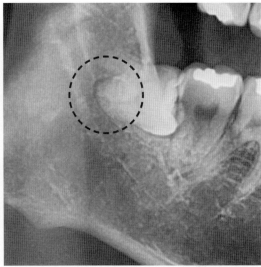

In my experience, appearance of Youngsam's sign meant that the roots were involved with the lingual cortical plate. You may not believe this as you haven't heard of this anywhere else, but remember I've extracted the most amount of third molars for the longest period of time in South Korea.

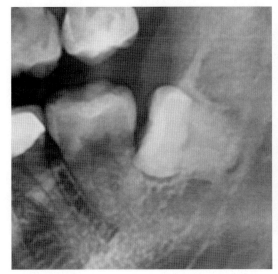 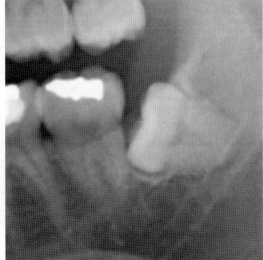

40-year-old female patient. Youngsam's sign is obvious on the apex of #38. We confirmed with a CBCT as well. The OPG to the right was taken 10 years ago with a different OPG machine which had lower resolution but you can still make out Youngsam's sign at the apex.

07
Variants of Youngsam's Sign ★★★

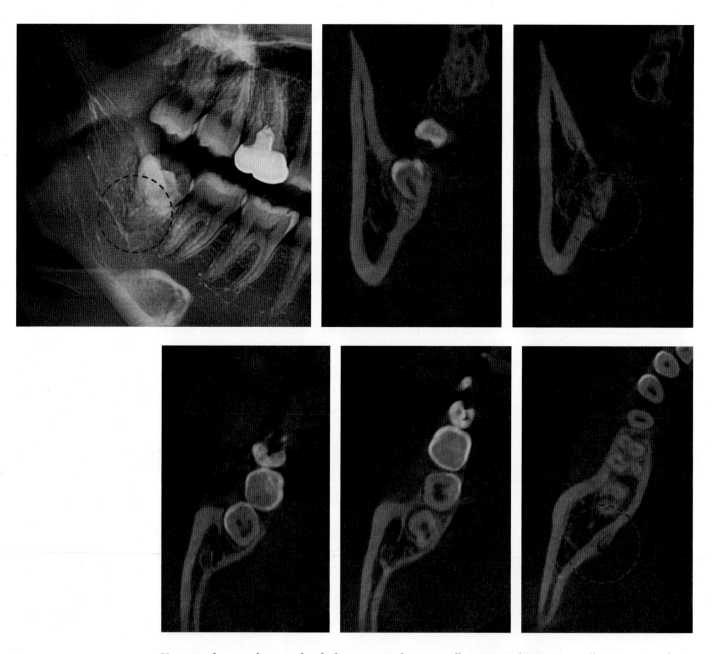

You can observe the apical radiolucency on the vertically impacted #48. You will see it more clearly on the included coronal and horizontal section of the CBCT. The apex has gone through the cortical bone and the PDL space within the cortical plate is enlarged. You have to be very careful if root tip fractures in the process of extraction, as it is very easy to dislodge the root tip into the sublingual space.

★★★

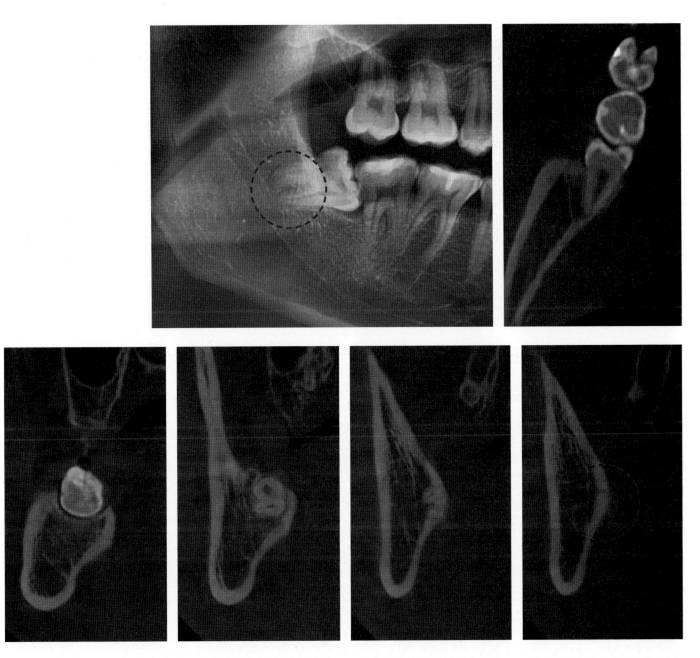

Horizontally impacted third molar with apical radiolucency on the distal root. On CBCT, the distal root was intruding into the lingual cortical bone and radiolucency is obvious. But even without the dark appearance on the CBCT, Youngsam's sign may still appear on the OPG if the roots are embedded into the cortical bone.

★★★

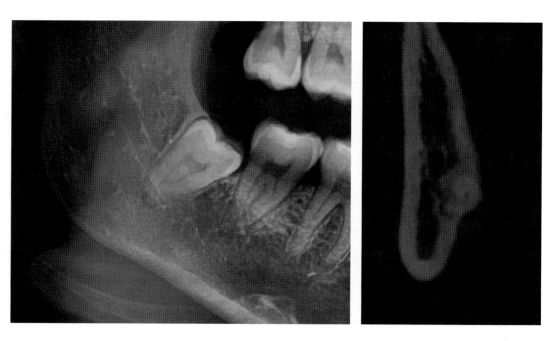

You can see the darkening of external outline of the third molar root apex on the OPG. Even on the coronal section of the CBCT, the apex is embedded within the cortical bone and there is dark radiolucency around it.

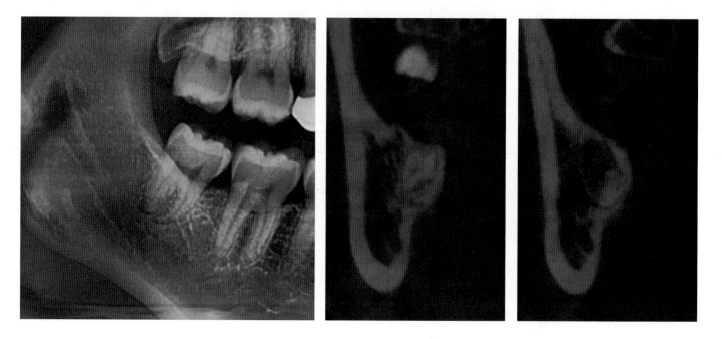

36-year-old female patient. Youngsam's sign on #48 root apex confirmed once again with the CBCT.

08
Extraction of third molars showing Youngsam's Sign ★★★

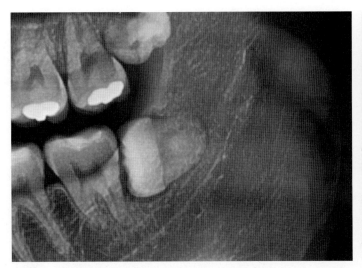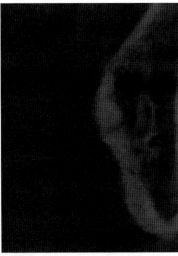

As mentioned earlier, I think chronic pericorinitis had applied continuous pressure to push the roots into the cortical bone. But I had colleagues who disagreed to my hypothesis so I will leave that decision up to you.

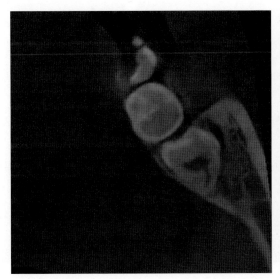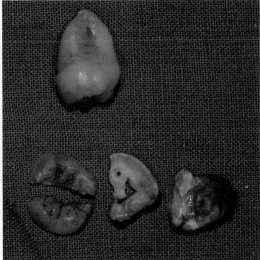

As I had mentioned earlier, it is not easy to predict how difficult a third molar extraction is going to be. But of all the other factors, Youngsam's sign is a reliable indicator of a potential challenge. Now I rarely have extractions that take longer than 5 minutes. But largest part of the cases where it does take longer are the cases with Youngsam's sign. If you read through the horizontally impacted third molar extraction part you will learn about how I've extracted this tooth and why the root had to be sectioned in half following removal of crown. Simply put, it means that the PDL space was too narrow to fit an elevator.

★★★

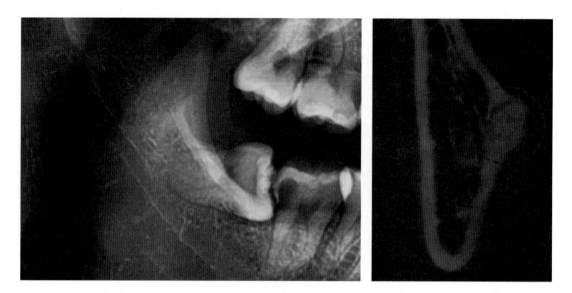

A relatively simple looking horizontally impacted third molar at first glance. But now that you know about Youngsam's Sign, you can guess that this extraction isn't going to be so straightforward.

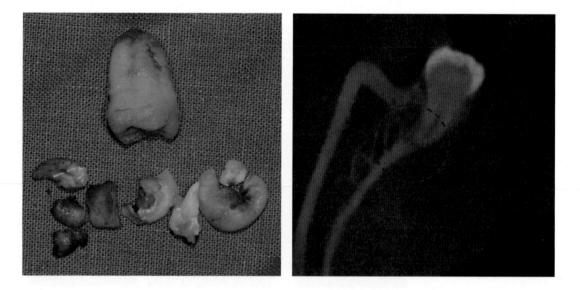

As you can see from the photo of the extracted tooth, it wasn't an easy extraction. If it wasn't for the apex being embedded in the lingual cortical bone, the root removal would've been only dont need a matter of one simple twist of the elevator.

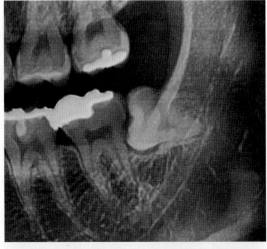

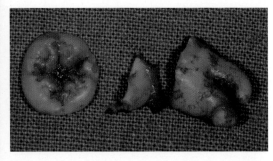

25-year-old male patient. Clearly visible Youngsam's sign around mesial root apex as shown on the OPG. On CBCT slice you can infer that the developing root had encountered the cortical plate and turned its course of development buccally. This case was quite challenging due to the chronic pericorinitis wedging the tooth in further. If any root tip fractures in cases like this, it will be best to forget about retrieving it.

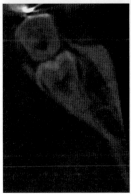

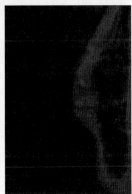

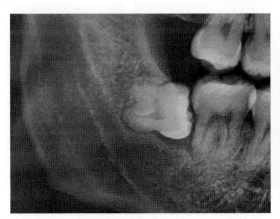

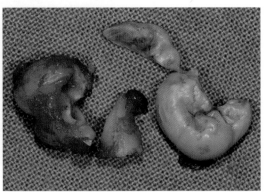

Similar to the case above, you can see Youngsam's Sign around the apex of the mesial root and the chronic periocorinitis had wedged the tooth in further. On top of that, we have the peanut (buttocks) shaped roots which is classically the most difficult roots to extract. I tried creating a little trench to extract it but the tooth kept fracturing. You can see the sign of struggle on the extracted tooth as I had to section this tooth multiple times.

★

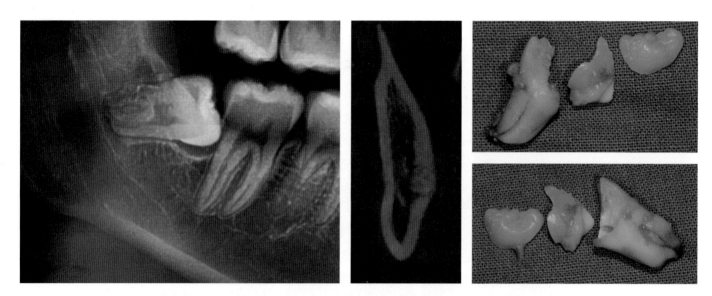

You can see Youngsam's Sign on the apex of the root as shown on the OPG. Again, CBCT confirms that the root apices were embedded in the lingual cortical plate. When you look at the buccal aspect of the tooth, you won't notice any anomaly of the roots. However, you can see that the lingual view of the tooth is similar to that of what is shown on the OPG. I think development of the roots were affected as they had encountered the hard, strong cortical bone. Again, it would be safer to leave the fractured root tips behind for cases like this.

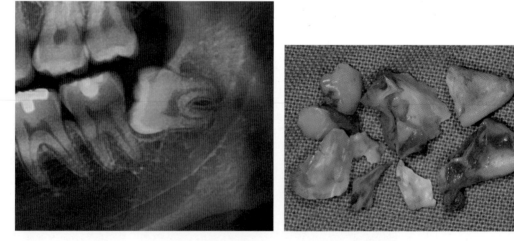

Again, Youngsam's Sign is visible around the apex of the roots on the OPG. It may not always be the case, but you will notice cases like these are more than likely to be challenging.

09
Precautions for extracting third molars with Youngsam's Sign ★★★

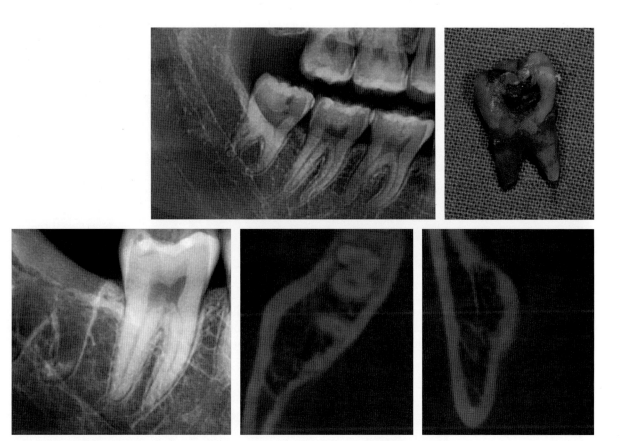

There isn't any different method of extraction when it comes to extracting third molars with Youngsam's sign. You approach it like any other case without one. However, things are little different when a root tip fractures. The root tips with Youngsam's sign are a lot more prone to fracture. Actually, if the root tip fractures allow quicker extraction of the tooth, it's a good thing. Because, when the cortical plate is tightly grasping onto the root tip, extraction can be quite challenging. The point is, you don't have to go out of your way to try and remove this root tip. I will go into more detail in the following chapters.

When I was younger, my motto was to "Leave No Root Tips behind" but now I am a changed person. Perhaps it's because I am getting old; my back is giving and I need my procedures to be quicker with less unnecessary risks. However, I really want to stress this to novice dentists in particular. If a fractured root tip requires more than a flick with an explorer or a probe, it's not worth it. If you try to engage something like a root pick, you're exposing yourself to the risk of dislodging the root tip into the sublingual space. When I was younger, I extracted these roots while stopping the roots from dislodging, using my finger to apply external pressure from the outside of the lingual plate. However, I don't think this is a good practice even for the patients. The roots are part of our body and it's made to stay in our body for our entire lifespan. Therefore, it's not like the broken root wasn't supposed to be there in the first place. It also hasn't caused any problems for the patient yet, so why not leave it behind? We will discuss this in more detail in the next chapter.

★

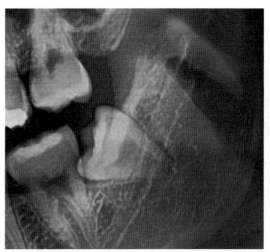 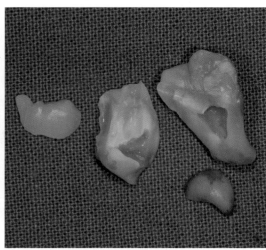

You can see Youngsam's sign on the distal aspect of the root apex. Approached the tooth as I normally would but it wasn't easy. If you didn't know about Youngsam's Sign, you would've assumed this case was easy as well. The tooth wouldn't move a single bit and I decided to section the tooth in half. The root tip was fractured in the course of delivery but was removed safely.

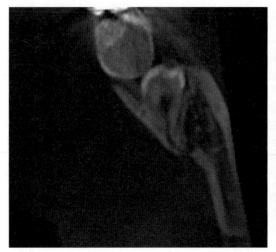 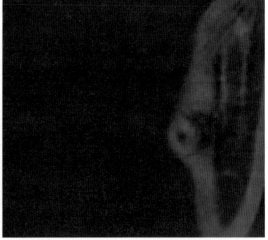

You can see that the root tip was intruding the lingual cortical bone on the CBCT slice. You could be wondering why I tried to remove this root tip contrary to what I've said before. When you look at the OPG, you can't see any anomaly from the morphologies of the root and the IAN canal and you can only notice Youngsam's Sign on the apex. Therefore, it's safe to assume that the IAN canal travels buccally to the root and without any contact or involvement to one another. Usually you would approach the broken root tip from the buccal side when you try to remove it and knowing that there is a safe distance between the root and the nerve, I thought it would be worth a try. But as I've warned you time and time again, please be mindful that there is always elevated risk of dislodging the root tip into the sublingual space.

10
Enlarged PDL space due to advanced caries ★★

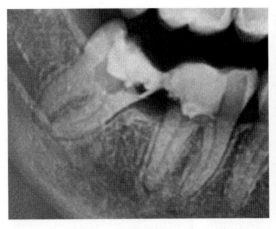
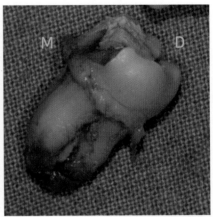

Patient visited a dental clinic near his home for pain from the third molar but apparently the clinician just extirpated the 47 and asked the patient to have the #48 removed elsewhere. You can see what appears to be Youngsam's sign on the apex but it could also be periapical periodontitis from irreversible pulpitis. It seems 47 distal root has similar appearance as well. I checked the apex following the extraction and although part of the interseptal bone was removed with the tooth, it was evident from the attached infectious soft tissue that the radiolucency was from irreversible pulpitis. You may find the third molars with periapical periodontitis to be easier to extract. But in my experience, this wasn't always the case. On average, the third molars with severe caries were harder to extract. The photo of the tooth above was taken by one of my staff. She thought she was taking a photo of the buccal aspect but she got confused. You are actually looking at the lingual aspect. Mesial and distal are as marked on the photo.

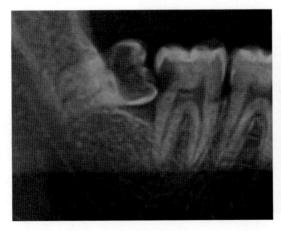
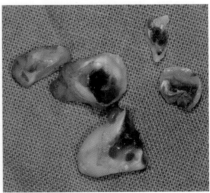

This was another case where we had to extract the third molar due to severe carious lesion. The radiolucency around the root apex isn't your typical presentation of the periapical periodontitis. As expected, the extraction was challenging. In particular, the mesial root with PDL space widening was harder to extract. The root tip actually fractured as it was embedded into the lingual cortical bone. I've concluded that the radiolucency shown on the OPG is more a Youngsam's sign than periapical periodontitis.

11
Periapical periodontitis or Youngsam's Sign? ★

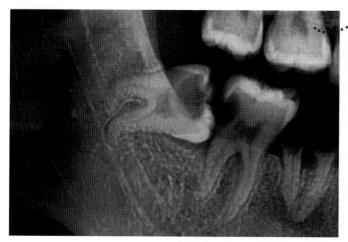 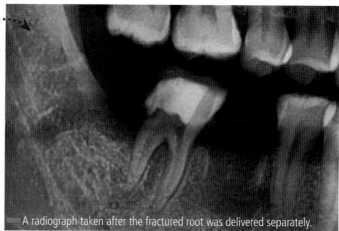

A radiograph taken after the fractured root was delivered separately.

Another case of severely carious #48 which needed extraction. In cases like this, it will be very challenging to localise the source of pain, as it may as well be coming from the irreversible pulpitis of the #47. I usually just start off with extirpation of #47 to reduce the pain level prior to extraction of the #48. It was very difficult to differentiate whether the periapical radiolucency was a result of PA periodontitis or a Youngsam's Sign. But something didn't sit right as the root tip fractured in the process of extraction. I had to make a decision whether to leave to root behind or not. In the end I decided to take a CBCT to confirm whether the root was fractured due to severe curvature or if the root tip was intruding into the cortical bone. Let's take a look at the slices.

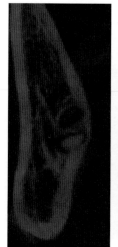 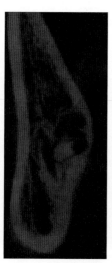 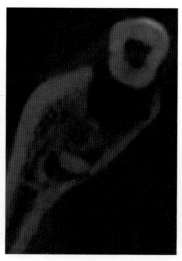 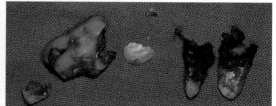

On the CBCT, you can see that the root was wedged into the lingual cortical bone. Therefore, in theory, you could leave this root behind as it is more likely to be a Youngsam's sign than inflammatory tissue. But I decided to remove it carefully anyway. Again, what I consider to be the most important guidance factor with root removals is the pain level the patient is experiencing. If the IAN canal is travelling immediately buccally, then the risk of nerve damage is very high. You must be extra careful and always consider leaving the roots behind.

12
Differentiating Youngsam's Sign and Immature dentition ★★

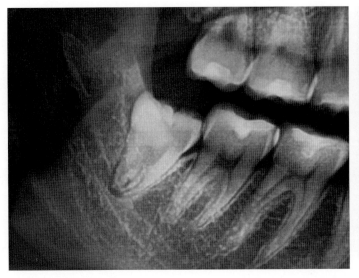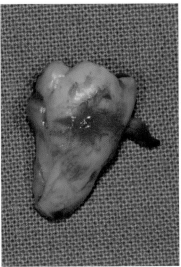

19-year-old female patient. You can see that the root apex hasn't closed yet. If you consider the patient's age, it should be easy to decide whether it's a Youngsam's Sign or a developing root.

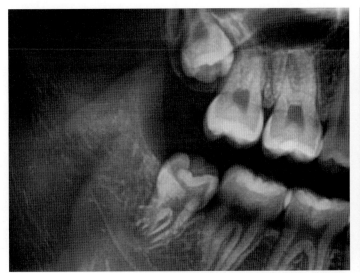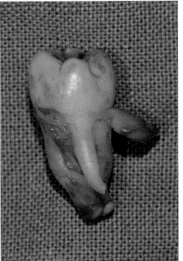

22-year-old female patient with immature root.

13
It may seem like a Youngsam's Sign but... ★

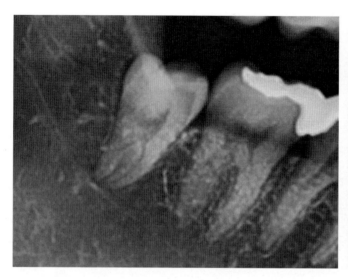 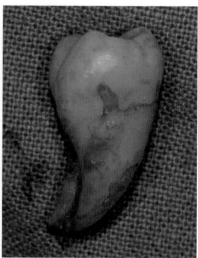

27-year-old female patient with a Youngsam's Sign on the apex of #48. Extraction procedure was uneventful and was carried out using an elevator as I would for any other cases like this. But what if the root tip had fractured? Should you have left it behind as you can see a Youngsam's Sign there? Or would you attempt to remove it? Each case is different and other factors like how busy you are on the day may affect your decision making but take a look at the CBCT below. You may think twice about it.

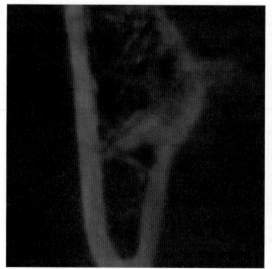 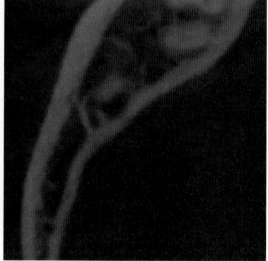

You will see how reckless it would've been to attempt to remove the fractured root. This is another false negative case of Youngsam's Sign. Most cases you will see that the IAN canal is travelling buccally, but it isn't always the case. If the canal travels lingually and you approach the root tip from the buccal aspect than you may push the root tip into the IAN canal causing damage to the nerve. Let's discuss what we are going to do with fractured and retained root tip in the next chapter.

Wisdom Tooth Coronectomy

Chapter 03 translated by

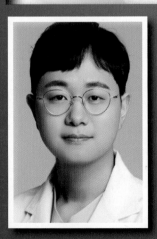

Dr. GiTae Kwon DDS

Instagram - @tooth.stagram
Faculty of GIIA - Gangnam International Implant Academy
DDS - New York University College of Dentistry

Dr. Gitae Kwon has been a faculty member at GIIA since 2019. He is a perfectionist and has an insatiable passion for dentistry, including wisdom teeth extraction and dental implant surgery. You will be able to find him on Instagram (@tooth.stagram) or in person with Dr. Youngsam Kim for the GIIA live surgery seminar held in Tijuana (Mexico).

01
First of all, what is coronectomy? ★★

Coronectomy is a procedure where the crown of the tooth is removed while the root of the tooth is left behind. It is usually called 'Intentional Coronectomy' as it is intentionally carried out when it is difficult to remove the root, or the risk of nerve damage is high with root removal. The principle is to leave the root behind if there are no major complications unless it gets exposed or is likely to cause problems in the future.

Coronectomy was surely performed unintentionally for many years, however the history of studying coronectomy is rather short and most studies were published in this century.

This is actually related to the introduction of MTA. Many practitioners believe that MTA must be used after coronectomy, however, I do not believe that it is necessary and I do not personally use it. In fact, it is practically not easy to use MTA for coronectomy.

Anyway, why is coronectomy gaining more popularity in recent years? Is it because human evolution is creating more impacted teeth in our mouth and they are more dangerous to remove? May be, is it related to CBCT becoming more widely available?

CBCT and intentional coronectomy

I believe that the reason coronectomy is getting more popular in recent years is due to the availability of CBCT. In the past, before the CBCT era, clinicians removed third molars without realizing the danger of damaging the nerve, but with the CBCT images nowadays, clinicians can identify the position of the nerve in relation to the root of the third molars and perform coronectomy when the risk of nerve damage is high. For example, in the past we may have just assumed that 1% of third molars extraction will have nerve damage; however, now with CBCT, we can identify them even further and can say that the risk is 0.1% or 10% instead and choose to do coronectomy for those with higher risks.

So how was it done in the past?

Wait!

Tips from my senior colleagues on third molar extraction and ★★★ roots??

There are 3 main tips I have received from my senior colleagues.

- When the root is left behind, anything under 5 mm in length gets absorbed (Some say 3 mm). Remaining roots are part of my body. Don't worry about it.
- If there is any pathology around the root, then remove it.
- If the root is luxated, then remove it. If it's not luxated, you may leave it.

These are the important advice I got from my senior colleagues when I became a dentist 20 years ago. And time has passed, now I have done more third molar extraction than anyone else in Korea and here are my advice based on my own experience.

The size of the remaining root does not affect the outcome.

What matters is how well the remaining root is surrounded by the bone, not the size of the root remaining.

It is very rare to see the wisdom tooth (third molar) root with periapical pathology.

I have done more third molar extraction than anyone else, yet I have not seen many with periapical pathology (well… at least in Korea where access to care is easy due to low-cost government insurance). Also if it has the periapical pathology is present, usually the extraction is easy and if the root is left after the crown is removed, it is likely to find its way out itself.

The position of the remaining root is important but whether it's luxated or not is not the consideration.

Even if the root has been luxated, it does not have to be removed. Once the blood clot forms, the fact that it's been luxated does not make any difference. Usually, after a month, enough bone formation occurs and as long as the root does not find its way out before that, the root will stay inside the bone.

02
Dr. Youngsam Kim's rules on leaving the root behind ★★★

Based on the aforementioned information, I leave the root behind in following situations.

✓ When the root is thin and curved

✓ When the nerve is close to the root and the patient is complaining of pain during extraction

✓ When the patient is complaining of pain even if when the nerve is not close to the root

✓ When the remaining root is likely to be positioned within the lingual cortical bone (Youngsam's sign)

✓ When the patient has underlying medical condition such as hypertension

✓ When I am too busy

Yes, the last one is a joke. My point is that you don't need to be afraid of leaving the root behind. You don't need to think that removing the whole tooth is 100% success and leaving the root is half success. You are doing the perfect procedure by leaving the root behind if you have reduced the complications which may have happened if you attempted to remove the root.

It is important to deliver the complication-free extraction by leaving the root behind than attempting to remove the whole tooth and cause more serious complications. Leaving the root behind is not a failure. What you have done is simple and safe extraction. But don't forget this important point. The remaining root must be surrounded by enough bone.

Now knowing that leaving the root behind is a safe procedure, do I do it often? Not really.

In fact, I get questions on this topic so much, sometimes I intentionally leave roots behind and follow up. I sometimes intentionally break the root and leave it when the root is close to the nerve or Youngsam's sign is seen. Whether to remove it or not is decided by the condition of the remaining root. Sometimes I ask this question to myself.

Did I intentionally leave the root behind or was I forced to do so?

At the end of the day, it does not matter and has no impact on prognosis.

03
Your situation justifies your action ★

Up until 2014, I rarely left the root behind. Not because my skill was great, but because I worked together with other dentists and usually had more time to perform third molar extraction. I only had very few extractions where the root was left behind. When the extraction took more time than required, my colleagues usually looked after my next patients. Also at that time, my pride did not allow me to leave the root behind.

But since 2014, I am the only one doing extraction in my new coffice. Sometimes I see dozens of third molar patients a day and was forced to leave the root behind. There was no way that I could perform extraction as I used to do and do other procedures as well (By the way, third molar extraction occupies around 50% of my day in average).

Not only that, I have ankylosing spondylitis and other chronic spinal problems. I had surgery twice, but I can't move like others and find it very difficult to move my neck around. I take anti-inflammatory drugs all the time and on some busy days, I must take steroids.

In 2015, I was asked to do a lecture on intentional coronectomy and tried to find cases. As I mentioned earlier, I usually get my staff to take photos whenever I do third molar extraction. However, I struggled to find cases where I left the root behind. Among the few cases I found, follow up was not easy as the majority of patients did not feel a need of coming back to get it checked especially because many of my patients come from other parts of Korea and even overseas. Anyway, I could confirm that majority of these cases where I left the root behind did not cause any problems. As I used as a title here, I think these situations allowed me to open my mind on the concept of coronectomy.

These days, I tried to stick to my philosophy (ESSE) and perform extraction as easy as possible.

Since I have enough skills and experience to perform extraction well, I do not need to do coronectomy most cases, however as everyone's situation is different, I recommend you to have a good read on this chapter and make your own principles on this topic.

Let's have a look at some cases now.

Leaving the Root behind ★★★

What should we do with the root left behind due to crown fracture?

I have found a few cases among my patients where extractions were done in other clinics in the past. Some were done recently but some were done decades ago. Some patients knew that roots were left behind from the beginning and some were told by other dentists later. Regardless, none of these patients had any issues.

When I first started seminars on third molar extraction, I lectured on how to remove remaining roots. I showed some amazing heroic cases and felt good about it. And now I am teaching on why it is ok to leave it behind. As I mentioned earlier, cases we see on lectures should be something we can perform ourselves (Dental seminars should not be like David Copperfield's magic show or Cirque du Soleil where we will be wowed but cannot perform it ourselves). I can tell you that you will be reassured to see my cases here. Anyone can leave the root behind easily!

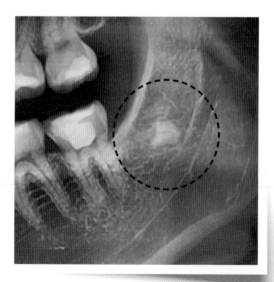 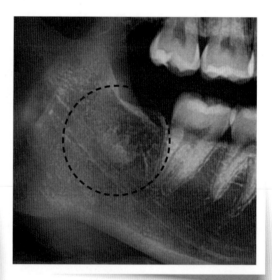

▬ 32 y.o female patient said that she had wisdom tooth extraction couple of years ago

▬ 26 y.o female patient said that she had wisdom tooth extraction 5 years ago

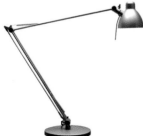

01
Roots left behind from other clinics long time ago ★

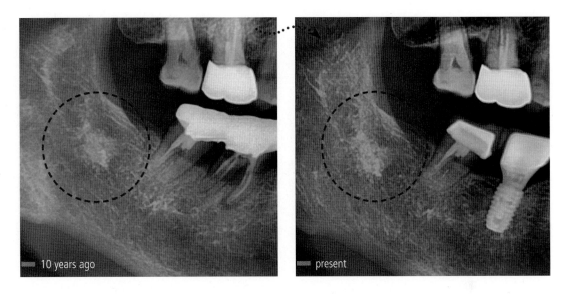

58 y.o. female patient. She comes to see me for more than 10 years now. According to the patient, she does not remember exactly when it was removed as it was done a long time ago. I have been reviewing this for more than 10 years now and there are no changes at all. The nice looking implant on 46 is done by me. ^^

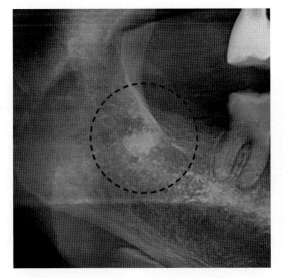

70 y.o. female patient. The patient said that the tooth was removed long time ago.

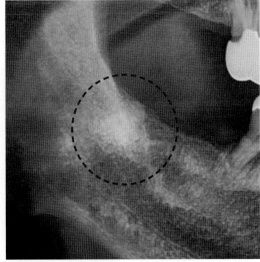

66 y.o. male patient from Japan. According to the patient, it was removed when he was younger and he is aware of the fact that the root was left behind.

★

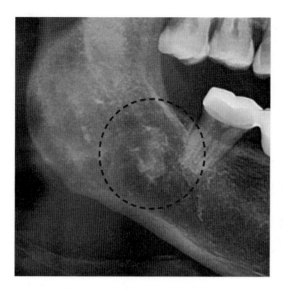

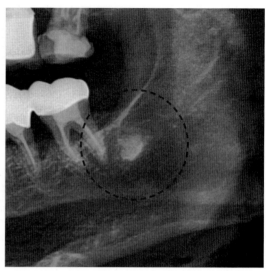

67 y.o. female patient. The patient does not remember having the wisdom tooth removed for at least last 20~30 years. Maybe it's not the root left behind from wisdom tooth extraction?

55 y.o. female patient. The patient said that the wisdom tooth was extracted 30 years ago.

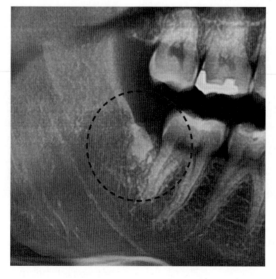

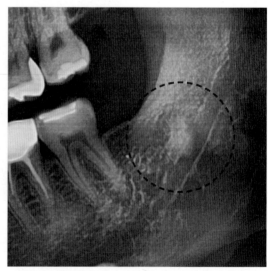

24 y.o. male patient. According to the patient, the tooth was extracted 14 months ago. He was informed about the remaining root then.

44 y.o. male patient. The patient had the extraction done 20 years ago and is aware of the remaining root.

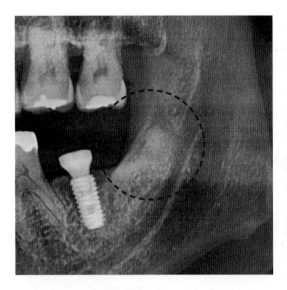

43 y.o. male patient. The patient had the extraction done 15 years ago and is aware of the remaining root.

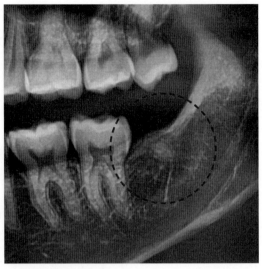

26 y.o. male patient. The tooth was removed around 3~4 years ago.

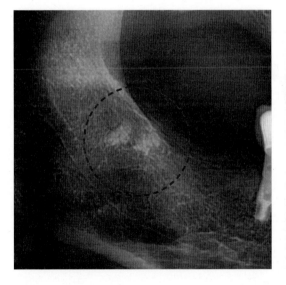

63 y.o. female patient. The tooth was removed 10 years ago.

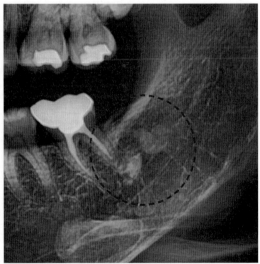

41 y.o. male patient. The tooth was removed 20 years ago.

02
Teeth are even used for bone graft these days… ★

This picture is an advertisement of dentin grinders in a Korean dental magazine.

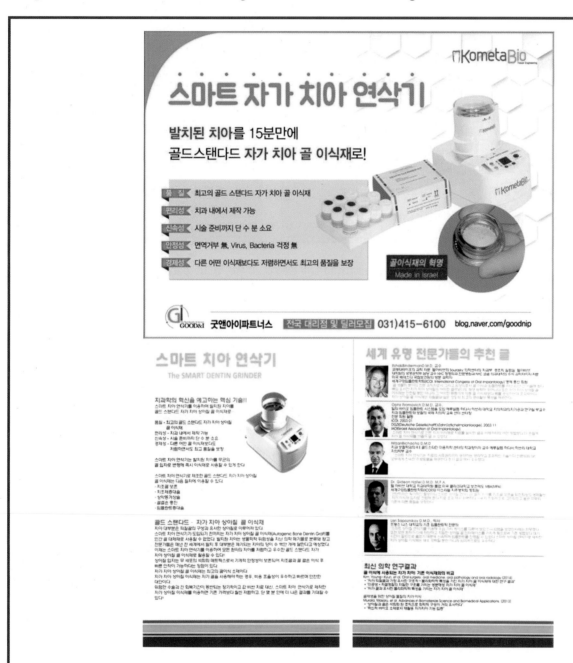

Tooth processing machine for bone grafting advertised on a dental newspaper

As shown on previous cases, one's own tooth does not cause problems. It seems that they are suggesting this idea as one's own tooth does not cause inflammatory reaction or rejection as it's a part of one's body once it's sterilized. It also doesn't seem to be completely resorbed and retain its structure. I have never used this but if they claim that one's own tooth can be safely placed inside the jaw, what problems would small root cause? ^^ (yes I understand that they perform special treatment on the tooth before grafting) Of course, you should study yourself to learn exact mechanism and how to use this.

03
A root left behind 6 months ago from another clinic ★

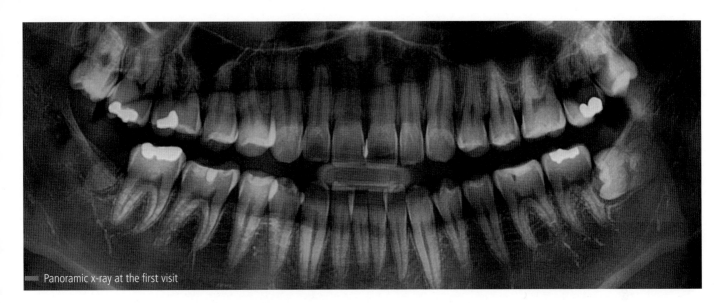

Panoramic x-ray at the first visit

27 y.o. female patient visited our clinic to get the tooth #38 removed. Panoramic x-ray showed a remaining root on #48 region. When asked about it, she said that it was done at another clinic 6 months ago. I have requested a copy of pre-op x-ray.

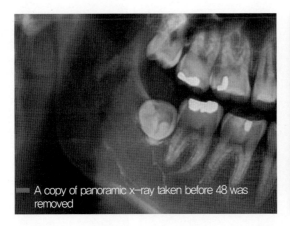

A copy of panoramic x-ray taken before 48 was removed

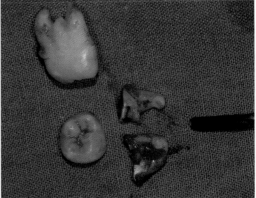

It seems that they could not remove the root due to severe impaction towards lingual. These days CBCT gives a clear picture of the situation, but when only the panoramic x-ray was available, this was very difficult to assess. From my experience, this wisdom tooth seems to be impacted towards lingual. Anyway, I regard this as a successful extraction.

The picture on the right is tooth #28 and #38. You can see the elevator in this picture as well. What this picture means is that after sectioning the crown, the elevator was inserted between two roots and used to fracture the root as the distal surface of the second molar prevented it from coming out. You will see more pictures like this one later.

04
Follow up of roots left behind by me <1> ★★

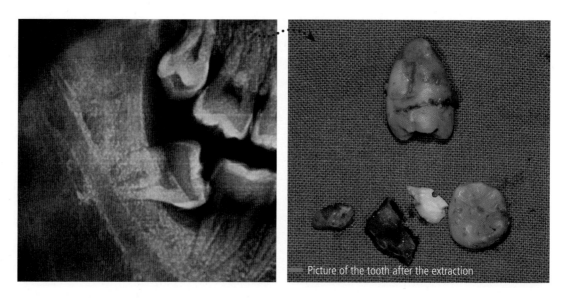

Picture of the tooth after the extraction

You can see the Youngsam's sign from this pre-op panoramic x-ray. During the procedure, both roots were fractured. Distal root was removed but the mesial root was left behind as patient was complaining of pain even on a gentle touch of the root. Probably the lingual nerve was running close to the root.

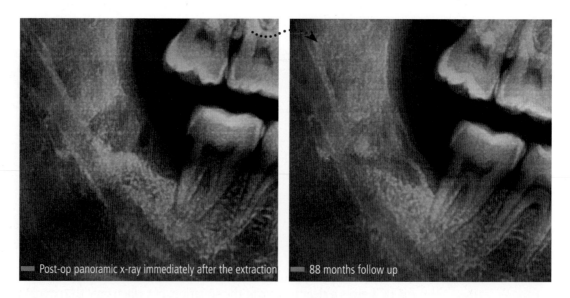

Post-op panoramic x-ray immediately after the extraction | 88 months follow up

Many patients at my clinic do not come back for the follow-up. This patient came back 8 months later to get the other wisdom teeth removed and we could review the root. You can see that the remaining root slightly migrated mesially. Remaining roots tend to migrate 1~2 mm towards the center of the healing socket only during the first month after the extraction. When the size of the socket is large, they tend to migrate more. We often see this migration even when the root is stuck in the strong cortical bone.

Follow up of roots left behind by me <2> ★

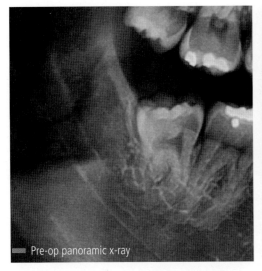
Pre-op panoramic x-ray

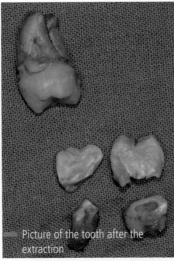
Picture of the tooth after the extraction

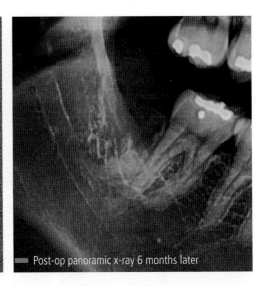
Post-op panoramic x-ray 6 months later

The mesial root of this #48 was thin and curved, so I decided to leave the root behind (And yes I was very busy!!). I do not have a post-op panoramic x-ray immediately after the procedure. The x-ray on the right is the one that is taken exactly 6 months and 13 days later when the patient visited me again to get the other wisdom tooth removed. The other wisdom tooth also had a small fracture on the distal root but the root was not removed.

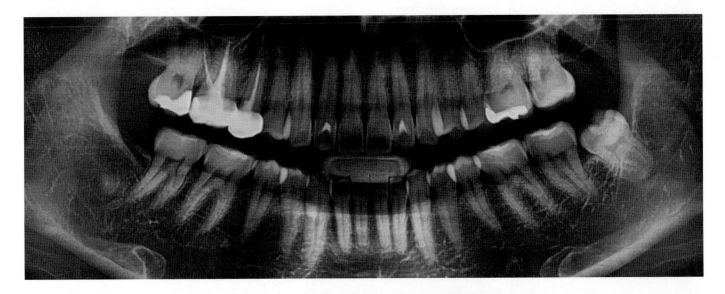

39 y.o. female patient who had her lower right wisdom tooth #48 removed by me 13 years ago. She came back to get the other wisdom tooth #38 removed this time. According to the patient, I have informed her that the small root portion is left behind after the extraction. There are no issues there. I guess she came back to me as she liked my extraction.

Follow up of roots left behind by me <3> ★

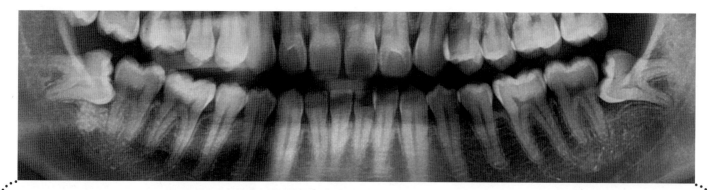

28 y.o. male patient's panoramic x-ray taken on his first visit. You can see Youngsam's sign on mesial roots of both wisdom teeth.

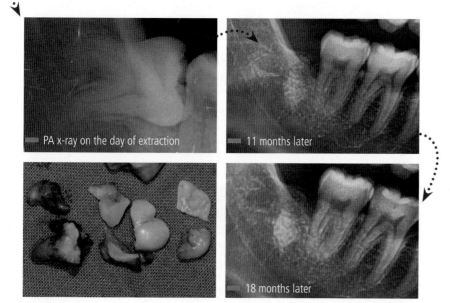

PA x-ray on the day of extraction

11 months later

18 months later

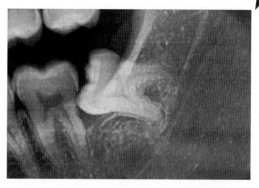

This is the panoramic x-ray taken 11 months later to check the remaining root of #38 and you can see Youngsam's sign here. I put this x-ray here to show you that Youngsam's sign can be seen differently even on the same patient.

I have removed #18 and #48 on his first visit. It is not clear on panoramic x-ray but you can see on this picture that mesial root is severely curved. When you look at the mesial root from lingual, you can see that the root is fractured. The x-ray taken 11 months later shows the remaining root.

This is the picture taken after #38 is removed. You can see that the root is curved and mesial root which showed Youngsam's sign is fractured. Post-op x-rays show that there is not much movement of the root after the extraction. Probably because of root's severe curvature.

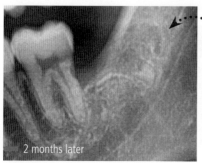

2 months later

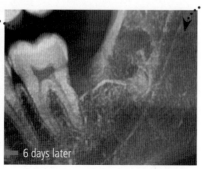

6 days later

Follow up of roots left behind by me <4> ★

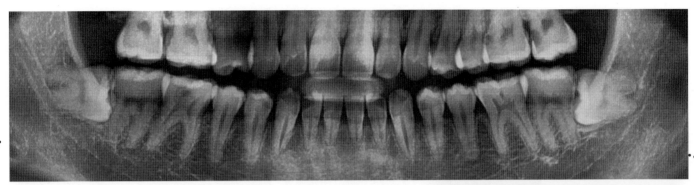

This panoramic x-ray was taken on patient's first visit. You can see Youngsam's sign on both wisdom teeth. I have decided to remove problematic #38 first and remove #48 later.

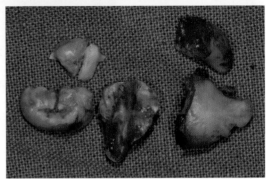

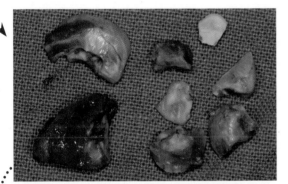

━ Picture taken after removing #48 2 months later

This is the picture taken after the removal of #38. I always remove the tooth in the same way so I can exactly tell how I removed this tooth just by looking at this picture. The top half of the crown was cut first and then the bottom half was cut and removed. Then I did an oblique cutting (more on chapter 7) to remove mesio-lingual part of the crown and some of lingual part of the root followed by separate removal of two roots. I think it took around 3 minutes to remove the tooth.

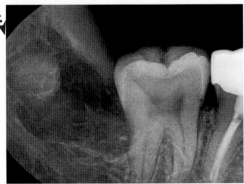

━ X-ray was taken 2 days after the extraction (I will talk more later, but it seems that I tried L extraction.

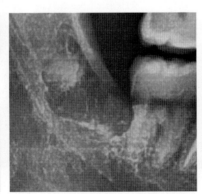

━ Panoramic x-ray taken 1 week later on a suture removal appointment

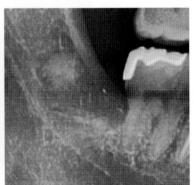

━ Panoramic x-ray taken 45 days after

Based on the observation so far, it is unlikely that the remaining root will cause problems later.

Follow up of roots left behind by me <5> ★★★

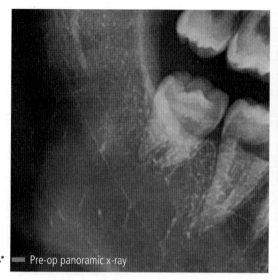

Pre-op panoramic x-ray

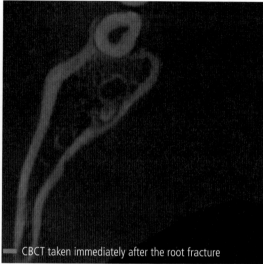

CBCT taken immediately after the root fracture

Pre-op panoramic x-ray shows Youngsam's sign. The patient who previously had CBCT done at another clinic requested CBCT this time as well but as it was not covered by the government's insurance, the procedure was performed only with the panoramic x-ray. After the extraction, the patient requested CBCT again when it was informed that the distal root is fractured. As expected, the fractured root was located within the lingual cortical bone and it appears to be slightly moved during the extraction.

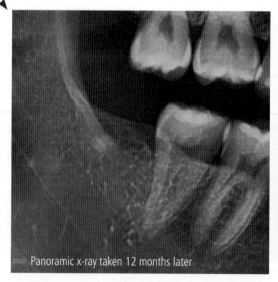

Panoramic x-ray taken 12 months later

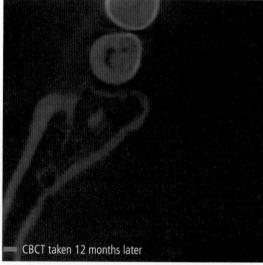

CBCT taken 12 months later

The patient visited me again 12 months later to get the other wisdom tooth removed. The patient requested CBCT again and it shows that the remaining root migrated towards the center of the bone. At that time, I was annoyed by the patient's demand to take CBCT but now I thank my patient as I can use these images for this book. ^^

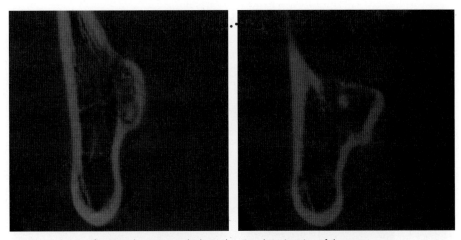

▬ Coronal view of CBCT taken 12 months later showing the migration of the root

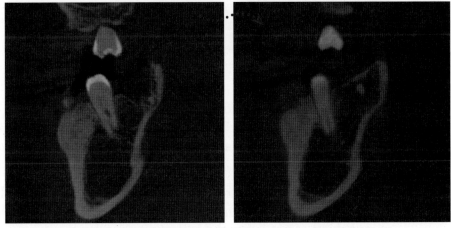

▬ Sagittal view of CBCT taken 12 months later showing the migration of the root

These are the coronal and sagittal view of CBCT taken 12 months later showing the migration of the root. The root migrated more than expected. You can see that cortical bone formation above the root.

Most of follow up pictures and x-rays were taken as patients came back to get other wisdom teeth removed. For most adults, I usually do not take panoramic x-rays within 2 years. However, patient's request allowed me to show you this wonderful case.

Please be aware...

The intention of this chapter is not to encourage you to leave the root behind. My message is that you don't need to be too stressed when you do not have any other option but to leave the root behind. Sometimes forcing to remove the root can lead to unpleasant outcomes. My conclusion is that leaving the root intentionally can be the appropriate option for both doctors and patients.

Intentional Coronectomy ★★

1. Intentional coronectomy

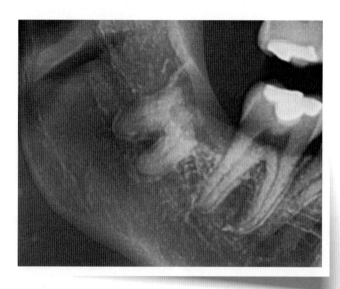

This is a picture of intentional coronectomy carried out due to dark band seen around the root. Probably this is the very first true intentional coronectomy I have performed. Most other coronectomy cases I have are due to many other forced reasons such as lack of time.

Previous cases shown are roots left behind due to fracture. So how do we separate between 'roots left behind' and 'intentional coronectomy'? Probably the intention to leave roots behind or not is not the important consideration here. I often leave roots intentionally. Most cases, I intentionally apply strong force to fracture the root.

This is not clearly defined in the literature, so I just made the rule myself. Well, my senior colleagues told me that roots smaller than 5 mm in length get absorbed, so they can be left behind (Well, in reality, those shorts roots do not get absorbed). So let's say that coronectomy is when the size of the single remaining root is over 5 mm. Let's also call it coronectomy when there are two or more roots left and the length of roots add up to be more than 5 mm.

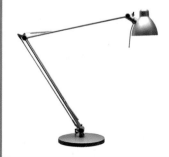

01
For the successful intentional coronectomy ★★★

Literatures show that the key to successful coronectomy is to have the top of the remaining root to be positioned at least 3~4 mm below the bone level and good primary closure. But I believe that as long as the crown is well removed, the position of the root and primary closure is not very important. As long as the crown is removed and the root is positioned 1~2 mm below the bone level, the blood clot can fill the socket well, there are not much pain or issues later and heal well. The socket is rounded and the bone level around the socket is not equal around. Therefore it is important to remove the crown portion well and make sure that the no part of the root is positioned above the bone level.

Some studies mention that intentional coronectomy is not for the beginners who are not good at extraction, but it is a procedure performed by experts to prevent the nerve damage. I would like you to read this chapter to become an expert.

Some conclusions I have made based on the literatures and my own experiences.

✓ It's good to remove the tooth 2~4 mm below the bone level.

✓ The removal of the remaining root is required around 5% of cases.

✓ The migration of the remaining root is reported to be between 14~81%

✓ Remaining roots migrate less than 3 mm in first 6 months and not much after that. Some suggest that there is no movement after first 12 months, but I think the movement stops well before that. It's probably better to say that the root does not move after the ossification of the socket.

✓ Some use orthodontic force to remove the remaining root safely or to encourage bone growth on distal of the second molar. But I don't think it's necessary.

✓ Remaining root from successful coronectomy never causes problems inside the bone.

✓ Coronectomy definitely reduces the risk of nerve damage (By the way, I have never experienced any nerve damage even with the extraction in general).

✓ Post- operative pain is less than normal extraction.

✓ There doesn't seem to be any correlation to dry socket.

✓ There are not many studies available. More sample numbers and studies are required.

✓ Coronectomy is not for beginners.

02
Coronectomy related studies...

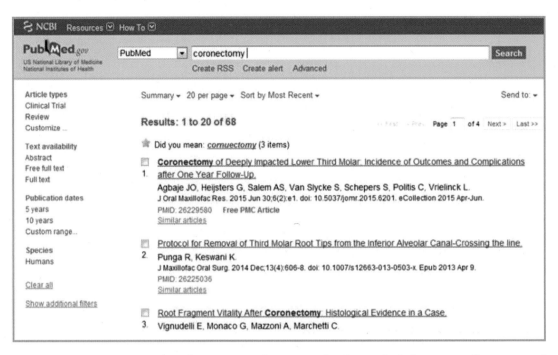

There are not many papers on this topic. And it is even harder to find them on well-recognized journals. I also could not find much information on textbooks used in Korea and overseas. Some did not even mention about coronectomy at all. Probably the principle taught is not to leave the root behind. I think we should develop the concept of coronectomy (intended or not) individually based on recent papers and my experiences discussed on this book.

Some helpful papers in my opinion

1. Br J Oral Maxillofac Surg 2005; 43: 7–12. A randomised controlled clinical trial to compare the incidence of injury to the inferior alveolar nerve as a result of coronectomy and removal of mandibular third molars

2. Oral Surg Oral Med Oral Pathol Oral Radiol Endod 2009;108: 821-827. Safety of coronectomy versus excision of wisdom teeth. A randomized controlled trial Yiu Yan Leung, BDS, MDS,a and Lim K. Cheung, BDS, PhD,b Hong Kong THE UNIVERSITY OF HONG KONG

3. British Dental Journal 209, 111 - 114 (2010) Published online:14 August 2010. Coronectomy – oral surgery's answer to modern day conservative dentistry

4. Inside Dentistry Published by AEGIS Communications. February 2013, Volume 9, Issue 2. Coronectomy of Mandibular Third Molars Case report describes a procedure in which the molars were in closerelationship with the inferior alveolar nerve. By Giuseppe Monaco, DMD | Giselle de Santis, DMD | Michele Diazzi, DMD | Claudio Marchetti, MD, DDS

5. Oral Surg Oral Med Oral Pathol Oral Radiol Endod 2004. Coronectomy (Intentional Partial Odontectomy of Lower Third Molars)

6. J Oral Maxillofac Surg 2004. Coronectomy: A Technique to Protect the Inferior Alveolar Nerve

7. International Dentistry. Coronectomy - An Alternative Therapy for the symptomatic impacted 3rd molar - Report of 9 cases

8. British J Oral Maxillofac Surg 2006. Is Coronectomy Really Preferable to Extraction?

9. J Oral Maxillofac Surg 2009. Clinical Evaluations of Coronectomy (Intentional Partial Odontectomy) for Mandibular Third Molars Using Dental Computed Tomography - A Case-Control Study

10. Oral Surgery, Oral Medicine, Oral Pathology,Oral Radiology, and Endodontology 2009. Safety of coronectomy versus excision of wisdom teeth - a randomized controlled trial

11. Oral Surgery 2010. A Review of Coronectomy

12. British Dental Journal 2010. Coronectomy – Oral Surgery's answer to modern-day conservative dentistry

13. Dental Update 2010. Coronectomy of a 3rd Molar with Cyst Lining Enucleation in the Management of a Dentigerous Cyst

14. Dental Update 2011. Coronectomy of Third Molar. A Reduced Risk Technique for Inferior Alveolar Nerve Damage

15. JOMS 2011. Coronectomy in Patients With High Risk of Inferior Alveolar Nerve Injury Diagnosed by Computed Tomography

03
Someone else's intentional(?) coronectomy ★★

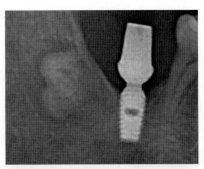

Male patient in mid-40s came to see me after losing his implant crown on #47. According to him, the wisdom tooth was removed around 10 years ago. There are no issues since.

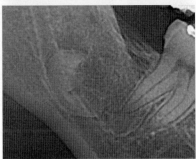

According to the patient, the wisdom tooth was removed around 4 years ago. I don't know the original shape of the tooth, but I can see how difficult the extraction would have been. I don't know whether the root was left intentionally or not, but I would say that this is the successful coronectomy.

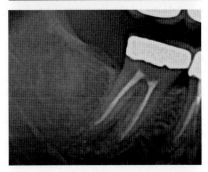

This is from 41 y.o. female patient and according to her the extraction was very difficult, but she does not remember exactly when it was done. She's been seeing me for last 5 years, and there were no changes to the root. I remember that the root canal treatment was difficult on this patient due to her long roots. I guess her wisdom tooth also had a long root.

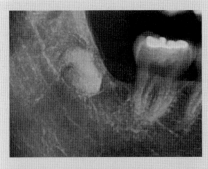

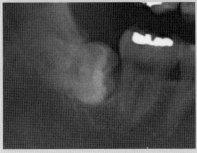

42 y.o. male patient and had his wisdom tooth removed 18 months ago at one of the university dental hospitals in Seoul. According to the patient, the instrument was fractured during the procedure, and they had to stop. The patient was my distant relative and I have asked him to get a copy of pre-op x-ray. I also know a colleague at the hospital and asked about the procedure and was informed that the extraction was performed by the most experienced professor at the hospital. I am emphasizing this here again that the coronectomy is not designed for the novice dentists as you can see in this case. It is not very clear on pre-op x-ray but you can clearly see Youngsam's sign on post-op x-ray.

★

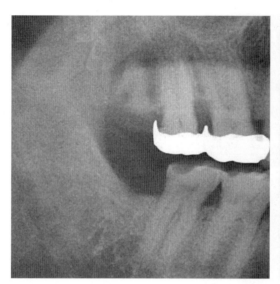 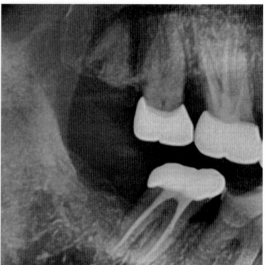

These are x-rays of 74 y.o. male patient. The left x-ray was taken in 2008 and the right was taken in 2016. I saw this patient since 2002 when I first opened my clinic as he was the building manager of the building where my clinic was located. At that time, I did not have digital panoramic x-ray and clinical records no longer exist. Now he is retired but still comes to see me. I remember removing his lower wisdom tooth but do not remember anything about the remaining root of #18 but he says that I have attempted to remove this tooth. Anyway, I remember that his lower wisdom tooth was one of two most difficult extractions I have done due to long and strong roots. Both of these two difficult extractions were done on well-built male patients over the age of 50.

Many dentists think that the indication for coronectomy is horizontally impacted wisdom tooth superimposing the Inferior alveolar nerve. But I would also add well-erupted wisdom tooth of mid-aged male patients to the list. I have worked together with a female oral surgeon for around 10 years. Her surgical skills were the best of all surgeons I have met. There are many surgeons who showed me some good cases, but with her, I could see all her cases myself and I can confidently say that she is really good.

But despite all her skill sets, she could not perform wisdom tooth extraction well in cases like this. Although the tooth may be well erupted, cases like this are difficult and require a lot of forces. In cases like this, it is a good idea to remove the crown of the tooth using 45-degree handpiece first and extract or perform coronectomy.

Intentional Coronectomy ★★

2. Vertically impacted lower wisdom tooth

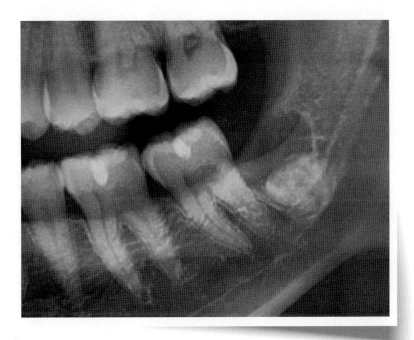

First, we will discuss vertically impacted lower wisdom tooth.

If you consider the success of coronectomy alone, completely impacted wisdom tooth where there is more bone around the tooth may show the better outcome, however, the process of removing the crown can be harder in this circumstance. Also, non-functioning impacted tooth is usually very easy to remove therefore unless there is a risk of nerve damage, intentional coronectomy is not usually performed. Rather, a fully erupted wisdom tooth can be harder to remove and therefore coronectomy can be more beneficial.

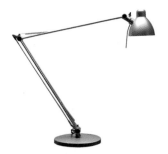

01
Intentional coronectomy of erupted wisdom tooth <1> ★★★

CASE 1

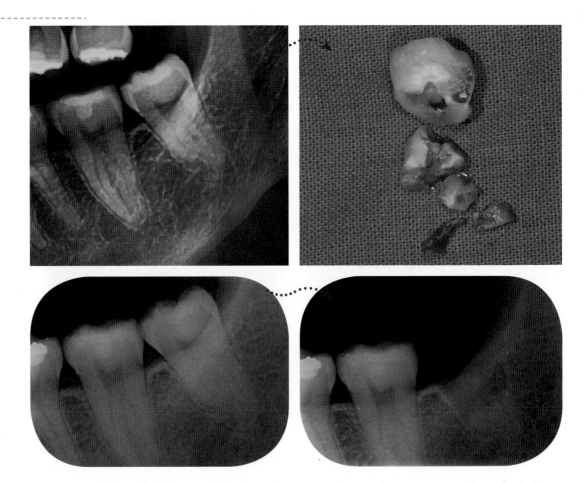

This is a well-erupted wisdom tooth where the roots appear to be superimposed on the Inferior alveolar nerve. Usually, forceps are used to remove the tooth, but the patient recently had angle trimming procedure done on the lower jaw and we could not use the forceps. Instead, 45-degree handpiece was used and coronectomy was performed. Also, the patient had another wisdom tooth to be removed later and follow up was possible.

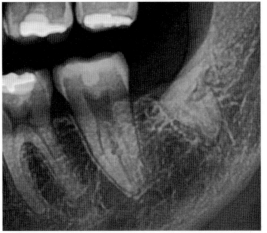

This panoramic x-ray was taken 3 months later and there were no complaints from patient and clinically showed good healing. Recent phone conversation with her (12 months after the procedure) also confirmed that there is no pain from the area. Let's see how the coronectomy was performed on this patient.

Coronectomy procedure

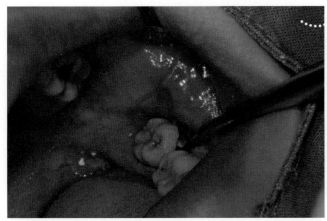

▬ Elevator was used to fracture and remove the crown after cutting mesio-buccal aspect using 45-degree handpiece.

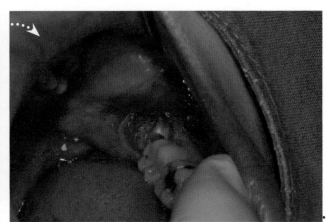

▬ After the removal of the crown

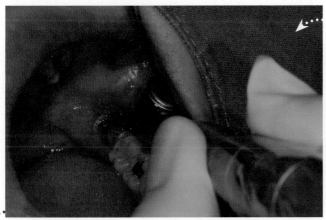

▬ Removal of more tooth structure on the lingual aspect to reduce the height in zig-zag motion.

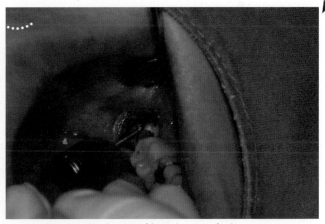

▬ For the vertical reduction of buccal aspect, further cutting was performed.

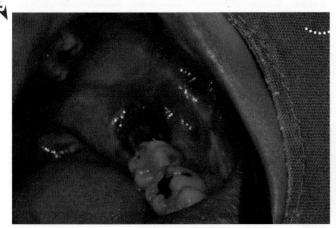

▬ You can see that the crown height is reduced.

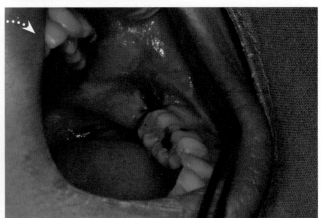

▬ I don't think the suture will help the success of coronectomy but it was performed anyway to maintain blood clot.

Intentional coronectomy of erupted wisdom tooth <2> ★★★

CASE 2

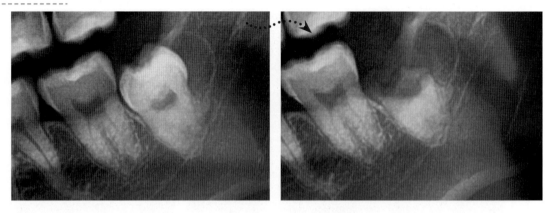

These are pre and post-op x-rays (immediately after the procedure) of 24 y.o. female patient. You can see the dentigerous cyst on the pre-op x-ray. The biopsy was suggested but the patient refused. It does not look very hard but why did I perform coronectomy here?

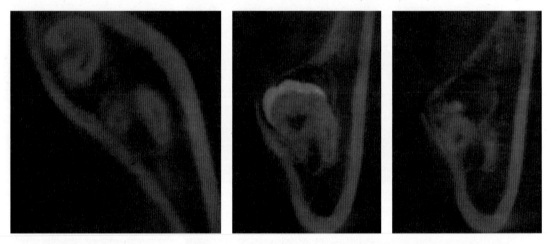

These CBCT images show that Inferior alveolar nerve is running between two roots. I would have removed the tooth if I did not know this but knowing this, I thought that this will be the perfectly right case for the coronectomy. Usually, in these cases, I use 45-degree handpiece to cut the buccal aspect of the crown and remove the crown.

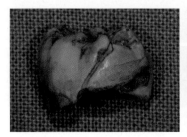 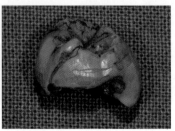

You can see how I used the handpiece in these two pictures. You will find that the crown can be removed easily without too much cutting. I have a few videos of this procedure so please keep visiting my youtube channel. My principle is to upload every video I take on my youtube channel, not just the good ones so you will see these cases there as well.

Intentional coronectomy of erupted wisdom tooth <3> ★★

CASE 3

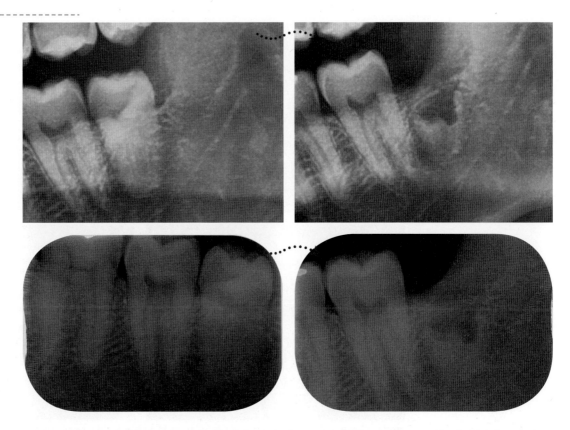

This is a case of 54 y.o. male patient with underlying medical conditions of high blood pressure, high cholesterol, and hypothyroidism. The patient suffered from pericoronitis and was glad that coronectomy will stop the inflammation. Due to the distance from his home to the clinic, he could not come back to see me again. In a case like this, I rarely remove the bone around the tooth.

CASE 4

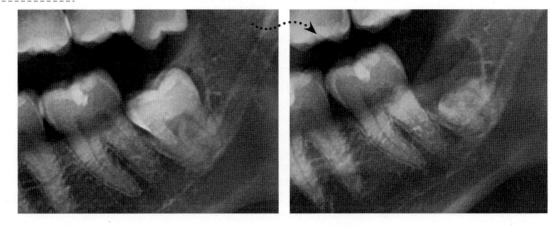

This is a case of 34 y.o. male patient. The tooth had roots superimposed on inferior alveolar nerve and coronectomy was performed. I could not follow up the patient. I have tried to ask him to come back but he said that there are no issues and refused to come back.

Intentional coronectomy of erupted wisdom tooth <4> ★

CASE 5

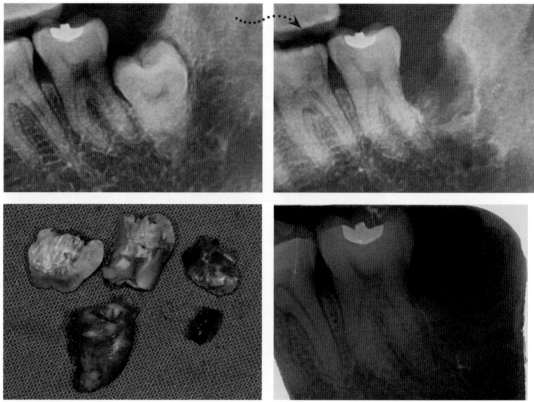

■ PA x-ray was taken a day after the extraction and you can see the small remaining root better on this than on the panoramic x-ray.

This is a case of 46 y.o. male patient who had previously experienced a traumatic wisdom tooth extraction and came to see me to get this one removed. According to the patient, he went to the university dental hospital for his previous wisdom teeth and it took 5 hours and 6 dentists tried to remove them. Not many dentists will be willing to do wisdom tooth extraction on a patient with such history.

The panoramic x-ray shows that the crown of the tooth is rotated by 90-degrees and the nerve is running on apical half of the root. The darkness on the apical root surface tells that the nerve is running there. As you can see on the post-op x-ray, I did the minimal bone removal, however, there was more than usual bleeding during the procedure and the procedure had to be temporarily stopped and continued later. I was thinking about stopping the procedure after sectioning the crown into 3 pieces and removing (to save the time wasted due to hemorrhage) but eventually decided to remove the most of the root as well. On the day of the extraction, intra-oral x-ray could not be done due to excess bleeding and a panoramic x-ray was taken instead. Panoramic x-ray may show that the whole root is removed but when the PA x-ray was taken a day after, it was confirmed that the part of the root was left behind (also can be seen on the clinical picture taken). When the extraction was done, I did not realize this so I should call this 'unintentional intentional coronectomy'. I have asked him to come back for a review, but he did not come back since then as he has no issues.

Intentional coronectomy of erupted wisdom tooth <5> ★

CASE 6

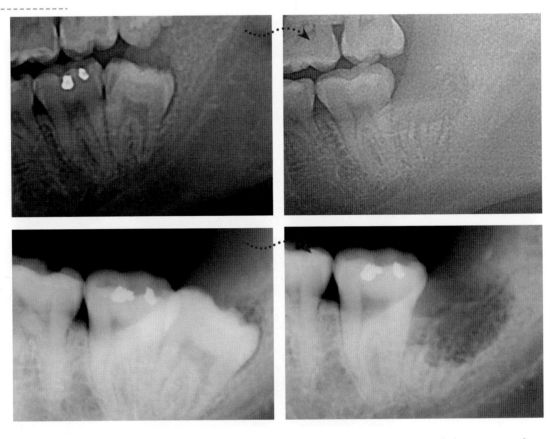

This was performed 5 years ago. I do not have immediate post-op x-rays and these were taken 8 months after the procedure. The patient did not come back since then.

CASE 7

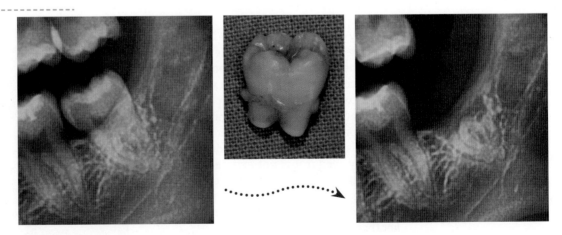

Roots were fractured during the extraction and I chose to leave them intentionally to follow up and see the prognosis. However, the patient did not come back since. I was advised on the phone that there are no issues.

Intentional coronectomy of erupted wisdom tooth <6> ★

CASE 8

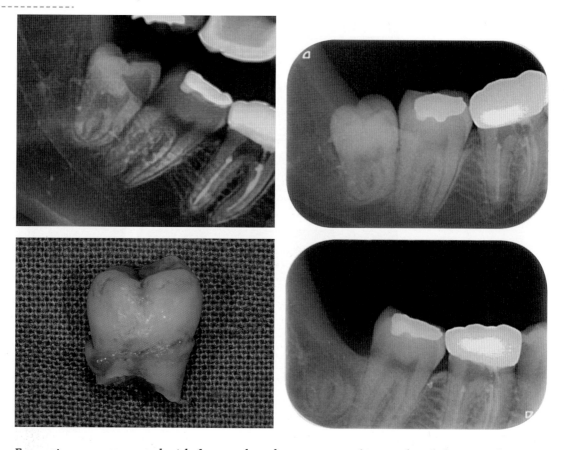

Extraction was attempted with forceps, but the crown was fractured and the procedure was stopped. All the above x-rays were taken on the same day of the extraction. You can see that the roots are thin and curved, and touching the nerve.

The x-ray on the right was taken 10 months after the procedure when the patient came back to get the opposing wisdom tooth removed. Considering that the x-ray beam was angled to take PA x-ray on the day of the procedure, the root has only moved around 1mm. I often get a question, if it is required to remove the root when it is confirmed that the root is migrating coronally even if it is not exposed. I don't believe that it is required to remove it but at the same time as the removal will be simple due to migration, it will be beneficial to remove it earlier than later.

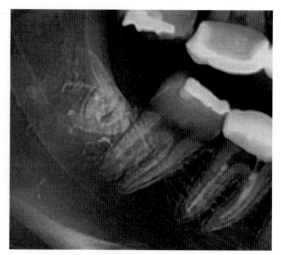

Intentional Coronectomy ★★

3. Horizontally impacted wisdom tooth

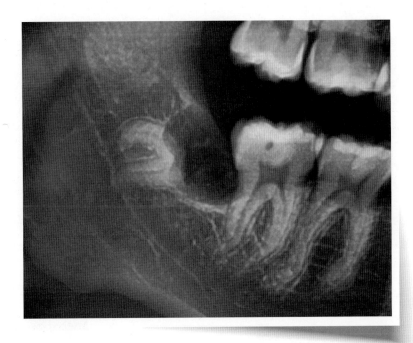

There is no special method of performing coronectomy on the horizontally impacted tooth. The top part of the horizontally impacted tooth is easily accessible and therefore the removal of the crown part of the tooth is simple. The key to success is to remove the crown completely, especially the bottom part of the crown... More specifically the mesio-lingual aspect of the crown. If you are reading this chapter first, I suggest you skip after understanding the basics of coronectomy first. If you read the later chapter of the horizontally impacted tooth, you will easily understand how the crown and the coronal part of the root are removed. If you follow my technique of removing the horizontally impact-ed tooth, you will see that the coronectomy is basically stopping half way.

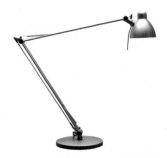

01
Coronectomy of horizontally impacted wisdom tooth <1> ★★★

CASE 1

This is a case of 25 y.o. male patient. You can see Youngsam's sign and curved roots on x-rays. You can guess that when the roots were forming, they contacted the lingual cortical plate and ended up being curved. As the extraction was predicted to be difficult, coronectomy was performed.

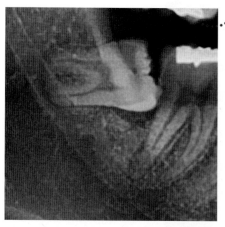

— You can clearly see Youngsam's sign on this pre-op x-ray

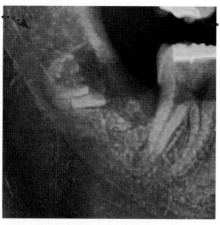

— Immediate post-op Panoramic x-ray

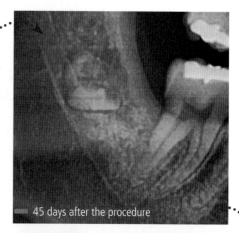

45 days after the procedure

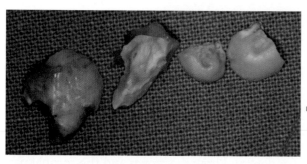

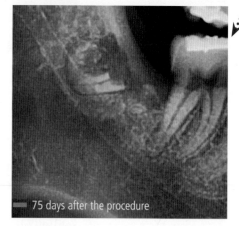

—Post-op picture of the crown part of the tooth. These are one of the most difficult extractions.

75 days after the procedure

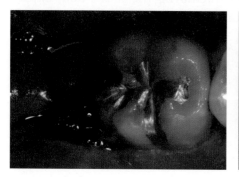

—1 week after the procedure

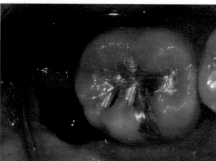

—18 days after the procedure

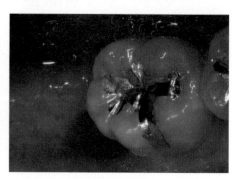

—35 days after the procedure

Coronectomy of horizontally impacted wisdom tooth <2> ★★★

CASE 2

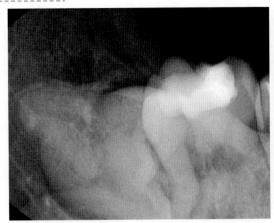 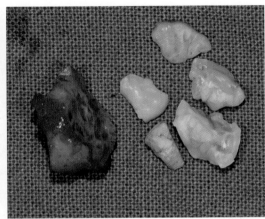

You can clearly see the Youngsam's sign on pre-op x-rays. Since the root is curved upwards, it's likely that the cortical plate is present underneath it on lingual aspect.

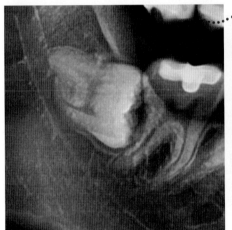 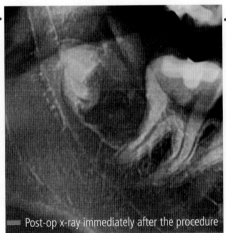 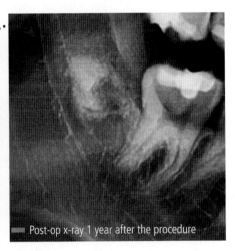

Post-op x-ray immediately after the procedure

Post-op x-ray 1 year after the procedure

Unlike panoramic x-rays, the PA x-ray clearly shows the Youngsam's sign on the mesial root. Sometimes Youngsam's sign appears differently even on panoramic x-rays taken on the same day. When you see this sign at least once, you should assume that it can be a risk factor. Also in a case like this, there is a risk of damaging the inferior alveolar nerve during the crown removal, therefore it is suggested to section enamel only from the distal of #7 and remove the crown in multiple pieces followed by removing the middle part after performing disto-cervical cutting which will be explained further in the later chapter on removal of horizontally impacted wisdom tooth.

The patient came back a year later, and the panoramic x-ray was taken. The root does not look as clear, possibly got resorbed and surrounded by well-formed bone. The soft tissue has healed well.

Coronectomy of horizontally impacted wisdom tooth <3> ★

CASE 3

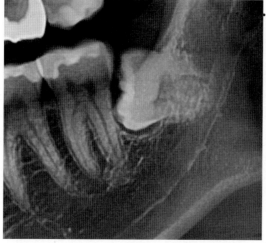 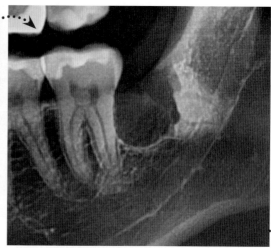

 Pre and post-op x-rays taken immediately after the procedure. You can clearly see where the bur touched the root.

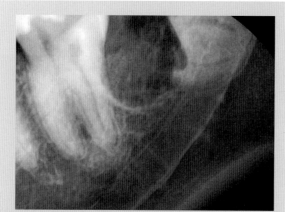

 This PA x-ray was taken during the procedure to decide whether to continue or stop the procedure. You can see that the cutting was done very close to the nerve

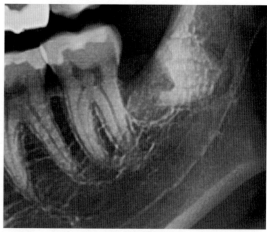

 Panoramic x-ray taken 5 months later. You can see the slight mesial migration of the root.

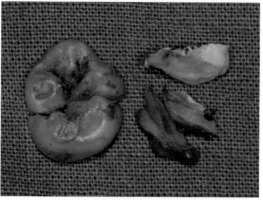

 Post-op picture of the tooth. You can see that the root is fractured in many pieces but it did not come out completely.

This is a case of 30 y.o. male patient. The tooth kept breaking and the removal of the root was not easy. At that time I was testing some coronectomy cases, I decided to leave the root behind intentionally. The crown was removed by horizontal division, and to remove the middle part, I have done the oblique cutting and disto-cervical cutting which will be discussed further in the later chapter. I have strongly suggested him to come back for the follow-up and managed to take a post-op x-ray. Soft tissue was fully healed without any signs of issues.

Coronectomy of horizontally impacted wisdom tooth <4> ★

CASE 4

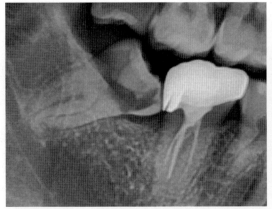 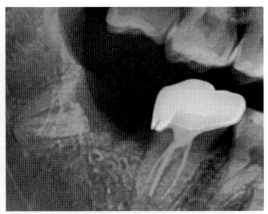

▬ Pre and post-op x-rays taken immediately after the procedure. You can clearly see where the bur touched the root.

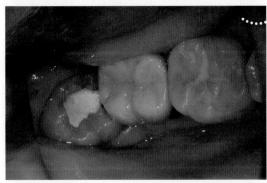 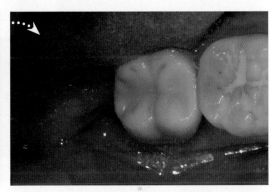

▬ Clinical pictures taken pre-op and 34 days post-op

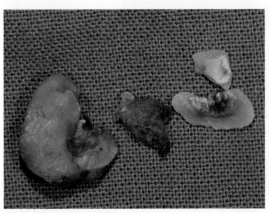

▬ Picture of the tooth removed. You can see the cotton from the pulp chamber space

▬ Post-op x-ray taken 34 days after the procedure. You can see that there is much movement of the root

This is a case of 32 y.o. female patient who previously saw another dentist with wisdom tooth pain. Instead of removing the tooth, the dentist performed pulpectomy as the pain was caused by tooth decay. You can see the cotton present inside the tooth. I have performed coronectomy as I was curious about the prognosis of the tooth which has the history of tooth decay. The patient was planning to come back a month later to get another wisdom tooth removed so the follow up was expected. Two last images are a clinical picture and panoramic x-ray taken 34 days later.

Coronectomy of horizontally impacted wisdom tooth <5> ★★★

CASE 5

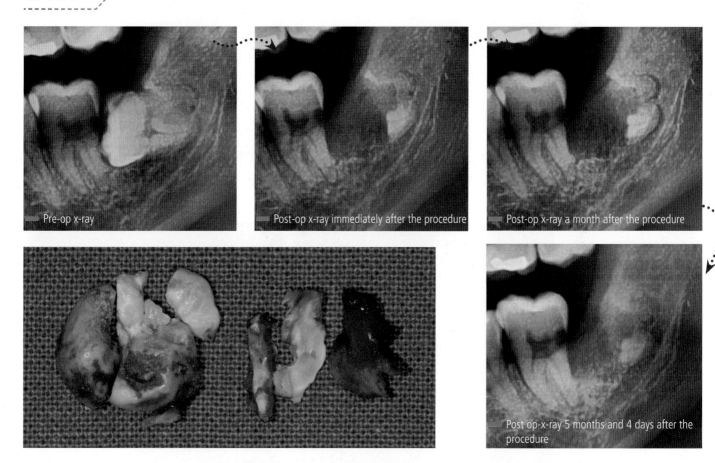

This is a case of 34 y.o. male patient and you can see Youngsam's sign on pre-op x-ray. The post-op x-ray shows the remaining root. You will understand better how the roots are left like that once you read the chapter on horizontal wisdom tooth extraction. I usually remove the wisdom tooth on another side about a month after. The post-op x-ray was taken when the patient came back for another wisdom tooth extraction. In most cases, the root migrates about this much in the first month and there is not much movement after that.

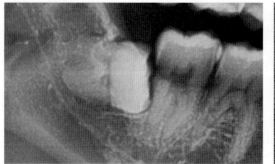
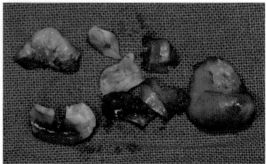

This is the extraction of #48 on the same patient. You can see from the picture that the roots were not removed easily.

Coronectomy of horizontally impacted wisdom tooth <6> ★

CASE 6

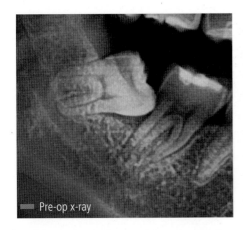

Pre-op x-ray

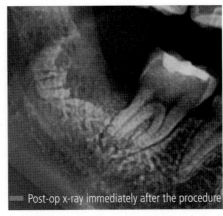

Post-op x-ray immediately after the procedure

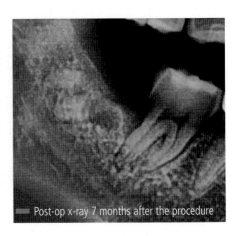

Post-op x-ray 7 months after the procedure

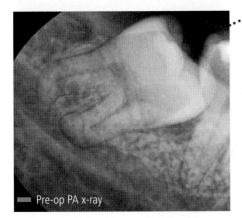

Pre-op PA x-ray

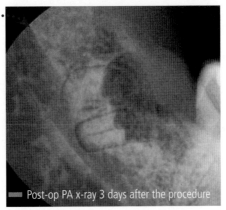

Post-op PA x-ray 3 days after the procedure

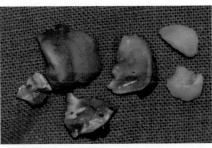

Post-op picture of the wisdom tooth

This is the case of 35 y.o. male patient. You can see pre-op and post-op x-rays and a picture. Both panoramic and PA pre-op x-rays show Youngsam's sign. There was not much movement observed on the post-op x-ray taken 7 months later. Soft tissue was healed well.

02
Coronectomy on older patients <1> ★★★

CASE 1

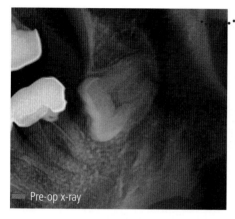

Pre-op x-ray

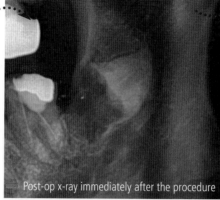

Post-op x-ray immediately after the procedure

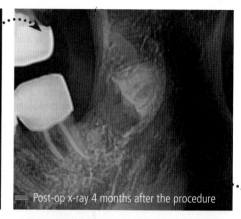

Post-op x-ray 4 months after the procedure

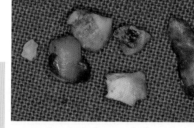

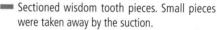
Sectioned wisdom tooth pieces. Small pieces were taken away by the suction.

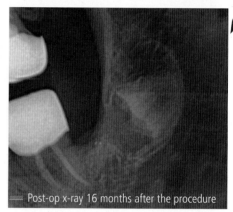

Post-op x-ray 16 months after the procedure

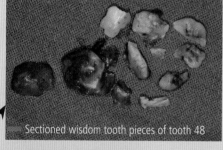

Sectioned wisdom tooth pieces of tooth 48

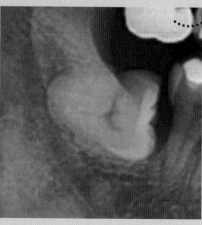

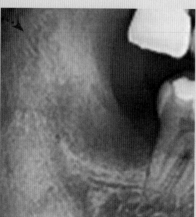

58 y.o. female patient found me after trying other clinics for help. The nerve canal was pressured by the tooth and there was severe pericoronitis. I have removed the crown in pieces. Due to her age and chronic inflammation around the tooth, enamel on mesial aspect of the crown was ankylosed to the bone. Due to the busy schedule, I have stopped the procedure there. The patient showed the trust in me with the fact that I have attempted the extraction for her and wanted to get other treatments done by me as well. Later, all her family members came to see me as well and the follow up was possible.

After removing the tooth #38 and other general dental procedures, the patient wanted the tooth #48 to be removed as well. This tooth also shows Youngsam's sign and due to chronic pericoronitis, the tooth was pushed distally and the extraction was not easy. But as I approach every case in the same manner, the extraction was completed within 10 minutes.

Coronectomy on older patients <2> ★

CASE 2

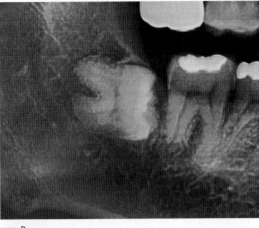

■ Pre-op x-ray

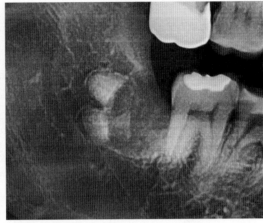

■ Post-op x-ray immediately after the procedure

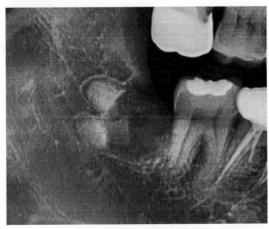

■ Post-op x-ray 25 days after the procedure

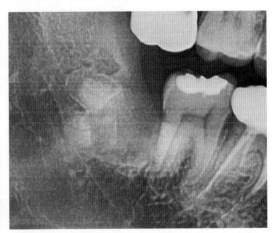

■ Post-op x-ray 4 months and 16 days after the procedure

This is the case of 46 y.o. male patient who was suffering from chronic pericoronitis. He had tooth #38 removed 4 years ago which was supposed to be easier than this tooth to be removed, yet it took a long time to be removed and the post-op pain was bad. Due to his high blood pressure, he was initially reluctant to get this removed, but the recurrent pericoronitis made him decide to come see me all the way from city of Sokcho. The root kept breaking, and I suspected possible ankylosis of the root. I stopped the procedure due to the pain and bleeding although lingual part of the middle part of the tooth was still intact. He did not come back since then but it was confirmed by phone conversation that there are no issues.

03
Coronectomy on elderly patients ★

CASE 3

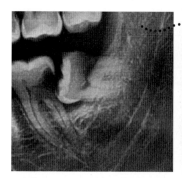
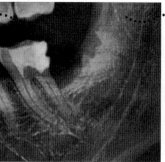
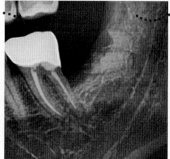
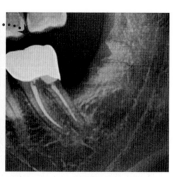

- Pre-op x-ray
- Post-op x-ray immediately after the procedure
- Post-op x-ray 1 month and 5 days after the procedure
- Post-op x-ray 2 months and 8 days after the procedure

This is the case of 50 y.o. male patient. The tooth kept breaking during the procedure and the root removal was difficult. The patient was my acquaintance, and I easily got the permission to perform coronectomy and regularly review. I feel that I could have made the remaining root surface to be smoother however soft tissue is covering it well and there are no issues.

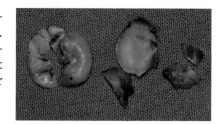

CASE 4

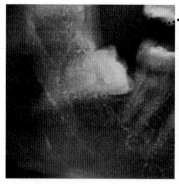
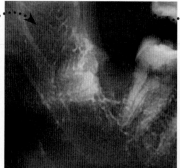
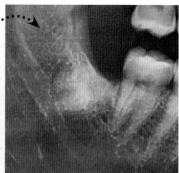

- Pre-op x-ray
- Post-op x-ray immediately after the procedure
- Post-op x-ray 11 months and 17 days after the procedure

This is the case of 44 y.o. male patient with pre and post-op x-rays and a clinical picture. The root looks to be ankylosed to the bone and the distal root shows Youngsam's sign.

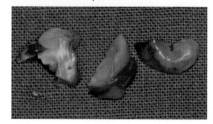

04
Intentional coronectomy cases without follow-ups <1> ★

CASE 1

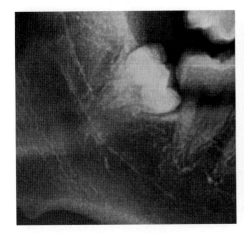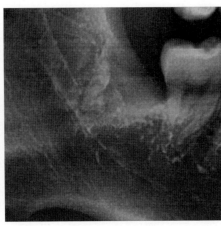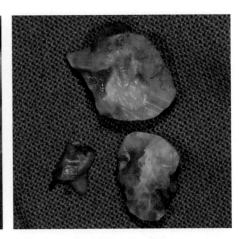

This is the case of 26 y.o. male patient. From the pre-op and 3 months post-op x-rays, it shows that the root is blurred and Youngsam's sign is slightly seen. I suspect that the tooth has multiple roots and one of them might be placed within the lingual cortical bone. You can see that the one root (Mesiolingual) is removed completely.

CASE 2

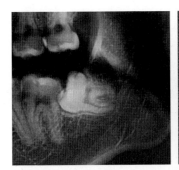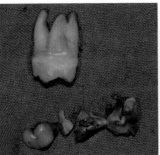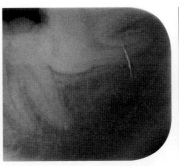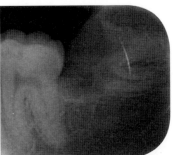

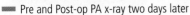
Pre and Post-op PA x-ray two days later ▬ Intentional coronectomy cases without follow-ups 2

This is the case of 22 y.o. male patient. Most coronectomy cases do not get reviewed easily and this patient also did not come back after the suture removal. Some patients do not even come back for the suture removal so I thank him for at least coming back for that. Since my clinic is located in downtown Seoul, most patients come from a far distance and once their chief complaints are dealt with, many of them do not come back. That is why I try to do more cases. I don't try to remove the ones which do not need to be removed and try to perform coronectomy safely. Unless I intentionally do them, these cases represent only 0.2% of all extraction cases.

Intentional coronectomy cases without follow-ups <2> ★

CASE 3

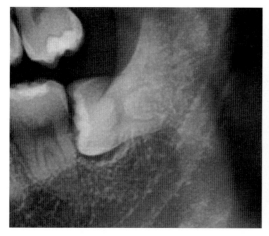 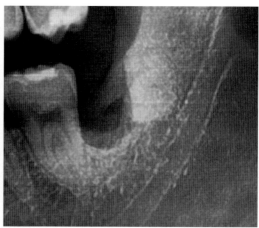 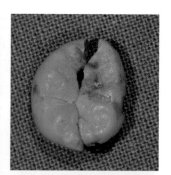

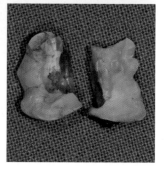

Since the follow up of coronectomy was not happening well, I have performed series of coronectomy procedures number of times. The most recent series of coronectomy was performed in early 2017. This is the case of 30 y.o. male patient and you can see the pre and post-op x-rays taken 7 days after the procedure. As discussed earlier, this is the case of ankylosis of the tooth due to pericoronitis. This shows the vertical division which I perform often to section the crown. The more details will be discussed on horizontal impaction chapter. This is why I suggest you to read this book more than once. When you read this chapter again after finishing the book at least once, you will see these pictures differently.

CASE 4

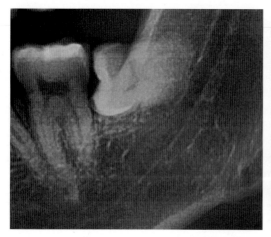 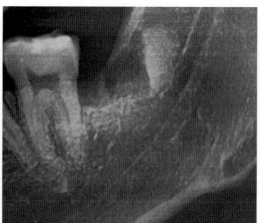 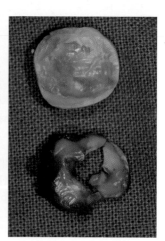

This is the case of 36 y.o. male patient. You can see the pre and post-op x-rays and a clinical picture. This is the intentional coronectomy performed around at same time as the previous case. There was no follow-up after the suture removal.

Intentional coronectomy cases without follow-ups <3> ★

CASE 5

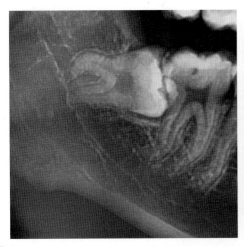 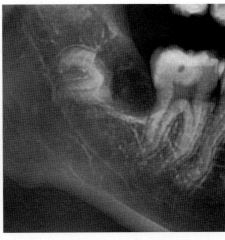 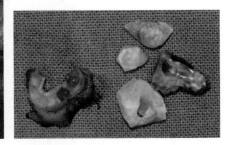

This is the case of 25 y.o. male patient. Intentional coronectomy was performed due to same reasons as before but did not come back for the follow-up. There were some restorations to be done as well but he decided to go to another clinic close to home. No issues were informed.

CASE 6

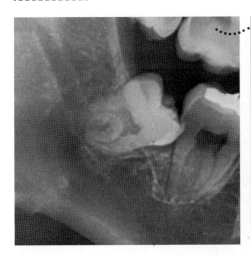 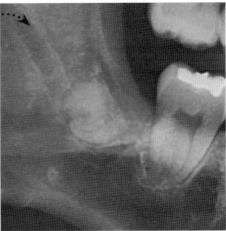 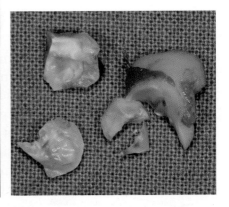

This is the case of 30 y.o. male patient. You can see the pre and post-op x-rays and a clinical picture. He came from the other parts of the country and wanted the same day extraction. You can see the dark band around the distal root. The removal of the root was attempted; however I had to stop due to patient's train schedule back home. I have not seen him again for 2 years, but he text messaged me saying that everything is ok.

Intentional Coronectomy ★★

4. Impacted maxillary wisdom tooth

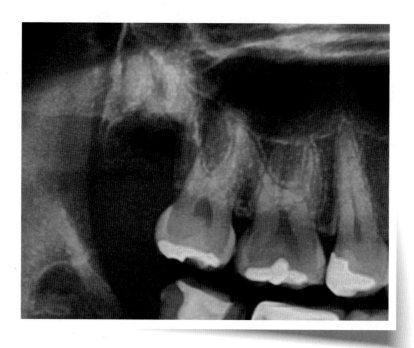

I have called it 'impacted' however there will be more 'non-impacted' cases with maxillary wisdom teeth. Usually, in a case of fully impacted maxillary wisdom tooth, the full flap will be raised and bone removal will be performed so the root is usually removed completely.

Based on my experience, if the root is fractured and it is located within the bone, I advised you not try to remove it. Especially, an inexperienced dentist should not try it. When it is not approached correctly, the root may move into the maxillary sinus and cause more problems. Also using the high-speed handpieces or straight slow speed handpieces are difficult in maxillary extraction cases. Therefore, unless the root can be removed simply just by using explorer, you should consider leaving the root behind.

Maxillary wisdom tooth extraction is usually easy, so I am not going to spend too much time on this topic but if you find it difficult to remove the whole tooth, coronectomy should be considered. Of course, even this may be difficult to the inexperienced clinicians.

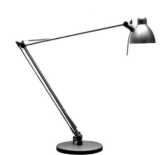

01
Intentional coronectomy of maxillary wisdom tooth <1> ★★

CASE 1

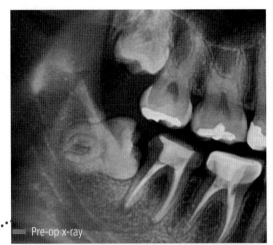

Pre-op x-ray

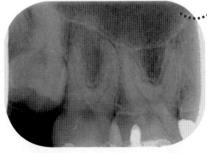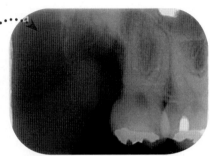

Pre and Post-op PA x-ray of maxillary wisdom tooth

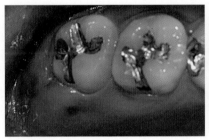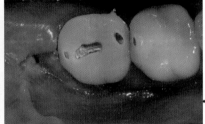

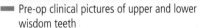

Pre-op clinical pictures of upper and lower wisdom teeth

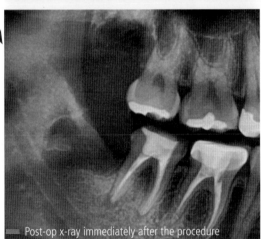

Post-op x-ray immediately after the procedure

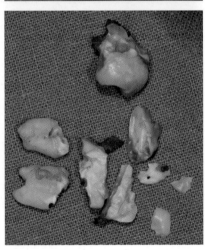

This is the case of 28 y.o. female patient who visited me a few days before moving to the USA. She was referred by another dentist as the patient wanted to get her wisdom teeth removed before she departed. The dentist who referred the patient to me was an oral surgeon who did not have time to see this patient due to the busy schedule. Although it was hard to believe, tooth #47 recently had a new crown cemented with a temporary cement. Since it was a temporary cement, I removed the crown before the extraction. The x-ray showed Youngsam's sign slightly and the extraction was difficult and took a long time to finish. The removal of upper wisdom tooth was not necessary in my opinion, however, the patient requested it to be extracted as she was worried about the high cost of wisdom tooth extraction in the USA. Since I spent too much time trying to remove the lower wisdom tooth and many patients were waiting for me, I stopped the procedure after removing the crown of the maxillary wisdom tooth. This was the first intentional coronectomy of the maxillary wisdom tooth and there are no issues since.

Intentional coronectomy of maxillary wisdom tooth <2> ★

CASE 2

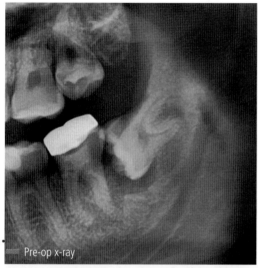

Pre-op x-ray

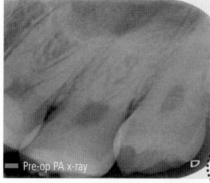

Pre-op PA x-ray

This case was presented on the previous chapter. As previously mentioned, this is the case which I will remember for a long time, it will be discussed again at later chapter of horizontally impacted wisdom tooth. Let me explain why this case is presented in this chapter as well.

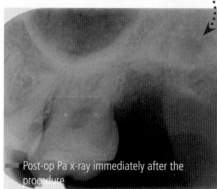

Post-op Pa x-ray immediately after the procedure

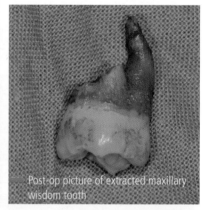

Post-op picture of extracted maxillary wisdom tooth

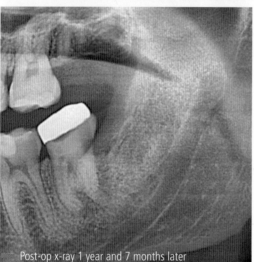

Post-op x-ray 1 year and 7 months later

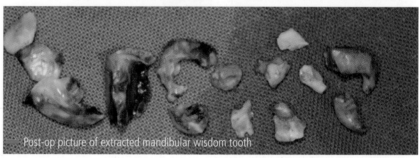

Post-op picture of extracted mandibular wisdom tooth

This is the case of 27 y.o. male patient who came to see me with his brother just to get his wisdom teeth removed. Tooth #38 was pushed distally and showed signs of ankylosis due to pericoronitis and the curvature of the root made the extraction difficult. This extraction took the longest time among all the extractions I have done in 2015. In 2015, I was working by myself and there were many patients waiting but my pride did not stop me from finishing the treatment. I expected the maxillary wisdom tooth to be simple, however, the root was fractured. Due to my delayed schedule, I had to stop the procedure after getting patient's consent. To check the remaining root, I asked him to come back, however, due to the distance from his home, he emailed me a copy of panoramic x-ray taken at his nearby clinic 1 year and 7 months after the procedure. The remaining root is not causing any issues and positioned at the same spot. The lower wisdom tooth's socket is healed very well too.

Intentional coronectomy of maxillary wisdom tooth \<3> ★

CASE 3

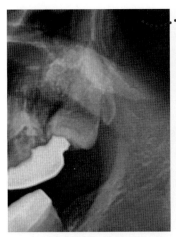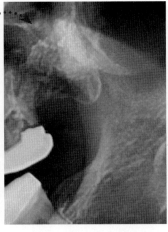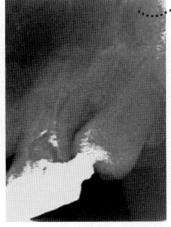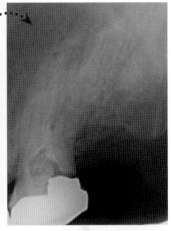

▬ Pre and post-op panoramic x-rays taken 2 days after the procedure ▬ Pre and post-op panoramic x-rays taken 2 days after the procedure

This is the case of 29 y.o. female patient and I usually approach these cases from buccal by using slow speed handpiece. However, on this day, my assistant gave me the high-speed handpiece as I usually do for mandibular wisdom tooth extraction. Maybe she also thought that amalgam removal was required as well. As mentioned, if I was using the slow speed, I would have removed the crown by approaching it from the buccal aspect however since it was a high-speed handpiece I was using, I did it in the same way as the mandibular wisdom tooth extraction. I usually do not use high-speed handpiece for the maxillary wisdom tooth extraction but when the flap does not need to be raised, it is sometimes used. I will discuss further on this topic on later chapter of maxillary wisdom tooth extraction.

As the crown was fractured, I stopped the procedure. After the procedure, I also polished the amalgam overhang of tooth #27. The patient did not come back, however, no issues were reported on a phone conversation. I would have removed this tooth only using an elevator if the amalgam removal was not required.

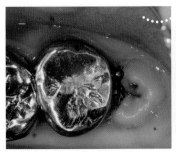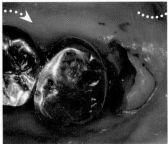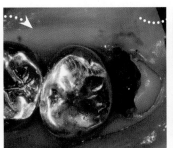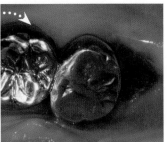

▬ Two days after the procedure

These are clinical pictures taken during the procedure and two days after.

Intentional coronectomy of maxillary wisdom tooth <4> ★

CASE 4

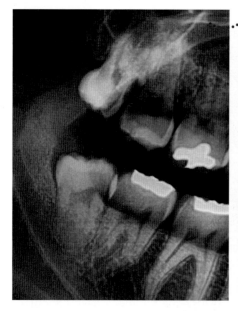 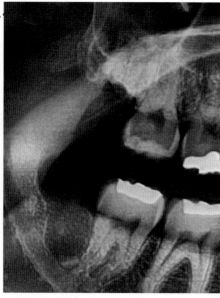 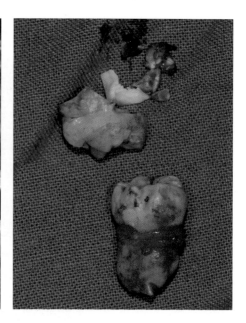

This is the case of 29 y.o. male patient. His wisdom tooth crown was unusually large and another tooth was fused to the lingual to it. As you can see in the clinical picture, the bucco-lingual width was large, and I could not grasp the tooth with forceps. It also had multiple curved roots. The extraction was not easy, and I decided to remove the crown using 45-degree handpiece and review. I have taken a post-op panoramic x-ray immediately after the procedure to check the remaining root. You can also see the small remaining root portion of the mandibular wisdom tooth. The patient did not come back since.

The Removal of the Remaining Root ★★★
after Intentional Coronectomy

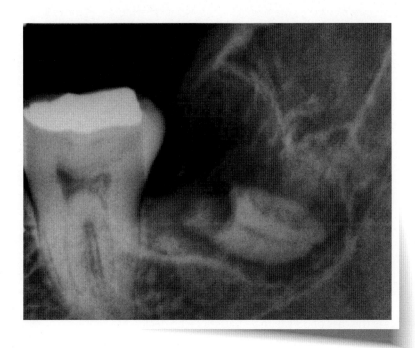

There are two main reasons of intentional coronectomy.

First, the removal of the root is dangerous so we are aiming to bury the root permanently. Second, the removal of the root is not appropriate at this stage but we are aiming to remove it in future. In this instance, to remove the remaining root safely, sometimes addition treatments are done such as orthodontic intervention.

However, when the intentional coronectomy is performed correctly, the remaining root should be removed only when problems arise. In most problematic cases, usually the root is migrated to the favorable and safe position for removal; therefore, the removal can be performed easily.

Therefore, in my opinion, both leaving the root behind without complications and removing the remaining root later can be considered to be successful intentional coronectomy.

01
The removal of the remaining root after coronectomy <1> ★★

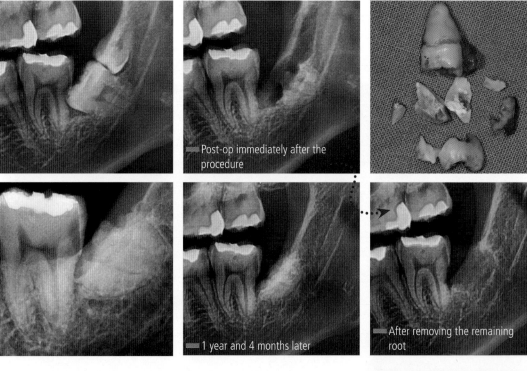

Post-op immediately after the procedure

1 year and 4 months later

After removing the remaining root

This is the case of 33 y.o. male patients who decided to remove both 3rd and 4th lower molars on the same day. I have extracted supernumerary 4th molar first then attempted to remove the third molar. However, after removing the crown, the root could not be removed easily, and the patient was complaining of pain so it was decided to leave the root behind. No issues were noted on the day of suture removal. The patient and I were satisfied with the result. However, the patient came back after 1 year and 4 months complaining of discomfort from the area. The panoramic x-ray showed that the root has migrated coronally, and the remaining root was removed on that day but it was not simple. It was just like doing another difficult

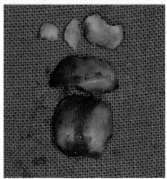

extraction. Since then another year has passed, and the patient has no issues at all. I consider this as a successful coronectomy.

However, we need to think about why the remaining root migrated. I think it is probably due to the 4th molar (or distomolar). The remaining root should be surrounded by healthy bone, however, due to the 4th molar's socket space, the root was exposed to the soft tissue and migrated coronally.

The reason why the extraction was difficult initially can be answered by looking at the shape of the root. The hip shaped roots are the most difficult ones to remove.

The removal of the remaining root after coronectomy <2> ★★

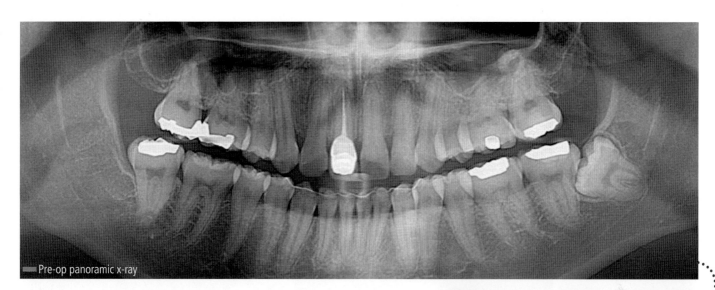

Pre-op panoramic x-ray

This is the case of a female patient in her late 20s who works at the dental laboratory I use. She wanted to remove the tooth #38 although the tooth was not bothering her. She came to see me as she was satisfied with my extraction of her tooth #48 I have done. I checked the pre-op x-ray of #48 as well and wondered why I removed the tooth back then.

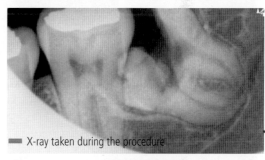

X-ray taken during the procedure

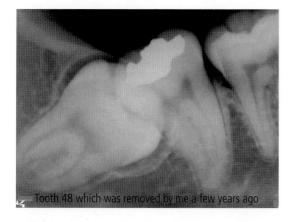

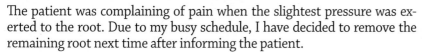
Tooth 48 which was removed by me a few years ago

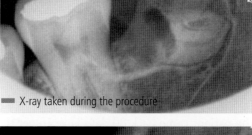

X-ray taken during the procedure

The patient was complaining of pain when the slightest pressure was exerted to the root. Due to my busy schedule, I have decided to remove the remaining root next time after informing the patient.

The 40 days post-op x-ray taken 40 days shows that the root has migrated within the socket.

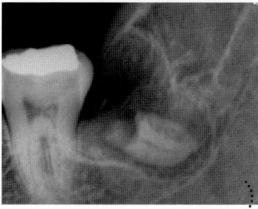

Post-op x-ray taken 40 days after the procedure

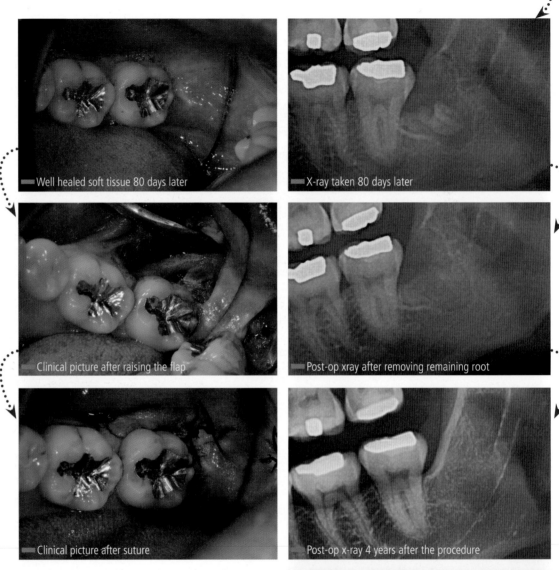

Well healed soft tissue 80 days later

X-ray taken 80 days later

Clinical picture after raising the flap

Post-op xray after removing remaining root

Clinical picture after suture

Post-op x-ray 4 years after the procedure

The patient came back 80 days later to get the remaining root removed. She was not experiencing any major discomfort and did not want to get it removed, but I wanted to remove it. The clinical picture shows that the socket is healed well.

The removed root shows where the inferior alveolar nerve passes (arrow). Since the root was removed only after 80 days, it is hard to predict how the remaining root would have reacted if left untouched, however, I feel that it may have stayed without causing any issues. This was the case done 5 years ago and at that time I had a principle of not leaving the root behind, I would probably have left it if the patient came to see me now. It may not be correct due to the angle of the x-ray beam but it appears that the wall of the canal is not very strong. Therefore the slight touch of the root caused the severe pain in my opinion.

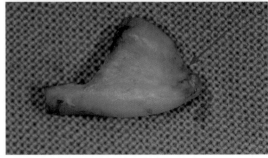

Clinical picture of the root

The Removal of the Remaining Root from ★★ the Extraction Done at the Another Clinics

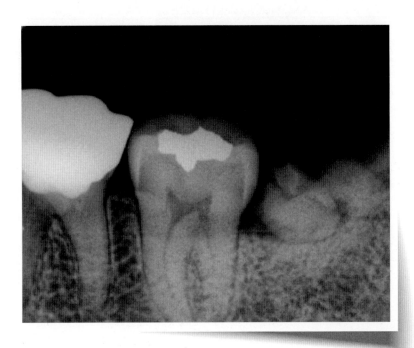

The previous two cases show the removal of remaining root after attempting to remove the tooth by myself. But I also have cases where the extraction was initially attempted at the other clinics.

Some of the cases presented here are the ones where the patient was informed that the extraction is completely done. I have performed so many wisdom teeth extractions, but there are not many cases where the remaining roots cause problems. However, seeing so many cases from other clinics where the remaining roots are causing problems made me think that it may be due to the different philosophies on this concept rather the differences in skill levels. As previously mentioned, it is a philosophical matter on how to leave the root. Let's have a look at some cases. These cases will lead you to next chapters on actual complete extractions.

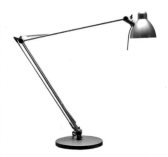

01
The removal of the remaining root from the extraction done at the other ★ clinics

CASE 1

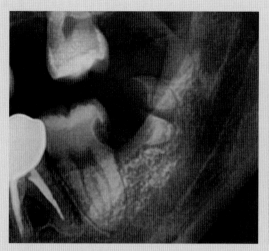 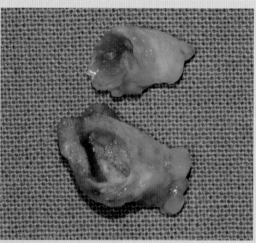

This is the case of 30 y.o. male patient who had his wisdom tooth extracted 6 months ago. His chief complaint was severe pain from the area. The remaining root was removed. I considered to get the pre-op x-ray from the other clinic but decided not to at the end.

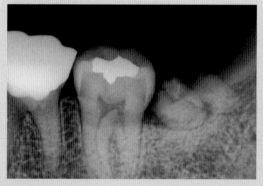 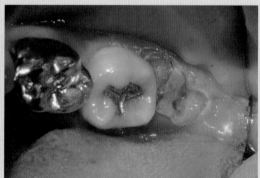

This is the case of a female patient in her thirties. She does not remember when the extraction was done but came to see me as she was getting pain from the area. The picture was taken after removing the root. I wanted to see pre and post-op x-rays of the extraction but could not request it from the patient.

However, the root was removed safely without any nerve damage so I will consider it as a successful coronectomy.

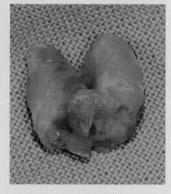

★

CASE 2

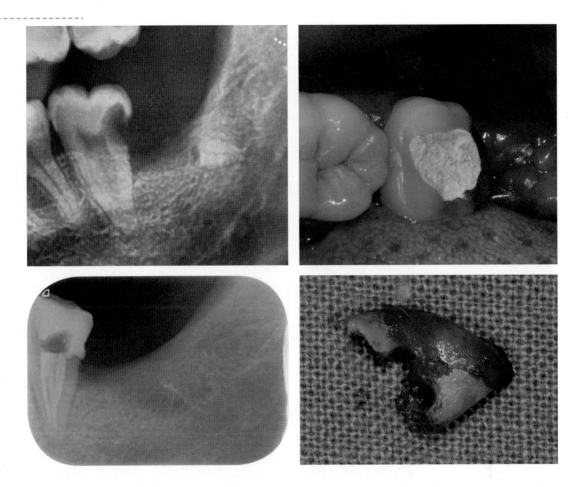

This is the case of a male patient in his forties. He had his wisdom tooth removed a couple of months ago and came to see me due to severe pain from the area. I have explained to him that the cause of the pain was from the tooth #37, however, he insisted on removing the remaining root as well. After completing the root canal treatment on #37, I have removed the remaining root as well. I personally don't think that the removal of the remaining root was necessary. Although the root looks small, it was bigger than expected bucco-lingually and the removal was difficult. There was bone present coronal to the root so the bone was removed using high-speed handpiece.

★★★

CASE 3

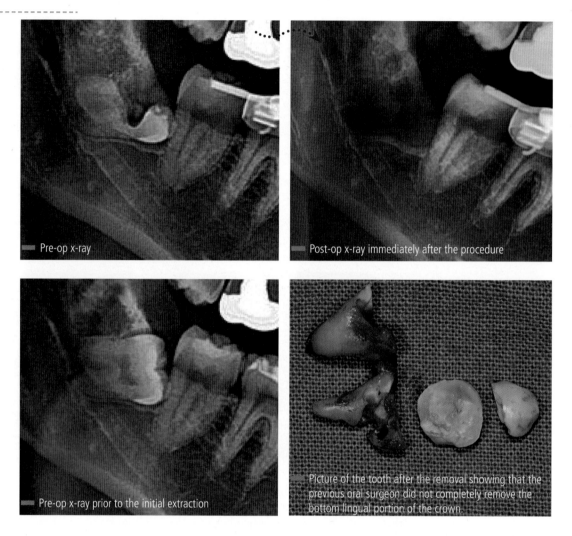

Pre-op x-ray

Post-op x-ray immediately after the procedure

Pre-op x-ray prior to the initial extraction

Picture of the tooth after the removal showing that the previous oral surgeon did not completely remove the bottom lingual portion of the crown.

The dentist who referred me this patient initially referred the patient to the nearby oral surgeon for the removal of teeth #18 and #48 prior to the orthodontic treatment. But as you can see the outcome from the first extraction was not ideal. The dentist asked the oral surgeon if the extraction is complete and the answer from the oral surgeon was yes. It was done in the city in the another province and usually, when the extraction is referred to a surgeon for the orthodontic reasons, the referring dentist usually cannot demand to the oral surgeon too much due to the low cost of extraction in Korea under its national insurance. So when the patient came back to the dentist like this, the dentist could not tell the oral surgeon that he is not happy with the outcome, and instead, he referred the patient to me. I am not intending to criticize anyone just based on the story from one side and understand that anyone can make a mistake. Probably I have made similar mistakes as well in the past. However, this is clearly not coronectomy as the crown of the tooth is not properly removed. If the crown were properly removed, I would say that this is a successful extraction as the patient would not be in any pain and the orthodontic treatment would have been possible. I will discuss more about extraction of such tooth in the later chapter on the horizontally impacted wisdom tooth. Anyway, the most important factor in intentional coronectomy is the complete removal of the crown.

★★★

CASE 4

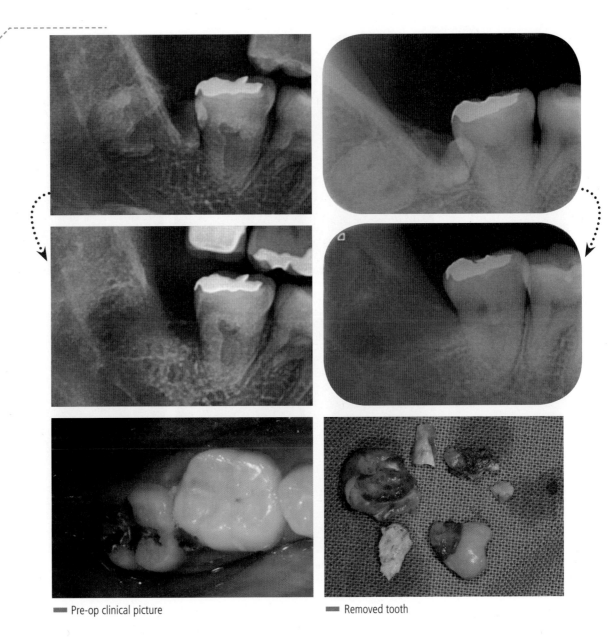

Pre-op clinical picture

Removed tooth

This case was mentioned in chapter 1. This case will probably appear three times in this book. We tend to learn more from other's mistakes.

The patient had the extraction done somewhere else but came to see me due to severe pain from the area. As you can see from the pre-op picture, clinically there doesn't seem to be any major issues. However, the pre-op panoramic x-ray shows that the crown is not completely removed. I will discuss more on how to remove such tooth in the later chapter on the horizontally impacted wisdom tooth. The x-ray also shows Youngsam's sign, suggesting that the removal of the root may not be easy.

It seems that the previous dentist could not remove the lingual aspect of the crown as the tooth was tilted toward lingual too much. I cannot over-emphasize this. The most important factor in intentional coronectomy is the complete removal of the crown.

★★

CASE 5

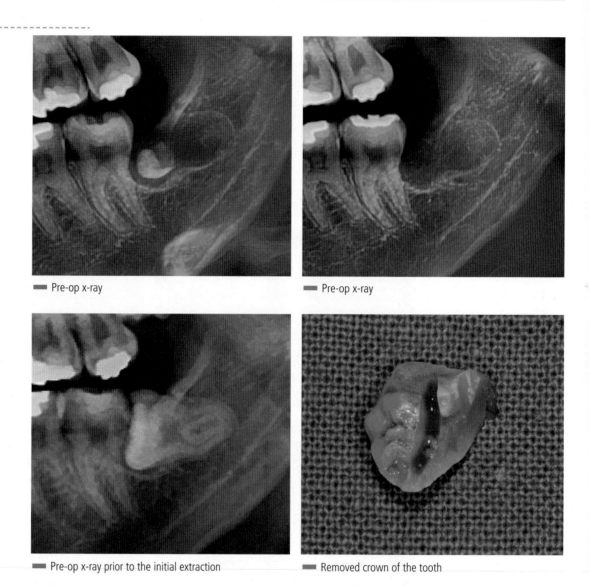

■ Pre-op x-ray

■ Pre-op x-ray

■ Pre-op x-ray prior to the initial extraction

■ Removed crown of the tooth

This is the case of a female patient in her twenties. She had the extraction done 4 days prior to the visit to my clinic. The patient did not have any major symptoms other than what would be generally expected after the wisdom tooth extraction but the panoramic x-ray showed that the mesial part of the crown is left behind. After anaesthetizing the patient and removing suture, I have managed to remove the piece and I realized that it was the mesio-lingual aspect of the crown, the most difficult part of the crown to be removed during wisdom tooth extraction! By looking at the tooth, it seems that the long shank fissure bur was used. I don't think that it was done intentionally. There are many ways of removing the tooth without removing the mesial part (especially the lingual aspect) of the crown. When using the fissure bur, straight handpiece must be used. Probably after removing the top part of the crown, slow speed was used to section the crown in half. Then this part of the crown can be left behind. Anyway, the remaining crown part usually causes problems, so I chose to remove it.

Anesthesia, Incision, Surgical Flap Design, Suture for highlighted all other Wisdom Tooth Extraction

04
CHAPTER

Chapter 04 translated by

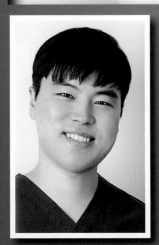

Dr. Jong Yoon DDS

University of California - San Francisco, School of Dentistry
- Owner Dentist at Borderview Dental in Blaine, WA

Ever since I met Dr. Kim, I learned so much from him and was amazed by his unique and efficient extraction techniques. I sincerely appreciate all he has done for me in improving my skills in dentistry. It is an honor for me to participate in translating and editing a chapter of his wisdom tooth extraction book, and I have no doubt that every dentist can learn from it.

01
Dr. Youngsam Kim's basic philosophy on extraction - Be afraid of failure ★★★

Easy, Simple, Safe, and Efficient (ESSE) Extraction

Now, let's enter the world of extraction. Before we start, let's review my important philosophies on third molar extraction.

Be afraid of failure more than success.

Even if you achieve success in 99% of extraction cases, it is much more agonizing to have 1% of cases that fail. Once you feel defeated, it takes a long time to recover your confidence. To achieve a steady improvement in your extraction skill, you need to avoid making any frustrating cases. There are plenty of cases for you to do.

Do not mess with the lingual side~

It is better to not attempt an extraction than to mess with the lingual side. The incision must be made 90-degree towards the buccal side and buccal side only. Make an incision and cut the tooth or bone only in the safe area.

Extraction is not about strength- learn the skill that fits your style (especially on strength and perceptual ability)

Discover your own method. Everybody rides a bike differently. Even a major league athlete plays baseball in an individualized style that fits him. Instead of mimicking someone blindly, find the posture and method that are unique to your strengths and perceptual ability.

Use the instruments that are familiar to you.

If you learn to play golf or baseball for the first time, you need to first get used to the basic equipment. Using a variety of advanced tools is good only after you have attained a certain level of mastery. First, let's learn to use one basic instrument properly.

Every patient is different. Every case is different. I only use the instruments that are familiar to me. If you have a new tool that you want to use, you need to first practice using it in simple cases.

Now, let's take a look at the instruments that are familiar to Dr. Kim.

02
Extraction tray at various dental hospitals' OMS clinics <1> ★

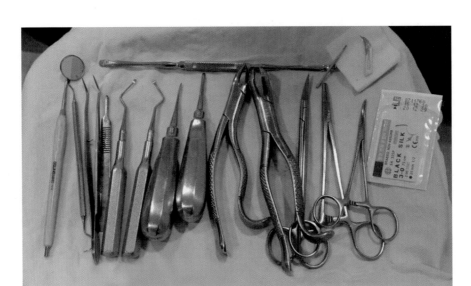

Gangnam Severance Hospital OMS Surgeon's Extraction Instruments

As an educational institution, there are many instruments in the extraction tray. But it is not realistic to have so many instruments in the private practice. For someone like me who does tens of extractions per day, it is not easy to prepare a tray like this all the time.

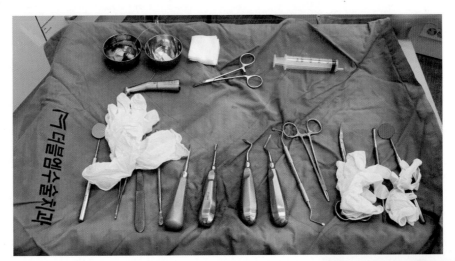

Kwang-Ju Double M clinic: A private dental practice that is famous for third molar extractions in South Korea

This is an extraction tray from an OMFS office that focuses on third molar extractions. In this relatively simple extraction kit, you can also find 1:5 electric handpiece. You can refer to the next chapter for this 1:5 electric handpiece.

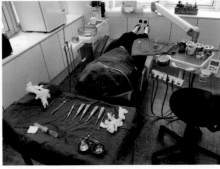

Extraction tray at various dental hospitals' OMS clinics <2> ★

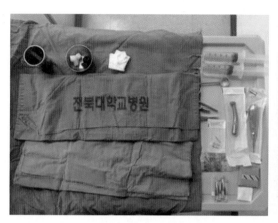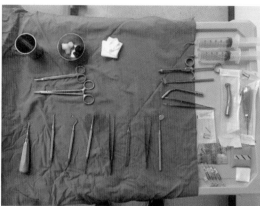

Chonbuk National University, Dental Hospital, Extraction Tray

This is an extraction tray at my alma mater. This setup is simple, and is similar to my personal extraction tray setup at my office. Of course, I learned my fundamentals from school...

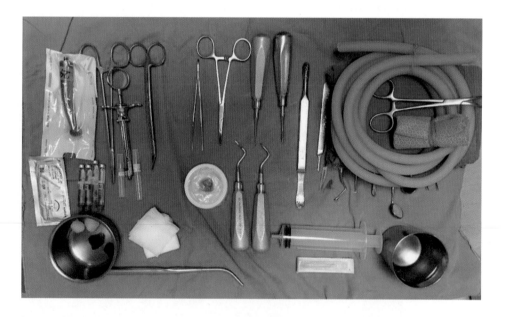

Seoul National University, Dental Hospital OMS Clinic, Extraction Tray

No one would deny that the extraction tray at the Seoul National University is the mother of all extraction trays in South Korea. But I heard that each professor has very distinct style at SNU. Nevertheless, it is still useful to know what instruments are being used at the university that launched dentistry in South Korea.

Extraction tray at various dental hospitals' OMS clinics <3> ★

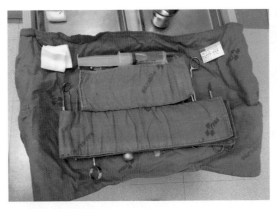

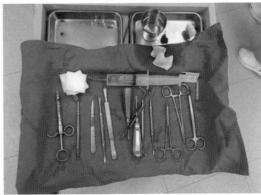

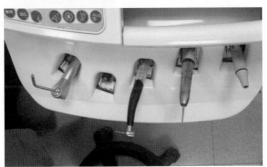

Pusan National University, Dental Hospital OMS Clinic, Extraction Tray

Considering that this is an oral surgery residency clinic, there are very few instruments in the tray. Of course, there are pros and cons on having many instruments vs. few instruments. But since the oral surgery department is an educational institution, it would be beneficial to have various instruments to learn their usage and to find the one that fits one's style. Even though the tray looks simple here, you can still bring out more instruments as you go. Therefore, I think it is fine to have just a few instruments in the basic extraction tray.

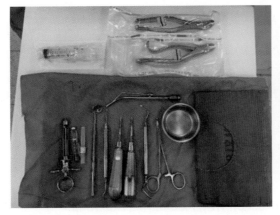

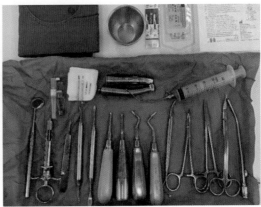

Kyung Hee University, Dental Hospital, Extraction Tray

The left photo seems to be the simple extraction tray, and the right photo seems to be the surgical extraction tray. Forceps are already prepared. You can tell that these instruments have gone through the hands of many dentists. Unlike at a national university, you can see a lot of "made in South Korea" instruments at a private university. As a side note, I am reminded that university dental hospitals still have a far superior sanitary standard compared to that of local practices.

03
Extraction trays at other foreign countries ★

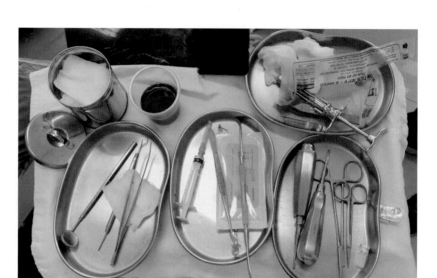

Hue University, College of Dentistry, Vietnam - Extraction Tray

This extraction tray is from the Hue University, College of Dentistry, in Vietnam. If they need an additional instrument, they add in sterilized instrument in the tray. Like in other Asian countries, they use a high speed handpiece and a fissure bur.

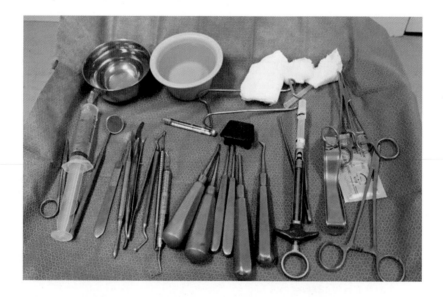

A Private Practice Extraction Tray, Melbourne, Australia

I saw this extraction tray when I visited an Oral Maxillofacial private practice in Melbourne, Australia. The dentist had excellent surgical skills. Just like in a typical OMS treatment room, there were not many additional instruments at the chair, and he used a portable low speed handpiece. I took a photo of the handpiece because it is made in Korea. The same motor is also used for the implant surgery, so it can spray water within the handpiece, but the dentist had his assistant irrigate saline as he skillfully performed the extraction. He normally removes all four wisdom teeth in one appointment.

04
Some universities ban high speed handpiece use ★★

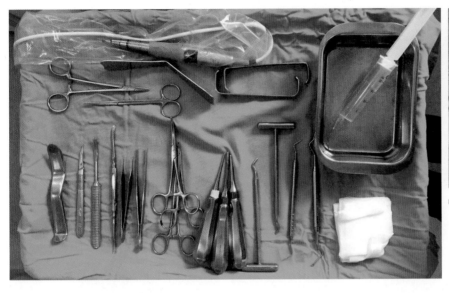

University of Barcelona, College of Dentistry. OMS Surgeon's Extraction Instruments

I took this photo when I visited the University of Barcelona OMS clinic. All instruments were sterilized. This is almost impossible in private practice setting in Korea.

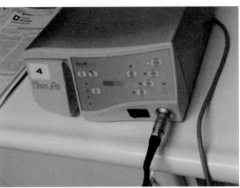

The low speed handpiece system at the University of Barcelona, College of Dentistry, OMS clinic.

This separate system may be suited for a specialized extraction clinic but it seems unnecessary for a GP office providing various procedures. It lacks power but newer improved versions are coming out into the market.

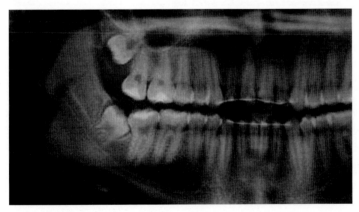

As mentioned, it is still debatable whether we should use high speed handpieces for extraction. In South Korea, only 1 out of 11 dental schools exclusively use low speed for extraction (Yonsei University). Surgical department at the University of Barcelona only teaches extraction using a low speed handpiece. However, the surgical department at Barcelona seems to be the only one with this belief.

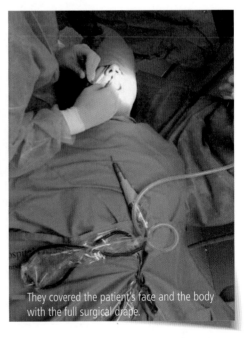

They covered the patient's face and the body with the full surgical drape.

Since it is a university hospital, they strive for the best infection control standard. They do not even use chair attached handpiece for complete infection control of connection line.

05
Extraction done by an oral surgery resident at Barcelona dental university

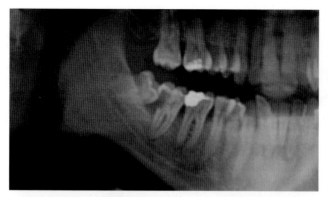

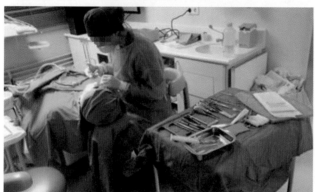

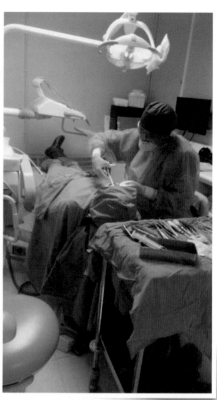

Despite my strong preference for using a high speed handpiece for extraction, I still learned a lot from watching others use a slow speed handpiece at the University of Barcelona. The extractions were done slightly more aggressive including considerable bone removal. It may be because they are residents and relatively inexperienced. Many extractions were done with a full flap, bone removal, and consumed a considerable amount of time. They would have only taken me average 3 to 5 minutes to complete. They were able to extract despite these difficulties. However, they were done with considerable amount of bone removal.

I have worked with an oral surgeon who exclusively used the low speed handpiece, and I myself have used the low speed handpiece in many cases. But I believe that the high speed handpiece is more appropriate for extraction. However, there is one thing that I certainly learned from observing at the University of Barcelona OMS. You can remove a lot of bone during an extraction. ^^ This trip boosted my confidence in extraction.

My Spanish dentist colleague, Dr. Xavi Costa, invited me to this satisfying Barcelona trip where I spent most of my time learning the extraction style of the University of Barcelona and no time for famous Gaudi. Three years later, when I returned for Xavi Costa's wedding in Barcelona, I spent most of my time seeing Gaudi architecture. ^^

06
Extraction tray at the MeiKai University Dental Hospital ★

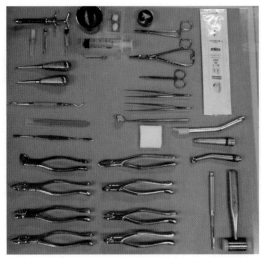

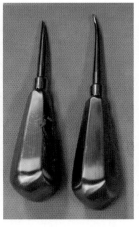

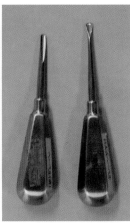

Each basic extraction kit has a straight and a curved elevator.

Japan. These instruments are similar to those used in most East Asian countries. However, one notable characteristic among Japanese dentists is that they prefer techniques that are widely proven and safe. Also, they mostly follow techniques learned in school or in study groups. Overall, the extraction technique was similar among all Japanese dentists.

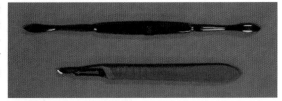

Like in most other OMS, the No. 15 blade was mainly used.

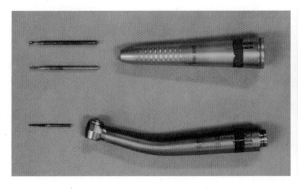

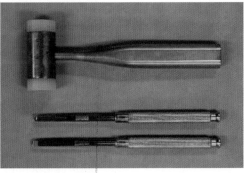

Fundamentally, Japanese dentists like to use a high speed contra-angle handpiece for extractions. Sometimes, I observed them using a 45 degree handpiece or a straight handpiece, but a high speed contra-angle handpiece was mainly used. Also, they were not particularly concerned about chip air or emphysema. In most cases that I observed, the fissure bur was mainly used, and the diamond fissure bur was used occasionally. Japanese dentists used a straight low speed handpiece in addition at times. As you can read in the other chapters of this book, it is difficult to section the tooth delicately with the fissure bur. Therefore, the straight low speed handpiece often needs to be used together.

One unique extraction technique that I observed in Japan was that the dentists often use the chisel and the mallet. The chisel and the mallet were used to remove the bone above the maxillary third molar or to create a space to place an elevator. In Korea, the Kyung Hee University College of Dentistry often uses this technique.

07
Extraction tray at the Peking University Dental Hospital ★

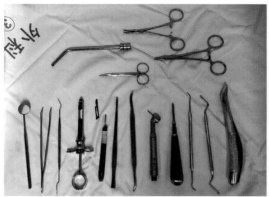 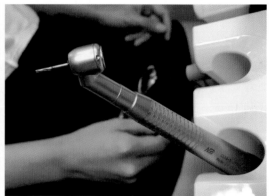

Extraction tray at the Peking University OMS department in China. This tray setup looks pretty much identical to the ones in Korea and Japan. Perhaps because China is such a big country, there are many differences among dental clinics across different regions. But, fundamentally, extraction technique was similar to that of nearby countries such as Korean, Japan, Taiwan, and Hong Kong.

In China, it seems like dentists most often use a 45 degree handpiece. Occasionally, there were handpieces that did not provide chip air, but most 45 degree handpieces that I observed provided chip air (creating a mist at the terminal end of the handpiece). Among the 45 degree handpieces that I observed at the Peking University, especially in the Operating Room, there were handpieces that did not provide chip air and only provided water.

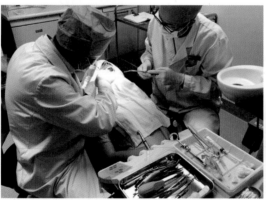 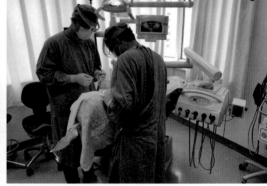

Photo of dentists extracting third molars in the regular treatment room. It was impressive to observe the dentists staying in the same chair to perform serial extractions. It seemed that the number of chairs was lacking compared to the number of patients and dentists.

Photo of dentists extracting third molars in the Operating Room. Dentists do perform basic third molar extractions here without sedation, but extractions with IV sedation seemed more routine. I did not see much difference in the equipment or instruments compared to that of the other East Asian countries.

The technique for disinfecting oral cavity and facial skin, and using sterilization drape were similar to the techniques in Korea. However, I noticed that they often take digital radiographs and not use them while providing patient care in the chair. I was able to observe a plethora of cases due to a large volume of patients. This is the clinic that I most recently visited. They treated me very kindly, and it was great to observe so many extraction cases. I would like to visit the place again to gain even more experience.

08
University of California at Los Angeles (UCLA), Dental Hospital OMS Clinic, Extraction Tray ★

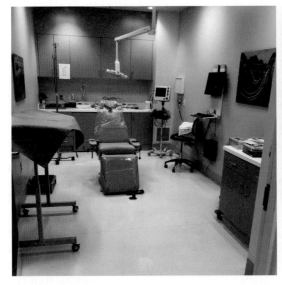

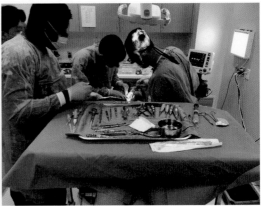

UCLA College of Dentistry OMS Outpatient Operating Room. Most third molar extractions are done here. There are 4 rooms like this in the clinic.

This is a photo of surgery in the Outpatient Operating Room. Just like in the typical operating room, they performed surgery while standing. Like in the other parts of the U.S. and in Australia, they performed surgery without putting the sterilized towel or disinfection on the patient's face.

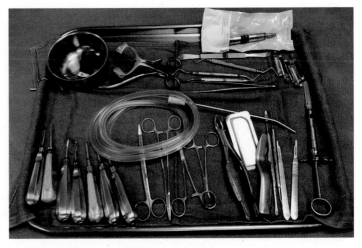

This is the basic third molar extraction tray setup at the UCLA College of Dentistry's OMS clinic. There are many instruments on the tray. It makes sense because, in the U.S., they tend to extract all 4 third molars in one appointment. Like in many other U.S. dental offices, they use the mouth opener and the tongue retractor. One unique thing is the bone rongeur that is placed under the mouth opener. I use the bone rongeur very rarely when the upper third molar is fully impacted in the bone. Also, it is notable that the upper small forceps is included in all extraction trays. I noticed that they use this forceps like a mosquito forceps to grab small pieces. Because it is beneficial for the residents to use a variety of instruments, they have many kinds of periosteal elevators. There is a surgical curette with sharp, curve ends and a root picker that is long and thin. However, I rarely saw them being used, and, in many instances, the sharp ends were broken.

There are two blade holders, but I rarely saw #12 blade being used. Most times, they used #15 blade or similar instruments.

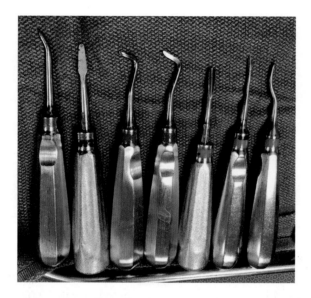

These are basic elevators in the extraction tray. From the right side, there is a curved elevator. I noticed that it's common to see at least one very curved elevator in the extraction tray. For me, very rarely, I use the curved elevator when it's difficult to approach the tooth in the maxillary arch.

Next to the curved elevator, there are one thick and one thin elevators, and there are right and left curved elevators. These curved elevators are, in my opinion, rarely needed except for removing a large piece of broken root. You cannot put too much force on these curved elevators. I rather prefer using a thinner, longer root picker. I even rarely use a root picker. I normally remove root fragments using an explorer with a mirror. Out of so many instruments in this tray, they are missing a mirror and an explorer.

More than anything, there is no EL3C elevator, which is my favorite. If there is an opportunity, I'd like to give EL3C elevators to the incoming 1st year OMS residents as gifts.

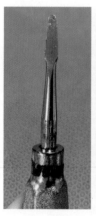
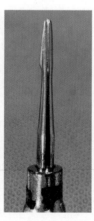
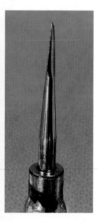

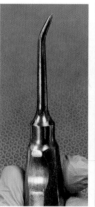
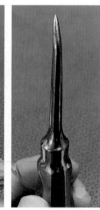

This is Cogswell A elevator from Hu-Friedy. This instrument is used to break the tooth after sectioning the tooth with the low speed handpiece. When I extract the vertically impacted tooth with the low speed handpiece, I usually do hemi-section from the buccal surface, and you can use this instrument to break the tooth. For me of course, I like to use the EL3C elevator or the EL5C elevator to do the same.

This is similar to Cogswell B elevator from the Hu-Friedy, but I don't think this is a Hu Friedy brand. This instrument can be used in the furcation to pull the tooth or it can be used in the notch made on the root to pull the tooth. Rarely, I've seen others putting the instrument between the second and the third molars to create movement. Even though this practice is normal in the OS world, I personally oppose using the elevator in between teeth.

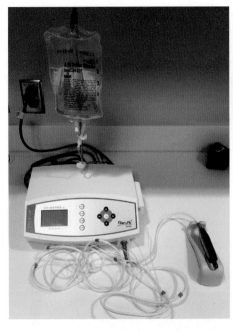

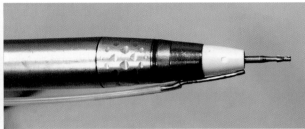

For bone removal and tooth sectioning, portable motor with a handpiece that sprays saline is normally used. In U.S. and Europe, many use a low speed straight handpiece for the extraction. In Korea and Japan, they use a high speed handpiece in the chair, but since an operating room does not have a high speed handpiece, it is common to use a low speed handpiece in the OR. Either handpiece will spray saline or an assistant can irrigate saline from the side. For me, when I perform implant surgery, I prefer to have an assistant irrigate saline to gain better visual field.

Portable low speed handpiece is set to 80,000 RPM for extractions. With high torque, it is very easy to section the tooth.

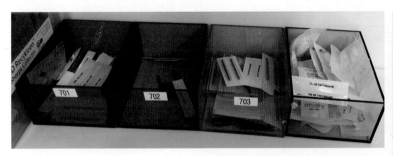

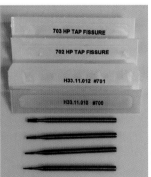

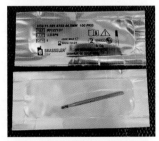

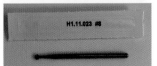

There are various kinds of burs next to the motor. Normally, a tapered fissure bur is used, and a #703 bur (thickness is similar to that of a round bur size #6) is routinely used for the tooth sectioning. The burs vary in thickness, and thin burs can be used to remove the root tip.

I saw some individually wrapped burs.

Also, there are some round burs, but they are rarely used. For alveoloplasty procedure, they use a thick and large bur similar to a denture carbide bur.

Anyhow, they use a low speed handpiece for extractions. Professors and residents have minor personal preferences, but there was no big difference in extraction style across the clinic. It was interesting that professors were very kind and friendly, so the program atmosphere was very friendly. Residents seemed to be proud of one another in the harmonious environment.

09
Dr. Kim's extraction tray for third molar ★★★

I like to use the same tray for all extractions. Not only for very complex cases, but also for very simple cases, I use the same tray. There is only one reason. I have so many patients who need third molar extractions, and it is impossible to customize a tray for each individual case. At my office, it is very rare to take radiographs ahead of time and we offer same day exam and extraction. Therefore, there is no time to assemble individualized extraction trays.

It is good to utilize various instruments to customize each extraction case, but it is also good to use the same instruments for variety of cases. It is similar to feeling more comfortable to ride your old bike than to ride a new bike. I recommend that you get used to using one instrument. Let's get accustomed to my extraction instruments and methods.

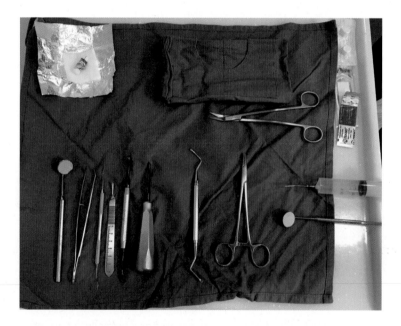

This is my extraction tray. Instruments include a mouth mirror, cotton pliers, explorer, blade handle, periosteal elevator, elevator, surgical curette, needle holder, and scissors. The black-coated elevator instrument in the photo is a new instrument from Hu-Friedy. I only have one, and I happened to take a photo of it. Anyhow, this is enough if you just add suture needle, gauze, and sterile drape. Excluding the forceps, I usually perform extractions using only these instruments 98% of the times.

Except for the elevator (Hu-Friedy EL3C), you can substitute any other instruments that look similar to these instruments, but I have a habit of using the same instruments that are familiar to me. Let's take a closer look at them individually.

10
3 essential extraction instruments ★★★

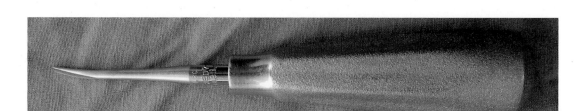

Hu-Friedy EL3C

I use this elevator most often, and I sometimes complement with an EL5C that is wider. You need to use good quality instruments especially when an instrument needs to be thin and load bearing. Good quality means instruments are less likely to break over time, so that they could prove to be economical in the long run.

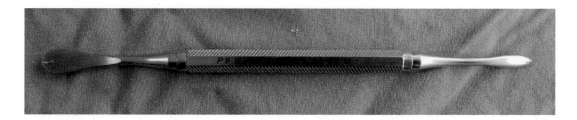

Hu-Friedy P9

I use this periosteal elevator most often. Unlike with other instruments, if you can find an instrument that looks similar, I do not mind using other brands. Recently, I have been using instruments that are made in Korea or in Pakistan that are less expensive.

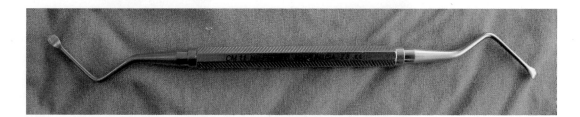

Hu-Friedy CM 11

I use this surgical curette most often. Rather than using it to clean out the socket after an extraction, I use this instrument more often to reflect the soft tissue that covers tooth towards the lingual surface, to break off a crown piece after sectioning, and to take out sectioned tooth pieces. If you can find an instrument with a similar size, I do not insist on using this brand only. Especially, if you are a seasoned dentist who is comfortable doing extractions, you will not use more than necessary strength when using a surgical curette; so do not worry so much about breaking the instrument. But if you are a new dentist, it is very common for you to damage instruments by using them inappropriately. Some would say that new dentists should buy cheap instruments as they are likely to break things, but I would suggest that Hu-Friedy instruments have excellent quality and economical advantage in the long run. Anyhow, I like surgical curettes with 2-2.5 mm diameter of any brand.

11
Should we curette out the socket aggressively after an extraction? ★★

Is it necessary to clean out the extraction socket with the surgical curette after an extraction? Recent trend states that remaining periodontal ligament can help with recovery and therefore need not be removed. But you need to completely remove the dental follicle that used to encircle the impacted crown. If you want to keep the socket clean, I recommend you to irrigate the site and the surrounding with sterile saline. It is especially important to rinse with sterile saline if you sectioned the tooth or if there was infection around the third molar.

I mainly use the surgical curette to release the gingiva from the coronal crown for a vertically impacted tooth and to remove soft tissue that encircle the crown after the extraction.

I sometimes hear complaints from the new dentists that they cannot put force on the surgical curette because it has a small handle. Do you think a dental manufacturing company did not know that? The reason for the small handle in the surgical curette is so that you don't use too much force. Sure, I have seen curettes with thicker handles, but curettes with thin handles are made to not put much force on the instrument.

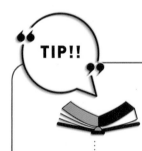

TIP!!

My ESSE Implant Tray

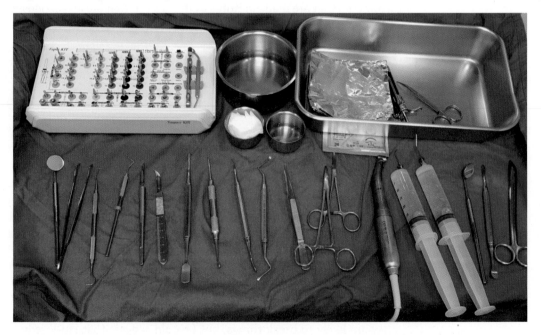

This is my implant tray. There is not much difference compared to my extraction tray other than this tray having assistant's instruments.

Anesthesia for the Third Molar Removal ★★

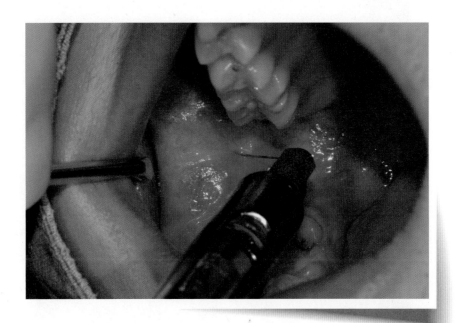

I debated a lot whether to include a chapter on anesthesia. Because those who read the book or those who attend my seminars for third molar extraction would have given enough anesthesia in their lives. However, if you cannot anesthetize the area sufficiently, it is hard to focus on third molar extraction. When I host live-surgery seminars, I have a participant give anesthesia, and one of the hardest things is when the patient complains about pain during the extraction. One needs to focus on tooth sectioning, bone troughing, positioning of elevators and forceps, controlling the force, etc.; yet, when a patient complains of pain, we have to stop what we are doing, and we lose flow of the treatment.

Even though I have habit of starting the extraction right after delivering anesthesia, I rarely have patient complaining of pain during the treatment. My average extraction time is 2~3 minutes, and patients are anesthetized during then. Maybe there is 1~2 out of 100 patients that I have to give additional anesthesia during the treatment. Sometimes, I make a bet with my staff members about this, but there is maybe one out of 200 third molar extraction cases where a patient complains of pain. It is not to boast that I am good at delivering anesthesia. It is just that, as a dentist who does a lot of third molar extractions, I get good results without complications... let's find out the difference.

01
Dr. Kim's anesthesia instruments for third molar removal ★

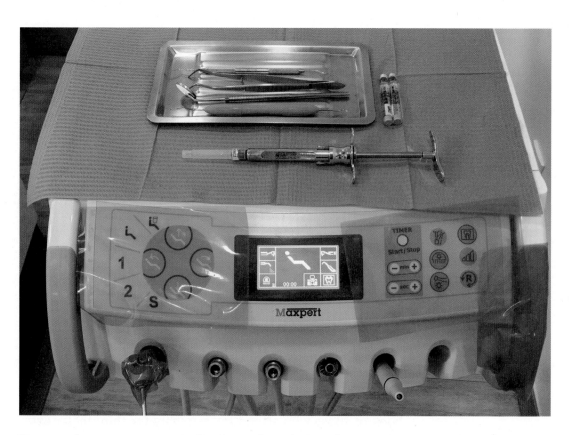

These are basic instruments for local anesthesia before the extraction: a mouth mirror, cotton pliers, explorer, and scaler. The scaler is for removing the calculus around a third molar and nearby teeth. I think scaling teeth is the best antiseptic method for third molar extraction. Whatever antiseptic medication you use, it is impossible to kill all bacteria in the mouth. Therefore, it is most important to clean the area physically. Often times, patients come due to inflammation around the tooth, so it is important to clean around the third molar. In fact, if you scratch around third molar and second molar with an explorer, often times, you can see heavy plaque or even calculus. If the plaque/calculus enter the extraction socket, they can cause inflammation, so it is recommended to remove them.

Remember. It is impossible to sterilize the mouth, but you can clean the extraction site mechanically and physically. You cannot kill all oral bacteria; in fact, you should not. You can only reduce the bacterial load.

Wait!

Debates regarding the third molar extraction #1

What to use to clean "the" mouth?

There are various opinions on whether it is necessary to clean the mouth before extraction. So many dentists and dental hospitals have their own opinions. I found out that most widely used antiseptics are <Potadine, H_2O_2, Chlorhexidine>. I don't think using Potadine has actual antiseptic effect other than making patients feel better. Potadine is an extra-oral antiseptic to clean the facial skin where sterile towel drape cannot cover, and you have to wait 30 minutes for it to dry after applying on the facial skin, so it is not very realistic. I only use Potadine for implant surgery. H_2O_2 may have antiseptic effect, but I am not sure if there is much meaning in using it. You can't kill all bacteria in the mouth. To reduce bacterial load, Chlorhexidine is used most commonly. However, I normally don't use Chlorhexidine other than for putting gauze after extraction, because it is troublesome.

If you need to clean intraoral area before an extraction, I would highly recommend that you have a scaler ready to use. Prior to implant surgery, I ask my hygienist to do prophylaxis and remove as much plaques as possible. Killing all intraoral bacteria is not possible and should not be done. More than anything, use a scaler to clean the surgical area so that bacteria-ridden plaques don't get into the extraction socket and the surgical area.

I rarely have patients getting inflammation after extraction, and I give a big credit to using

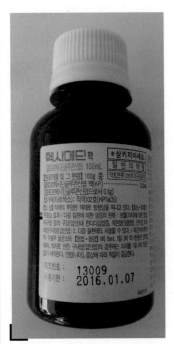
Chlorhexidine, selling in Korea.

the scaler. If you are extracting third molar or performing oral surgery, it is important to keep the nearby tooth physically clean.

One of my colleagues at a seminar told me to emphasize this part. Sometimes he sees patients who have a lot of plaque in their mouth, yet they decline to get teeth scaling and only want to get extraction. If you meet a patient like that, I recommend that you have the patient read the following letter.

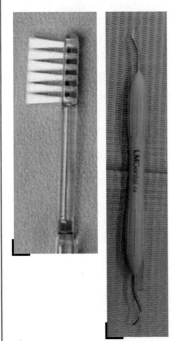

Dear patients who need third molar extraction,

If you fall down and get a thorn stuck in your arm, would you only take out the thorn?
Would you not remove the dirt around the thorn, clean out the area, then remove the thorn in order for the wound to heal well? As much as it is important to extract a third molar, it is also important to clean the area. It would be wise to take your third molar extraction as an opportunity to start getting teeth cleaning and improving oral hygiene at home.

02
Dr. Kim's dressing set ★

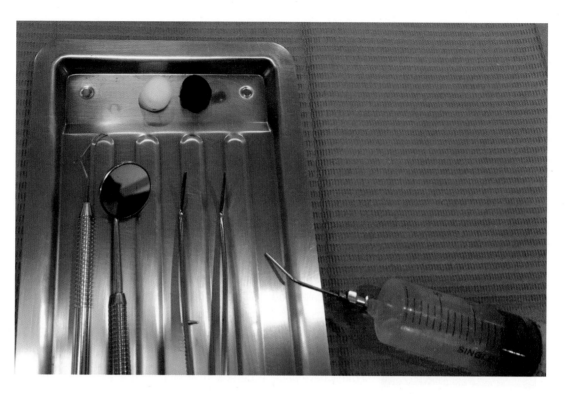

This is my dressing set. Just like other South Korean dentists, I use hydrogen peroxide (H_2O_2) and Potadine (Povidone Iodine Solution). To be honest, Potadine gauze is just for show. Potadine is an antiseptic for external skin, and the solution is effective as it dries and releases Iodine over a period of time, so it is not much effective inside the mouth. To be effective in reducing bacteria, it would be wiser to physically remove plaque with gauze. If you want to use it, it would be suitable to apply Potadine on the facial skin before extraction or implant surgery.

But sterile saline solution is very important. Not before extraction, but during or after extraction, it is very essential to wash away any debris or pus. Here, sterile saline solution is effective as a physical mechanism, rather than as a chemical mechanism.

Remember... The best method to reduce the number of bacteria in the mouth is to rinse the socket with a sufficient amount of sterile saline solution.

Gossip

When I visited an OMS department at a dental hospital in a foreign country, I saw them irrigating the site with Potadine diluted with sterile saline solution. I am not sure if mixing the solution makes the irrigation more effective, but I can understand the intention. Anyhow, I have hope that it may work, and out of habit, I have been using the mixed solution as my irrigant.

03
Which needle to use? ★

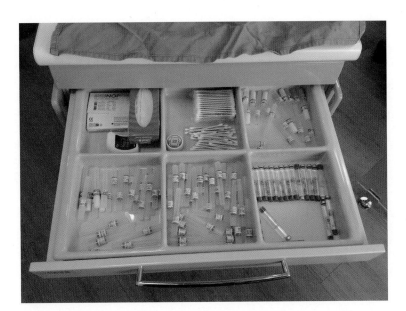

In the top drawer in the mobile cart, there are various needles and lidocaine. Note that there are plenty of needles in case I need to get a new one.

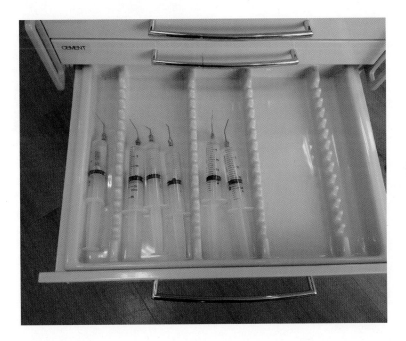

In the mobile cart, there are a plenty of 30 cc irrigation syringes that are sterilized to be used by my assistants. I would like to sterilize these syringes and put them in the extraction set just like in implant surgery, but due to very low extraction fee in my country, it is unrealistic. But, for tips, I use single use tips or autoclaved metal tips.

04
My go-to needle ★

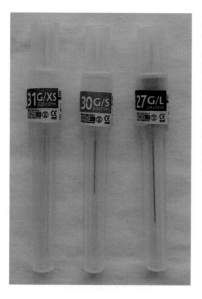

My dental office has many types of needles. I currently prefer to use the 30-gauge 25 mm long needle. When I was a new dentist, just like how I learned in school, I used the 27-gauge long needle for giving blocks, so I can get a feel while delivering anesthesia. For infiltration, I used the 30-gauge short needle to reduce pain. But, in order to perform as many third molar extraction as possible, it is very efficient to use one needle. For my ESSE, I only use the 30-gauge long needle. It is good to know how to properly use many instruments, but it is also good to use familiar instruments in familiar ways.

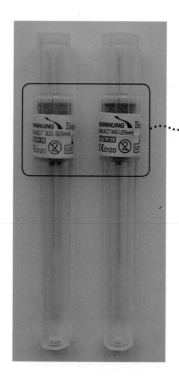

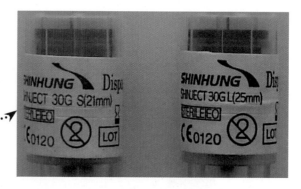

The needle on the right side is the 30-gauge 25 mm needle that I use most often. If the needle gets bent or broken after delivering a block, then I switch to the 30-gauge short needle for delivering infiltration. If you use a thin 30-gauge needle, there are less pain and damage to the tissue. I like to give enough infiltration on the lingual side, so I do not use thick 27-gauge needle for the fear of lingual nerve damage.

05
How I use the needle

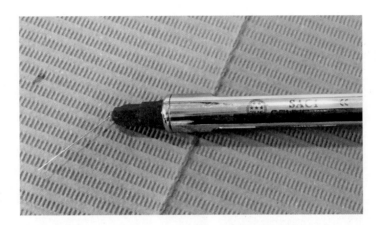

Due to my back pain, and out of habit, I like to bend the needle like the above and insert the needle as perpendicularly as possible in the area that is superior and frontal to the mandibular foramen. Also, I do not aspirate the needle. Rather, I insert the needle as if delivering infiltration. That is because I think you can cause damage to the nearby tissue by aspirating. This is just my thought solely based on my experience. Therefore, I encourage you to deliver anesthesia just as you have been doing. I am just writing down my style of delivering anesthesia because other dentists have asked me during their visits.

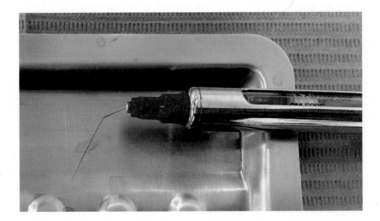

If contact angle is difficult when anesthetizing mandibular lingual surface or maxillary palatal surface, I bend the needle one more time and insert the needle as perpendicular as possible. Like I mentioned above, this is my style, and you don't have to do it this way. But if you are using a long thin needle like me, be careful that the needle does not break and be buried in the soft tissue. If you bend the needle, the needle usually enters the tissue very perpendicular, and it is very rare to go deep in the tissue. Even if needle breaks, it is easy to remove the broken part with the cotton pliers.

06
How I deliver inferior alveolar nerve block anesthesia ★★

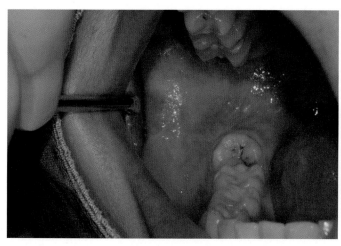 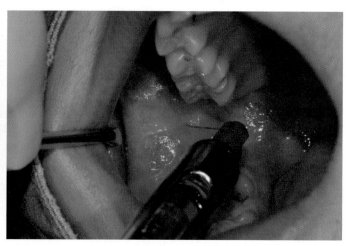

■ This is how I deliver mandibular nerve block. I usually do not use finger; I use mirror. I use a mirror to press hard on the anterior border of ramus, instead of feeling the area with finger, and I estimate the soft tissue thickness to be 1 cm, and I place needle in front of the mandibular foramen.

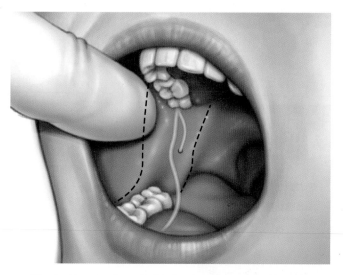

■ Standard travel pathway for inferior alveolar nerve and lingual nerve.

I try to minimize giving block anesthesia. I like to use one carpule to give an accurate anesthesia. To be honest, I think most third molar extraction can be done with an infiltration. But because delivering block anesthesia ($5) compensates better than delivering infiltration anesthesia ($1.50), and for unexpected circumstances, I deliver block anesthesia. But I never use the thick 27-gauge (about 0.4mm) needle as I believe using it to contact the bone and to aspirate can cause too much tissue damage. I do 10,000s of third molar extractions, and I think I would have gotten lingual nerve damage or similar side effects if I deliver anesthesia like that. I know this is a controversial issue. As I mentioned before, I think you should deliver anesthesia in your own style. Like I said, I wrote this section only because other dentists have asked me about my technique.

Even for one in 10,000 chances, I would like to avoid any complication. This is why I only use only 1 carpule with 30-gauge (about 0.3 mm) long needle.

But I do not force using my injection technique to other dentists. If you are a dentist, you should have your own injection technique. As long as you have great anesthesia effect and no side effect, I think that's fine.

07
Anatomical differences are common… You can cause tissue damage ★

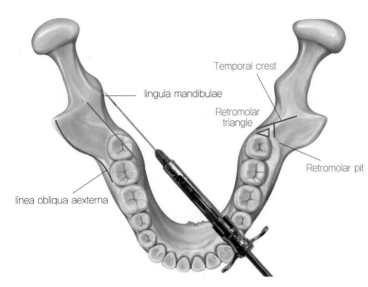

This illustration shows the pathway of the needle in the mandible. The angle of the syringe is similar to the angle of the inner surface of the mandible.

According to the research by Moris et al, out of 44 cadavers, they placed the needle like in traditional inferior alveolar nerve block anesthesia, and while keeping the needle in place, they performed dissection around the insertion area, and they measured the distance between the needle and the lingual nerve/lingula, as well as measuring the width of lingual nerve/inferior alveolar nerve. They measured that the distance between the needle and the lingual nerve is 0.73 +- 0.70 mm (0.00-3.00 mm). Out of 44 simulation cases, the needle went through the lingual nerve in 2 cases (4.5%), and needle traveled within 0.1mm of the lingual nerve in 7 cases (16%). Also, in this research, the average diameter of the lingual nerve near the lingula was 3.42 +- 0.38 mm (1.95-4.15 mm), and the average diameter of the inferior alveolar nerve is 2.53 +- 0.29 mm (1.95-3.25 mm).

<Moris CD, Rasmussen J et al. J Oral Maxillofac Surg 2010;68:2833-2836>

According to the research by Stacy et al, there is 78% chance of getting barbed tip as a result of needle bending during an inferior alveolar nerve block anesthesia (1994). More than 2/3 of barbed tips show "Outward facing barb," and this barbed tip can cause big physical damage to the nerve when being removed after delivering block anesthesia.

<Stacy GC, Hajjar G et al. Oral Surg Oral Med Oral Pathol 1994 Jun;77(6):585-8>

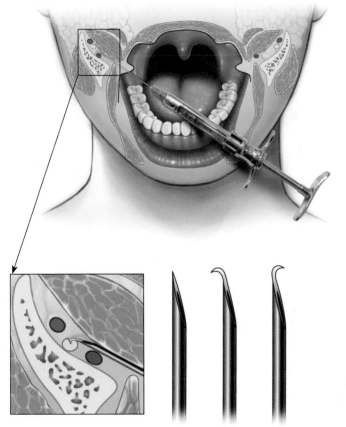

This illustration shows that there can be damage to inner structures in the mandible during block anesthesia.

I did my best not to reference too many research papers in this book, but I read and referenced above papers after reading an article by Dr. Sang-hoon Cho at the Good Jaw Dental Clinic in Ulsan, South Korea.

When you practice dentistry for a while, you forget all anatomical knowledge that you learned in dental school. Maybe it is just me... So, whenever I feel like I've fallen into mannerism, I open up an anatomy textbook. We learned to inject the needle 1cm above the occlusal plane in the anterior portion of the ramus of mandible, coming from the opposing first molar. And in order to anesthetize the lingual nerve or the long buccal nerve, we were told to move the needle as it is already inserted.

But we have to remember two things.

First is that the insertion area has many important anatomical structures such as mandibular nerve and other nerves, artery, and vein. Also, there are many anatomical variations.

Second is that depending on the angle of the mandible, the needle cannot contact the periosteum from the insertion angle. Any dentist would have this experience. In order to contact the bone with the needle, one inserts the needle several times or moves the needle while inserted. This is very dangerous in my opinion.

08
Deliver sufficient local infiltration anesthesia to the lingual surface ★★★

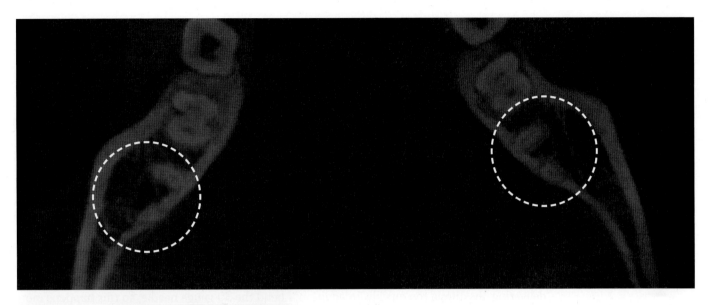

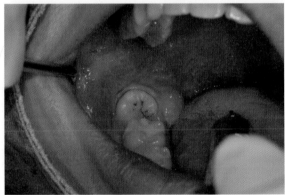

For third molar extractions, you need to deliver enough local infiltration anesthesia to the lingual surface.

Every dentist has experienced difficulty anesthetizing mandibular second molars. I have extracted thousands of third molars as well as treating mandibular second molars, but I rarely have had difficulty achieving profound anesthesia. I think it is because I give enough anesthesia on the lingual surface. Mandibular second molar is hard to get numb, even if you give enough anesthesia on the lingual surface. The reason is that up to a mandibular second molar, teeth are surrounded by thick cortical bone on both buccal and lingual surfaces, and it is hard for local anesthetic to reach the apical foramen. On the other hand, let's take a look at the wisdom teeth in white circles in the photo above. Third molar is usually located near the lingual cortical bone because there is not enough space for its roots. Also, cortical bone on the lingual side is thinner than that on the buccal side. As I mentioned in the chapter for radiographic interpretation, research paper shows that 30% of wisdom teeth have roots that pass through the mandibular lingual cortical bone. Therefore, it is essential to give enough local infiltration anesthesia on the lingual surface to achieve painless third molar extractions.

I have already discussed in the earlier chapter about third molar roots being located within the lingual cortical bone, how it looks like on the panoramic radiograph, and what to watch out for when tackling these cases (see the figures above). So I will pass on the details here. Some dentists have told me that the reason they do not give sufficient local infiltration anesthesia on the lingual surface is due to the fear of lingual nerve damage. I would like to tell them to trust my experience. I have never had a single lingual nerve damage, even though I have extracted tons of third molars. However, you have to use a thin needle for lingual local infiltration. This will minimize the damage even if you happen to inject near the lingual nerve. Considering the thickness of the lingual nerve (3~4 mm), you don't need to worry about the 30-gauge needle (0.3 mm) doing much damage.

09
When you put too much force… ★

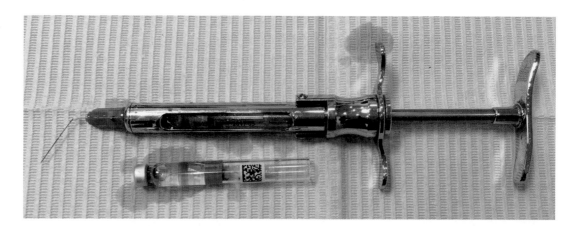

I broke two carpules in a row while delivering anesthesia. I am not sure if I'm too strong or if these carpules are defective… This might be a rare occurrence for others, but I experience this situation quite often. Since I have a very short time to do many extractions, I developed a habit of delivering anesthesia too quickly. In addition, I bend the 30-gauge needle, so this happens more often.

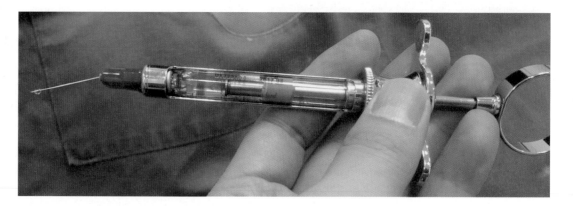

I think I push the syringe harder than other dentists do. I break anesthetic carpules sometimes, but I even puncture the rubber inside it sometimes (see the photo above). When I used to work with other dentists, I could not always get the instruments set up that I like, so I would get into those situations quite often using other dentists' syringes.

I'm not telling you these things to copy what I do, but to illustrate that I put a lot of force when delivering local infiltration anesthesia. Also, I used to remove the hook from my syringes. Nowadays, I feel lazy and just purchase syringes that do not have the hook, so that it is impossible to aspirate. I will tell you why in the next page…

10
Metal syringe that I use-note that the hook is removed ★

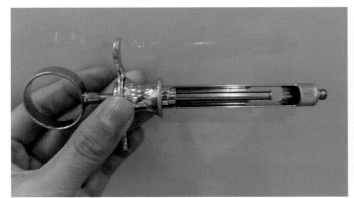 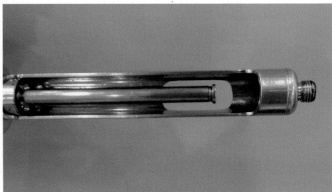

Whether tooth is in the maxillary or mandibular arch or impacted, my philosophy is to start extraction right after delivering anesthesia. Because I have too many patients, I have to use the same instruments and the same extraction trays for all patients.

I do not aspirate when using the 30-gauge thin needle. For the past 20 years of practicing dentistry, I don't think I ever aspirated except when I was in school, and I never had a problem. I think that moving the needle around near mandibular foramen can rather cause nerve damage.

Reason I use aspiration syringes with a finger loop even though I do not aspirate is because I can push the back side of the finger loop to forcefully deliver anesthesia. If you have large hands like me, you will understand. But if you use syringe with the hook, the rubber may get stuck or even get punctured, causing trouble. So I like to remove the hook like in the photo above.

I think it is best to deliver anesthesia in the way that is the most familiar to you, but just keep in mind this is how I do mine.

Anyhow, I believe moving around a thick 27-gauge needle within the tissue and delivering anesthetic can cause tissue damage, and the more often you do it, there is higher chance of causing nerve damage.

Caution

I know my anesthesia technique may be controversial. So I never force others to do the same. Every dentist should have his or her own technique. So please understand and regard my technique as a reference.

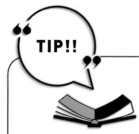

TIP!!

If you cannot achieve profound anesthesia during third molar extraction?

 Tip 1

If it is a vertically impacted tooth, you can place an elevator in the buccal surface to make a room, then perform PDL injection using the 30-gauge thin needle. This is as if you are delivering PDL anesthesia when you are having difficulty numbing a mandibular second molar for endodontic treatment. Since the third molar will be extracted, you don't need to worry about causing trauma to the periodontal ligament. So place an elevator on the buccal surface and deliver anesthesia to achieve profound anesthesia.

 Tip 2

Just like in endodontic treatment, deliver pulpal anesthesia. When you section an impacted tooth, patient may complain of cold pain. As in endodontic treatment, you make a hole to the pulp chamber, and deliver anesthesia to the pulp. Normally, it is easy to anesthetize periodontal ligament, but pulp may not be anesthetized, if anesthetic does not reach the root surface. If patient is in pain even after delivering sufficient amount of anesthetic around the third molar and the periodontal ligament, I suggest delivering pulpal anesthesia. Then, you can continue on with your extraction.

 Tip 3

<Target the cervical area>. You cannot make a hole on the cervical area during endodontic treatment, but it does not matter in third molar extraction. The cervical area is very close to the pulp, so even with simple cutting, pulp can be reached. Even for a horizontally impacted tooth, target the distal cervical area.

11
Delivering pulpal anesthesia ★★

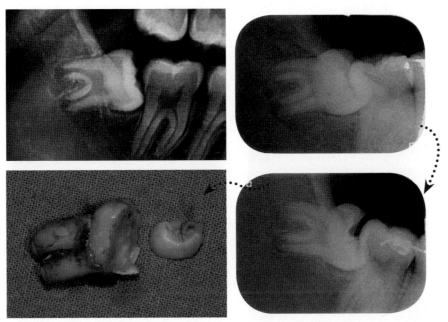

A 16 yo male patient was referred for third molar extraction while on braces. I was sectioning the mesial crown, and he complained of pain. Additional anesthesia was ineffective, so I performed disto-cervical cutting, and delivered pulpal anesthesia. Because the patient is young and had large pulp chamber, slight cutting of distal cervical surface allowed easy access to the pulp chamber.

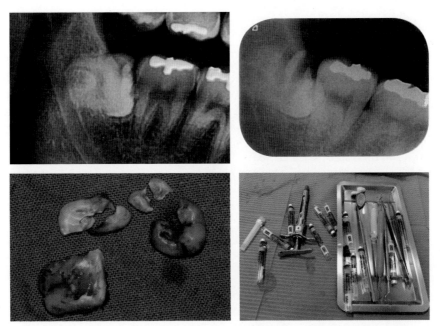

I could not achieve profound anesthesia on this 27 yo male patient, so it was hard to continue on sectioning mesial surface of the crown. After trying different anesthesia techniques, I ultimately did disto-cervical cutting and delivered pulpal anesthesia, just like the case above. I took a photo to commemorate using the greatest number of needles (3) and lidocaine carpules (13) in recent few years.

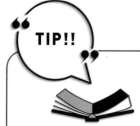

TIP!!

Inferior alveolar nerve block and lingual nerve damage

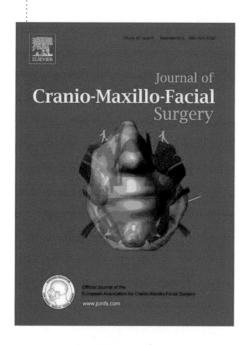

In the article <Clinical Investigation into the Incidence of Damage to the Lingual Nerve Caused by Local Anaesthesia> in the Journal of Craniomaxillofacial Surgery published in 1994, they administered mandibular block to 12,104 patients. 72.4% of patients received crown prep and/or operative treatments, 27.13% received periodontal treatments, and the remaining 0.3% received other dental treatments. Only 18 patients (0.15%) experienced abnormal sensation on the tongue, and 17 of these patients recovered completely within 6 months. Only one patient (0.008%) had persistent slight abnormal sensation in the tongue after a year. Likewise, you cannot completely eliminate the possibility of lingual nerve damage in the block anesthesia, but you do not have to worry too much about it. -Dr. Jae-wook Lee.

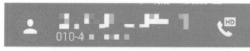

The left figure shows a text message that I received from my senior colleague who has 20 years of clinical experience.

The above research paper said it is very unlikely to cause nerve damage after mandibular nerve block, but you still have to be careful as you see in this text message. Even though it is 1 in 10,000 chances, this can happen to a dentist like me who does tons of extractions. So, in order to minimize tissue damage during block anesthesia, I use thin 30-gauge needle.

Senior :
Hey, Young-sam. Sorry for contacting you out of the blue. I recently delivered mandibular nerve block to do a crown prep, and the patient stated that he has no sensation on his tongue and his lip. I never had this happen before. Can you suggest any treatment please?

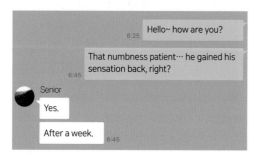

Towards the end of finishing this book, I asked my senior colleague how that patient is doing, and she told me the patient recovered his senses completely.

Incision and Suture for Third Molar Extraction

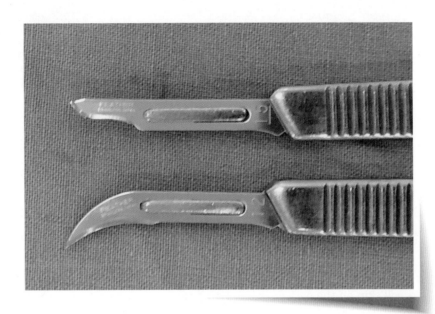

I normally use the No. 12 blade and the No. 15 blade. During an implant surgery, to perform delicate incision, I use the No. 15c blade, but that is not the case for the extraction. I use the No. 15 blade for the extraction. For implant surgery, I prepare both blades (#12 and #15c). To incise up to the distal surface of the tooth adjacent to the surgical site, I use the No. 12 blade. During a third molar extraction, if the third molar is not erupted and gingiva covers over 2nd molar's distal surface, I use the No. 12 blade.

For your reference, the cost for the blades are: (each box has 100 blades) the No. 15, No. 12, and No. 112 are 22,000 won ($22) per box; 220 won ($22 cents) per blade, the No. 15c is 54,000 won ($54) per box; 540 won (54 cents) per blade. It is not that expensive, but I don't think you need to use more expensive blades.

Since the topic of incision and suture is already mentioned in so many other books and lectures, I will just briefly mention my opinion according to my ESSE philosophy.

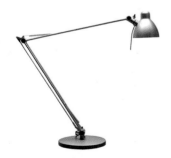

01
Dr. Kim's blade of choice

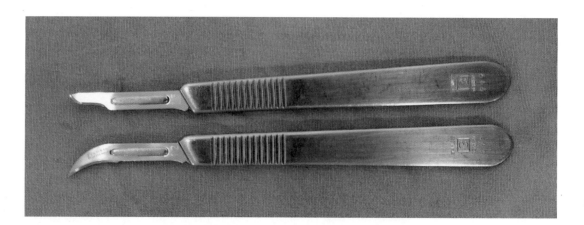

If a third molar is not visible at all in the mouth, in order to make a clean incision to the distal surface of #7, I use the No. 12 blade. For all other cases, I usually use the No. 15 blade. Also, if you have to make a vertical incision, I recommend the No. 15 blade. For a third molar extraction, I normally use just one blade. This is not because I'm trying to save the cost of the blades, but because I do not make that many incisions. But if you're a new dentist, use what you like to use.

I will skip on the basic incision, flap design, and suture procedure, as many other text- books already covered the topic. But I want to emphasize that you need to incise to the periosteum for third molar extraction. Maybe you should think that you only need to cut to the periosteum, as mucosa would be cut along with it. Incision and suture for third molar extraction need to be made to the muco-periosteum.

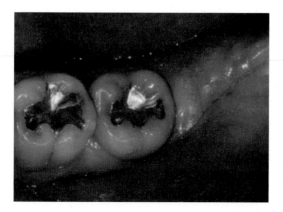

This is when I normally use the No. 12 blade. You can see that gingiva covers over the im-pacted third molar up to the distal surface of #7.

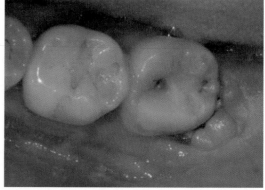

This is when I normally use the No. 15 blade. You can visualize a part of the third molar. Of-ten, even if there is more gingival coverage, I would use the No. 15 blade if I need to make a vertical incision.

02
Dr. Kim's incision ★★

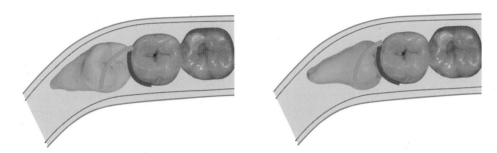

When the crown is not visible at all, I use the No. 12 blade to make a clean incision to the distal surface of #7(see the Green line). Red line usually gets incised upon reflecting gum tissue, but I recommend new dentists to use the No. 12 blade to make incision along the Red line. I will talk about extending the incision line to the mesial surface in the next page.

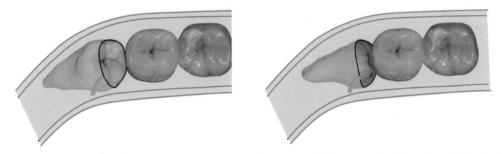

If you can see less than half of the crown, I use the No. 15 blade instead of the No. 12 blade. With the No. 15 blade, I think about how I would have made an incision if I could not see the tooth at all. If you extend the Green line (towards lingual surface), incision line looks similar to the case when the third molar is not visible at all.

The No. 12 blade has an irregular cutting surface, so it feels unstable using it at times. The No. 15 blade is much more comfortable to use to make a vertical incision, if necessary. But if I have to use just one blade for an extraction, it would be the No. 12 blade.

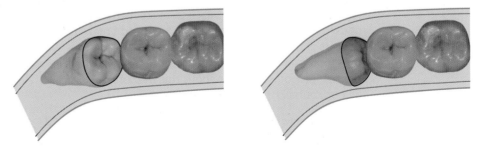

If you can see more than half of the crown, I do not make an incision. In rare cases, when an extraction is complicated, I make an incision and reflect flaps to gain a wide visual field. I try to minimize making the incision, and it is my own philosophy.

03
Dr. Kim's philosophy on making an incision <1> ★★★

It is better to make an incision than to have torn tissue

For a new dentist, what is more important than an easy, speedy extraction is whether you can extract the tooth or not. So it is important for beginners to make a wide incision and surgical flap when necessary. 'Minimal incision' is to make an effort to minimize incision and flap when you can afford to do so. For new dentists, it is important to obtain skills to make clean incisions/flap, as this skill is important in implant surgery as well. Until that skill is achieved, I recommend practicing making a wide incision and surgical flap like oral surgery residents do.

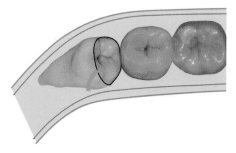

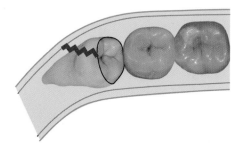

━My favorite incision technique is to make a small buccal incision like the Green line. I usually use the No. 15 blade. If I can see the crown, I don't have to use the No. 12 blade to make an incision close to the distal surface of #7, so I use the No. 15 blade. I also recommend the No. 15 blade to make a vertical incision.

━I normally do not make an incision, but if you don't make an incision, the lingual gingiva can get torn like the Purple line. This is the area that I don't want it torn. The most important philosophy in making an incision is that it is better to incise than to get torn tissue. According to my experience, even though tissue is not torn, if the gingiva or soft tissue gets too much tension and gets damaged during an extraction, there is more post op pain and swelling than when a clean incision is made. Also, there is a risk of lingual nerve damage when the lingual gingiva is torn, so one needs to be very careful.

When I was a new dentist, I used to make many incisions. I learned to make incisions. But once I got used to doing more extractions, I noticed I make less incisions. But what I have realized over the years is that if you do not incise at all, you may get torn tissue in an unwanted area, or even if not torn, you can cause trauma to the tissue beyond its elasticity. Therefore, I started making minimal incision. I will talk about this in more detail in the later chapters (Extraction of vertical and horizontal impacted 3rd molars).

Let's imagine which would be more traumatic – making a 1 cm incision in the middle of the gingiva and suturing it versus stretching the gingiva by 2 cm and putting it back. Making an incision will cause minimal trauma limited to the incised area, but stretching the tissue by 1 cm would cause damage to the whole tissue.

It is better to make incision than to get a torn tissue!!

When I extract a tooth, often times my staff comment that I extract a tooth like giving birth to a child. Then I regret that I incised the tissue too little. I try to minimize making an incision, but it is never good to go beyond the elastic limit of gingival tissue. When you make an incision, the incised tissue heals. But it is never good to stretch or retract the tissue too much because your incision was too small. I will make a good example here. Some of you may have heard of incision in the perineal region for child birth.

The Perineum: the area between the anus and the vulva

Have you heard of perineotomy?

Perineotomy is performed to make a surgical incision of the perineum by 3~4 cm after visualizing 3~4 cm of a newborn's head, to quickly enlarge the opening for the baby to pass through. Many OB-GYNs recommend performing perineotomy before childbirth. Why? Because it is better to make incision than to get torn tissue. It is to prevent laceration in an unwanted area and damage to the urethra, rectum, anus, or anal sphincter. Of course, women are designed to give birth naturally without having perineotomy, so there is a recent trend among expectant mothers not receiving perineotomy. In fact, the perineum very elastic, and does not need to be incised if given enough time to stretch. Its muscle has great elasticity.

Nevertheless, many OB-GYNs recommend perineotomy. On the other hand, periodontium is not created for child birth. Periodontium is made to strongly encase a tooth. Therefore, you need to make an incision not only for achieving a good visual field, but also for letting the third molar come out through the gingiva. If you don't incise sufficiently, you may get torn tissue in an unwanted area, and it could be on the lingual surface. We should always be careful around the lingual surface, so it is helpful to secure enough space for the tooth to come out on the buccal surface.

When I use this example in a lecture, some people say I'm too eccentric. But in a lecture, I think it's very important to listen and understand right away. Therefore, I like to use a shocking example.

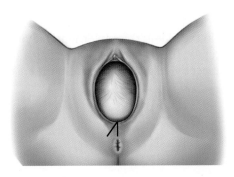

■ What is perineotomy?

It is to make an incision in the perineum like in the photo. Incision could be in the center or it could be sideway towards inside or outside. After child birth, suture is placed.

04
Extending the incision line to the mesial surface ★★★

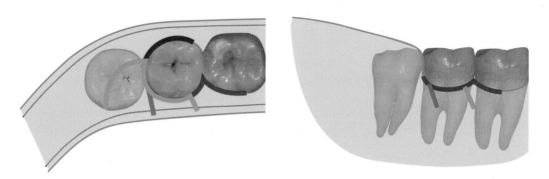

When you don't see the crown at all or when the third molar is buried deep vertically, I like to extend my incision to the distal surface of 2nd molars using the No. 12 blade. I try not to extend incision to the mesial surface of the 2nd molars. But on very busy days or when the third molar is located buccally and I need a wider visual field, I extend the incision line to the mesial surface of 2ND molars and create a flap.

There are 3 ways to extend incision line to the mesial surface:

- **Blue line:** Making a vertical incision at the distal surface of the 2nd molars

- **Green line:** Making a vertical incision at the mesial surface of the 2nd molars

- **Red line:** Extending incision into the interdental papilla between the 1st and 2nd molars

I often make a vertical incision at the mesial surface of 2nd molars like in the Green line. But this method could be tricky for the beginners. Also, it is time consuming to suture a vertical incision, and it is not easy especially if you are using a large size needle like I do. Though I am used to placing a suture this way, I do not insist on recommending this method to the new dentists. On the other hand, there are some other dentists who do not place sutures, and their reason is to prevent post-operative swelling.

But, sometimes, because the No. 12 blade is not useful for making a vertical incision, I like to extend my incision like in the Red line. If you are using a large size needle like me, it is easier to suture interdental papilla than to suture a vertical incision. Interdental papilla can be reflected using a periosteal elevator, without using a blade. I always like to place a suture here, but some dentists like to leave the flap alone to prevent hematoma. I suggest that you try these different incision methods and choose the best method based on your experience.

Some people incise and reflect the lingual surface of 2nd molars, but I never do it. For me, the lingual surface is like the Atlantic Ocean in the European Middle Age. I would like to keep my fear of the lingual surface as an unknown world. Even though there might be gold beyond the ocean, I would like to stay in the Mediterranean Sea. But, if you gain some confidence, you can try reflecting the lingual gingiva. The real problem is getting a torn tissue. It is not a big problem to make an incision and reflect the lingual gingiva from the crestal ridge.

05
Dr. Kim's philosophy on making an incision <2> ★★★

Never mess with the lingual surface

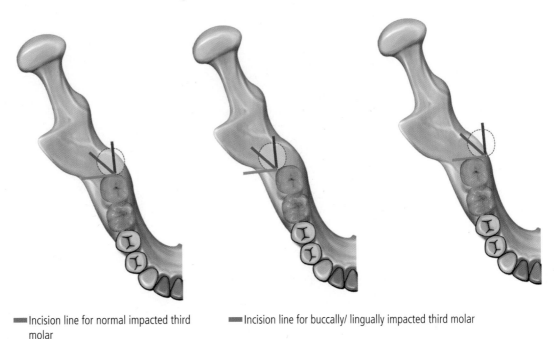

━━Incision line for normal impacted third molar

━━Incision line for buccally/ lingually impacted third molar

To perform a safe third molar extraction, I find it most important to extend incision buccally. In the picture above, I like to incise along the Green line (rather than along the Red line). It would be better to incise along the Blue line, but it may be dangerous due to the unpredictable nature of the lingual nerve. It is especially dangerous if the third molar is located deep distally or lingually.

Some new dentists attempt to incise along the distal surface of the third molar, and their blade ends up dropping deep in the tissue. The distal area to the third molar is not to be trusted.

Just like how Europeans in the Middle Age used to think that there was a cliff beyond the Atlantic Ocean, lingual surface should be that cliff. The reason I have not had any lingual nerve damage is because I never messed with the lingual surface during extraction.

Using a mirror or finger, you have to retract cheek and tissues buccally as much as possible then make an incision on top of the bone. Be sure to remember this. Incision is to be made as much buccally as possible on the periosteum, as you are retracting the tissue in the buccal direction.

06
Dr. Kim's philosophy on making an incision <3> ★★

Incise from the buccal surface as much as you can

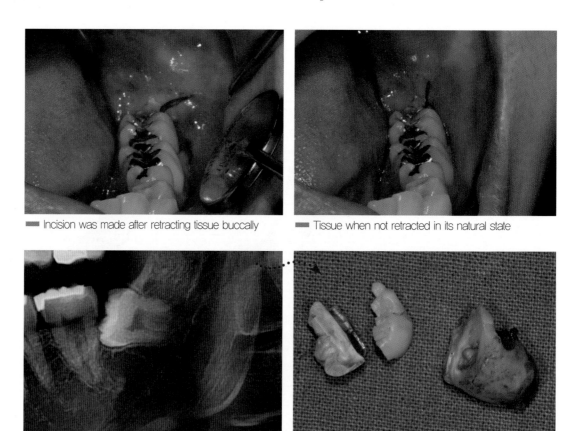

◼ Incision was made after retracting tissue buccally

◼ Tissue when not retracted in its natural state

◼ This patient's Panoramic radiograph

◼ Extracted tooth

This incision line was made to extract a fully impacted tooth. When you make an incision, you need to retract the tissue and make an incision on the mucoperiosteum and not on the movable tissue. As seen in the above photograph, even though one thinks the incision is made buccally, the incision line may go back to the lingual surface once you let go off the retraction.

Please remember this. Never incise on the lingual surface.

Incision must be made on the buccal surface, after retracting the buccal tissue, on the hard periosteum. Soft tissue incision must be extended to where it is connected to the hard tissue. The purpose of the incision is to incise on the periosteum on top of the bone.

07
Pathway of the lingual nerve

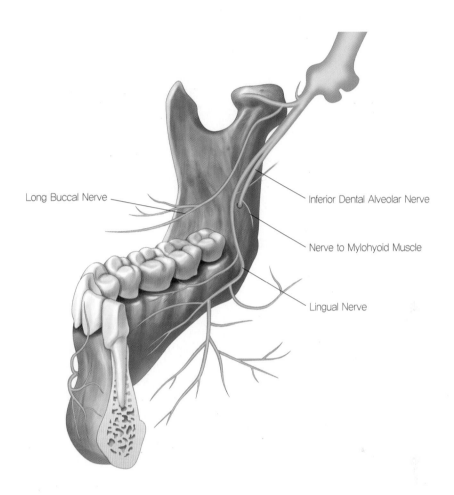

Long Buccal Nerve

Inferior Dental Alveolar Nerve

Nerve to Mylohyoid Muscle

Lingual Nerve

Nerves around mandible and lingual nerve pathway

Because the lingual nerve is highly variable, it can get damaged at any time. Usually, dentists are very careful around the inferior alveolar nerve during an extraction, but the inferior alveolar nerve is not easy to damage. Rather, it is more common to damage the lingual nerve by a brief moment of inattention. So I never mess with the lingual surface.

I am yet to have any patient who experienced nerve damage even after extracting so many teeth. This is because I do my best not to make even one case that will make me sad.

08
The lingual nerve has very diverse pathways ★★

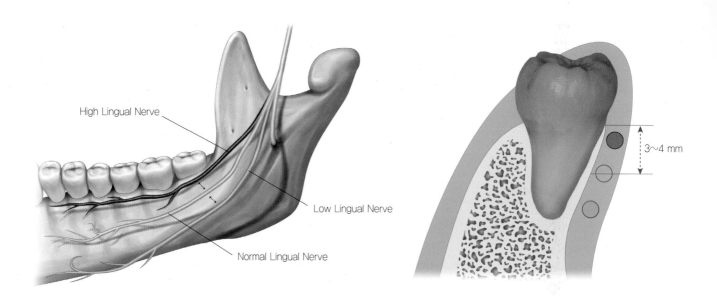

High Lingual Nerve

Low Lingual Nerve

Normal Lingual Nerve

3~4 mm

Clinically speaking, normal pathway of the lingual nerve is the Yellow Line. But the pathway can vary like the Green Line (nerve located inferior to the normal position) or like the Purple Line (nerve is very close to the third molar or the second molar crowns). I read articles to gain more anatomical knowledge, but the pathways are still observed to be varied greatly. It is probably because the lingual nerve travels through soft tissue, and there are various methods for research and evaluation. Still, I can make a conclusion that lingual nerve is generally located 3~4 mm near the lingual crest around the third molar. Most research paper says within 3mm, but some research papers report an average of 8 mm, so I wrote 3~4 mm. But this standard deviation is very large, and there is 7.5~17.6% chance that the lingual nerve is located above the lingual crest. Horizontally speaking, the lingual nerve is 2~3 mm away from the lingual crest, but 22~62% of the time, the nerve is touching the lingual crest. As I mentioned before, every research paper has different measurements and different standard deviation, so we just need to know the approximate outline. Just be sure to remember that the lingual nerve varies its courses quite a bit, therefore, you should never touch the lingual area of a third molar during extraction. According to the article by Behind et al., they studied 669 lingual nerve pathways among 430 fresh cadavers, they observed that 14.05% (94) of the time, the lingual nerve travels above the lingual crest; in one case, they observed a lingual nerve that travels along the retromolar pad (0.15%). Also, they observed lingual nerves that physically touch the lingual crest in 22.27% cases (149).

But there is good news - see the next page.

09
Incision pathway from the distal surface or near the lingual surface of third molar

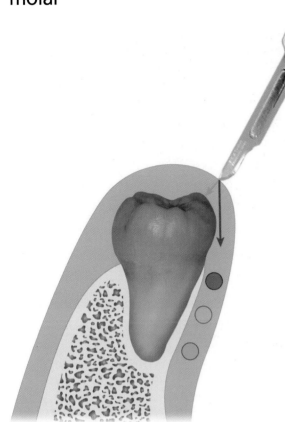

When you make an incision on the distal surface or near the lingual surface of a third molar, you need to angle your blade handle towards the lingual surface. Like shown above, you need to incise like the green arrow. If you incise like the red arrow, you may sink into a pit. There might be more severe undercut than the picture above, so you should never incise the distal surface or near the lingual surface of a third molar. If you suspect an undercut or you lack confidence, make an incision as much towards buccal as possible.

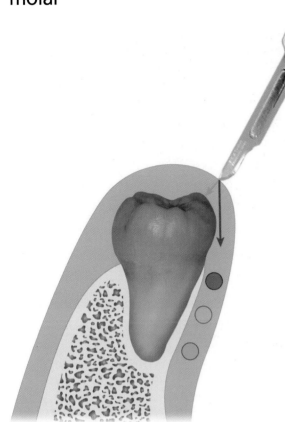

치과의사신문 | 제119호 2017년 4월 17일 월요일　　　**종합뉴스 3**

사랑니 발치 전 부작용 및 주의사항 설명 필요

대법원 "발치 후 감각 이상 신체적 특이점 있다면 치의 책임 없다"

사랑니 발치 후 혀가 마비됐더라도 보통 사람과 다른 환자의 신체적 특이점이 원인이라면 치과의사에게 손해배상 책임이 없다는 대법원 판결이 나왔다.

대법원 민사2부는 사랑니를 빼고 난 뒤 혀가 일부 마비된 박모(44) 씨가 치과의사 진모(63) 씨를 상대로 낸 소해배상 청구소송(2014다10113)에게 원고승소 판결한 원심을 깨고 최근 사건을 전주지법으로 돌려보냈다.

재판부는 "고도의 전문지식을 필요로 하는 의료행위는 의사의 주의의무 위반과 손해발생 사이에 인과관계가 있는지 여부를 밝혀내기 극히 어려운 특수성이 있다.

수술 도중 발생한 결과에 대해 개연성이 담보되지 않은 사정들을 가지고 막연하게 의사에게 무과실의 증명책임을 지우는 것은 허용되지 않는다"고 밝혔다.

그러면서 "박 씨의 장애가 발치를 위한 마취 과정에서 진 씨가 주사침을 설 신경 방향 쪽으로 잘못 찔렀기 때문에 발생했을 가능성도 있지만, 박 씨의 설 신경이 설측 골판에 밀착해 지나가는 등 그 해부학적 원인 때문에 발생했을 가능성도 있다"며 "해부학적 원인에 의한 불가항력적인 손상의 발생 가능성도 있는데 막연히 진 씨의 과실을 추정해 손해배상책임을 인정한 원심은 잘못이다"고 말했다.

박 씨는 2008년 5월 진 씨가 운영하는 치과에서 사랑니 발치 수술을 받고 열흘 뒤 혀가 마비되는 증상이 나타났다. 박 씨는 종합병원에서 신경이 손상됐다는 진단을 받자 "진 씨가 사랑니를 발치하는 과정에서 마취 주사침 등을 신경을 훼손시켰다"며 소송을 낸 바 있다.

1심에서 재판부는 "진 씨가 진료 상 주의의무를 다하지 못했다기보다는 박 씨의 혀 신경 위치가 남들과 달라 나타난 불가항력적인 합병증"이라며 "다만 의사로서 시술 시 일어날 수 있는 부작용을 환자에게 미리 설명했어야 하는데 진 씨는 이 의무를 위반했으므로 300만원을 배상하라"

며 원고일부승소 판결했다.

2심은 "박 씨의 신체적 특징이 사고의 원인이 됐다고 보기 어렵고, 혀 마비 증세가 사랑니 발치 시술 후 일반적으로 나타날 수 있는 합병증의 범위 내에 있는 것도 아니다"라며 "손해배상금액을 1,500여만원으로 대폭 올렸다.

한국의료분쟁조정중재원 관계자는 "사랑니는 매복 정도가 깊을수록 발치과정에서 주변조직에 손상을 줄 가능성이 높은데 사랑니 발치 전 부작용과 주의사항을 듣지 못했다면 자기결정권 침해에 따른 설명의무 위반 여부 등을 두고 다툴 수 있다"고 말했다.

구명회기자 nine@ddsnews.co.kr

A verdict from Korean Court of Justice in a Korean dental magazine.

The verdict is about how lingual nerve damage after third molar extractions could happen because of wide range of variations in the lingual nerve location in different individuals. Hence, if informed consent, which includes possible complications and risks, was fully explained before the surgery and the dentist made an attempt to prevent possible lingual nerve damage during the surgery, the dentist is not guilty, even if the patient ended up getting paresthesia after the extraction.

10
Is this the lingual nerve? ★

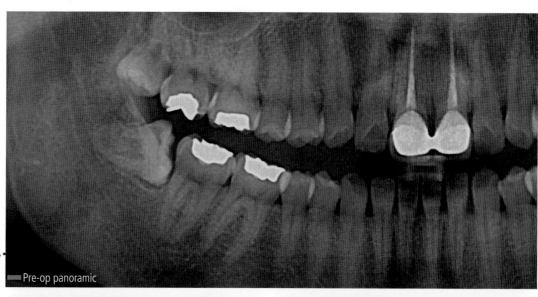
Pre-op panoramic

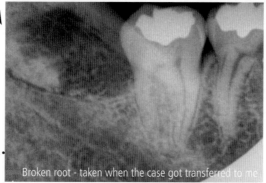
Broken root - taken when the case got transferred to me

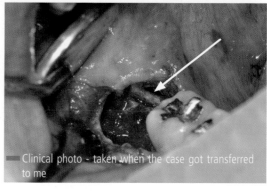
Clinical photo - taken when the case got transferred to me

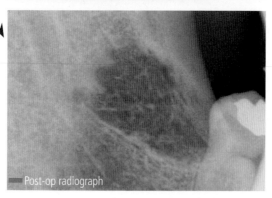
Post-op radiograph

I received an SOS from a resident who could not finish extracting a tooth because the patient was in severe pain. Panoramic radiograph shows a remaining root tip. Clinical intra-oral photo shows the incision line is towards the lingual surface, and the lingual nerve is exposed. Patient complained of severe pain when touched around the area. It is a great relief that the lingual nerve did not get cut along the incision line.

11
Accessory instruments ★★

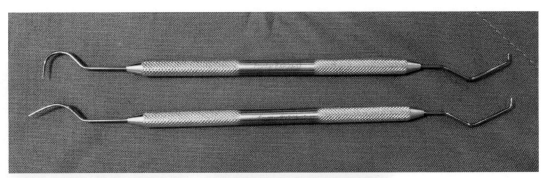

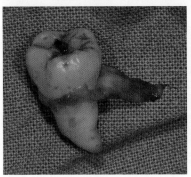 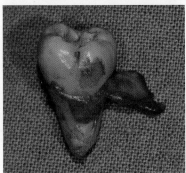

To cut the periodontal ligament around third molar, I recommend using an explorer instead of a blade. I recommend using a standard explorer after bending it (see video). I do not use an explorer much anymore, but I highly recommend a new dentist to try this method. When I was an associate dentist, I instructed my staff to cut the periodontal ligament around the third molar with an explorer before I enter the room. Cutting the periodontal ligament with an explorer will be a big help to a new dentist. If you extract a tooth without cutting the periodontal ligament-it feels as if you are playing a tug of war and a dog helps to pull the robe of your opponent. And if you extract a tooth without cutting the periodontal ligament, it is common having to pull this tissue away as it holds the tooth in place. The periodontal ligament tissue is especially strong in vertically erupted third molar.

This video shows cutting the periodontal ligament before extraction, after anesthesia

This video shows how easy the extraction goes when you cut periodontal ligament around third molar

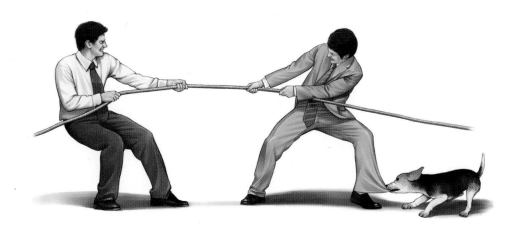

12
Case study - after extraction, I had to use a blade to remove the periodontal ★ ligament attached to the distal surface of third molar

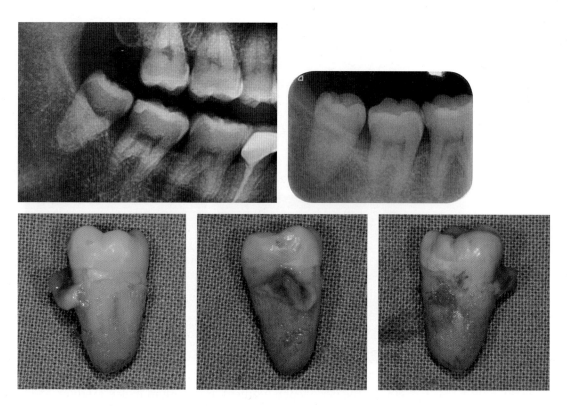

Even if you don't remove the periodontal ligament attached to the distal surface of a tooth, periodontal ligament usually gets removed during an extraction process. If a third molar was functioning normally, periodontal ligament is thickened, and it would be strongly attached to the tooth. Instead of removing the tissue after the extraction, I prefer to remove it with clean incision before starting.

Anyhow, fibers in the periodontal ligament must spread deep into the gums. The fact that the periodontal ligament and the associated fibers are removed along with the third molar during extraction means that we are causing huge trauma to the soft tissue. In order to minimize postoperative pain, to expedite the recovery, and to keep the distal surface of 2nd molars healthy, we should be careful not to pull on the periodontal ligament that comes with the third molar.

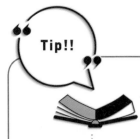

Tip!!

How to remove root tips? ★

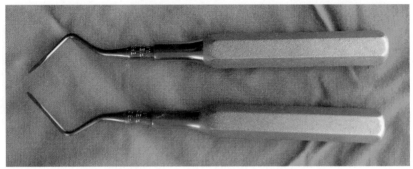

My Root tip picks - Hu-Friedy (U.S.)

I use this instrument when the root tip is strongly embedded in the socket. I am sure that whoever invented this instrument made it bent and thin so as not to put too much force. My experience tells me that you don't need to put a lot of force to remove root tip. So I rarely use even this instrument.

Remember, new dentists - You should not spend too much time and energy removing the root tip in the socket. That is why I have a chapter dedicated to coronectomy in the beginning of the book. When you have more experience with extractions, removing root tips gets easier. If you cannot remove the root tips easily, do not remove it - simply monitor. Because new dentists may make big mistakes while attempting to remove root tips.

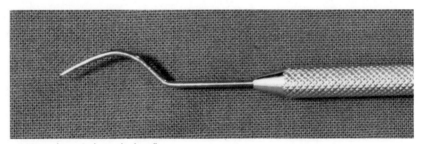

My explorer tip (note the bend)

I normally use an explorer. Most root tips can be removed simply by creating a gap between tooth and the socket. In 90% of my root tip cases, I use an explorer. Except when I am very busy or when I want to observe for educational purposes, I rarely leave root tips. Also, I use the explorer to cut the periodontal ligament around the root before performing extraction.

13
Suture that I use

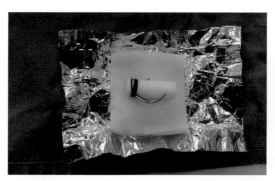 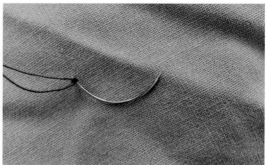

Like in the photo above, I always have the suture prepared in my tray. I use the reverse cutting 3-0 3/8 circle needle tied to silk. This is to save the cost of suture because extraction fee is too cheap in my country. Also, this needle is big and is resistant to bending. Therefore, I can suture quickly [10 units of needle in 1 box: 5,000 won ($5). 500 won ($0.50) per needle. 24 packs of 3-0 black silk in 1 box: 33,000 won ($33). 1 pack has 17 units of 45cm silk. 81 won ($0.80) per silk]. Anyhow, except for working on the maxillary anterior area or maxillary labial surfaces, I only use the above suture needle for all extractions.

Some may recommend the 1/2 circle large needle for suturing after extraction, but I will not talk too much about suturing technique here.

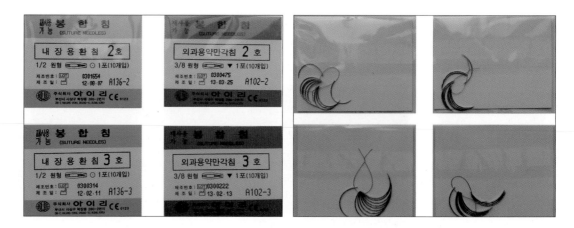

There are a variety of types and sizes of needles. I advise you to find your own suturing style.

14
Nylon suture that I use

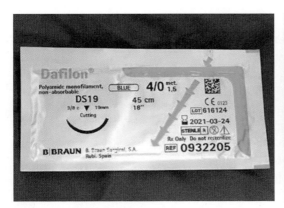
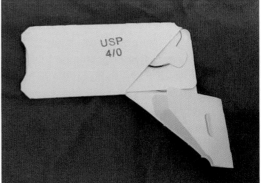

This is the suture that I use most often for implant surgery. I will not talk much about suturing technique in this book. Your own style would be just fine for the purpose.

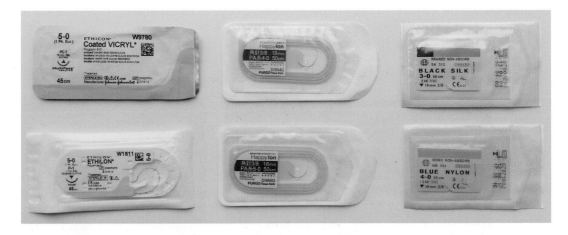

Other sutures in my stock. But except for suturing extra-orally or suturing for flap/implant surgery, I rarely use these sutures. But I advise new dentists to have a variety of sutures available. It's not too late to find your style after using a variety of sutures. I would not force you to follow my anesthesia, incision, and flap technique. I just like to share my technique with you as I discuss my extraction cases in the following chapters.

Wait!

Finger rest on mandibular anterior teeth is a must for the ★★★ mandibular teeth extraction

When I lead the hands-on CE course for third molar extraction, it makes me most nervous when the participants are not using finger rests. It is common to see participants using the handpiece like the photo on the right, even though they probably learned about finger rests so many times in school. If you are a new dentist with less than 15 years of working experience, I highly recommend you to change your posture as you have many more years to practice dentistry. Finger rests on mandibular anterior teeth is a must for quick and safe dental treatment. Whether using a blade for incision or placing implants, finger rest is mandatory. I am also known for placing implants efficiently, and I think this is due to my finger rest. Whether placing multiple implants at the same time or changing angulation of implants, stable finger rest in the mandibular anterior teeth is a must. I owe not having a single big accident despite extracting a lot of wisdom teeth to my stable finger rests on the mandibular anterior teeth.

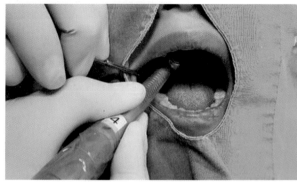

■ Unstable finger rests is blocking the clinician's visual field as well. This posture will not allow the accurate sectioning of a tooth.

Some dentists tell me that they cannot place finger rests due to the bite block in the mouth. But I believe that finger rest on the mandibular anterior teeth is still possible with the bite block in the mouth, and finger rest is still a must even if you need to give up the bite block.

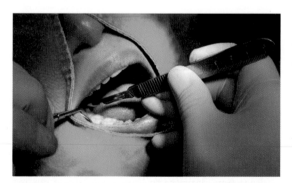

■ Correct finger rests for the blade in the lower right quadrant

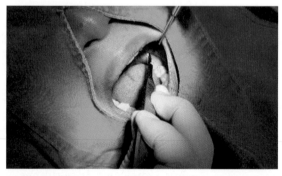

■ Correct finger rests for the blade in the lower left quadrant

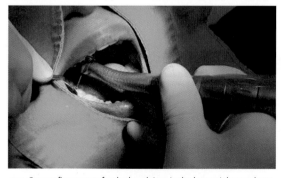

■ Correct finger rests for the handpiece in the lower right quadrant

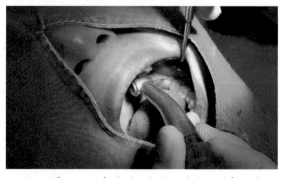

■ Correct finger rests for the handpiece in the lower left quadrant

Incision and Suture Cases for Third molar ★★ Extraction

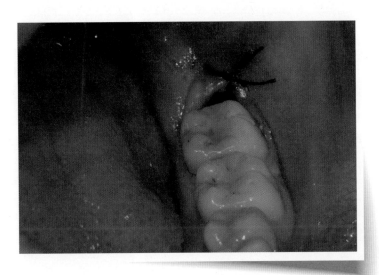

As I perform more and more implant surgeries, I find it very important to obtain primary stability and primary closure. In surgery, there is nothing more important than closing a wound with sutures. What about in third molar extraction? My conclusion is <Do not stress out too much>.

Some dentists may try to suture as precisely as possible after extraction, just like in implant surgery. Some may place a drain, and some may cut a triangle in the gum distal to 2nd molars and let the blood escape through it. Some may reflect the interdental papilla between 1st and 2nd molars and do not place a suture. Not placing a suture is not a bad idea. But in South Korea, placing simple sutures is necessary to receive 10,500 won ($10) for the follow up visit (to remove sutures), and to convince patients to return for the follow up. Most private practitioners like me place sutures for that reason (of course, it is also helpful for patients to get follow up visit). For this reason, I place a figure 8 suture to prevent food impaction or an interrupted suture in the middle or distal surface.

I don't normally place a drain. I try to place sutures, as minimally as possible so that gingiva can hold its natural shape.

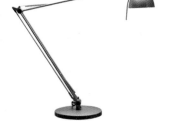

01
Case 1 - No vertical incision was made on the mesial surface ★

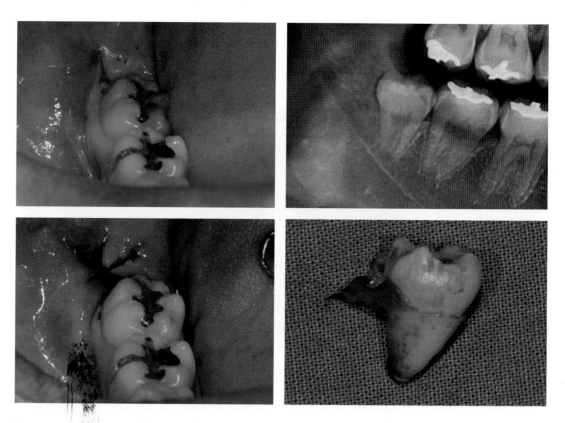

You can only see a small part of the crown, but crown size is small and it is placed near the occlusal plane. Therefore, I just placed a small incision on the buccal surface and extracted the tooth without placing muco-periosteal flap or removing bone. I barely touched the distal surface of the tooth and started the extraction, so you can see that the distal surface of the extracted tooth has the periodontal ligament attached. I think it's important to tell apart PDL from the follicle that was used to surround the tooth.

Like in the above case where I could visualize a part of the crown, I usually place sutures, but I do not place sutures for the part that showed the crown initially. My needle size is very big and is cumbersome to suture small incisions, but I try my best.

When I make a large incision because I cannot visualize a third molar at all, I still try to suture according to the natural gingival position. Unlike in implant surgery where I try to place sutures without having any exposure, here I place sutures loosely leaving a slight opening.

02
Case 2 - No vertical incision was made on the mesial surface

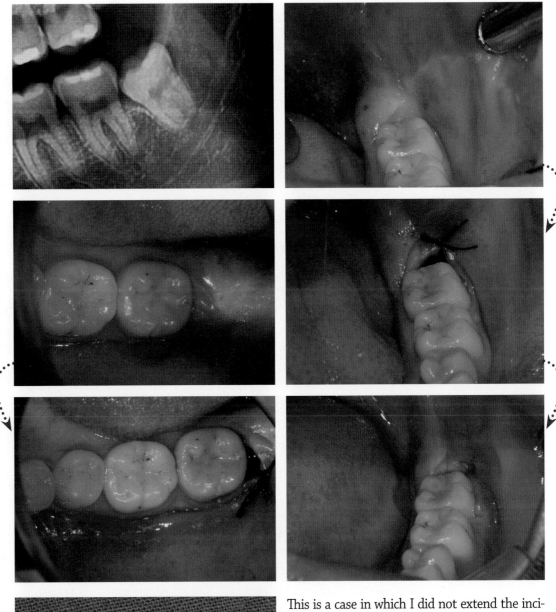

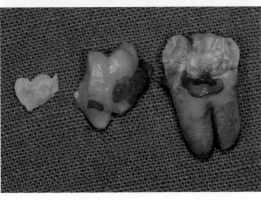

This is a case in which I did not extend the incision line to the mesial surface. After a week, I took a photo after removing sutures. You can check the condition of the buccal gingiva of #7 that had been reflected during the surgery. In this case, I sectioned the mesial surface of the crown, and sectioned the lingual surface to extract. We will discuss the detail in the later chapter on vertically impacted third molar. Because I expected some swelling, I made loose sutures. You can see that gingiva distal to 2nd molars is slightly opened and holds its natural shape.

03
Case 3 - No vertical incision was made on the mesial surface ★

TIP!!

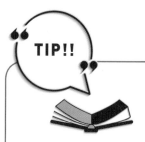

I'm worried that you may think I'm a pervert making an example like this, but I think this analogy will stick to your head so here I go… remember the episiotomy before child birth? Where do OB-GYNs place sutures? Only the incised area…

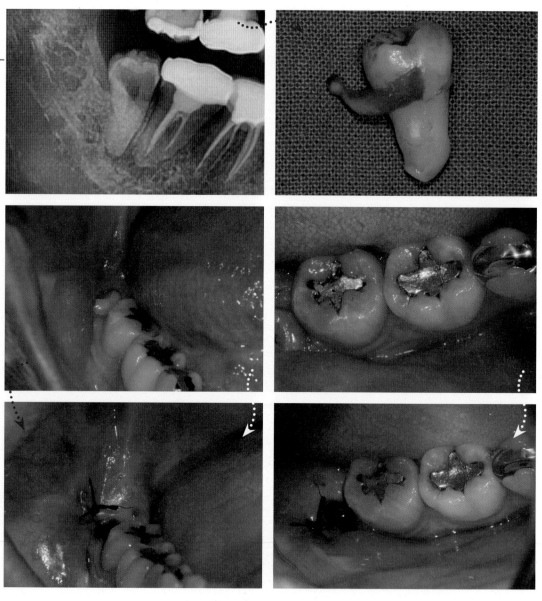

In vertically impacted third molar cases, if I can visualize the tooth slightly, I only make a small incision to the buccal surface in 90% of the time.

Because I'm too busy, I minimize making an incision, surgical flap, and suture, so I prefer making an incision and suture like this. You can barely see the crown in this case, but because the tooth is located high vertically, I did not extend my incision to the mesial surface, and I made a small incision to the buccal surface. I placed a suture where I made an incision, so there is a natural opening on the 2nd molar's distal surface, which is good to prevent swelling. I think this amount of opening is great. New dentists may place sutures in the socket instead of suturing the incision line, but I recommend to suture only the incision line. Recently, I came to think that the suture technique like the above is helpful to keep the periodontal ligament of the 2nd molar's distal surface healthy.

04
Case 4 - No vertical incision was made on the mesial surface ★

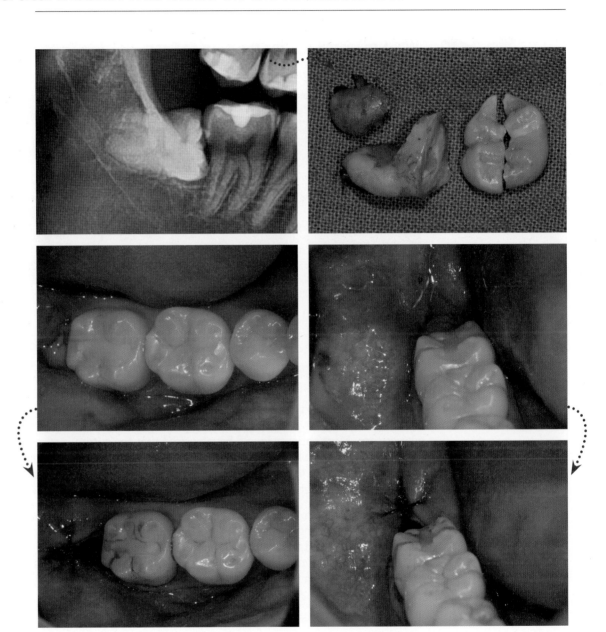

For horizontally impacted third molars, except for cases where you cannot visualize the tooth at all, I do not extend my incision line to the 2nd molar's mesial surface.

For this horizontally impacted third molar, there is no need to make an extensive incision as I rarely remove buccal bone. I can easily extract the crown and root by making a minimal incision. Of course, patient is less likely to get post-operative swelling and pain.

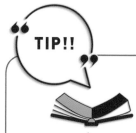

TIP!!

What to watch out for the new dentists

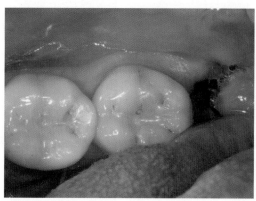 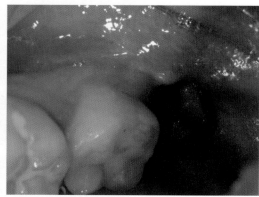

▬ A new dentist placed sutures and the patient came back for suture removal after 1 week. Often, buccal suture is already torn.

Most notable characteristic of sutures placed by a new dentist is that buccal suture is always torn.

I lead third molar extraction hands-on courses once a month, and I am the one removing sutures placed by the participants during post-op visits. And I notice that buccal sutures are always torn. Most patients would have noticed that the suture is torn after a day or two, living very uncomfortably, then coming back to remove it. Sometimes, patients return without having any suture in the mouth. Sometimes I tell the new dentists that if your suture skill is not that great, it is better to remove the suture in 3~4 days, instead of waiting for 1 week.

It's very important to place sutures in the full thickness. The problem may be that incision and flap are not being done in full thickness. If you make a clear buccal full thickness flap, your suture may be stable too, but if you make a shallow incision, your suture may also be too shallow. Since I perform the minimal incision and flap design, I place sutures as deeply in the tissue as I can, and I avoid putting too much tension in the suture.

Remember that as a new dentist, buccal sutures may get torn easily, so try to prevent it from happening. Just as you need to make an incision to the periosteum, you need to place a suture to the periosteum.

05
Extending incision line to the mesial surface - Case 1. Making vertical incision★ on the distal surface of #7

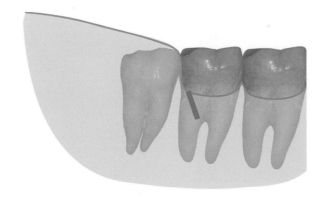

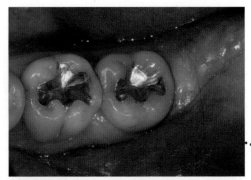

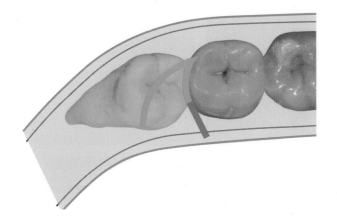

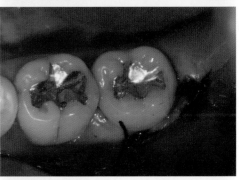

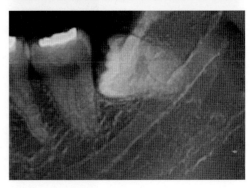

When the third molar is not clinically visible, I use the No. 12 blade for the incision near the distal of a 2nd molar.

But it is not easy to make a vertical incision with the No. 12 blade, so I usually extend the flap to the distal surface of a 1st molar to avoid vertical incision. If I have to make a vertical incision with the No. 12 blade, like in the case above, it is easier to place one in the distal surface of 2nd molar due to the angle of the blade handle, but I rarely do this. I have only done few cases like the above. If I have to place a vertical incision, I normally place it on the mesial of 2nd molar.

In the case above, it may appear that a vertical incision was made in the middle of a 2nd molar and not on the distal surface of a 2nd molar. But the incision was made diagonally from the distal of a 2nd molar to the mesial surface of a 2nd molar.

New dentists may have difficulty suturing after making a vertical incision. It is especially hard with the long, thick suture needle. But know that unlike elsewhere, if you place a good suture in the distal surface, it is not a big deal to not suture the vertical incision. Vertical incision must be made diagonally to avoid possible long buccal nerve damage.

06
Extending incision line to the mesial surface - Case 2. Making vertical incision ★ on the distal surface of #7

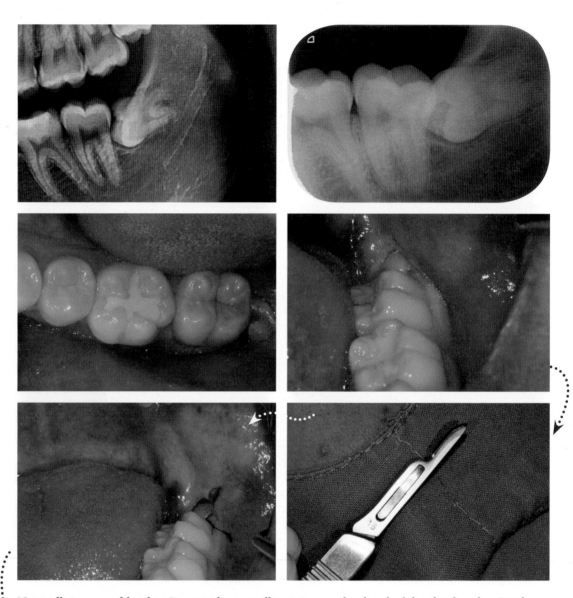

Normally in a case like this, I just make a small incision on the distal of the third molar. But here, the third molar is located towards the buccal surface and I thought it would be useful to lay a mucoperiosteal flap. Therefore, I made a slight vertical incision on the #7 distal surface. Without the vertical incision, you can pull the tissue too forcefully towards the buccal surface and place too much tension even to the 2nd molar's mesial surface.

I normally don't make this kind of incision, but as I was finishing writing this book, I met a dentist who told me that this is the most preferred incision method for the OMS surgeons. It may be true among his surgeon colleagues, but my experience tells me that this incision is preferred by more GP's, and the OMFS surgeons prefer to make the bigger incision. Unless we make a scientific study over this, it is better to find your own method. But if you are making a buccal incision from the 2nd molar's distal surface, you have to avoid cutting the long buccal nerve. This is especially true when the buccal vestibule is shallow. Some say it doesn't matter to damage the long buccal nerve, but it is better to prevent it...

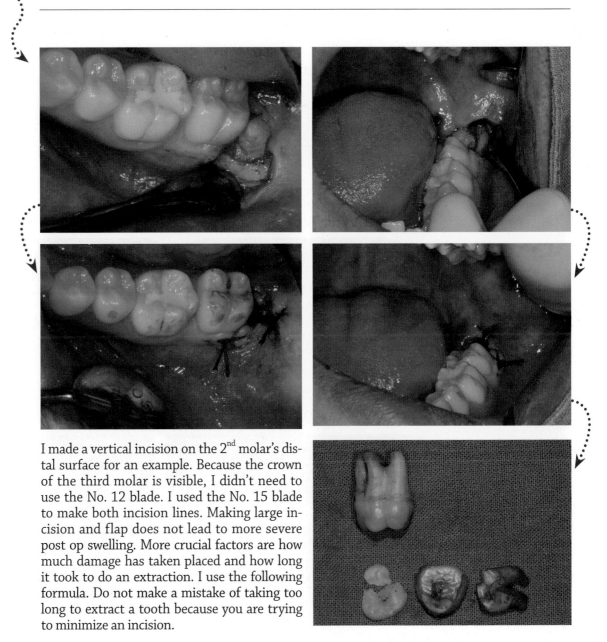

I made a vertical incision on the 2nd molar's distal surface for an example. Because the crown of the third molar is visible, I didn't need to use the No. 12 blade. I used the No. 15 blade to make both incision lines. Making large incision and flap does not lead to more severe post op swelling. More crucial factors are how much damage has taken placed and how long it took to do an extraction. I use the following formula. Do not make a mistake of taking too long to extract a tooth because you are trying to minimize an incision.

Post-operative swelling and pain =
amount of damage due to incision, flap, sectioning, etc ×extraction time

07
Extending an incision line to the mesial surface - Case 1. Making vertical incision on the mesial surface of #7 ★★★

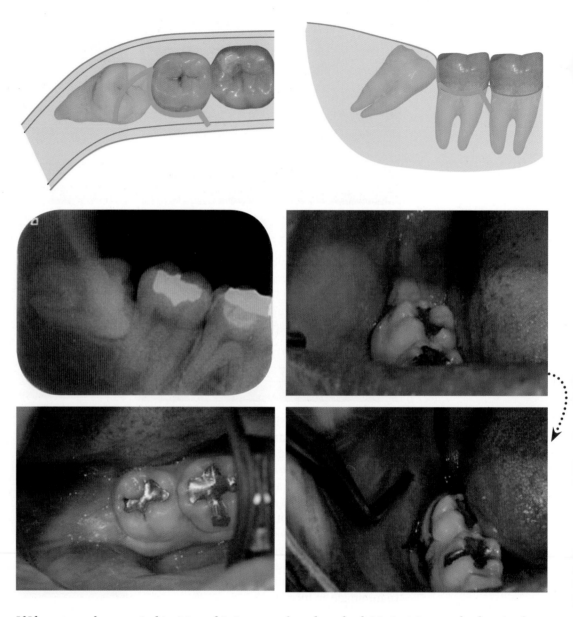

If I have to make a vertical incision, this is my preferred method. My incision method varies from day to day depending on my mood and situation, but if I have to extend an incision line toward the front, I would make an incision on a 2nd molar's mesial surface. Rather than extending the incision to the distal surface of a 1st molar, making a vertical incision on a 2nd molar's mesial surface provides a better visual field, more stable flap reflection, and better coverage for the suture.

08
Extending an incision line to the mesial surface- Case 2. Making vertical incision ★ on the mesial surface of #7

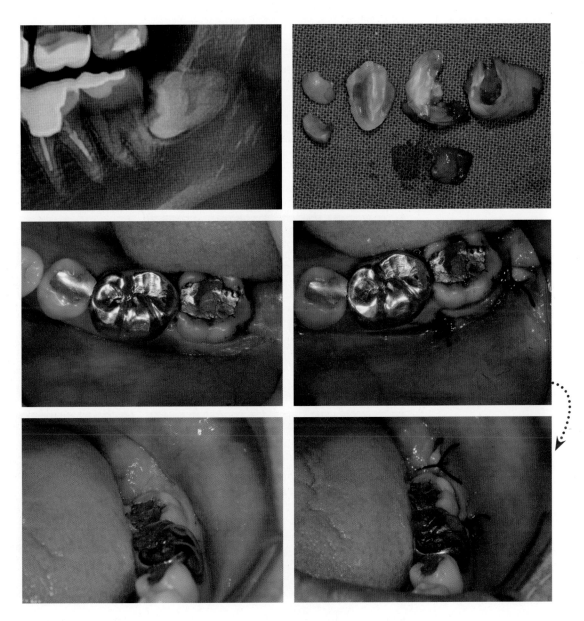

This is my most preferred incision method- I use the No. 12 or No. 15 blade. If I only need to make a vertical incision, I use the No. 15 blade. But if I use the No. 12 blade to make an incision on the distal of a 2nd molar, I also use the No.12 blade to make a vertical incision on the mesial surface. In fact, I took these photos as an example for this book, and this is not necessarily my best case. I hope you understand that I could only take photos on slow days on my acquaintances.

09

Extending an incision line to the mesial surface - Case 1. Extending incision ★ line to include interdental papilla between #6 and #7 ────────

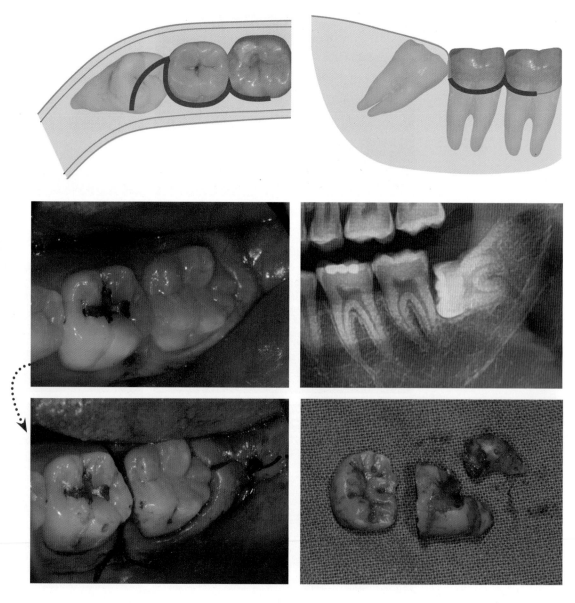

I use this incision method when I'm in a hurry. Usually, I make a small incision just near the third molar and extract the tooth. But if the third molar is located far buccal or requires a wider visual field, I use the sharp end of the periosteal elevator to reflect the flap from the 1st molar disto-buccal interdental papilla to the 2nd molar disto-buccal incision line. Some dentists do not place a suture in the interdental papilla between 1st and 2nd molar to prevent swelling, but I rather prefer to place a loose suture on the 2nd molar's distal surface.

10
Extending an incision line to the mesial surface - Case 2. Extending incision ★★ line to include interdental papilla between #6 and #7

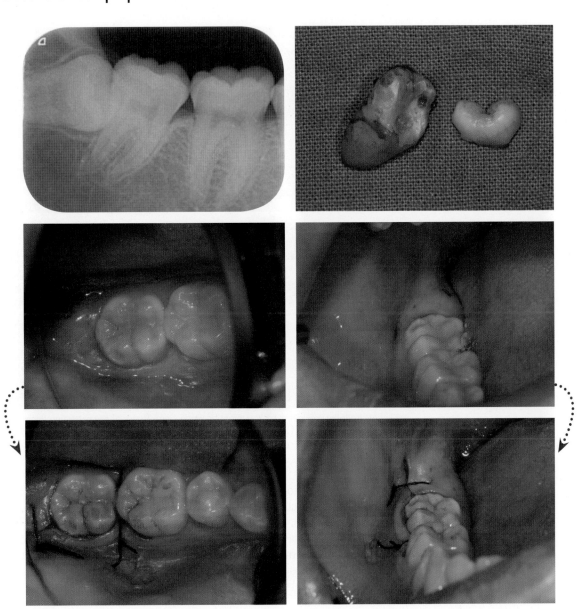

I had not planned on extending an incision line to the mesial surface due to small crown size, but because the third molar was located on the buccal surface, I made the incision line to the buccal surface and extended the line to the mesial surface. I reflect the interdental papilla between 1st and 2nd molars using a periosteal elevator without making an incision, but it is helpful for new dentists to use the No. 12 blade. If you are using a periosteal elevator that has a round end, I think it is necessary to use a blade to incise the sulcus.

I think it takes practice to make a muco-periosteal flap. Through my years of experience of leading extraction seminar, it takes a while to get used to this simple movement. For new dentists, it is necessary to repeatedly practice making basic incision, flap, and suture through performing third molar extractions.

11
How far to extend a mucoperiosteal flap after making an incision? ★★★

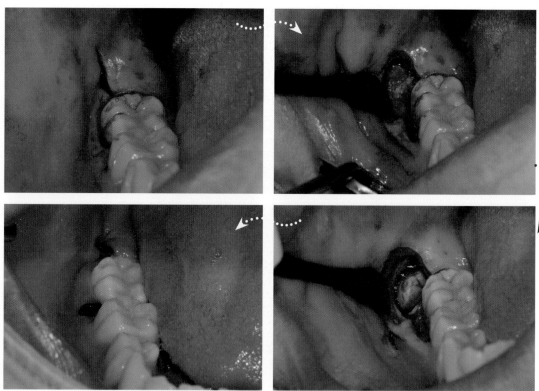

■ Photos from the previous case. You might be wondering - How was the extraction done after that incision? To what extent were the flap and bone sectioning done?

"It would be correct to say that the nerves of the alveolar bone are all located in the periosteum. Especially as it gets closer to the basal bone and not the alveolar bone, the importance of the periosteum increases. My philosophy is to do a minimal incision, flap, and bone removal. Therefore, I usually never lay a flap unless absolutely necessary. In cases such as above where most of the third molar cannot be visualized, I reflect a flap and remove the buccal bone to gain a better visual field. My philosophy is to always try to minimize making a mucoperiosteal flap and minimize removing buccal bone.

Performing the mucoperiosteal flap naturally improves as one gains more experience. This skill is also very important for the implant surgery. For a new dentist, I recommend that you don't focus on minimizing the mucoperiosteal flap. I recommend that you practice making sufficient incision and flap. But, as your skill improves, try to minimize making the flap.

Now, let's discuss the mucoperiosteal flap and buccal bone removal next.

Mucoperiosteal Flap and Buccal Bone ★★ Removal for Third Molar Extraction

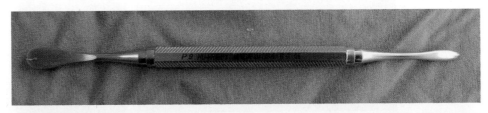

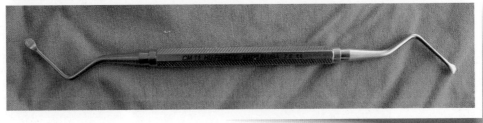

The above pictures are the periosteal elevator (Hu-Friedy P9) and surgical curette (Hu-Friedy CM 11) that I use most often. However, unlike an EL3C elevator, as long as the shape and size are similar, I do not necessarily only use these instruments from the same company. I have been using more made in Korea instruments recently that are less expensive.

Usually I start by using the surgical curette to incise once more and then widen the incision. Next, I use the sharp end of the periosteal elevator to start the flap, and I finish with the wide end of the instrument. When I need to retract soft tissue for tooth/bone removal, I use the sharp end and the wide end interchangeably according to the size of the tissue; however, I normally use the wide end for the retraction.

Because topics of mucoperiosteal flap and bone removal are often discussed in other literatures, I thought about skipping the topic but decided to mention it briefly. It is not necessary to follow my style - simply recognize that there are people that think like me.

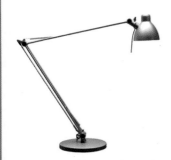

01
Dr. Kim's mucoperiosteal flap and buccal bone removal ★★

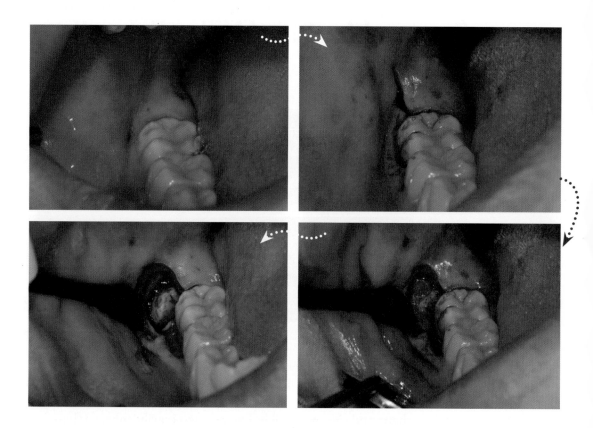

Pictures of the previous case after making incision, flap, and buccal bone removal

My philosophy is to minimize the flap size and buccal cortical bone removal. Most of the flaps and buccal bone removal are done to improve the operator's visual field for the extraction. If the tooth remains hard to visualize even after making the incision and flap, I use the high speed handpiece to smooth out the buccal surface of the third molar - this is not to remove the buccal bone, but it is rather to remove soft tissue around the tooth and to gain better visualization of the tooth.

However, the buccal bone must be removed sufficiently in cases that require it. Especially in cases where the third molar is located buccally or when the alveolar bone is located above the third molar's buccal height of contour, the buccal bone must be removed to a certain degree.

Also, most new dentists have difficulty sectioning the mesial part of the crown - the most common reason is that the buccal aspect of the crown was not properly removed. The lingual surface of the crown is often not completely cut with the bur as the remaining part is usually removed by fracturing it with an elevator. Therefore, it is necessary to section the buccal surface of the tooth completely. Experienced dentists are good at sectioning the buccal surface of the tooth, but new dentists often cannot completely section the buccal surface. For new dentists, it is important to completely section through the buccal surface (it is easier to visualize and is safer compared to the lingual surface) to help with removing the mesial part of the crown, even if there is not enough sectioning to the lingual surface. Especially for new dentists, I recommend removing sufficient buccal bone to the point that the buccal surface of the third molar is clearly visualized.

02
Mucoperiosteal flap and buccal bone removal method recommended ★★★
for the new dentist

As I mentioned before, visualization of the operating field is critical for new dentists. It is good to make an effort to minimize the amount of incision, reflection, and bone removal, but this effort must be made after becoming more experienced with third molar extractions. New dentists need to focus on whether they can extract the third molar or not, rather than focusing on making minimal incision, flap reflection, and bone removal. This effort should be made after gaining enough experience in extracting third molars. There is a phrase that I repeatedly tell my audience in implant lectures. <Flapless implant surgery is not for those who do not know how to make a flap. Rather, it is for those who are so proficient at making flaps.> Some new dentists get interested in the flapless surgery as they experience difficulty making flaps, but this is as dangerous as trying to fly when you cannot even walk.

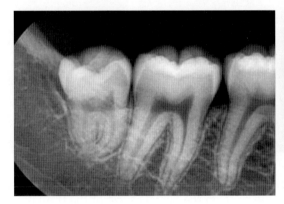 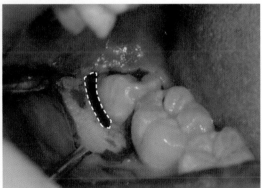

━ I do not flap like this, but you can observe see clean incision, flap reflection, and buccal bone removal by an OMFS surgeon

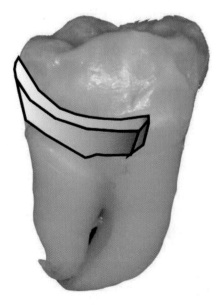

Above photo was taken from a lecture slide on third molar extraction by my colleague, who is an oral surgeon. If I were an operator, I would not have done the flap, buccal bone removal, or incision.

But for some cases, it is important to use the above method. Especially for the beginners, you can hone your surgical skills on incision, laying a flap, bone removal, and suturing by going through these steps. That is how OMFS residents learn to extract a tooth during their residency. Even for dentists who lack perceptual ability, the above method will make the extraction easy and successful. In the next page, we will observe another case by Dr. Min-Kyo Seo.

03
Mucoperiosteal flap and buccal bone removal method recommended by ★★ oral surgeons

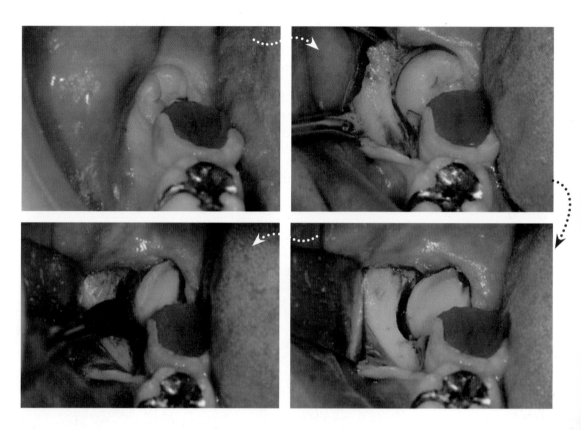

Let's focus on the elevator used in the above case. It is difficult to use a wide elevator like this one without removing the bone on the buccal aspect of the third molar. Because I use a narrow EL3C elevator, rather than removing the buccal bone to engage the elevator, I can simply remove enough soft tissue for the visualization of the operating field. For someone that uses a narrow elevator like me, it is good to remove buccal bone narrow and deep, if it needs to be done for visualization. A fissure bur is commonly used to remove the buccal bone. The fact that a fissure bur is great at removing the buccal bone may be the reason that oral surgeons commonly use it for surgical extractions.

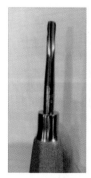
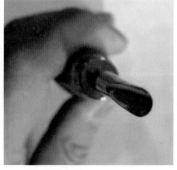

According to my experience, oral surgeons prefer to use this type of elevator. The elevator is usually short, wide, and strong with a very big arc of a circle.

However, such an elevator cannot be inserted between the alveolar bone and the tooth in their natural state, and therefore it can only be used when the surrounding bone is removed.

▬ Hu-Friedy EL4S: the elevator of choice by an oral surgeon, who is my long time colleague

04
Dr. Kim and third molar ★★

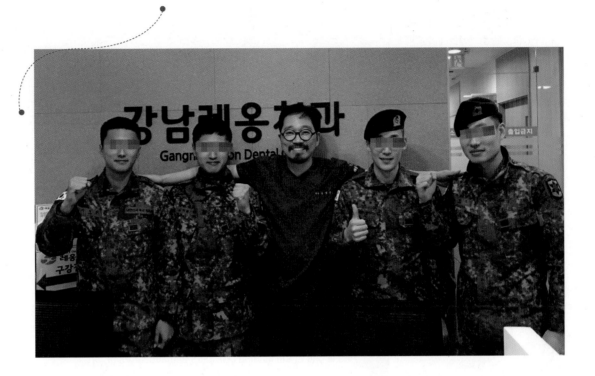

I enjoy third molar extractions. Not only because I had to perform them a lot as many try to avoid the procedure, but I also enjoy the procedure itself. I personally have a dislike toward prepping teeth. As such, I grew to be more interested in oral surgery and periodontics rather than prosthodontics.

The above picture was taken when a group of soldiers came to my office together during army leave for third molar extractions. I took a lot of pictures during this time as I had grown a beard for the first time in my life. Anyways, a couple of these soldiers ended up not getting extractions done as they wanted to drink during their break, but nonetheless, it makes me proud when the younger generation recognizes me.

For me, extracting a third molar is like fishing. Just like people who do not eat fish that still enjoy fishing, I cannot stop doing third molar extractions - not because of the profit but because of the 'tactile excitement.' What a blessing it is that I can enjoy that tactile excitement at the dental office I work at when others need to invest a lot of time to travel for that same experience? ^^

In the first chapter, I explained simply why I enjoy third molar extractions and why I ended up doing so many of them, as well as my philosophy regarding wisdom teeth extractions. You might wonder why I have written these random 'brags' about myself. I want you to know that the content of this book is the result of my experience performing countless extractions more than any other, and think of my 'brags' as a way for me to increase my credibility. Or, you can think that since I am a GP, I may have exaggerated my experience as I have a minor case of 'GP complex.'

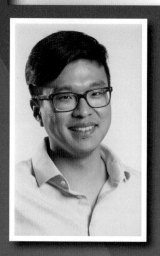

Dr. Scott J-S Park BDSc

Dr. Scott Park graduated from The University of Queensland in 2005 and worked in both public and private dental practices before joining Preventive Dentistry (Canberra, Australia) in 2008.
Scott's special interests are preventive, cosmetic, implant and sleep dentistry.
He is one of the leading providers and educators of Somnodent anti-sleep apnoea and anti-snoring appliances (Somnomed Australia Pty Ltd) in Australia.
With the power of three Trios 3 Intra-Oral Digital Scanners (3 Shape Pty Ltd), the practice has become the leading provider of digital dentistry in the Australian Capital Territory state.
He also enjoys sharing his knowledge and experience of digital dentistry and digitally guided implant placement with other colleagues.
Scott is the recommended dentist for five different diplomatic embassies in Canberra and also is a member for Australian Capital Territory, The National Unification Advisory Council Republic of Korea.
He is happily married with three young daughters, and he spends a lot of his spare time being a doting dad.

First of all, I would like to thank Dr. Youngsam Kim for imparting his wealth of knowledge and experience with our colleagues in Australia. I am now safe to say wisdom tooth extraction is one of my specialized interest.
ESSE (Easy, Simple, Safe, Efficient) principle makes sense to both patients and operators and this could also be applied to other areas of your dentistry.
Dr. Kim's book, Easy Simple Safe Efficient Minimally Invasive & Atraumatic Extraction of Third Molars, is now being translated into English and I sincerely hope it reaches many colleagues all around the world for improving their extraction skill and patient care. I am honoured to be a part of the translation process and recommend this book for every colleague with every experience level. There are many clinical tips that could be adopted and be put into practice very next day!

Chapter 05-1 translated by

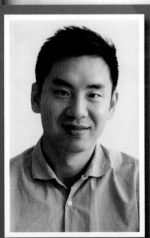

Dr. Ryan Dongchan Seo BDSc

I graduated from the University of Queensland, Australia in 2006. Upon graduation I started working at private practice in Brisbane CBD as an associate dentist. I was able to treat patients with complex treatment plan soon after the graduation under the good mentorship from the principal dentist. Our practice was one of the very first which had CAD/CAM technology and it has become one of my specialty. I have purchased the practice from the principal dentist 3 years ago and in the middle of expanding the clinic to deliver more treatment options to our patients.

It is a great honour to be able to participate in translation of ESSE Extraction of Third Molars. Surgical dentistry was not something I particularly enjoyed. Surgical extraction can be difficult to begin with, especially without the good mentorship. This book has details of the every step of extration and thorough instructions of how to use instruments. I belive this book will add confidence and knowledge to surgical extraction, which is a vital skill required by a general dentist. This book has changed how I approached wisdom tooth extractions. Thank you Dr. Kim.

Elevator for Wisdom Tooth Extraction

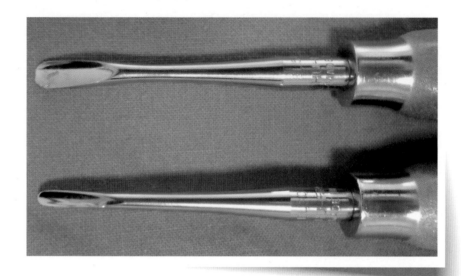

Elevator is very important in extraction of wisdom tooth. I didn't understand why this instrument was called an 'elevator' when I was at early stage of learning wisdom tooth extraction. I thought it was used to merely to create the gap between the root and the alveolar socket. I have learnt why the instrument was called an elevator as I did more and more extractions. It is used to 'elevate' the root of the tooth within the narrow alveolar socket. I have seen many luxators in the recent dental exhibition which is used to increase the gap between the root and socket. I don't stock any of those at all. Luxator is not necessary if you utilize elevator properly, especially thin curved elevator I use. Elevator can function as a Luxator initially to insert in between the tooth and alveolar bone and as an elevator when you 'lift' the tooth in the PDL space.

Let's have a look at more detailed use of the elevator.

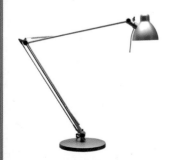

01
Dr. Youngsam's elevator ★★★

I personally love to use this particular elevator, Hu-Friedy EL3C. My extraction skill relies heavily on this elevator. Its thin and curved end is able to go into PDL space without removal of the bone. It is so precious that Kim youngsam's wisdom tooth extraction doesn't exist without this Hu-Friedy EL3C. I also have recommended this elevator to other colleagues and almost every one of them found it very satisfactory. It is also very durable.

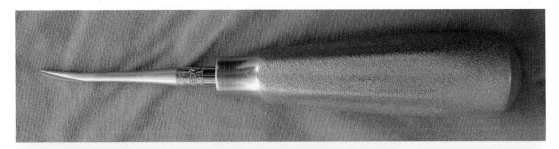

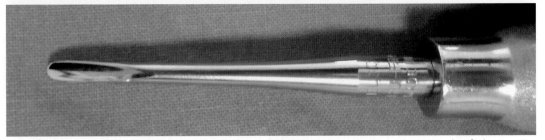

■ I call EL3C as an elevator but sales representative from Hu-Friedy call this Luxator. (In catalogue it is classified as Luxating Elevator). True elevators receive letter 'E' rather than EL. I have been calling EL3C as an elevator ever since I started practicing and most of the colleagues know them as an elevator. Hence in this book EL3C would be called an elevator. Due to the numerous implant and periodontal surgery, very fine and long luxators are on the market these days and to separate EL3C from those, I think it is wise to call it an elevator. Luxating elevator is still an elevator. :)

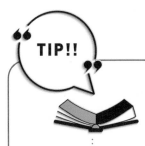

TIP!!

This is from Hu-Friedy from America. Model name is EL3C, 3 stands of 3mm (width of elevator) and C means curved. EL5C that I sometimes use is handy when there is increased PDL space or tooth is sectioned with thick round bur #6 (>1.6mm). EL5C doesn't belong to my extraction kit but rather keep it in a separate pouch so that I can use it only when necessary.

Another common elevator used by OMFS is EL4S, in which 4 means 4mm width of elevator and S means straight, as some of you might already have realized. This is how the most commonly used elevator is named.

02
Recommended elevator from my colleagues ★

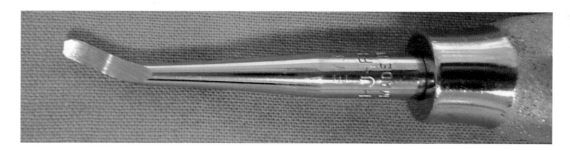

Some of my senior colleagues have strongly recommended this elevator. They have mentioned that it is quite useful for vertically impacted mandibular wisdom tooth. I would recommend EL3C over this elevator as we need to be equipped for left and right hand side separately and only can be used in selected cases.

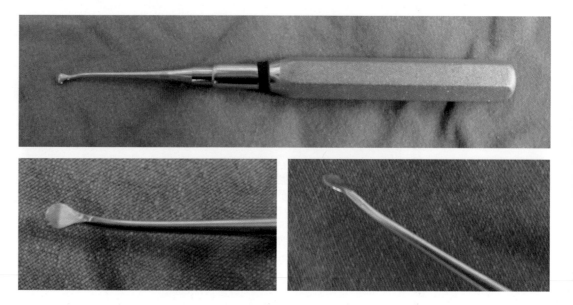

Fellow dentists have recommended this straight curette (Hu-Friedy CM2). It is quite thin, so that it is useful when inserting into PDL space without bone removal, but access could be difficult due to its straight end. Also it is more fragile. Though I have seen many colleagues who use this elevator in conjunction with other instruments.

Every instrument has pros and cons, but it is more important to become familiar with the particular instrument. I therefore think using various instruments can be disadvantageous in terms of getting familiar with your instruments. That is why I use Hu-Friedy EL3C most of the time and numerous dentists who use EL3C from my recommendation found it very satisfactory.

03
Elevators that I use at occasion

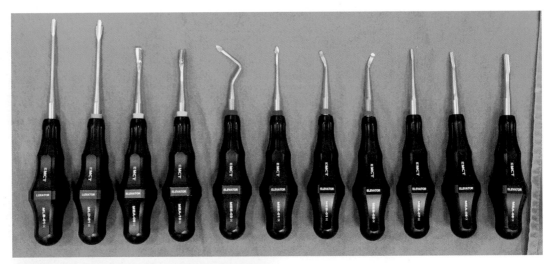

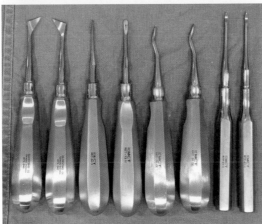

I do lots of extractions and sometimes I have to extract a wisdom tooth in unusual location and/or with unique root shapes. That's when I use these special elevators. However I don't use expensive Hu-Friedy instruments as its less frequent use means it is not cost effective. I stock varieties of elevators with mid-range price tags. You don't always need to buy the expensive instruments for every single item as cheaper one doesn't mean that it would break after a little usage. Those can be found on www.2875mart.co.kr

While extracting thousands of wisdom teeth over last 3 years, I rarely used any other elevators than EL3C. However I sometimes try other instruments on purpose to become familiar with them and for those cases I take photos of the wisdom tooth with the used instruments adjacent to it.

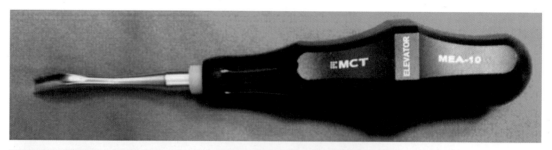

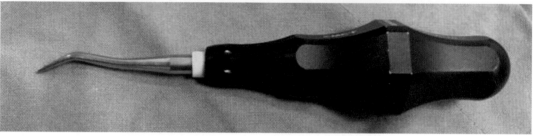

This is the elevator that I use for maxillary wisdom tooth sometimes. It is intended for canine; however, I use this elevator when there is no buccal access due to its vertical impaction. 97~98% of time I use EL3C and 1% of the case I use the above elevator. The rest and root picks make up less than 0.1%. I will mention remaining 2% in the following pages.

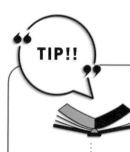

TIP!!

Principle of the lever

Leverage is very important principle. It is good to be reminded of following levers.

Raising a flap based on leverage principles

type 1

type 2

type 3

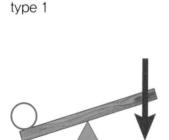

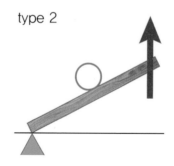

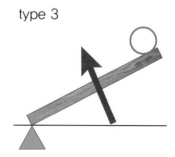

A picture explaining the principles of leverage. The clip is in Korean so just watch.

04
How to use elevator

Extraction relies on the technique, not on force. Of course it is better to apply the right force but extraction doesn't become all that difficult even if you don't have strength. Elevator is a lever that can exponentially increase the force you apply so as long as you know the principle, there is no extraction case that you couldn't complete due to lack of the force. Elevator makes extraction very easy. I think the most important principle during the use of elevator is to never insert the elevator into embrasure of 7's.

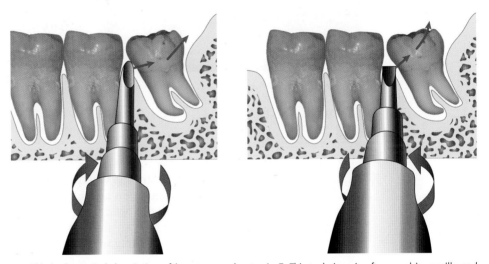

━━ This is the typical description of how to use elevator in 7. This technique is often used in maxilla and sometimes in mandible

It is very important not to insert the elevator on embrasure of #7 to extract #8. I can't emphasize more! A very common complication that leads many colleagues to giving up wisdom tooth removal is sensitivity on 7's. Not to mention 7's cracking during wisdom tooth removal, quite a few patients mention that #7 became sensitive after their 8's removed.

What causes this? It could be temporary damage to the ligament on #7, but when it lasts for several months it is due to the cracks or damage on cervical area of 7's caused by elevation like the above diagram. The pain might lead to root canal or extraction. Many dentists avoid wisdom tooth extraction not because of the bleeding or possible nerve damage but it is because of the patients complaining chronic continuing pain on #7. As there is no visible signs it can be quite frustrating. Some might assure saying it is due to the exposure of the distal surface but in many cases pain would not resolve by itself.

So where should I use the elevator on? And how?

05
The basis of extraction is lever principle ★★

Let's have a look at short video below

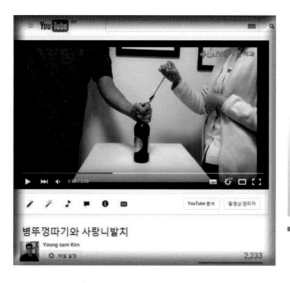

A clip, used can opening to show how the principles of leverage are utilized in wisdom tooth extractions.

This is what I have uploaded a few years ago when I started lecturing on wisdom tooth extraction. Let's consider a bottle cap. Even if you are very strong, it is very hard to remove a bottle cap with out the proper tool. It is easy to open using a bottle opener. Though I can open it quite easily if I have any hard, angled tool as I can apply lever principle. Same applies to extraction. It shouldn't have done as extracting something from the soil but rather should be done like taking magnet off the whiteboard. Extraction is similar to opening a bottle cap not extracting a carrot from the soil.

This is a story while I was giving a lecture and live surgery on wisdom tooth removal last month. I was demonstrating how to extract a wisdom tooth while explaining the lever principle. I emphasized how important it is to engage at a fulcrum and how easy it can be to extract a wisdom tooth with anchor being at the right anchor.

I said "If you have trouble extracting a vertically impacted wisdom tooth, it is because it is not engaged properly. You can exert enormous force as long as you have a good engagement on fulcrum."

One of the attendants was a little suspicious and asked 'what if it doesn't come out still? '

Then I answered back "As long as you get a proper engagement, the tooth will at least break even it is not extracted" At the same time, I engaged an elevator and applied the pressure, then the wisdom tooth came out half broken.

I think elevator can demonstrate much more force than forceps if you could utilize lever principle. If you break the coronal part of the wisdom tooth and finish the case off as it is, it is a successful coronectomy.

06
Elevator should never slip! ★★★

Using elevator relies on basic lever principle. It is the technique not the force. The most important factor for lever to work at its best is the fulcrum. Elevator must not slip inside the mouth and it depends if the elevator is fully engaged to avoid slippage. Where there is no bone removal during extraction, there is an increased chance of elevator slipping so the clinician must be very cautious. I caused 7~8 cm tear in larynx once to the patient while I was extracting #38 sitting on the right hand side of the patient. It wasn't long after I graduated from university and wasn't confident with suturing either. Fortunately there wasn't much bleeding and pain so I could finish off with a few simple sutures. From then I always check if the elevator is fully engaged at fulcrum before I exert any force and make sure that it doesn't slip. If you are using a sharp, thin elevator like El3C I use it is crucial to check if the elevator is stuck(?) at the point you would like to transmit the force. In addition I use my elbow and other hand to rest to minimize the damage in case it slips. I have heard worse scenarios where elevator got pushed buccally and pierced extraorally and caused worse tear on patient's larynx.

As residents are beginners they remove the buccal bone to create the 'gutter'. However doing so results in weakening of the alveolar bone where elevator is working on making engagement at fulcrum more difficult. I don't remove the bone in most of the time unless it is above the height of contour or occlusal surface. I rather remove part of the tooth within alveolar bone to create the space and extract. But if you are relatively new, it is not a bad idea to practice to use fissure bur (008 or 010) or round bur (less than size 4) to create the gutter? 'purchase point' needs to be removed from the sentence? so that elevator doesn't slip. Please refer to the previous chapter (extraction and removal of buccal bone).

Safety always comes first. Please do not make an incident that makes me sad.

Like many traffic accidents, clinical accidents happen when you think that you are more confident. That is why you have to always be cautious. I still pay attention to ensure the elevator doesn't slip while extracting.

07
I only use this… If I am only allowed a single instrument ★

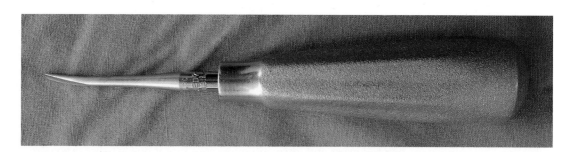

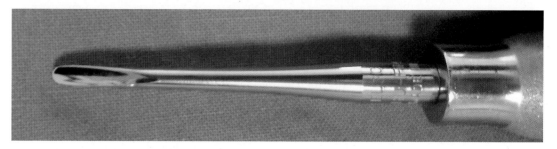

90% of my extraction skill comes from this elevator. You might wonder I repeat the same words over and over but that is how important this elevator is. You will be sucked into this Hu-Friedy EL3C which is thin, sharp and durable.

But due to its thin and sharp character, I would like to urge to be extra cautious at early stage of your clinical career. Instead EL5C with 5mm width could be a safer choice. Even for those experienced clinicians, I still strongly recommend to use these elevators. You can do most of the extractions without bone removal and its curved tip makes it handy for upper 8's.

Wait!

It is my principle to extract wisdom tooth on the day of ★ consultation

I have recently hired associates dentist which allowed a little bit of extra time. I still see average of 25 patients daily and half of them are either wisdom tooth extraction and implant. It is my principle to extract the wisdom tooth on the day of consultation as many patients come from distances or a day off at work to have the wisdom tooth extracted. Doing so routinely has resulted in increased efficiency and drew more patients for wisdom tooth extraction. In addition, doing wisdom tooth only would not make the practice very profitable at all and that is why I can't spend too much time on doing extractions even though I love doing them.

08
My humiliating story

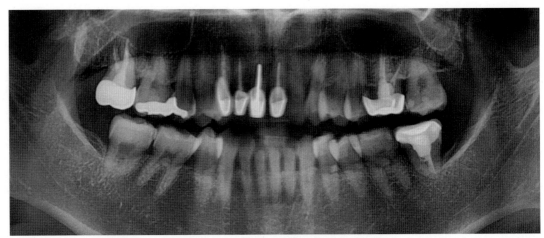

━ This is #37 replanted after the extraction 15 years. Considering the condition of overall periodontal status not being great, #37 is not doing bad in this case.

I have referred two patients in my entire career for the extraction. First patient was due to my severe back pain from scoliosis 7~8 years ago. I couldn't bear the pain due to the prolonged surgical time and had to refer to an oral surgeon.

The other case is a bit shocking. It was 15 years ago when I was straight out of school. My other colleague was helping me with horizontally impacted lower wisdom tooth, but he accidentally took out one in front. Fortunately it was replanted right away, had RCT and crowned. This patient is still my regular patient.

Wait!

I am still improving with my extraction ★

At the early stage of my career, I thought I was quite good at extraction. I found myself improving as I did more cases. I admit I was quite arrogant thinking I am the best and no one does better than I do. When I felt I was not getting any better I started preparing courses for wisdom tooth extraction. As I was preparing for the seminar I looked into how other practitioners were doing and found there were many other techniques. I started incorporating those techniques and found myself getting better. I was very humble at that stage.

There is a quote saying 'The best way to learn is to teach'. This is why I run the seminar every year and hope writing this book does the same.

09
Hu-Friedy EL5C with wider tip ★★★

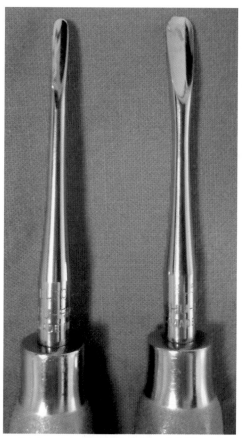

━ This is a photograph with EL3C and EL5C adjacent to each other. 5C is not quite twice as wide as 3C but it looks more than twice wider to my eyes.

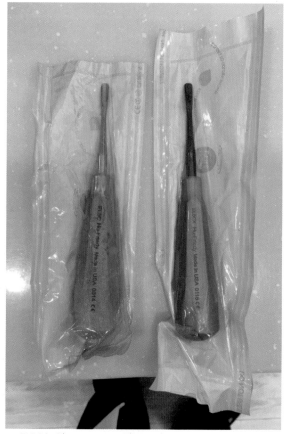

━ EL5C inside separate sterile pouch.

Due to higher frequency of usage, EL5C is in its own sterile pouch so that it can be used readily. As EL3C is very sharp, I advise to start with EL5C for beginners prior using EL3C. Normally straight elevator that is most commonly used is 4mm wide and for the dentists who are used to the straight elevator is recommended to use 5C before 3C.

This elevator is not in the extraction kit. It is always kept in separate sterile pouch and gets used only when necessary. When there is widened PDL space due to the inflammation around vertically erupted wisdom tooth or when tooth is sectioned with large bur of at least size 6.2% of the time I use this elevator EL5C. Black elevator from above photo is a new product from Hu-Friedy with a better surface treatment. I am very satisfied so far.

10
Comparison of width of elevators ★

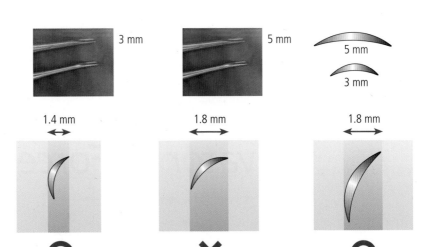

━━ This picture illustrates if 3 mm elevators goes into wider gap, it can idle. The different gaps are created from #4 bur and #6 bur. 3 mm elevator can be useful without bone removal in narrow space but if space becomes wider, it gets difficult to engage.

━━ This picture illustrates how 3 mm, 5 mm elevators work in wider gap. The gap has been created by #6 round bur but can be used in cases where the gap is too wide for 3 mm elevator to engage properly. I use 5 mm elevator to extract vertically impacted lower wisdom tooth where impaction is not too deep and there is buccal bone loss due to the inflammation making the gap too wide for 3 mm elevator.

EL3C elevator can not be used as a wheel if #6 round bur was used to section the tooth. Therefore #4 round bur is used to remove the coronal part of the tooth. If there is a widened PDL space or a large crevice that has been created from removal of part of the tooth, 5 mm elevator becomes useful.

Where there are not many wisdom tooth extraction cases, I recommend you equip 1 EL5C for every 3 EL3C whereas if you do it more often 1 EL5C for every 5 EL3C would be preferable. However if you do the bone removal more often or use a larger round bur, it would be wise to have more EL5C ready.

Wait!

Which do you prefer?

Elevator Vs Forceps

Most of the new clinicians think it is cool to use elevator for the extraction than forceps. Of course it depends on the professor/clinical demonstrator which instrument you were allowed and taught to use. This might have caused the elevators and forceps being completely contrary to each other but they aren't. Every instrument has its own use. I often use elevator but when the tooth can be extracted by forceps, I would use the forceps first. Forceps are used first especially in cases where lower wisdom tooth is near full eruption making buccal elevation difficult or for fully erupted upper wisdom tooth. If there is enough buccal bone to be used as fulcrum I would use elevator first but if you have to remove a buccal bone to create a fulcrum or use the adjacent tooth as a fulcrum, it is advantageous to use a forceps first. Throughout the chapters, I mentioned which instrument is better for which circumstances, so I wouldn't mention it again but the elevator and forceps are mutual supplementation not contrary to each other.

Forceps for Wisdom Tooth Extraction

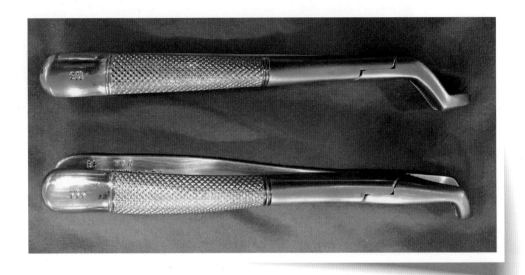

As I like to use an instrument that I am familiar with, the forceps I use most often are from Hu-Friedy even though it is pricey. Since the forceps are very durable and hard they don't break even after frequent use for 10 years that I did. The forceps I use are classified only for upper and lower not left and right, and more you use, more you become familiar with its proper use and where to be cautious. Teeth have various anatomy and different instrument is used for every different tooth with different anatomy, it will take along time to get used to the instrument. ?? OR

This sentence sounds more logical.

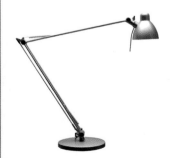

01
Dr. Youngsam Kim's forceps ★★★

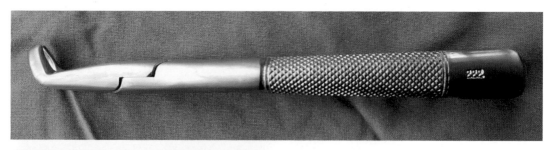

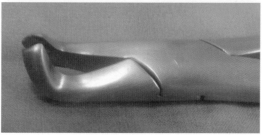

For lower, I use Hu-Friedy 222. I don't use a forceps with a beak since it is better to become familiar with a single instrument. Forceps with a beak doesn't make a good grip for a single rooted tooth or submerged wisdom tooth. I use this forceps as it can extract a tooth regardless of its root shape.

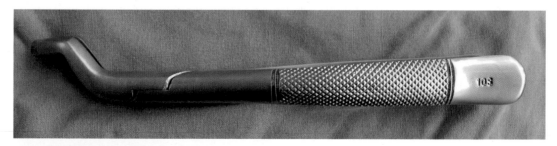

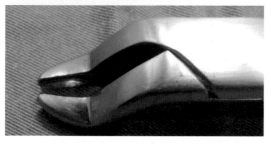

For upper wisdom tooth, I mainly use Hu-Friedy 10S. It is universal not left or right specific. There is forceps with a beak to fit into the furcation, but I don't use it for the same reason as mandible. Other than upper first molar, forceps with a beak has very limited use due to various anatomy of the wisdom tooth. I haven't had difficulty extracting a wisdom tooth with just these two forceps.

02
The comparison between rubber dam clamp and beaks of the forceps

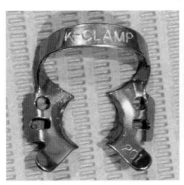 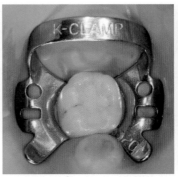 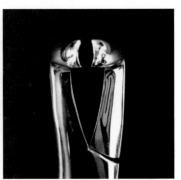

Why do rubber dam clamps look like this? The cross section of forceps look similar to that of rubber dam clamp, except that rubber clamp has the elasticity to prevent the damage to the tooth. It is because this shape allows the firm grip on the tooth just below the maximum circumference of the tooth. I use rubber dam clamp to check if there is a firm engagement before I decide to use forceps. It is key to use forceps prior to using elevator if rubber dam clamp gets a firm engagement.

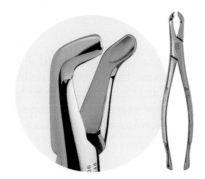 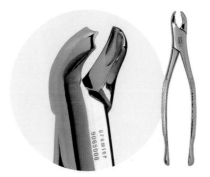

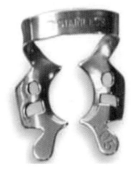

But some forceps have a beak in the middle. For mandibular one, there is one each on buccal and lingual surface whereas for upper there is a beak on buccal. They allow the firm grip all the way into the furcation. However unless there is a severe periodontal disease it is quite difficult for beak to extend into the furcation and even more difficult for third molar due to the high alveolar bone level.

Imagine if a clamp had a beak in the middle, it would interfere with engagement rather. That is why I use a universal forceps without beak. Many forceps with beak are limited to 6's and 7's according to the manufacturers. I never recommend to use these for 8's and even not for 7's as there are lots of variations and some do not have furcation. Even if a forceps has a 4 grip points (the corner of beak), it would only engage 3 points in most cases causing the forceps to slip when you try to mobilize the tooth.

I have a single forceps with beaks which I only use when there is extensive decay on the coronal part of the tooth with bone resorption which allows the forceps extend into the furcation area. I haven't used this for years whilst extracting thousands of third molars.

03
At the Dr. TaeHee Lee's clinic in Australia... ★

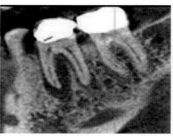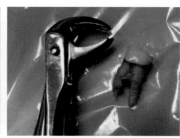

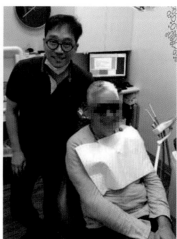

This is x-ray of the tooth that was extracted and extracted tooth with the forceps used. Photograph was taken with consent of the patients at Dr. TaeHee Lee's clinic.

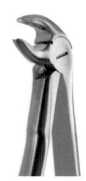

This forceps with beak was ideal for the tooth with above x-ray which had furcation and was crowned. However this kind of forceps designed for lower posterior wouldn't be ideal for third molar extraction.

Large manufacturer such as Hu-Friedy and Premier advised the clinicians to use these forceps case by case but I never recommend for lower third molar. Apart from the slipping issue, the direction where forceps move is not on the extraction path of the wisdom tooth. When misused it can damage distal surface of 7's.

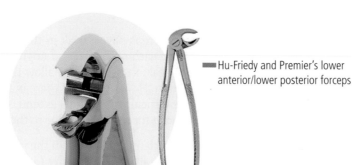

■ Hu-Friedy and Premier's lower anterior/lower posterior forceps

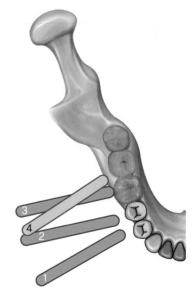

In number 1's case, and maybe for number 2, it could be possible. But for 3, it is impossible and it would look like number 4. This could lead to damage on distal surface of #7 while luxating. When using these forceps to extract premolar, it needs to be perpendicular to the buccal surface of the tooth. Ideally it would be best not to use like myself unless extracting lower anterior.

04
New products from Hu-Friedy ★

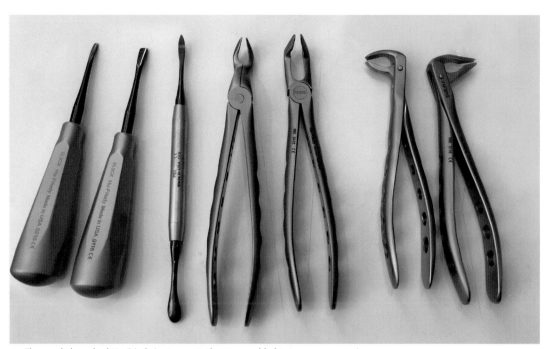

▬ The newly launched Hu-Friedy instruments that were added to my armamentarium.

In 2016, I was gifted new instruments from Hu-Friedy Korea. It was due to the promotional effect through my ongoing seminar, and they also were interested in reviews for those instruments from me. I actually want to express my thanks to Hu-Friedy for making good products and enabling easy extraction of wisdom teeth. There are many similar instruments but without Hu-Friedy I could have only been an ordinary dentist. Whether it is made of different material or just being new products, it has been getting good comments due to its sharpness. How and where to use still stay the same as the previous range.

But new forceps are quite different from the previous model. New forceps has a bit more elasticity so I wasn't very familiar with it but I am using it routinely when I need forceps with small beak. I will mention how it is used in more detail later in the chapter.

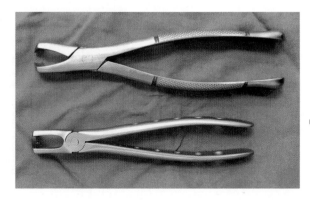

▬ Length comparison of new and older forceps. New forceps are a bit shorter. I think it is to prevent clinicians putting excessive force on it as it isn't as strong as previous model even though new forceps are made of special metal.

05
New forceps from Hu-Friedy with a small beak ★

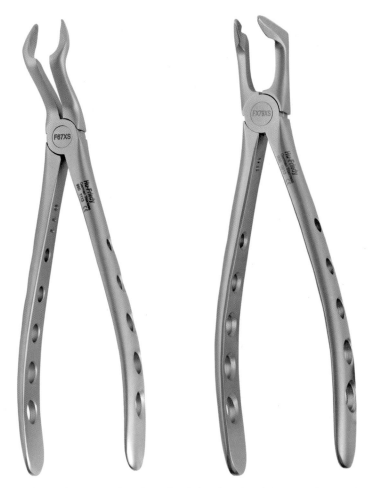

━New forceps from Hu Friedy with small and sharp beak (Model F67XS and FX79XS)

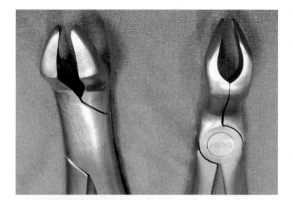

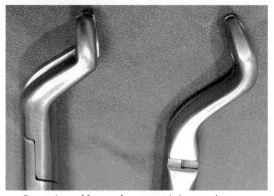

━Comparison of forceps for upper wisdom tooth

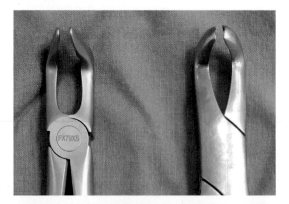

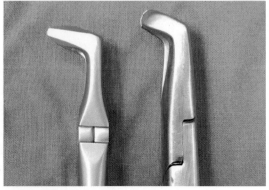

━Comparison of forceps for lower wisdom tooth

I didn't use these in the beginning, but I have found these very handy after a little while especially for upper wisdom tooth with slight vertical impaction or lower wisdom tooth after coronal/cervical removal. I was worried about its breakage due to elasticity but the Hu-Friedy assured that it is made of more durable metal and is very strong. It hasn't broken or bent yet. Even though I only use it at occasion it could still be used more frequently than other clinicians due to more number of extractions I do.

06
Basic principle of wisdom tooth extraction using forceps ★★★

▬ Take a firm grip on tooth

60% of the entire force needs to be used to get a firm grip on the tooth so that forceps don't slip. I wiggle the tooth back and forth with forceps not to luxate the tooth but to make sure it has a firm grip. If you are unsure whether the forceps have firm grip then you should never apply the force. If forceps with a beak slips, it can easily damage the adjacent tooth. Sometimes it bounces and damages the opposing tooth. When you extract with forceps, please don't forget to check if you have a firm grip before applying any force.

▬ Forceps are for twisting, not pulling

This is the first principle that I teach during the wisdom tooth extraction seminar. I point out straight away if a student tries to pull it. It might take some time to throw away the habit of pulling. I am pretty sure that some of the readers might be extracting in the same way. Doing so makes extraction more difficult but one day, the opposing tooth would be damaged.

▬ Please be aware of the opposing tooth!

When you grab the lower wisdom tooth, rest your finger on the opposing tooth before you apply the force. This will be explained in the later chapter. For upper wisdom tooth extraction, you can not only increase the efficiency but also can prevent the damage on the opposing tooth by twisting.

▬ When you twist and wiggle the tooth, limit the force on the tooth

One day, one of my assistant asked me 'How come none of your extraction patients complain of the TMJ pain after extraction with forceps? My previous dentist did less than 1/10 of what you did and still many of them complain of TMJ pain during or after extraction.' I simply answered ' It is important that the force doesn't become transmitted all the way to TMJ'. When you open a bottle cap, the force only needs to be transmitted to bottle cap. If force goes to the whole bottle, there is a problem. We will come back to this but when you wiggle and twist the lower wisdom tooth with a forceps, it is crucial to ensure minimal transmission of the force to TMJ. To do so, the tooth needs to in the centre of the rotation of the force from the forceps. Once you become familiar, you can divide the force onto different part of the tooth.

▬ When you twist the tooth, please consider the shape of the root

I have mentioned above as it is always mentioned in other books or lectures but I don't think it is as important as other principles. It is also important to luxate a tooth with the forceps, then considering the shape of the root can be helpful. When I have difficulty trying to extract with thea forceps or an elevator, I try by alternating two instruments and it can be helpful to luxate according to the shape of the root.

07
Have a firm grip on the tooth with forceps ★★★

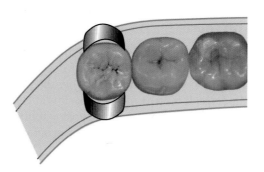 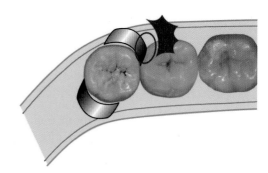

When you grab a tooth with the forceps, it needs to be very firm. If your entire force is 100% when you extract with the forceps, 60% of that should go to grabbing the tooth. That will prevent the forceps slipping like the diagram above. We often overlook the slipping force of the forceps. It can damage the opposing tooth due to the force of lever.

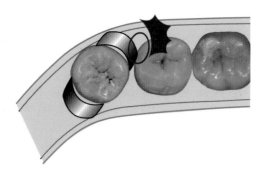 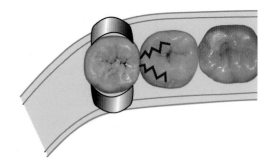

While wiggling wisdom tooth with forceps, the movement of the tooth can damage the coronal part of the adjacent tooth even without forceps slipping. Small wisdom tooth or severely rotated wisdom tooth can cause damage to adjacent tooth even with a little bit of movement. Let's not make one incident that makes me sad rather than make 99 incidents that make me happy.

Even though the forceps didn't slip or the wisdom tooth did not rub on it, adjacent tooth can still be damaged during the luxation of the wisdom tooth. Every force you apply should be directed away from the adjacent tooth.

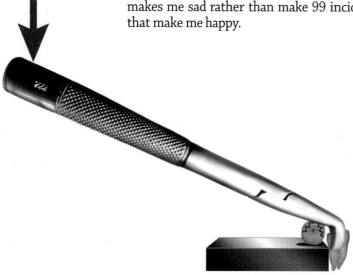

Like the diagram on the left, if you grab the wisdom tooth and push the forceps to the direction of the arrow with adjacent tooth in front, it would crack. When forceps slip, the edge of the beak is hitting the adjacent tooth much stronger than this. You need to be very cautious. If the adjacent tooth is sensitive to cold and hot after wisdom tooth removal, it could be also due to the damage from the forceps.

During the first session of lecture on wisdom tooth extraction, I always ask the attendants what made them to attend the course. One of them replied "While I was observing her senior dentist extracting the wisdom tooth with forceps, I saw the adjacent tooth cracking as the dentist started to twist the wisdom tooth. I thought there must be a better,and safer techniques". She realized it might not be as easy as she thought. I have heard the same opinions from my other colleagues and friends. Please be reminded that the dentists who don't take out the wisdom tooth are not doing so due to the fear of damaging the nerve. The technique we learn in the beginning is very important. Those incidents should not happen even once in many occasions but during our entire career. Let's not make one incident that makes me sad. We need to adhere to the principle.

Wait!

How good is Dr. Youngsam Kim at wisdom tooth extraction?

As I have mentioned, I can't really say that I am much better than any other clinicians in extracting wisdom tooth out. Those are better than myself in other fields of the dentistry so wisdom tooth extraction was likely to be out of their interests. The only and best way I can express is in number of the extractions I did. One day I received a phone call from 'National health audit office' They have told me that my clinic made the most claims for wisdom tooth extraction. At the peak, it was nearly as twice many as the clinic who did the second most extraction. I assume they called me due to the excessive number of the claims. But wisdom tooth extraction was a treatment that other clinics were not really keen to do, they didn't bother me after all. They were just curious I think.

Since my practice is located in Gangnam, many patients are without the national health insurance such as foreign resident and international students. So the actual number of extractions I did would be more than what national health audit office knows.

I have asked exact statistics from National health, but they could not give due to privacy issues. From analysis that I did for many years, my clinic did the most wisdom extractions from 2002 to 2011 (this is when the special wisdom tooth clinic opened up) and now roughly at between top 3 to top 5 due to more wisdom tooth clinics that started practicing. Recently I heard another dentist saying that he did the most wisdom extractions in Korea but the actual number was less than half of what I did. Anyway even if my clinic is ranked between 3rd and 5th in number of wisdom tooth extractions, I claim my clinic is the top clinic that has been extracting wisdom teeth consistently over the longest period of time. This is for extractions per clinic as extraction per practitioner is more difficult to find out.

08
Always consider the opposing tooth while using forceps ★★★

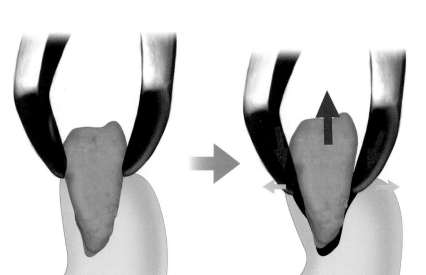

For lower wisdom tooth extraction, you must rest your finger on the opposing teeth before you apply any pressure. Forceps can bounce off by simply grabbing the tooth for some male clinicians. Extra caution is required for the wisdom tooth with small coronal size. When forceps bounces off, it is not molar that crack but rather anterior teeth can crack. When you are extracting premolars, you have to be very careful not to damage the upper anterior teeth.

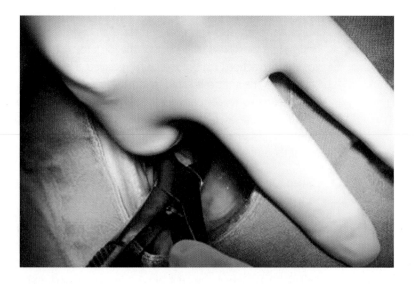

When extracting lower wisdom tooth with forceps, the finger should be rested on the opposing teeth after grabbing the wisdom tooth with just adequate force that prevents forceps slipping. You do not have to keep an eye while twisting and wiggling the tooth. As explained above, forceps and/or wisdom tooth can bounce off simply by grabbing and when wisdom tooth is extracted, it doesn't become extracted gradually but springs out of the socket.

09
Forceps is are to twist, not to pull ★★★

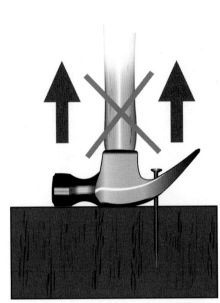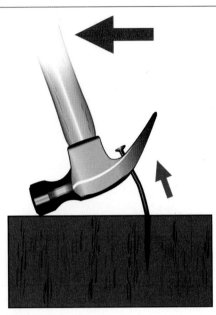

Forceps are for twisting, not for pulling.

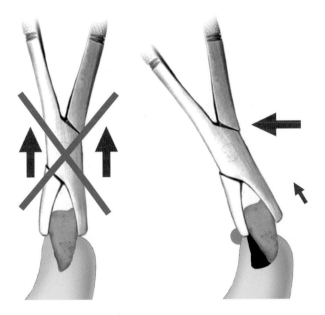

The above picture explains all. Wisdom tooth extraction is like pulling off the magnet from the metal board, not pulling off the nail. Therefore instantaneous force is critical than the gradual force. Shouldn't this be opposite? If you try to remove the nail from the wood by pulling, the foot should be resting on the wood to prevent it moving toward the same direction. All the force needs to be directed onto the nail and surrounding not onto the whole wood board. That is exactly why TMJ can become sore if you misuse the forceps during extraction as the result of excessive force being transmitted onto the TMJ.

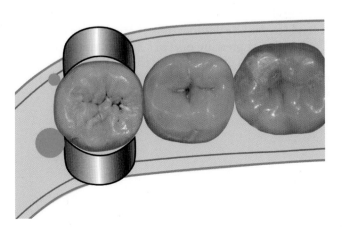

When you twist, make the centre of rotation on solid distal cortical bone like the green circles on the diagram. That makes the extraction much easier and prevents the damage on the adjacent tooth. I don't do luxation often and prefers to twist but if there is a trouble extracting by just twisting, I luxate a little just to have the right direction to apply the force.

10
Never put any pressure on TMJ ★★★

My long term time dental assistants have always said to myself how come my patients do not suffer from post op TMJ pain even with frequent use of the forceps. It is quite common during lower wisdom tooth extraction or after extraction using forceps. Even some tiny female dentists' patient suffers from TMJ pain during lower wisdom tooth extraction. In contrast I have solid biceps. I think where I place my centre of rotation is key to minimizing/eliminating the TMJ pain. I have seen many beginner associates grabbing the wisdom tooth with forceps and rotate/pull along the large axis. This will put enormous pressure on TMJ. The centre of rotation should be on the tooth and surrounding, as discussed in the previous page.

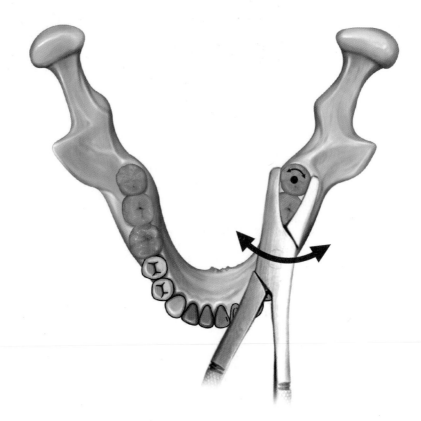

Dentists at the early stage of their career tend to grab the wisdom tooth with forceps and twist wide along the vertical axis. This can put quite a bit of pressure on TMJ. The force should be directed to the tooth, not TMJ. Please refer to explanation of how I pulled the nail out of the wood board and opening the cap of a beer bottle. The force is targeted onto the nail and the cap not onto the wood board and bottle. More extractions you do this would make more sense.

11
Twist depending on the morphology of the root ★

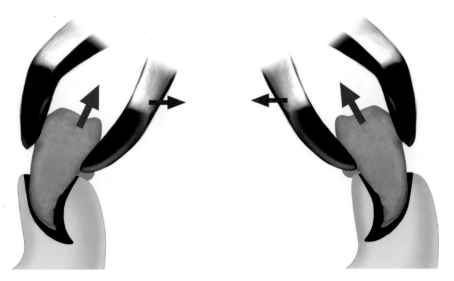

━━ Diagram explains the twisting should follow the root morphology

Depending on the root anatomy, Rotating and twisting the tooth is considered as a norm which I agree, but it should not be the only consideration when you start to twist the wisdom tooth. The radiograph is 2 dimensions whereas the root(s) are 3 dimensions. How elastic and dense the alveolar bone is around the roots should be considered prior to the shape of the root(s). Any practitioner can start to twist according to the shape of the root; however, the alveolar bone on that surface could be very dense making extraction very difficult. Extraction relies on the elasticity of periodontal ligament and alveolar bone. More importantly wisdom teeth that are functioning have much dense alveolar bone and ligament surrounding the roots, resulting in much harder extraction than impacted/non functioning wisdom teeth.

In conclusion, do not rely solely on the morphology of root(s) but apply the force toward various directions, luxate and feel which direction would be the best to apply the force.

By the way if there is no CT scan, coronal root morphology cannot be determined like the above diagram. Let's have a look at the picture on the right- hand side. If the alveolar bone on the left side is lingual, extraction can't usually be done in same way as above diagram. Rather it should be twisted toward buccal using hard buccal bone as fulcrum and elasticity on lingual alveolar bone.

12
Consider the centre of rotation when twisting with forceps ★

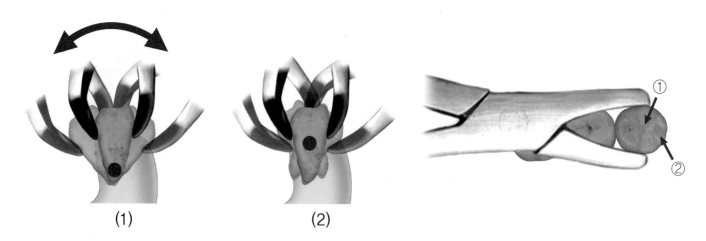

(1)   (2)

When wisdom tooth is wiggled, the centre of rotation needs to be controlled. More extractions you do, better you will be at finding the right centre of rotation. You will be able to focus the force onto the centre even while using a long, large forceps. When I am busy and the root is thin and curved, I break the crown on purpose with forceps then extract the root.

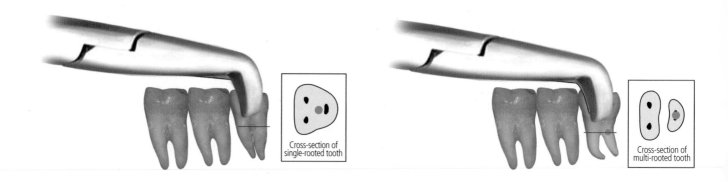

Cross-section of
single-rooted tooth

Cross-section of
multi-rooted tooth

How you will control the centre of rotation can be considered for single rooted tooth and multi rooted tooth. As you become more expert, breaking the crown can be done prior to extracting the root. It is impossible to explain this through the writing or diagram. You will need to improve yourself by doing more and more extractions. It is important to reach the stage where patients do not complain of any TMJ pain during/after extraction. Once you have achieved that stage, try to concentrate the force onto the root. But even with all these explanation, I don't think it is as crucial as other principles.

13
How to minimize the pressure onto TMJ ★★★

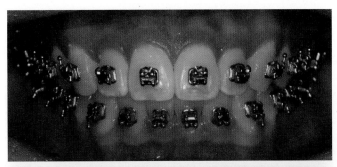

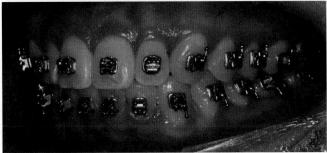

How should clinicians approach to minimize the pressure transmitted to TMJ? If we look at the brackets for orthodontics, this bracket can move the tooth even the root of it. During orthodontic treatment the entire force is applied to move the tooth. How about when we debond the bracket? We tried the best not to transmit any force to the tooth while debond. Same principle must be applied when extracting third molar tooth to prevent any excessive force transmitted onto TMJ. As mentioned on the previous page, tooth is being detached, not pulled out.

Not pulling... but twisting.

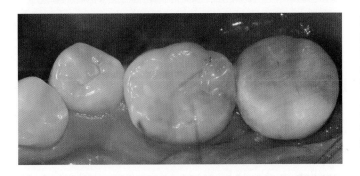

How about when removing a temporary crown with a forceps? Don't we all try to exert the force on the crown, but not on the tooth?

It is same principle for TMJ. The opposite side where being twisted acts as fulcrum of the lever.

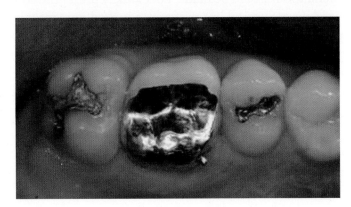

When we remove the temporary crown we exert the force only on single direction. If the temporary crown doesn't come off the tooth, we might apply the force to opposite direction but we never apply the pressure from the opposite direction at the same time.

To emphasize again, third molar is being detached, not being pulled out and if this can be remembered extraction would be smooth without any excessive force transmitted onto TMJ.

Every force that I apply to extract the tooth should be applied so that it doesn't go off the tooth.

Handpiece and Bur for Extraction of Wisdom Teeth

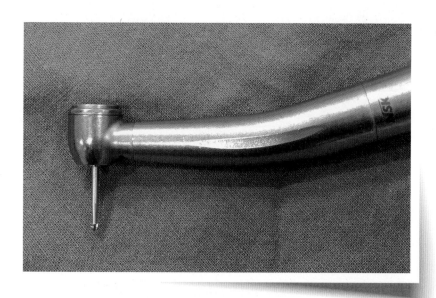

Primarily uses high speed handpieces and surgical round burs for surgical extraction. I will briefly explain why this is the case for most practitioners including myself.

However, there seems to be no significant difference between handpieces, whether it is high or low speeds, and also between various brands. Handpiece head sizes aren't as of great importance as long as it has sufficient power and fibreoptic lighting.

If a recommendation should be made, I personally prefer the cost and maintenance effective NSK handpiece. Surgical bur preference is predominantly long shank bur, and I will share the pros and cons compared to the fissure bur in this chapter.

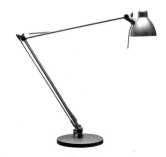

01
Dr. Youngsam Kim's handpiece ★

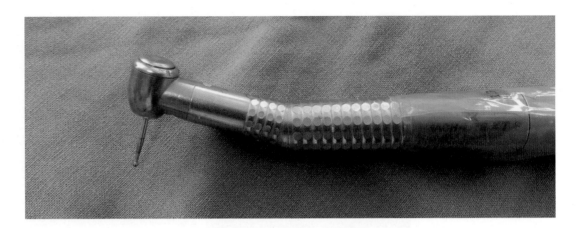

I don't have any preference over handpiece as long as it has a fibreoptic. I used to use Kavo (Germany), NSK (Japan) and Sirona (Germany). These days I mainly use NSK (Japan), Morita (Japan), W&H (Austria) and I prefer NSK (Japan) over other brands due to its cost effectiveness.

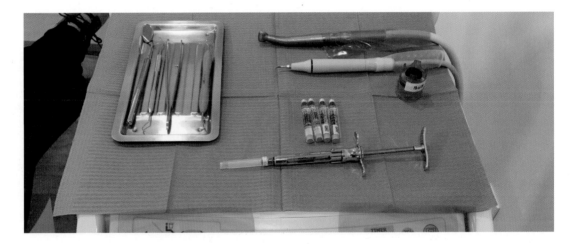

It is fundamental that every instrument goes through sterilization. However basic instrument sets, anesthetic syringes, handpieces, and ultrasonic scalers are placed on a single sterilization pouch? Comparing this to a world-class level, it can be seen as a compromised infection control standard. With having a particularly low fee for wisdom teeth extraction in Korea, this is regarded as a relatively high infection control standard. Handpieces and ultrasonic scaler tips are sterilized after every use and wrapped with an anti-microbial rubber ring for use. It would be nice to have the oscillating rod within sterilized as well, however it is little too early in Korea. Despite my best attempts, I often get opposition from dental suppliers based on a lack of system and demand.

Using an ultrasonic scaler for calculus-dense cases only as ultrasonic scaler could cause crack within enamel. The wisdom tooth surgery field should be clean and for that reason we routinely perform scaling unless the site is impeccable.

02
Looking back at the anatomy of high speed handpiece ★★

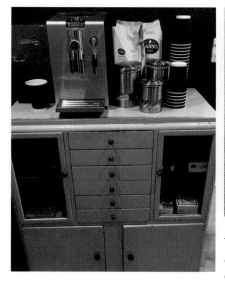

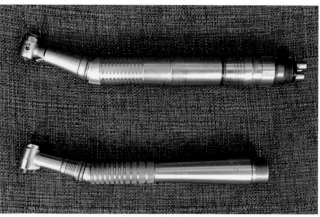

When I was in Australia to give a lecture on wisdom tooth extraction, I visited a dental clinic which was displaying old instruments on the reception area. Below is the comparison between old and new high speed handpieces.

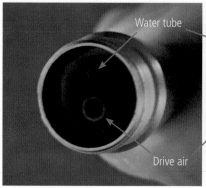

Water tube

Drive air

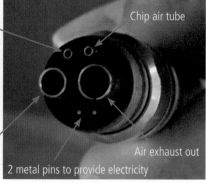

Chip air tube

Air exhaust out

2 metal pins to provide electricity

■ 2 hole high speed handpiece rarely used in developed countries but still being used in some other countries.

■ Modern high speed handpieces have 4 holes with international standard sizes and also has 2 pins to provide the electricity for the lightbulb.

In general high speed handpiece is air driven and water gets sprayed towards the bur. The very old handpieces did not have any tube for the air to exit. However relatively new hand pieces have separate air exhaustion tube through which all the air that rotates the bur exit to the rear of the handpiece. Surprisingly many dentists are still aware that air turbine which spins the bur gets sprayed at the same time as water spray. This air is called chip air which is separate to the turbine. There used to be only single spray of water jet when we prep the tooth however it has evolved to have three sprays to prevent the tooth to overheat and burn. We can turn off the chip air on the handpiece like we can turn off the water from triple x tip.

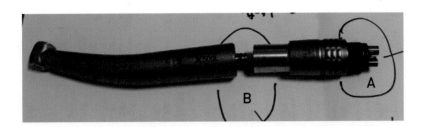

If the connecting part of the high speed handpiece looks like A, it would be quite difficult to connect to the main operating cable day to day basis. That is why handpieces these day have standards like B. Every company has different shape so it is crucial to check if the coupling is the one that matches the handpiece itself.

It is common to use high speed handpiece even after raising flap. Contra angled high speed handpieces are commonly used in Japan and Korea to extract wisdom teeth. However only slow speed straight handpieces are used in some countries still due to the risk of air emphysema. It might lead to court action if air emphysema occurs and to other complications. However I have never experienced or been reported any cases of air emphysema during wisdom tooth extraction with high speed handpieces. It happened few times while polishing class 5 cervical restoration or while blowing the air into the sulcus while taking impression.

I have extracted tens of thousands of wisdom teeth using high speed handpieces and yet to see an air emphysema. Even many dentists and periodontists in Europe and America use high speed even after raising flap.

It is quite safe to use high speed handpiece during wisdom tooth extraction. I have attached the photo to explain that air that turbines the handpieces does not get sprayed as same direction of the water. It is the chip air that gets sprayed. I have asked staff members to other surgery to turn off the chip air if there is a concern with air emphysema, however they said 'no' as it is air driven. Some clinicians use 45-degree handpiece saying that it is safe to be used air is discharged through the rear head of the handpiece. Air that rotates the bur discharges through the exhaust tube. There is separate air that helps water sprayed onto the site of the drilling called chip air. If there is a concern chip air can be turned off. Operating chairs these days have a switch to turn on/off the chip air. I don't think it is necessary but there is an option to switch the air off if you are worried. Generally 45-degree handpiece and low speed handpiece have chip air and some have the switch to turn off the chip air and it depends on each manufacturer.

Extractions are done on the chair, not in operating theatre in some university hospitals in Korea. They uses low speed handpiece for wisdom tooth extraction and use chip air to spray the water. If you use low speed handpiece to extract, a bigger flap is needed and more bone removal is necessary. In some cases, unnecessary bone removal could be required which could have been avoided if extracted using high speed handpiece. However I rarely use high speed handpiece on maxilla but there are many dentists who are not reluctant to use it on maxilla. The reason I don't use is emphysema is slightly more common on maxilla but it is rare that tooth sectioning is required for upper wisdom tooth.

03
Dr. Youngsam Kim's preferred bur ★★★

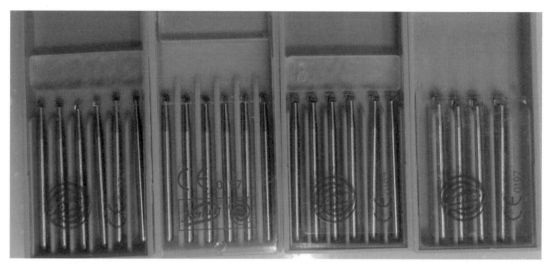

▬ The author's surgical long shank burs: in stock or used in the past - #4, #5, #6 & #8 from left

The author usually uses a long shank round bur. Size 4 (diameter 1.4 mm) was mainly used in the past, now size 6 (diameter 1.8 mm) is mainly used. Size 4 is now used as a supplementary and for vertically impacted wisdom teeth. The indication for each bur will be covered later in the chapter.

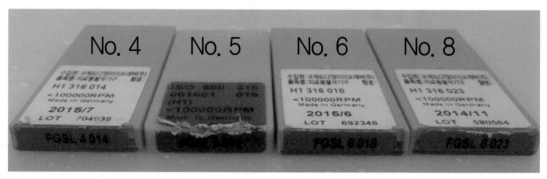

▬ Picture of labels with bur's number and diameter printed

Not sure about the significance of the diameter difference?

It's more significant than you think. The Author usually uses size 6 but occasionally size 4 is chosen.

If the primary purpose is cutting then size 6 is used, but for purchase point creation and for sectioning of the tooth size 4 is used. The author strongly recommends clinicians to have size 4 and 6 to be in their must-have repertoire. However, size 4 bur has a diameter of 1.4 mm which is smaller than width of its shank, it is not effective at cutting deep into tooth. With size 4, it is required to opening up its entry points at multiple levels or sectioning off drilled portion allowing shank to enter during extraction. It may not be easy to understand with words. Let's look at illustration.

04
Long shank surgical round burs: Their numbers and diameters ★

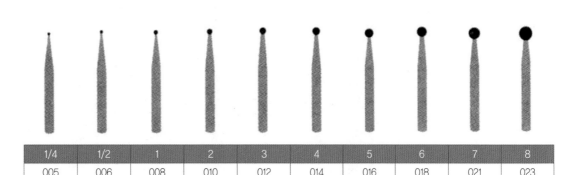

1/4	1/2	1	2	3	4	5	6	7	8
005	006	008	010	012	014	016	018	021	023

The number and diameter of the bur

Used size 4 (diameter 1.4 mm) round bur. It was thought to be only bur at beginner's level and later when experienced, I used it out of familiarity and now use more for finely sectioning tooth. However, as author's vertebrae suffers, started using larger bur instead. The occluding vertebrae has resulted decreased strength and endurance in author's arm. Size 4 round bur has smaller diameter to its shank diameter and it causes frequent locking during cutting hence greater force is required. For that reason, some dentists recommend size 8 bur (diameter 2.3 mm). With size 8 bur, cutting can be much easier with an expense of finesse. They probably have yet to personally pay for handpiece repair. Allowing some variation, it is accepted that wider burs have an increasing chance of handpiece cartridge damage. If the bur diameter is much bigger than the shank diameter, it increases the damaging effects on the handpiece cartridge. Based on my experience, the routine use of size 6 bur (diameter 1.8 mm) over size 4 bur will definitely result in more frequent handpiece cartridge damage. The exception would be with beginners using a size 4 bur with frequent locking into the tooth while cutting, which can result in more damage to the handpiece.

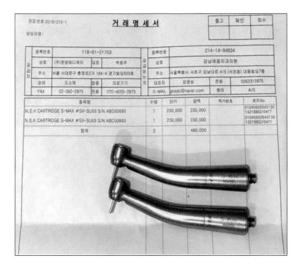

Handpiece Cartridge Replacement Price

The author's friend (who had worked at Shin Heung dental company for 10 years, now the owner of a different dental company) has been in business with me for past 16 years. The author may be taken advantage of here?? but this is how much it is for a simple handpiece repair. Considering the low fee for wisdom tooth removal, this is a big expenditure. This is why the author likes NSK handpieces for their low maintenance costs.

05
No.5 016 and No.6 018's difference is very important! ★★★

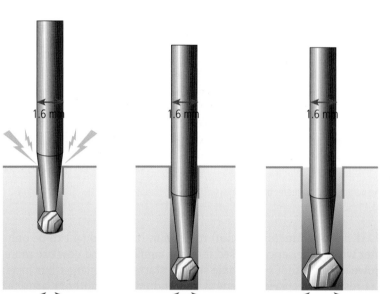

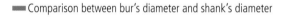
Comparison between bur's diameter and shank's diameter

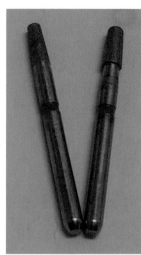
Authors preferred burs, 016 (left) and 018(right), for inlay preparation and this shows the difference in size.

Bur Shank's width is 1.6 mm, identical to No. 5 bur

Taking the bur's shank diameter into consideration, the diagram illustrates burs of No. 4, 5 & 6 in slightly emphasizing manners. No 4 bur is good for finely sectioning tooth, but it is hard to cut deeply due to its wider diameter of shank to bur. Therefore, it is recommended to use the wider diameter No. 6 bur for complete sectioning crown off in horizontally impacted wisdom tooth removal case. If the author has to remove a horizontally impacted wisdom tooth with a No. 4 bur, I often fracture the crown into multiple pieces each time locking happens.

Why don't we use No. 5 then? The mid-way is not a solution to every problem, the No. 5 bur has the negatives of both No. 4 & 6 burs. Some University Hospitals allow for the single use of burs, but it is impractical to many privately owned practices considering the low wisdom tooth extraction fee. Burs often get sterilized for reuse and staff at the practice may confuse the No. 5 bur with No. 4 or 6 burs. For this reason, it is not recommended to stock No. 5 burs at all. It is much easier to distinguish between No. 4 and 6 burs without the presence of No. 5 and this can create unnecessary mix ups in the practice.

Wait!

Various arguments associated with wisdom tooth ★★★ extraction #3

Which bur to use with high speed handpiece?

Round Bur Vs Fissure Bur

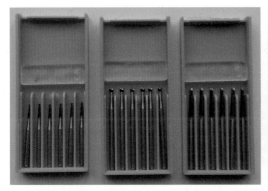
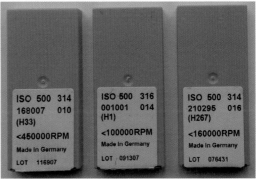

■ The oral surgeon's (OMFS's), who have worked with the author for a long time, extraction surgical burs (manufactured by Komet, German)

A pack of 6 price:
High speed short extraction carbide fissure bur: 16,150 won ($16)
High speed surgical round bur: 31,000 won ($31)
High speed long shank surgical fissure bur: 47,500 won ($47)

The author only uses surgical round burs for high speed handpiece. I have two oral surgeons whom have worked with me for a long time and one exclusively uses fissure burs, and the other uses both round and fissure burs in combination. Staff were accommodating of each operator's preference (In this book, the author calls burs that are not round and tapered metal burs 'surgical fissure bur' and the identical configuration in diamond burs is called 'surgical diamond bur').

The author's strong preference for round burs is because fissure burs can often be more damaging to surrounding soft tissue. My ESSE philosophy, with minimal incision and flap, can find the surgical bur abrading the surrounding soft tissue. Oral surgeon used to considerable incision length and full flaps being raised with every extraction, doesn't often run into impinging soft tissue, allowing for the use of a fissure surgical bur. It is recommended to use a round bur for more inexperienced general practitioners. Sometimes we often use the bur that we first learnt on out of familiarity and it stifles the use of other instruments. If you are relatively inexperienced, it may be a good idea to use both and compare. The author has had considerable experience with fissure burs and recently reused it for this book. However, the author finds that the round bur is the best answer.

The fissure bur often fractures preventing reuse, and a fractured fissure bur can be problematic when lodged into tissues.

06
Frequently used fissure burs ★

▶ Surgical Bur FG

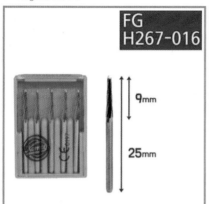

Komet company products which have been the author's longest companion and it makes up over 95% of the market in Korea. For this product, a 28 mm bur can be obtained and the author generally uses a 25 mm bur as an accepted general work-horse. The 25 mm bur compared to the 28 mm bur is less straining to the handpiece and causes less fractures. The shank diameter is equal to the widest part of the fissure bur at 1.6 mm and it tapers down towards the end. The narrowing is prone to fracture and breakage. If you do prefer the fissure bur, the author recommends the shorter 25 mm one over the 28 mm.

▶ Surgical Bur FG (Zekrya Bur)

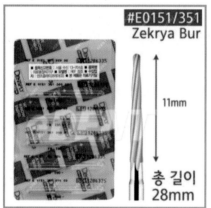

Dentsply products were introduced as the go to bur for a university dental hospital where I recently visited. After trailing it, the cutting ability was good but was very demanding to the handpiece. This probably contributes to fractures and breakages. The university clinic also commented they have to treat them as single use only due to its high incidence of fracture and breakage. For your information, this product range also sells a '5 mm shorter' 23 mm surgical bur. They sell in a pack of five and cost 33,000 won ($33). Due to its high fracture and breakage rate, it is thought to be selling at a cheaper price then other surgical fissure burs.

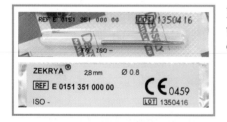

Dentsply burs are individually prepacked unlike those of Komet and these can be used without additional sterilization. This is a big advantage considering it is a surgical bur.

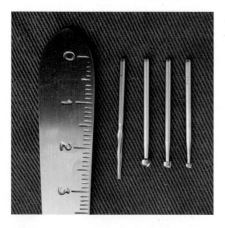

The surgical burs at author's practice and from left to right; Dentsply surgical fissure bur, Komet surgical round burs No. 8, No. 6 and No. 4 in order. Not sure whether round bur comes in 28 mm length as sometimes it is a struggle to reach extremely deeply placed horizontally impacted wisdom tooth due to its length. The practice stocks longer burs for these cases but it is only used in selectively as longer burs can create greater strain on the handpiece.

07
Utilizing surgical fissure bur - case 1 ★★★

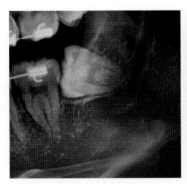 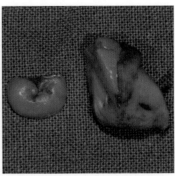 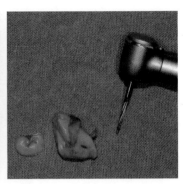

This is a case where an extraction was done utilizing a long shank surgical fissure bur. The author has a habit of taking postoperative photos with the instrument that's not routinely used.

This is a difficult case for operators with round burs where there is a considerable undercut at apical portion of lower 7's distal surface. The fissure bur is known for its cutting ability yet it is not more efficient in cutting speed when compared to round bur. Even though the mesial portion of crown is sectioned, the large undercut prevents the removal of sectioned crown. Therefore, sometimes it is necessary further cut the sectioned crown ..... ?

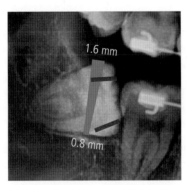

The undercut area is marked red, and the cutting surface is marked blue here. You can see why the sectioned crown fragment removal isn't easy here. The sectioned inferior crown portion was cut by the narrow end of bur due to its taper which is considerably smaller than the undercut area. Diameter of fissure bur's terminal tip is usually about half of it shank width, around 0.8 mm hence resulting in a very narrow cutting width.

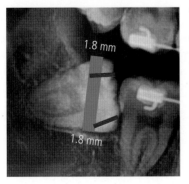

The sectioning of the inferior crown portion utilizing a surgical round bur is shown here. Compared to the fissure bur, No. 6 round bur (diameter 1.8 mm) can cut 1mm more at inferior portion hence is more effective for the undercut area. It is still smaller than the undercut area but is sufficiently compensated for by the lingual rotation upon removal of the sectioned crown fragment. Occasionally the sectioned crown fragment can be further cut vertically for ease of removal, it isn't discussed here as it will be covered in a later chapter. In conclusion, the difference at the inferior portion of the sectioned tooth by a round bur is much wider which eases removal by compensating for the undercut area.

Utilizing surgical fissure bur - case 2 ★

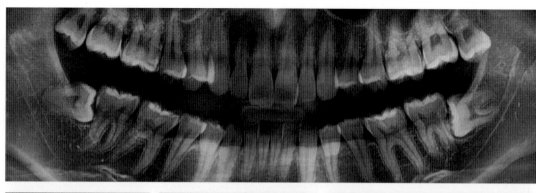

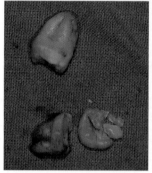 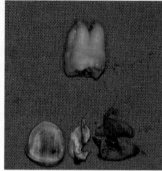 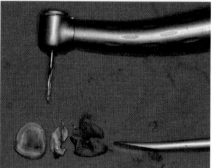

A 25 years old patient attended after watching the author's live surgery videos on YouTube. It is hard to satisfy a patient with high expectations but the surgery was relatively easy. The tooth #38 was removed by sectioning the crown, followed by subsequent sectioning of the root using elevators; no further tooth structure removal was done.

As mentioned, the author often takes photos of instruments used along with the extracted tooth for recording purposes as it may not get written onto chart. For this case, it was difficult to do distal crown cutting using a fissure bur without soft tissue hindrance.

If you have a strong preference for fissure burs, you may want to look into long shank, short cutting-end carbide fissure burs. However, these may also have a higher fracture risk in my opinion.

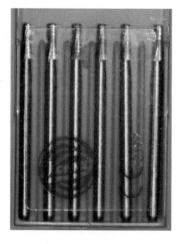

Two surgeons from 'Dae-Gu Cha Ahn Baek Dental', ranked within Top 5 dental practice in Korea, use these burs on high-speed handpiece. Author is trialling this bur for extraction based on the recommendation.

Utilizing surgical fissure bur - case 1 ★

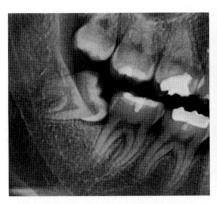
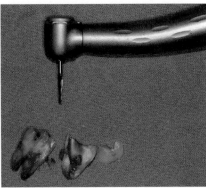

For this 21 year old male patient, the mesial crown cutting was initially performed yet the path of removal was hindered by the distal surface of the adjacent #7. Subsequent lifting and cutting was performed for this extraction. It would be recommended to use a fissure bur for these cases where the mesial portion of the tooth is slightly impacted against the distal surface of the adjacent #7.

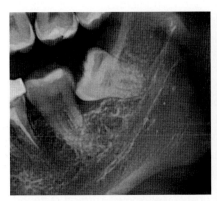
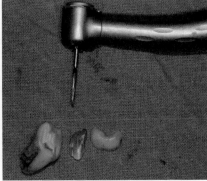

For this 30 year old female patient, fissure burs can effectively be utilized in this case of mild impaction to the distal surface of the adjacent #7. It was removed with oblique cutting and the tooth was turned the other way for the photo to show its lingual surface. Oblique cutting could be done with fissure bur, however, possible iatrogenic lingual and distal soft tissue damage must be carefully considered when performing oblique cutting, disto-cervical cutting, and others.

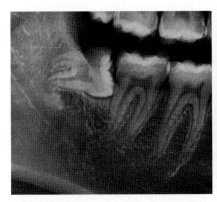
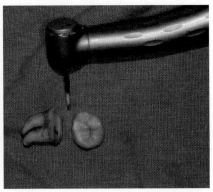

For this 22 year old male patient, the crown was easily sectioned and removed using a fissure bur assisted by the lack of undercut in 7's distal surface, and also the lack of bony enclosure around the crown.

Wait!

Various arguments associated with wisdom tooth ★★★ extraction #4

Which bur material to use?

Diamond Bur VS Carbide Bur

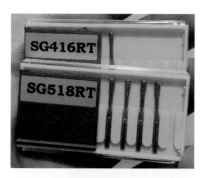

Diamond bur assisted wisdom tooth removal is often recommended for its superior cutting ability compared to carbide bur (the author doesn't agree with this). Also, because carbide burs often rebound causing adverse effects to the handpiece and could slip on cutting, resulting in possible soft tissue damage. However, there are few negatives compared to its numerous positives and this can be certainly overcome with operator experience. Tooth cutting is only a part of tooth extraction; hence use of a diamond bur can not be justified by its superior cutting ability only.

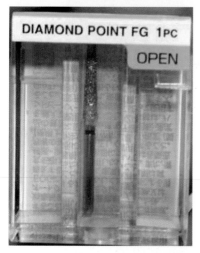

People with strong preference to carbide burs are concerned about possible diamond particles lodging into the surrounding tissues, and tooth particles may get wedged between surface gaps on the diamond burs causing sterilization problems. The author doesn't believe it is not an absolute contraindication and recommends a bur type that suits the operator's style and preference.

There are reasonably well-known surgical diamond burs for wisdom tooth extraction in Korea. They are reasonably priced at 19,000 won ($19) for a pack of 10 burs and it could be used as a single use only.

On the right is a Shofu (Japan) diamond surgical bur. It is a common choice in Japan and author thinks it is little too short. O Sung (Korea) makes burs with similar concept in 26.5 mm and 30 mm in lengths. The O Sung products are not as frequently used so the more commonly used Shofu (Japan) diamond surgical bur will be covered here.

In Japan, a diamond chamfer bur is often used for extraction and is not a general standard internationally.

For people who recommend diamond burs for its superior cutting ability, the author strongly recommends to use a carbide bur. The author likes to hear whether they could confirm their claim after using both diamond and carbide burs. Diamond burs often struggle to complete a tooth extraction and becomes almost unusable after second sterilization. Carbide burs can be used multiple times after repeated sterilizations. Also, diamond burs aren't easy to clean; removing lodged particles within the diamond gaps and it poses a sterilization risk hence some claims it must not be reused.

Despite of all these comments, it is most recommended to suit your own treatment philosophy and your hands.

08
Wisdom tooth extraction utilizing diamond bur – Korean ** Company

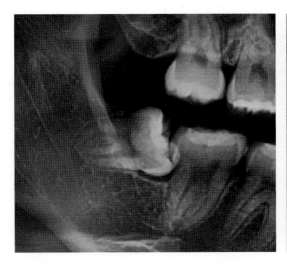
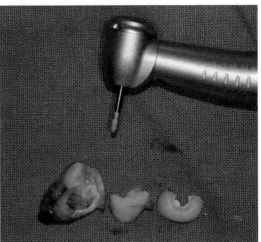

For this 22 year old female patient, the extraction was done utilizing Korean diamond fissure bur. The diamond bur was cutting very well in the first portion of the extraction but quickly became blunt caused difficulty in cutting. The tooth was luxated with subsequent lift & cutting for complete removal due to its bony enclosure surrounding the distal surface. The bur length was between conventional and long shank bur lengths, about 23.5 mm and it would be difficult to achieve deep vertical cutting.

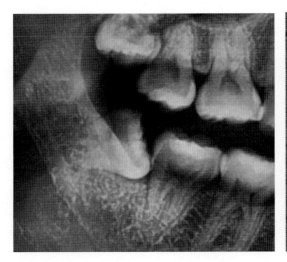
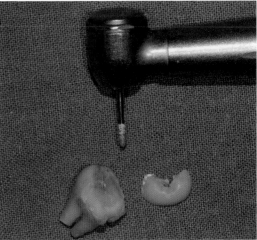

For this 25 year old female patient, mesial crown cutting was done for the extraction. The root fractured and the fragments were removed subsequently. With little cutting required as above, a diamond bur can be used but it is still recommended to be a single use due to its decreased durability. No rebound to the handpiece and minimal risk of bur fracture could be positives but this can be done with long shank surgical burs with some operator consideration.

09
Wisdom tooth extraction utilizing diamond bur – Japanese ** Company

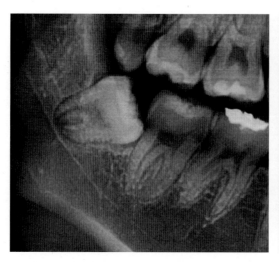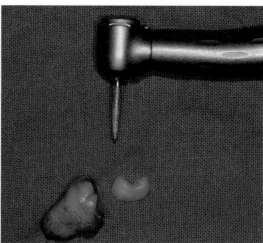

For this 23 years old female patient, a surgical diamond bur was used for the extraction. It is Japanese ** company product with 25 mm length, identical to conventional long shank surgical round burs and fissure burs. Diamond burs often cut smoothly through tooth structure until later stages where it gets blunt causing more difficulty in cutting difficult. The end of diamond bur is blunt out first and this is problematic for author's preferred surgical technique where multiple cuts are made for fracturing and delivering extracting tooth.

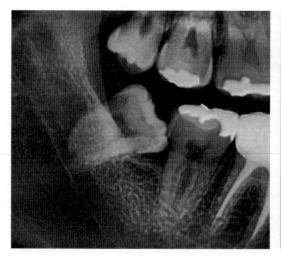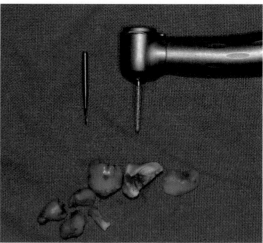

For this 28 year old male patient, it was initially attempted with diamond bur for mesial crown cutting but required subsequent lingual crown cutting. The root was surrounded by hard cortical bone which caused the crown to fracture upon lingual application of elevator. It is important to know that it's difficult to extract the roots of functioning wisdom tooth with whole crown exposed intraorally. The author used carbide fissure bur in addition to diamond bur while removing the roots.

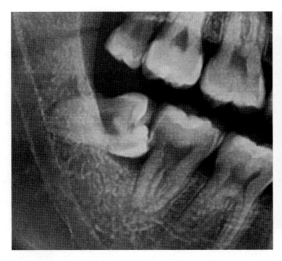 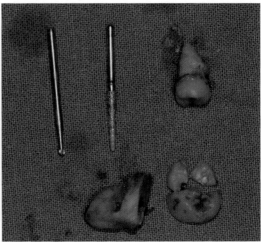

For this 27 years old male patient, the tooth was horizontally impacted with the whole crown above its surround alveolar bone. It is often difficult to just remove with lingual application of elevator. It was initially attempted with disto-cervical cutting with a diamond bur. As mentioned, diamond burs blunt out quickly, and it resulted in cutting multiple times for disto-cervical cutting. At the end, a long shank round #4 bur was used for cutting and creating a purchase point.

Wait!

Warning for possible soft tissue damage caused by surgical diamond bur ★★

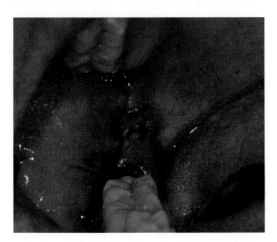

The soft tissue behind wisdom teeth can be damaged while performing disto-cervical cutting with surgical diamond burs. Surgical fissure burs in particular can be damaging as it can catch and tear soft tissue out. Most other diamond bur often abrade soft tissues upon cutting as shown here. High speeds exert constant water and air aiming at lower part of bur and this can create negative pressure gradient around bur in action resulting in pulling-in effect. Even though there was no soft tissue directly in contact with cutting bur, the damage was thought to be the result of soft tissue getting pulled into the bur via the negative pressure that was formed.

Regardless, the end-cutting round surgical bur is most suited for the author's philosophy of the least cutting, least smallest flap raise and multiple sectioning for removal.

10
Wisdom tooth extraction utilizing 30 mm long shank diamond round bur

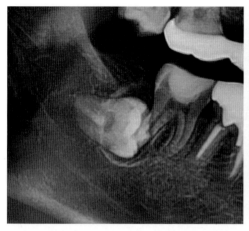
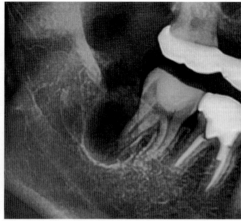
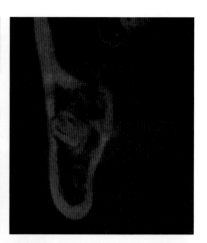

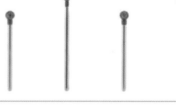
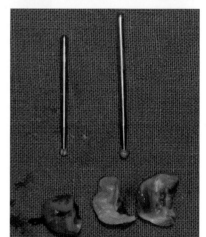

Ball Round				
Model Name				
Order Code	＊001ABR-S019C	＊001ABR-019C	＊001ABR-S029C	＊001ABR-029C
Head Length	1.76	1.76	2.66	2.66
Overall Length	25.0	30.0	25.0	30.0
Diameter	1.9	1.9	2.9	2.9

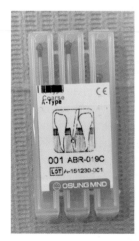
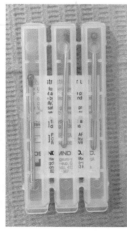

For this 25 years old female patient, she was referred by another dental practice. As per the author's preference to remove minimal amount of lingual bone, a 30 mm long shank bur was used to access from the occlusal all the way down to the bottom. As far as the author knows, it is the longest surgical bur in Korea. It is thought to be diamond rather than carbide to minimize strain applied to the handpiece cartridge by its extra-long shank. Long shank surgical round bur #6 was used for most of the cutting, and the deep apical portion was selectively cut with a 30 mm bur.

To be honest, the extraction could have been done without the extra-long bur. It would be nice to have one in your drawer for special circumstance. This is manufactured by O Sung Company, and I believe it can be ordered through various suppliers.

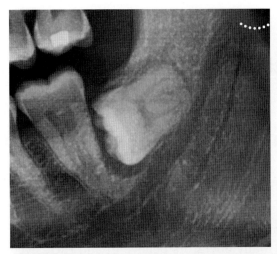
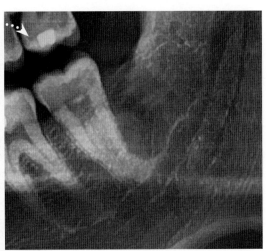

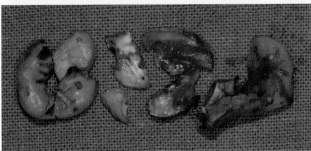

For this 30 year old male patient, he attended with the chief complaint of inflammation around the impacted wisdom tooth. In a few cases, the author's usual bur isn't able to reach to the full depth to section and may conduct supplementary lingual bone removal and attempt deliver sideways. The author may extract with the intention of using this long bur in rare cases.

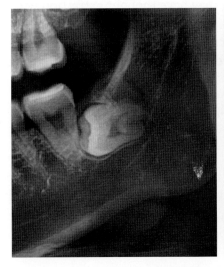
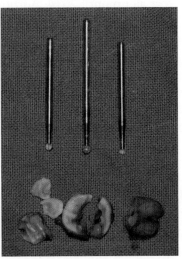

For this 27 year old female patient, she attended with her mother who is a dentist. With my growing experience and reputation, the author often gets self-referral and/or referred family members from many dentists. It is a lie if it doesn't cause a bit of stir inside. The extraction was easily done in 10 mins and the mother complemented.

Wait! **Various arguments associated with wisdom tooth ★★★ extraction #5**

Which handpiece to use?

High Speed VS Low Speed

It has been a long consideration whether to use high speed or low speed handpieces for wisdom tooth extraction. Many operators believe in and exclusively use their preferred instrument. Based on the author's survey, ** university exclusively use low speed handpieces for wisdom tooth extraction and other universities primarily used high speed and low speed as supplementary. Many oral & maxillofacial surgical offices do not have high speed handpiece set up and use slow speed handpieces for extraction. It is estimated about 10% of the world utilizes slow speed for prevention of surgical emphysema. In Barcelona University in Spain, the surgical department firmly believes slow speed must be used for extraction whereas the periodontic department does extraction utilizing high speed handpieces. The author doesn't believe we necessarily have to neither criticize nor follow anyone's opinion. It is most important to use your preferred instrument more effective and correct manners.

Author primarily use high speed handpiece and selectively use low speed handpiece for remaining root fragments of horizontally impacted wisdom tooth. Low speed wasn't used at all up until 2014. Author may have thought extraction with low speed is more for inexperienced and unskilled. Author also thought better extraction is one with fewer instruments were used. Since then author has changed his mind set and started to use various instruments and did extractions using low speed handpiece for a while.

The speed was a concern compared to high speed handpiece and what's more concern to high extraction volume operator like author was increasing fatigue associated with its use.

Many ** university graduates convert to high speed on their transition to private practices. Author strongly recommends to use high speed handpiece especially for relatively inexperienced wisdom tooth seminar attendees. Low speed handpiece is even more unaccustomed instrument as most of private practices often use high speed handpiece.

11
Dr. Kim's round burs for low speed handpiece ★★

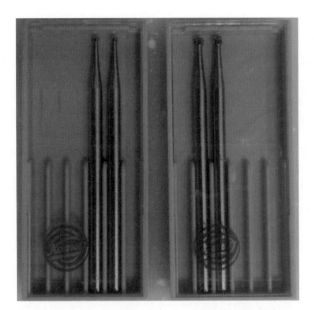

I also use round burs for low speed handpieces. As mentioned, low speed isn't often used and often selectively used to create a purchase point to very small root fragments. For that purpose, Size 4 or smaller size bur is preferred and it is a suited combination with author's chosen Hu-Friedy EL3C elevator. If you have to exclusively use low speed handpieces, it wouldn't be bad to use fissure burs with greater cutting ability.

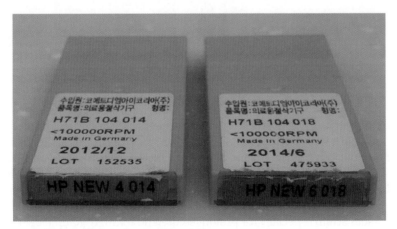

━━ Kim's surgical burs for low speed handpiece

Of course, bur size is identical to high speed ones.

Author also use size 4 (diameter 1.4 mm) round bur for low speed.

12
Fissure bur for low speed handpiece ★★★

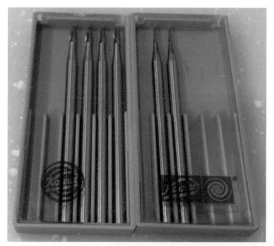 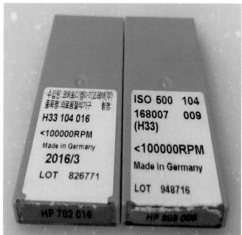

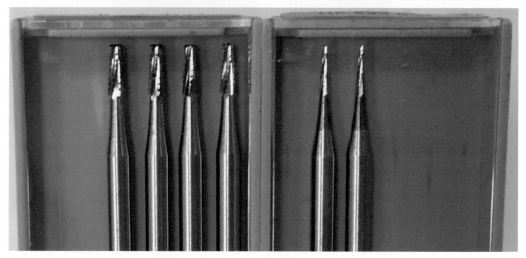

Operators with exclusive use of low speed handpieces often use fissure burs for their greater cutting ability. 016 or thicker bur is indicated due to reduced cutting ability of low speed. This bur also is smaller than its shank thickness (2.35 mm) and requires additional widening of the entry point upon deep, complete sectioning of the tooth. Slow speed fissure burs have a shorter cutting body length than high speeds resulting in a much lesser possibility of soft tissue damage. Narrow fissure burs on the right could be used to create a flat-head driver like groove at remaining root fragment of horizontally impacted wisdom tooth. There seems nothing like a highspeed round bur in speed and safety. More force requires using low speed for extraction due to its reduced cutting ability. It could result in accidental cutting of the lingual plate and rapidly build up wrist and shoulder strain especially for prolonged use and for high-volume operators like myself. Operators with a high volume of wisdom tooth extractions often start with low speed but eventually transition into a high speed handpiece.

Wait!

Dr. Youngsam Kim's Extraction Style?

Rather than relying on my own view, I have consulted with students and dentists over a long period of time. As mentioned, they all similarly agreed that my extraction style is simple and effective.

My wisdom tooth extraction style, based on the opinions gathered, could be described that it is not too different whether it is a difficult or basic wisdom tooth extraction. The author applies his own technique and principles according to needs.

I have my own method and philosophy using the elevator, the handpiece, and the forceps; I almost always move straight onto the next method if first attempt is not immediately successful. Based on my great deal of experience, I determine which method is more effective at each case.

From this book let's learn about the author's methods one by one. The secret may also be from using proficient instruments. The instruments used for basic and hard extractions are almost identical. For high volume of safe wisdom tooth extraction without complications, I solely use the best-suited instruments and methods to my own hands. Above all, I suffer progressive stiffness and chronic inflammation in my back further complicated by the surgical complication sustained previously. It has qualified as a disability. Therefore, I try to do rapid extractions avoiding the same damaging posture for a prolonged time. My constant, uniform extraction instruments and methods may be because extraction is often done at one position with a standardized posture due to my inability to look down and move freely.

Extraction of Wisdom Teeth using Low Speed Handpiece

05-2

Chapter 05-2 translated by

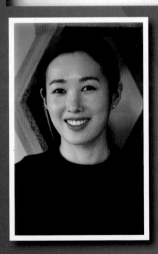

Dr. Min Ji Kwon BDSc

Dr. Min Ji Kwon completed her Bachelor of Dental Science degree with Honors Class IIA at the University of Queensland in 2013.
Since then she has worked in Sydney gaining valuable experiences and exposures to all facets of dentistry and is currently working in regional New South Wales. Dr Kwon enjoys all aspects of dentistry but has particular interest in wisdom teeth extractions and cosmetic dentistry.

It is a great honour to be able to participate in translation of ESSE Extraction of Third Molars. Surgical dentistry was not something I particularly enjoyed. Surgical extraction can be difficult to begin with, especially without the good mentorship. This book has details of the every step of extration and thorough instructions of how to use instruments. I belive this book will add confidence and knowledge to surgical extraction, which is a vital skill required by a general dentist. This book has changed how I approached wisdom tooth extractions.
Thank you Dr. Kim.

Extraction of Wisdom Teeth using Straight Low Speed Handpiece ★

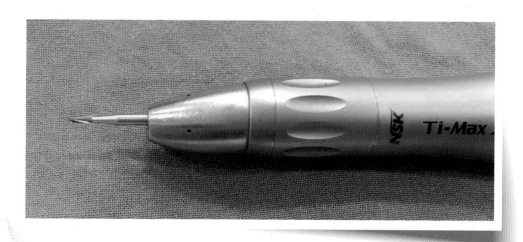

As author fundamentally uses high speed handpiece for extraction of wisdom teeth, wisdom teeth extraction using low speed handpiece will not be discussed separately. In fact, low speed handpieces are mainly used as an auxiliary equipment in removing root tip or buccal alveolar bone and are not used as a primary equipment for wisdom teeth extraction except in particular university dental hospitals. Nevertheless, wisdom teeth extraction only using low speed handpiece is common in the operating room (OR) setting where high speed handpiece is not available.

Extraction using low speed handpiece will only be briefly discussed in this chapter with no further elaboration in this book. It is advised for beginners to move on to the next chapter.

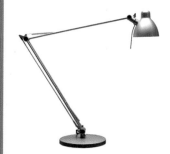

01
Common wisdom teeth extraction technique using low speed handpiece ★★

1. Horizontal Division

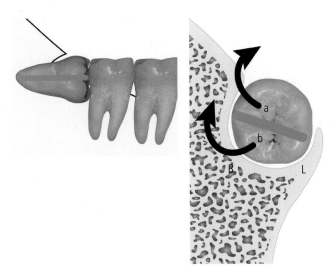

This is a technique where a tooth is sectioned horizontally to remove the upper half followed by the lower half of the tooth. This technique, however, involves removal of significant amount of buccal bone and the tooth. Dentists who lack in spatial ability seem to find this extraction technique challenging and often result in excessive buccal bone removal. Author has also done numerous extractions in this technique within a reasonable working time. However, author finds this technique unsuitable for a large number of wisdom teeth extractions over a long period. Additionally, this extraction technique is often accompanied by post-operative bleeding, swelling and nerve damage. Author is yet to have cases with such post-operative complications but these complications are certainly more commonly reported by other dentist following such extraction technique.

2. Crown Cutting (Vertical Division)

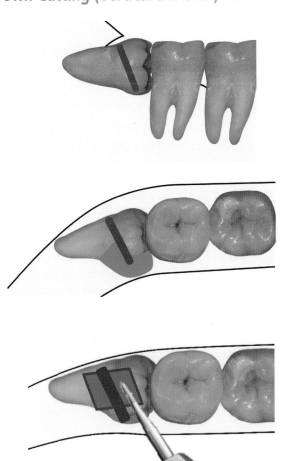

The crown of a tooth is removed first then the buccal bone is removed without any horizontal division. However, as the bur and the body of low speed handpiece lie in a parallel line without an angle, excessive buccal bone removal is required during tooth division, and this consequently leads to post-operative complications such as bleeding, swelling and nerve damage. Occasionally, dentists with lacking spatial ability struggle with tooth division using straight handpiece and end up removing the most of superior bone to expose the tooth for extraction. Crown cutting technique can be used separately but is more often used adjunctively during horizontal division extraction. Straight handpiece may be helpful in extraction of horizontally impacted teeth with presence of significant alveolar bone superior to the tooth or that are impacted deep in the alveolar bone. However, as extraction using high speed handpiece becomes more familiar, straight hand piece can be replaced with high speed handpiece in these cases. Author often uses this extraction technique for maxillary impacted wisdom teeth.

Attention

This diagram illustrates the amount of the tooth removed, access angle and the direction of the tooth removal. Blue indicates the amount and the direction of tooth removal while sectioning horizontally and red indicates those when sectioning vertically (crown sectioning). To prevent damaging lingual artery/nerve it is mandatory not to leave a little bit of the tooth structure on lingual.

02
Crown cutting (vertical division) extraction technique using straight ★ handpiece

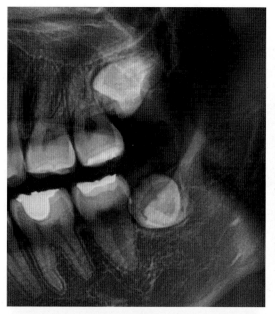
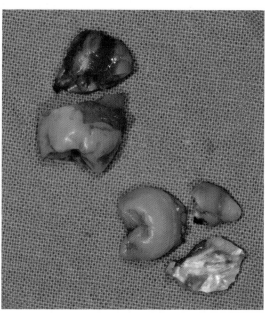

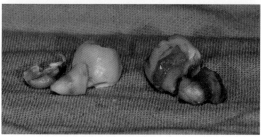

In this case, straight handpiece that was used to extract maxillary impacted wisdom tooth was also used to extract mandibular wisdom tooth to minimize the number of instruments used. Author rarely uses high speed handpiece for maxillary wisdom tooth extraction and occasionally uses straight handpiece in selective cases. However, straight handpiece is rarely used for mandibular wisdom teeth and even when it is used, it is more for horizontal division and not for crown cutting as the case shown. However, straight handpiece can be very useful where the crown of the wisdom tooth is lingually impacted. However, this technique has drawbacks as it is not a versatile technique that can be used in different clinical situations and also involves more buccal bone removal. Although some clinicians may have different opinion depending on their preference and extraction style, based on author's experience, this is not the most practical technique. This technique seems to be more commonly used by inexperienced dentists lacking spatial ability as they remove excessive buccal bone. This can certainly be author's personal opinion. This technique is more frequently used in maxillary wisdom tooth extraction as removal of buccal bone cannot be avoided or is not significant. This will be discussed further in maxillary wisdom teeth extraction part of this book.

03
Horizontal division extraction technique using straight handpiece <1>

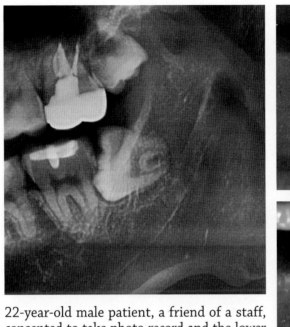

22-year-old male patient, a friend of a staff, consented to take photo record and the lower left wisdom tooth was extracted using straight handpiece.

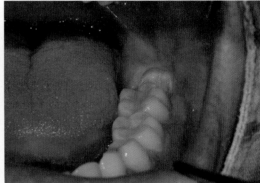

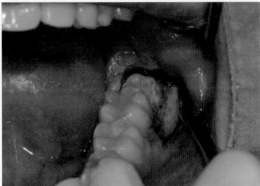

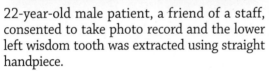

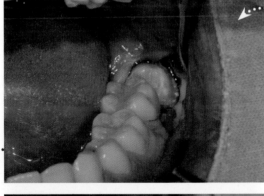

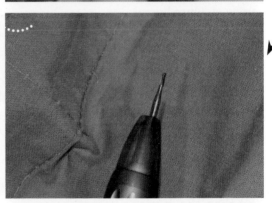

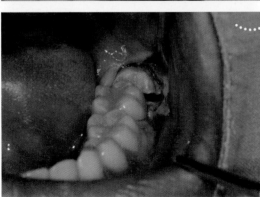

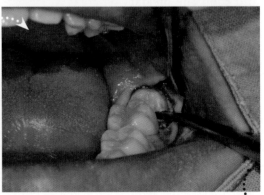

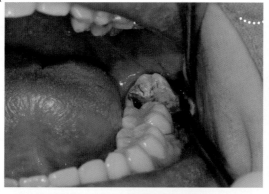
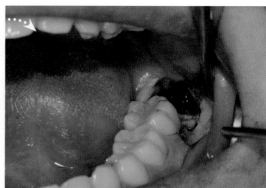
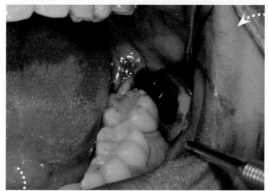
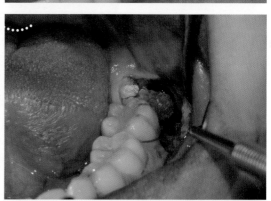
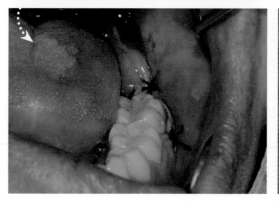
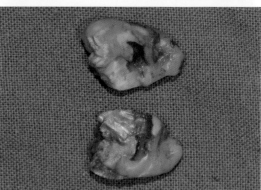
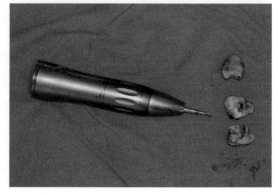

In general, a wisdom tooth extraction using straight handpiece require an incision past the mesial aspect of the second molar. Moreover, unless the tooth only has a small degree of impaction, removal of buccal bone is necessary and the deeper the tooth is impacted the more the buccal bone that needs to be removed. Once buccal bone is removed, the tooth is sectioned bucco-lingually and is separated into mesial and distal half segments using an elevator. The distal segment of the tooth, which does not lie in the undercut of the second molar distal region, is removed first and then the mesial segment of the tooth is removed. In clinical situations, different variables may arise. This technique is largely used for wisdom teeth extractions in operating room (OR) setting where high speed handpiece is not available. But with practice, wisdom teeth can also be easily extracted by this technique in clinical settings. However, in circumstances where there is a high patient flow, this technique can result in overwhelming stress to the wrist and the shoulders for the clinician and post-operative bleeding for the patient due to significant buccal bone removal. Furthermore, a potential risk of damaging lingual cortical bone also exists if excessive force is applied when sectioning the lingual aspect of the tooth. The distal aspect of the second molar is also at a risk of damage due to the direction of the bur during sectioning and the force applied during elevating the lower mesial segment of the wisdom tooth.

Horizontal division extraction technique using straight handpiece <2> ★

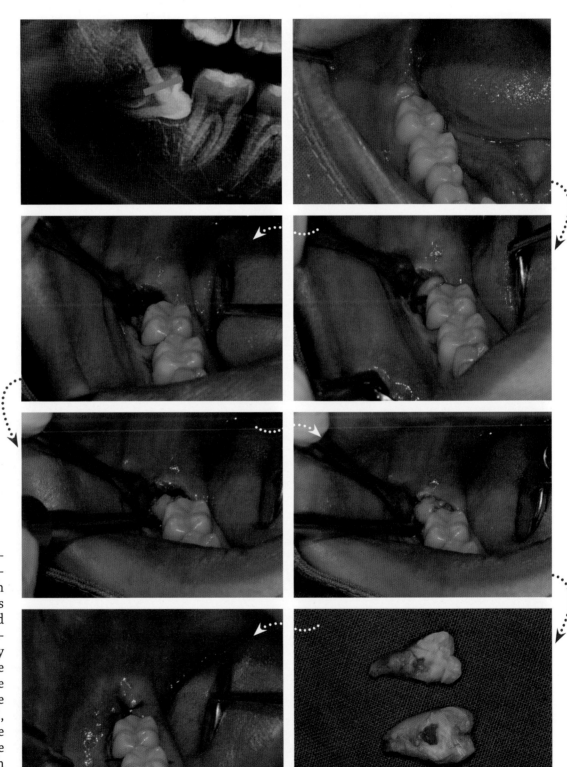

This technique certainly involves substantial force which puts significant stress on the shoulders and the wrist, but the author may feel this way due to infrequent use of this technique. If the wisdom tooth is more apically positioned, extensive buccal bone removal cannot be avoided as the tooth needs to be horizontally sectioned to the furcation point.

Horizontal division extraction technique using straight handpiece <3> ★

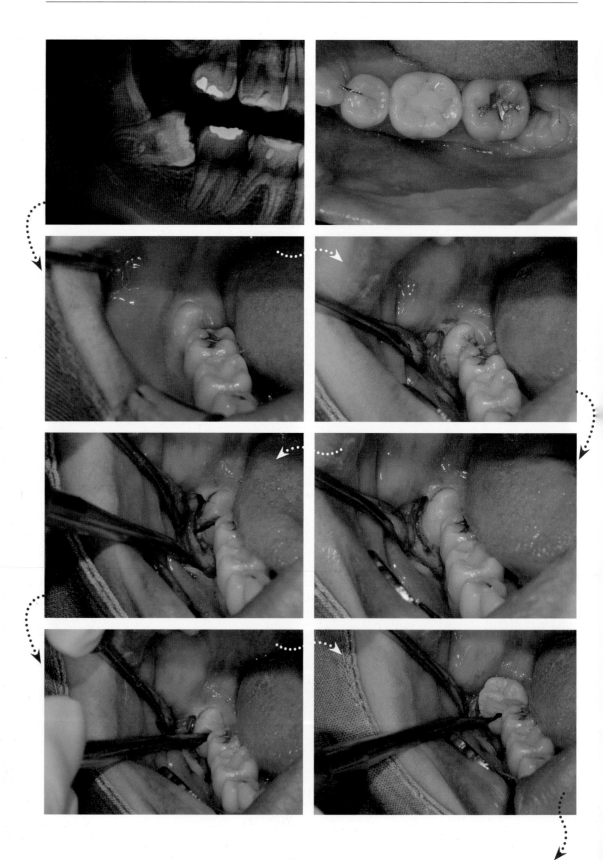

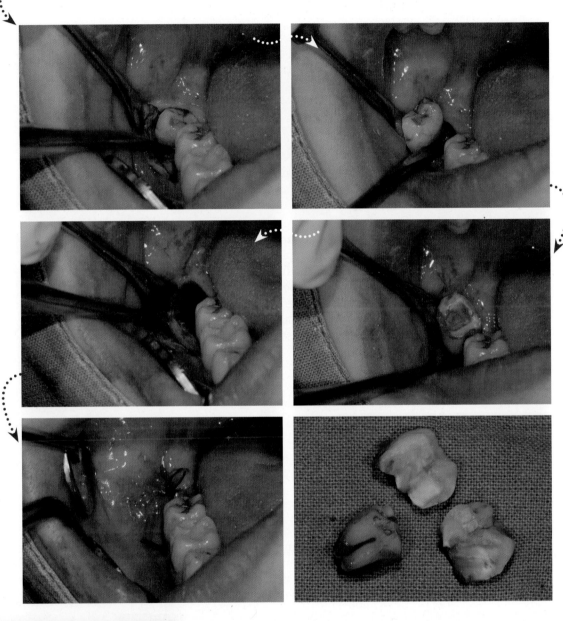

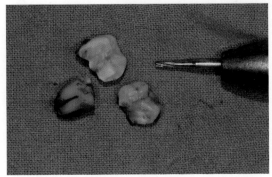

Lower right wisdom tooth on a 22-year-old female patient, a friend of a staff, was extracted using straight handpiece for the purpose of acquisition of photo records. As the tooth appeared to have two separate roots on the radiograph, horizontal cut was first made using straight handpiece to section the tooth in half. However, the crown fractured off as the roots were in fact jointed and the tooth was not sectioned completely to the furcation. On most occasions, such unexpected variables are accompanied during extraction using straight handpiece. There are many factors to be taken into considerations such as the shape of the roots, undercut in the second molar distal region and disto-buccal alveolar bone. If necessary, the crown and the root are intentionally separated to extract the tooth like this case.

04
A case of a wisdom tooth extraction using straight handpiece by another ★ dentist

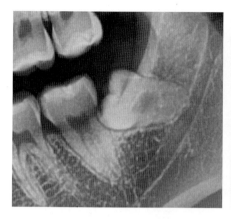
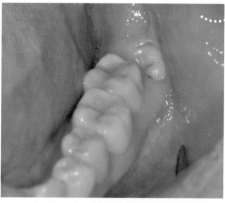
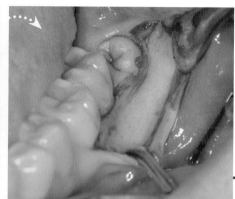

Extraction of a horizontally impacted wisdom tooth using straight handpiece requires further tooth sectioning towards the furcation point and for this reason, the flap has to be extended towards the first molar and involves more buccal bone removal. The more the tooth is horizontally inclined, the more the buccal bone removal is necessary.

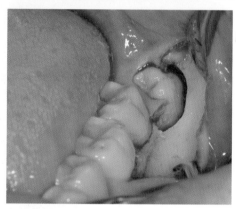

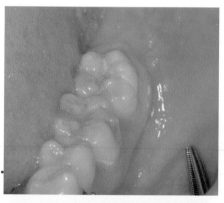

Frequently, straight handpiece fissure bur is used for sectioning of roots but round bur is preferred when removing alveolar bone around the crown as shown above. With this case, separation of periosteum and buccal bone removal is almost inevitable to extract #38.

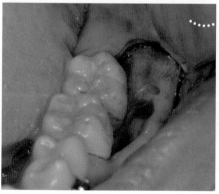
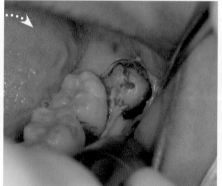
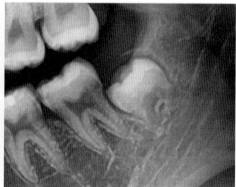

05
Horizontal division extraction technique using straight handpiece Case 1 ★

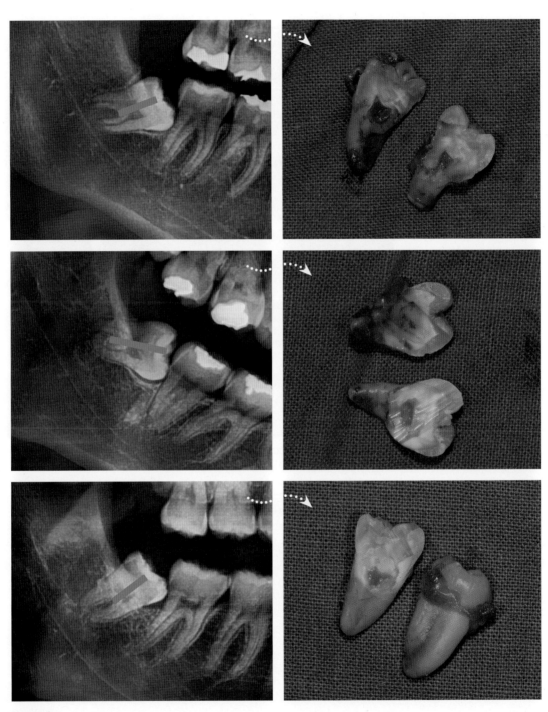

Dr. Jaewook Lee's comment

Case selection is crucial in extraction using straight handpiece. Especially for inexperienced clinicians, forceful application of an elevator on the mesial root following the removal of distal root can lead to post-operative discomfort on the distal surface of the second molar. Additionally, clinicians need to consider that incomplete tooth division will lead to fracture of the mesial portion of the crown from its root leaving the mesial root behind.

Horizontal division extraction technique using straight handpiece ★
Case 2

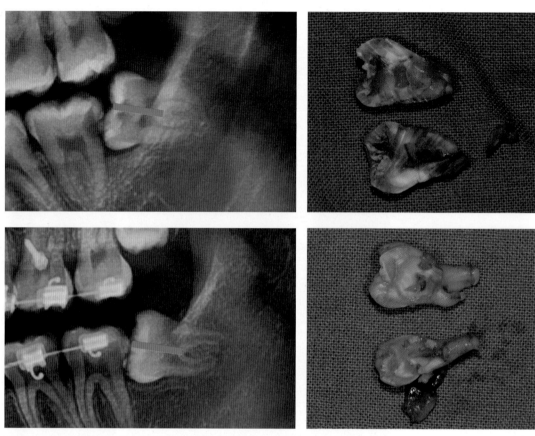

Case where wisdom tooth extracted in standard horizontal sectioning.

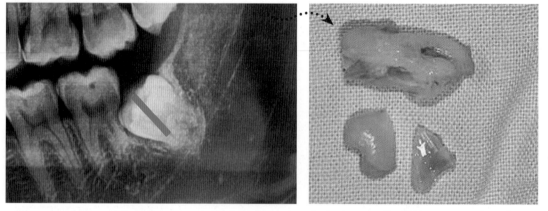

Case where facies mesialis dentis was removed horizontally from buccal using low speed handpiece to remove the undercut.

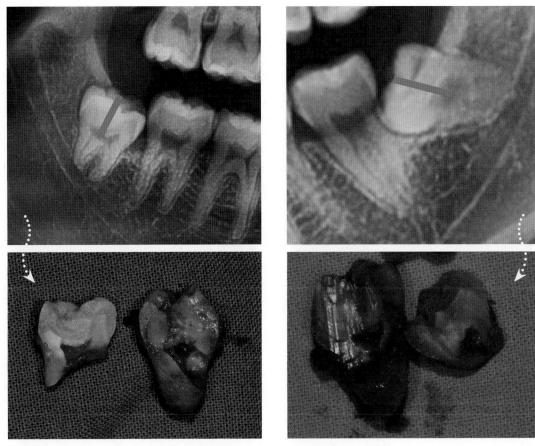

A case where horizontal division was made from the buccal aspect using the straight handpiece to first remove the distal part of the tooth in order to eliminate undercut in the distal alveolar bone.

As shown in the two cases above, a tooth cannot be sectioned perpendicularly to the occlusal surface using straight handpiece and the maximum angulation that can be achieved using straight handpiece would be what has been demonstrated in the photos. Comparing to the use of high speed handpiece, inconvenience needs to be endured particularly for extraction of wisdom teeth that are not horizontally impacted. Wisdom teeth that are upright with slight impaction to the distal alveolar bone or are slightly mesially impacted can easily be extracted with minimal tooth cutting using high speed handpiece. Furthermore, except for dentists who only perform extractions, contra-angle handpiece is the most frequently used handpiece for the majority of dental treatments including implant surgeries and therefore one may favour to use the same equipment throughout different dental procedures. For dentists, including author, who become comfortable using high speed handpiece in wisdom teeth extractions, achieving access for implant placement of the second molar can also become easier.

06
Extraction cases using combination of horizontal and vertical division

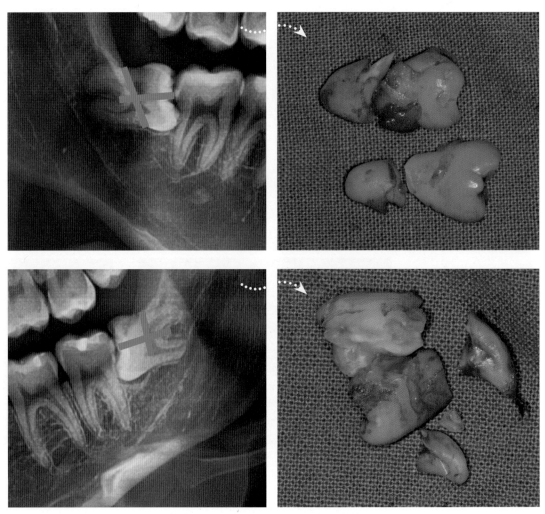

Horizontal and vertical division are frequently performed together for extractions

Author certainly finds extractions using straight handpiece as above more challenging. Maxillofacial surgeons who are used to such technique yet easily carry out extractions using the technique. However, this particular technique normally involves extension of the flap to the first molar and excessive buccal bone removal, particularly for those with higher degree of impaction. Therefore, it is not generally recommended except for extractions performed in surgical operating rooms where high speed handpiece is not accessible. It is possible to extract a tooth by removing its crown first without a horizontal division, but it still is challenging and inconvenient. Author suggests to use high speed handpiece as the primary choice to avoid excessive bone removal and unexpected variables.

Occasionally, 45-degree high speed handpiece is used to perform extractions just like a straight handpiece.

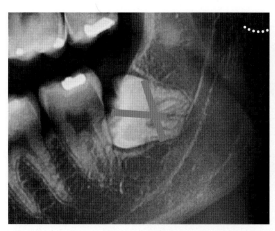
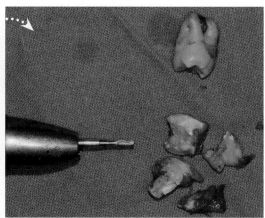

This was a lower left wisdom tooth extraction case on a 23-year-old male patient. Due to the presence of a large undercut and close proximity of distal alveolar bone to the distal surface of the second molar, removing mesial and distal segments was difficult. The tooth was then further divided vertically for its removal.

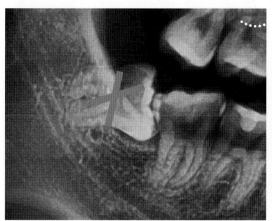
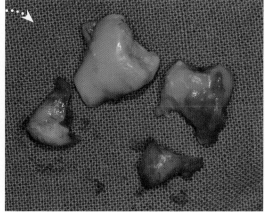

As the roots were apically facing, the tooth was once again divided vertically to be removed in four segments.

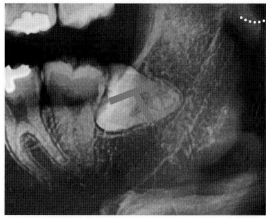
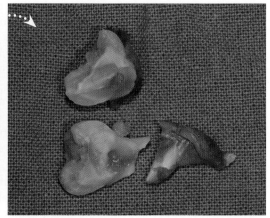

This is a similar case as the case above. To remove an already luxated wisdom tooth, vertical division was made.

07
What to look out while crown sectioning ★★★

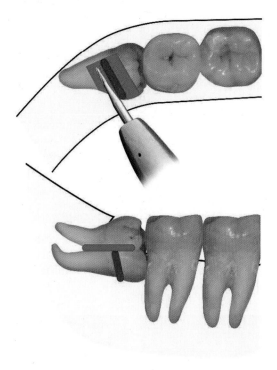

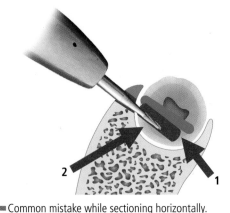

■ Common mistake while sectioning horizontally.

Blue illustrates the amount of bone removal when sectioning horizontally and red does for that while vertical sectioning.

■ Standard horizontal sectioning (blue) vertical sectioning (red).

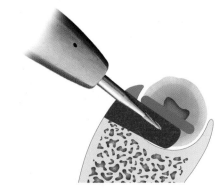

■ Removal of buccal bone to section the tooth vertically. Buccal bone needs to be removed adequately for good access for sectioning.

In general dentists have difficulty extracting the tooth when using contra-angle handpiece due to inadequate removal of the tooth towards lingual or due to the undercuts created while sectioning. Even with experienced hands it is difficult to section all the way to lingual without creating an undercut nor anyone should even attempt to do such sectioning. It could become more difficult when using low speed straight handpiece. Due to its lower cutting power (some say not) it can slip due to excessive pressure, or it can slip through the crown to the lingual bone after the entire crown is sectioned due to the difference in density. Clinicians should remember that sectioning should be stopped prior removing all of the crown at the lingual and crown needs to be broken off from the root. The problem can occur when the crown of third molar has deep vertical impaction like above diagram creating undercut just below the maximum circumference of second molar. In this situation crown is removed vertically (red line) whether hemisection is done or not and undercut will still be present after sectioning on the mesiobuccal area. So if straight handpiece is going to be used it is important to remove all the buccal and section mesiobuccal part of the crown entirely. This would ensure simple extraction even if section is stopped just prior reaching lingual. Incomplete removal of buccal portion of crown can lead to unplanned sectioning and undercuts and make it quite difficult to extract sectioned crown. Some clinicians might attempt to section further to lingual and it can be dangerous! This is why I recommend contra angle handpiece.

08
Dilemma of an anonymous periodontist

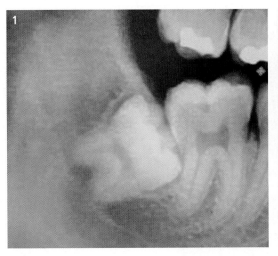

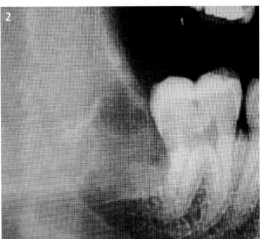

I had a call from a periodontist last year. Among 11 dental schools in Korea, one of them teach the fellows extraction using low speed straight handpiece. He was from that dental school and only learnt extraction using low speed straight piece... He confessed it was very difficult and inconvenient doing extractions in such a way. The above x-ray is from him with his writing.

He extracted the tooth in order as written on x-ray 3. Excessive bone removal was not avoidable to extract in such way and he thought it was just too much and not necessary. As a periodontist incision and elevation were straight forward for him but due to the excessive buccal bone removal, patients suffered from bleeding, pain and post op swelling. When he was at the university hospital, he wasn't overly concerned but since he started working in private clinic, it wasn't efficient to extract in such traumatic way. It wasn't cost effective and patient did not return to him for other treatments.

■ X-rays from a periodontist

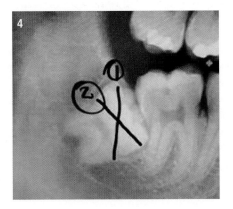

Consequently he decided to use high speed handpiece for wisdom tooth removal. He has asked what different approach he could take for the same case when using contra angled handpiece. Similar case to x-ray 4 has already been mentioned on this book but to summarize, section like line 1, not line 2.

In conclusion, using low speed handpiece extraction requires more bone removal.

09
If you approach using low speed handpiece... ★★★

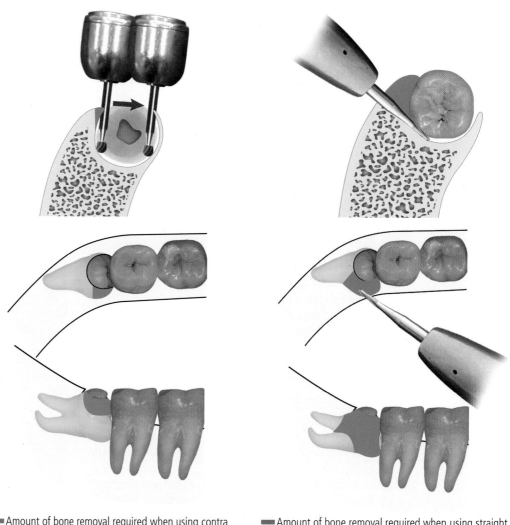

■ Amount of bone removal required when using contra angled handpiece

■ Amount of bone removal required when using straight handpiece

The above diagrams illustrate difference in amount of bone that is needs to be removed when using two different handpieces. This could be controversial and dependant on clinicians. Some clinicians using high speed handpiece might still remove quite a bit of bone around the tooth, if someone would like to do in minimally invasive way like myself, removal like the diagram on the left would suffice. However if lowspeed handpiece is to be used, it would be difficult to be minimally invasive as access needs to be from buccal. In addition it would lead to fatigue due to more pressure required for sectioning and would be difficult to perform multiple extractions like I do. Damage to the distal surface of #7 could also happen more commonly with low speed handpiece. These are the reason that I prefer high speed handpiece. Sectioning with low speed forces clinicians to elevate from mesiobuccal area to remove mesial crown or mesial root/s but this can increase the risk of nerve damage. I regard lever principle very important and like to use hard distobuccal bone as fulcrum, and this can reduce the risk of nerve/bone damage. I always try to minimize elevating on mesiobuccal bone.

Extraction of Wisdom Teeth using 45-degree ★ Handpiece

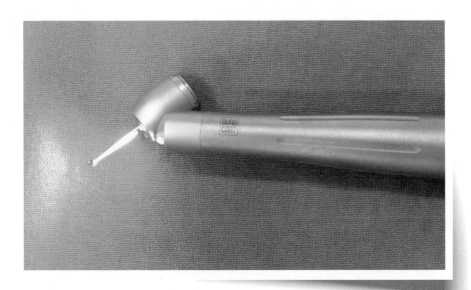

45-degree handpiece becomes useful during separation of the crown of a wisdom tooth which is vertically erupted or significantly lingually inclined. Access to mandibular wisdom teeth with regular handpiece is limited by the lateral ramus of the mandible and therefore 45-degree handpiece is used in these cases. The crown of the wisdom tooth can be easily removed by cutting the mesio-buccal aspect with 45-degree handpiece and fracturing off the segment using an elevator. For this reason, author strongly advises to stock at least one of 45-degree handpiece in the office. Author also has one available in the office, and it is frequently used in removing the crown of functional upright wisdom tooth in male patients with dense bone profile. This will only be briefly discussed in this section as it will be explored again in later chapter (extraction of vertically impacted wisdom teeth).

Consequently he decided to use high speed handpiece for wisdom tooth removal. He has asked what different approach he could take for the same case when using contra angled handpiece. Similar case to x-ray 4 has already been mentioned on this book but to summarize, section like line 1, not line 2. In conclusion, using low speed handpiece extraction requires more bone removal.

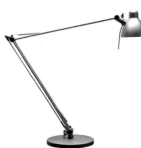

01
45-degree high speed handpiece? ★

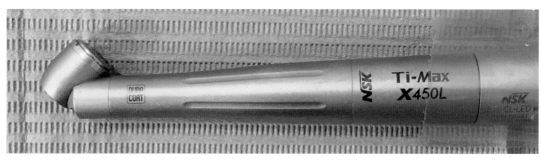

■ 45-degree handpiece used by author (NSK Ti-Max X 450L)

45-degree handpiece was not readily available in Korea at the time of purchase, so this was sent from a colleague from Japan. It is now officially imported to Korea. It is advised to contact NSK Korea for those who wish to purchase.
Due to the fact many dentists use this handpiece for extraction… These handpieces come with on/off function to switch chip air or no chip air at all depending on the manufacturer. This is designed for extraction only and doesn't have chip air.

This handpiece has a button to switch on/off the chip air. Please click the link (Insert QR code)

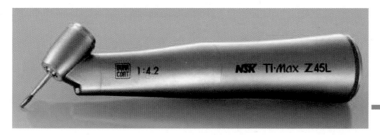

■ NSK 45-degree 1:4.2 low speed handpiece. Recently imported to Korea.

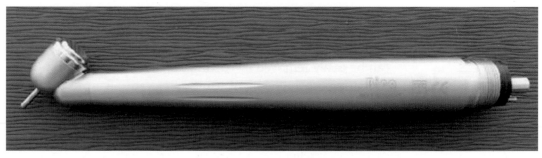

■ 45-degree handpiece purchased directly from China used to cost 1/30 of the price of that in Japan or Germany and the manufacturing cost in NSK China was only 1/10. The adoption configuration of the handpiece to the coupling must be checked prior to purchase.

As discussed earlier, 45-degree handpiece can be used in replacement of straight handpiece during horizontal division technique. Author finds this inconvenient as 45-degree handpiece is not routinely used. Rather it is more useful in vertical division extraction technique, and there are dentists who use 45-degree handpiece in such way. This would be an alternative approach in wisdom teeth extractions for clinicians lacking in spatial ability.

But I don't see much point of using this handpiece apart from the neck cutting(목치기) on vertically impacted tooth or lingually tilted wisdom tooth. But there are many dentists doing extractions only with this handpiece worldwide. If you are comfortable using contra angled handpiece I would rather recommend straight handpiece. Using different handpieces could be not familiar on clinicians' hands and access would be quite awkward when sectioning vertically impacted tooth.

02
Horizontal division extraction technique using 45-degree handpiece ★

Extraction technique using 45-degree handpiece is similar to that using straight handpiece. Either the tooth is sectioned horizontally from the side or the crown is sectioned off. The lower left wisdom tooth was extracted through horizontal division technique in this case for the purpose of demonstration but would normally be approached from the superior aspect with a handpiece. This will also be explored in more detail in later chapter (extraction of mesially impacted wisdom teeth).

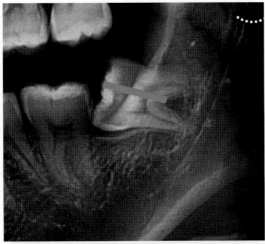
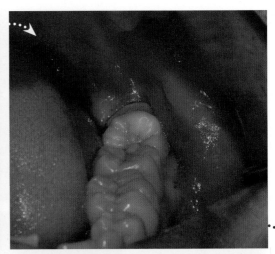
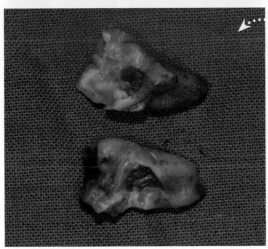
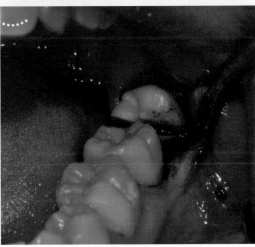

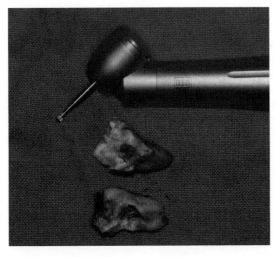

Due to time constraints during working hours, taking photo records and arranging them is a task. For this reason, author has a habit of taking photo with the instruments used for that particular extraction. If there is any instrument in the photos, it means that the particular instrument was used for the extraction case. Instruments that are repeatedly used for wisdom teeth extractions are not normally shown in photos. Author's extraction style is very consistent; therefore, instruments are observable only in the photos of exception cases.

03
Crown division extraction technique using 45-degree handpiece ★

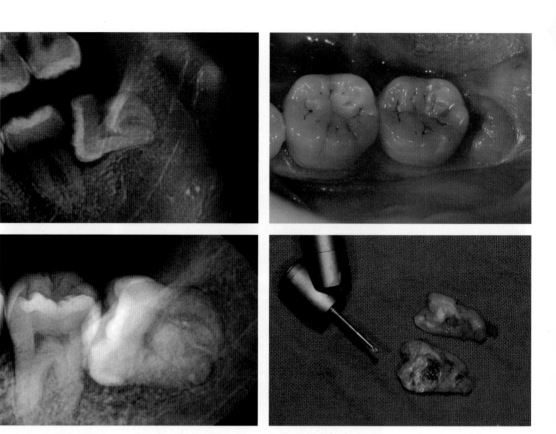

In the case above, the tooth was horizontally sectioned to the upper and the lower half as if the straight handpiece was used. However, for inexperienced clinicians, this technique can be difficult and also dangerous. If the handpiece is approached from the occlusal aspect instead of the buccal aspect, a part of the tooth may fracture off rather than being completely sectioned to two segments. Because it is not an everyday handpiece, it seems difficult to locate exactly where the tooth is sectioned. Furthermore, unlike straight handpiece, 45-degree handpiece has a major drawback that it does not allow sectioning to be made far enough for complete tooth division. Author predominantly uses 45-degree handpiece for the purpose of cutting off the mesio-buccal part and then fracturing off the rest using an elevator to remove the crown of the tooth (cervical cutting technique).

The reason why complete horizontal division is difficult will now be discussed.

04
Single or joint rooted teeth are not easily sectioned to two segments ★

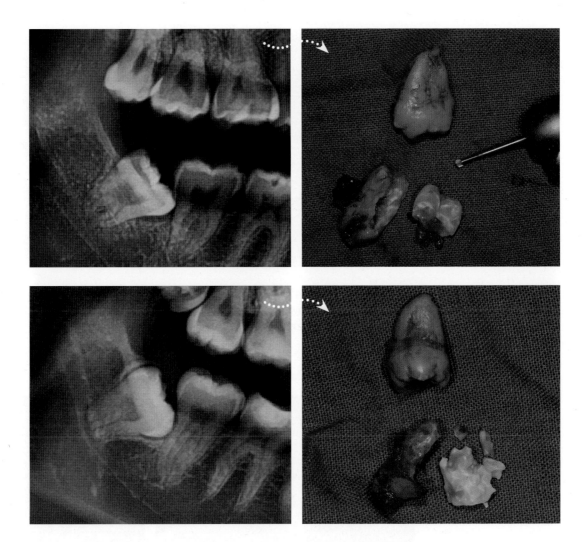

Single or joint rooted teeth cannot be easily sectioned unless significant buccal bone is removed and access for division towards the apical portion of the tooth is more restricted compared to using a straight handpiece. At times, distal portion of the tooth is fractured off first, and this allows removal of the rest of the tooth. This is a similar to the technique using straight handpiece where the distal portion of the tooth is removed first regardless of its proportional size following sectioning of the lateral aspect of the tooth. However, access pathway is more limited with 45-degree handpiece and because of that, the remaining tooth segment following the division may become trapped by the undercut in the mesial region. After all, clinicians must use the techniques that they feel comfortable and confident in performing. Author uses 45-degree handpiece in unavoidable situations where there is no other sterilized handpieces available at the time of extraction.

05
Crown cutting technique using 45-degree handpiece ★

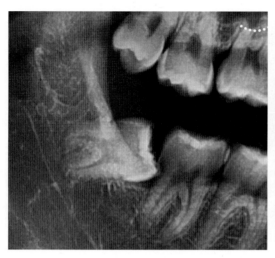 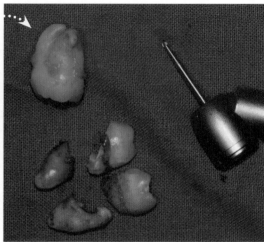

This is a case where 45-degree handpiece was used for crown cutting technique. Even through the tooth did not show significant bony impaction, access angulation made it difficult to remove the sectioned crown and therefore horizontal division was additionally made.

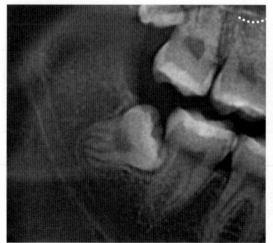 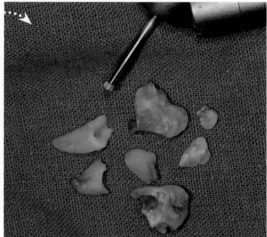

For those with more bony impaction, removal of sectioned segments can still be challenging without an adequate buccal bone removal. Therefore, the tooth is often divided further into multiple fragments.

06
Cervical cutting technique using 45-degree handpiece ★★

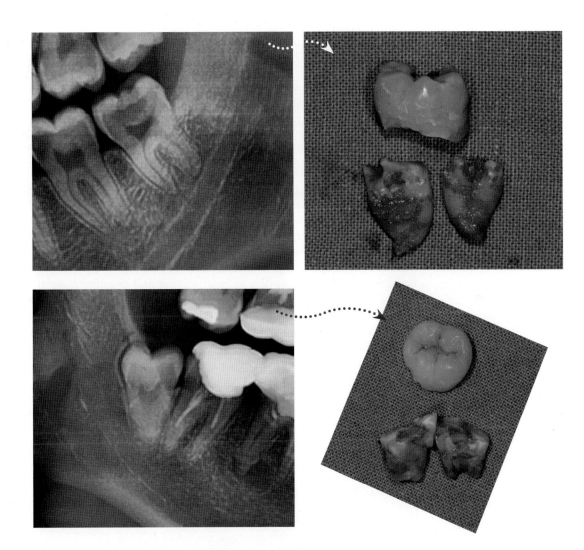

45-degree handpiece is rarely used in cervical cutting technique in extraction of horizontally impacted teeth as this requires excessive bone removal. However, in extracting vertically erupted wisdom teeth, approach with a regular handpiece for tooth cutting from the buccal aspect is limited by the ramus of the mandible and 45-degree handpiece can come in useful in this situation. More details will be explored in later chapter where extraction of vertically impacted teeth is discussed.

So I think if you intend to do numerous extractions of wisdom teeth it is ideal to equip a 45-degree handpiece. Even I do many extractions day to day, only have two 45-degree handpiece-one high speed and one 1:5 low speed.

07
Extraction using contra-angle slow speed handpiece ★

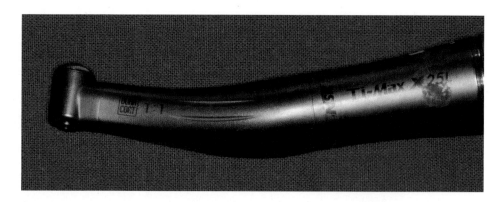

This is the most commonly used contra-angle slow speed handpiece by author. Earlier version of slow speed handpieces were air driven handpieces where the bur was secured by a latch and the head of the handpiece was detachable at the bend. However, this type of contra-angle slow speed handpiece is more susceptible to malfunction and requires more maintenance. They are now largely replaced by electric slow speed handpiece. The initial expense may be higher but is more economical in long term as its maintenance is easier and cheaper. Use of slow speed handpiece has become more convenient with installation of optic light and internal irrigation in newer models. The average speed of air driven handpiece is approximately 30,000 RPM where as that of electric handpiece is over 40,000 RPM. On NSK handpieces 1:1 sign is printed. This means that if the average maximum rotation speed is 40,000 RPM, the handpiece has the capacity to produce that maximum speed. In general, 20:1 sign is written on implant engine handpiece and this means that its rotation speed reduces by 1/20 and as a result it produces rotation speed of 2,000 RPM.

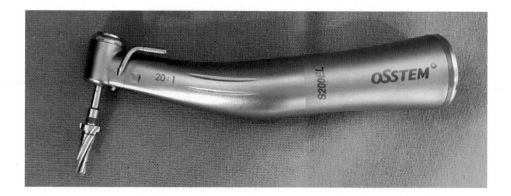

This is an implant slow speed handpiece with 20:1 reduction engine. Implant handpiece with that particular speed reduction engine would have been designed as it does not normally take more than 1,200 RPM to remove bone for implant placements. For handpieces designed for endodontic treatments, the reduction engine used to vary between 16:1 and 64:1. Rechargeable endodontic engine is not favoured in the modern days but was once widely used. A majority of the handpieces owned by author is NSK handpieces, and they perform well and are also cost effective. NSK handpieces reported to be leading the world market ahead of Kavo.

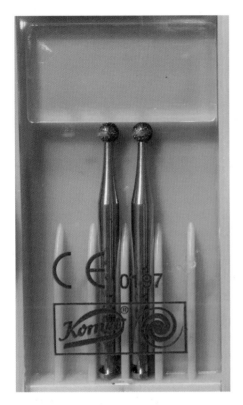

Is a handpiece with 40,000 RPM adequate for wisdom teeth extractions? Author managed to obtain 26 mm long shank oral surgical bur produced by Komet. The diameter of the shank was 2.35 mm, same as regular latch type burs, and the diameter of this diamond bur was 2.1 mm. Long-shanked burs generate significant vibrations in handpiece cartilage and so having diamond type bur head allows for smoother cutting. Although this bur was initially designed for oral surgeries, it is probably used more for bone removal during apicoectomy and tuberosity reduction surgery. If there is a clinician who is strongly resistant in using high speed handpiece in wisdom teeth extraction, slow speed handpiece may be an alternative option. In early days where high speed handpiece was not available, extraction using slow speed hand piece may have been attempted. Author has tried using a regular slow speed bur with a short shank but had to stop because of its short length. However, author rarely uses high speed handpiece for maxillary wisdom teeth extraction and using slow speed handpiece instead may be considered for simple tooth or bone removal or in the worst circumstances where straight handpiece cannot access the tooth.

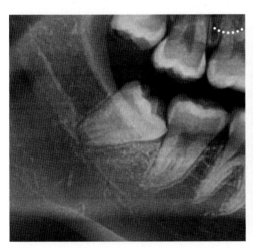
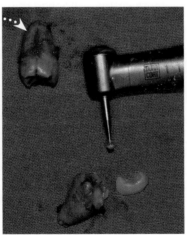

This was a lower right wisdom tooth extraction case in a 22-year-old female. The extraction procedure was foreseen to be straightforward, so NSK internal irrigation slow speed handpiece was tried. Removal of the tooth using slow speed handpiece was not practical as the bur quickly abraded and the speed and the torque of the handpiece quickly dropped down. The large diameter of the bur also made precise cutting difficult towards the lingual side. Above all, the handpiece continued to stop operating because of rapid fall in the torque and the speed. In general, using slow speed handpiece does feel adequate in removing caries; however, cutting the tooth through the enamel was a laborious process. A few more attempts were made but author had to change to a high speed handpiece as it was overly time consuming. Most importantly, author mainly uses long shank round bur with high speed handpiece, but this type of bur is not available with slow speed handpiece. Even if a similar bur was to be manufactured, the diameter of the bur is 1.8 mm whereas the diameter of the shank is 2.35 mm which means the shank is likely to become caught inside the tooth. What about a friction grip electric handpiece to which high speed bur can be adopted?

This is a friction grip slow speed handpiece which adopts high speed bur. This type of handpiece was once widely used and is still being produced by various manufacturing companies, predominantly as electric integral 1:1 type. However, author mostly used the same high speed bur on a high speed handpiece at a low speed to refine cavity preparation or crown margins. There are still dentists who favour using this handpiece but as they become more experienced and skilled, the frequency of usage certainly decreases.

What about using high speed bur on 1:1 reduction speed handpiece for teeth sectioning and wisdom teeth extractions? The rotational force is very poor that tooth removal is extremely time consuming. This type of handpiece was initially developed for the purpose of minimal tooth cutting with low rotational speed and using such handpiece in procedures involving substantial tooth removal would not be rational. In cases where use of high speed handpiece is not desired because of its air release or difficulty with access, then using slow speed handpiece may be considered. However, low rotational speed is still a big barrier in tooth cutting.

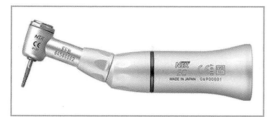

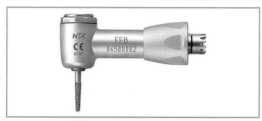

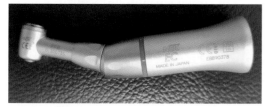

It was this reason why 1:5 increasing slow speed handpiece was developed. In general, the rotational speed of an electric slow speed handpiece is around 40,000 RPM so 1:5 increasing handpiece can generate rotational speed up to 200,000 RPM. This is a comparable rotational speed to that of high speed handpiece which has average rotational speed of high speed handpiece is 300,000~400,000 RPM. Author used to have an issue of high speed handpiece coming to a stop when a high force was applied during tooth cutting, although this may be mechanical problem of author's own high speed handpieces. It seemed that the torque was not sufficient for its high rotational speed. Then author decided to try out 1:5 increasing slow speed handpiece. The handpiece was attached to the regular 1:1 slow speed hand piece line and high speed bur was used for extractions. The torque was a little low but it was possible to extract a wisdom tooth. However, the manufacturing company strongly advised not to use the handpiece in such way as it puts excessive stress on the motor. The handpiece performs well without a torque problem when it is connected to a line with the motor specifically designed for 1:5 increasing slow speed handpiece. Although the handpiece has a great efficiency and are installed with internal irrigation and optic light, there is still a downside of its heavy weight.

◾A photo of reduction speed slow speed handpiece commonly used in the past

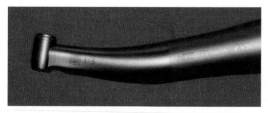

◾A photo taken by author

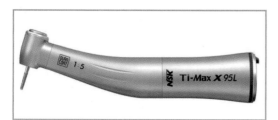

◾A photo from NSK catalogue

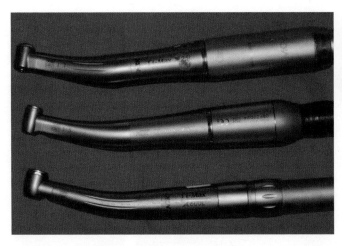
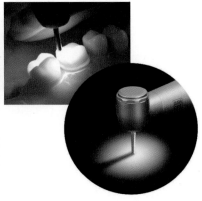

The first one on the top is a regular slow speed handpiece used for general dental treatment and the last one on the bottom is a regular high speed handpiece used for general dental treatment and wisdom teeth extraction. The middle one shown in the photo is the new NSK 1:5 high-torque slow speed handpiece where high speed bur can be adopted. The handpiece is now also manufactured in titanium material has and is a light- weight awith great speed and performance. Similar handpieces have already been in the market in Europe and Japan for 7 to 8 years, but it was introduced in Korea only 2 years ago. The handpiece was not widespread as it required installation of a separate line and the cost was high. However, this type of handpieces gained its popularity in recent years as dentists started to seek handpieces that can effectively cut through zirconia crowns. Manufacturing companies, however, warn inexperienced clinicians to be aware of potential damage to tooth structure when applied with a strong force as this high-torque slow speed handpiece does not stop during rotation due to its high speed and torque. It is also reported that increasing number of dentists in Japan use this type of handpiece with high speed bur for wisdom teeth extractions. Author has also installed the line for this handpiece on one of the chairs in the office for the purpose of wisdom teeth extractions. This type of handpiece has not been on the market long enough to discuss its durability but this may become the answer to the problem of having to frequently replace high speed handpiece cartilage after a constant use of long shank burs.

08
Using 1:5 increasing slow speed handpiece <1> ★

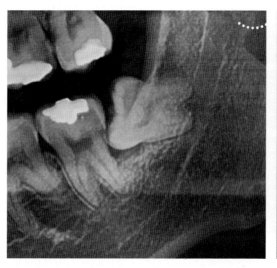 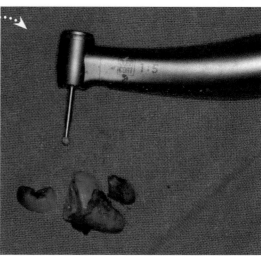

For extraction cases using 1:5 increasing slow handpiece, the photos are normally taken with instruments sitting in the direction that it was actually used for the procedure but a staff has taken this photo oppositely to show '1:5' sign written on the handpiece. Although photo records are not taken frequently anymore, there are some photos from simple extraction cases where the handpiece was first being tested out.

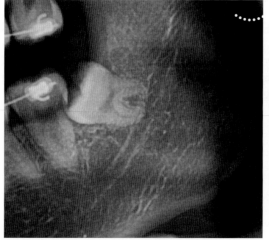 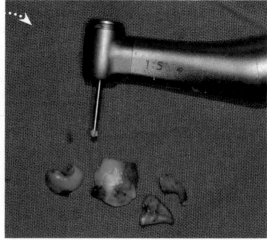

Same as the case above, the photo was taken in reverse by a staff to show '1:5' sign. This was an extraction case where a L extraction technique became 3 segment extraction. Author advises the readers to cover this book in sequence as recommended in the introduction (following the start signs) and the following content will be easier to comprehend.

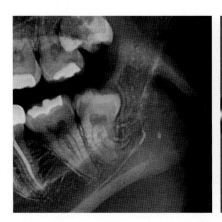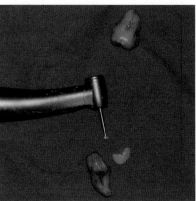

This is a case where a lower left wisdom tooth with an acute apical curvature was extracted using distal crown cutting technique. It was a relatively simple extraction case but photo was taken for demonstration purpose. It is not shown in the photo but there was also a small curved root in disto-lingual aspect which was either left in-situ or evacuated into suction. The fragment could also have been left out by the staff while taking the photo.

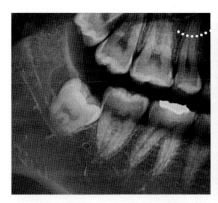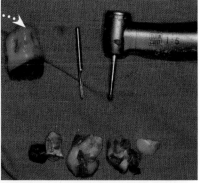

Even though this was a vertically impacted wisdom tooth, because of the severity of impaction, the lingual fragment was first removed through mesial crown cutting followed by lingual crown cutting. Distal crown cutting was additionally made to remove distal crown as the access was not large enough. Author has a principle of minimizing bone removal during extraction and therefore tooth often are sectioned into multiple fragments to be removed from a small access. In the case above, fissure bur was used for mesial crown cutting and round bur was used for the other sectioning. On the radiograph, radiolucency, which appeared to be a cyst, was evident on the distal region and was removed for biopsy. Histological examination came back benign.

Overall, 1:5 increasing slow speed handpiece can perform comparably to high speed handpiece.

Using 1:5 increasing slow speed handpiece <2> ★

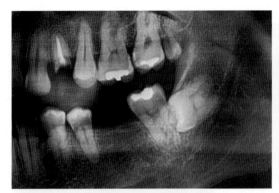
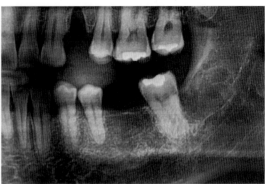
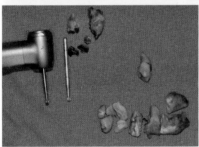

A 36-year-old patient was referred from another dental office for extraction of mandibular left wisdom tooth prior to orthodontic treatment and implant placement. The tooth was extracted through the technique discussed earlier but by using 1:5 increasing slow speed handpiece. #4 round bur was used here to allow for further sectioning of the tooth as the roots were in close proximity to the inferior alveolar nerve. L cutting was first made but the crown fractured off and the remaining segment was removed by cutting a groove into the mesial root.

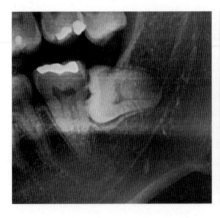
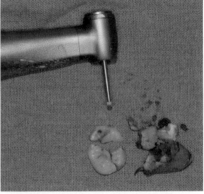

Usual technique was used to extract a mandibular left wisdom tooth on a 27-year-old patient. Elevator was applied on the buccal aspect of the tooth following removal of mesial crown; however, tooth could not be removed and disto-cervical cutting was additionally made. Multiple disto-cervical cutting also had to be made as the tooth continued to fracture off. Youngsam's sign evident on the apex of the root explains why the extraction was challenging.

09
Ncreasing supply of 1:5 increasing slow speed handpiece

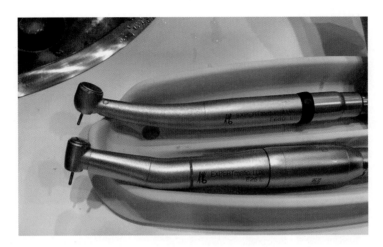

Majority of handpiece manufacturing companies displayed 1:5 increasing slow speed handpiece with red band as their main advertising product at a dental material exhibitions that author recently attended. This is likely to be due to increased popularity of the handpiece among dentists as more zirconia crowns are being placed as the price of gold continues to increase. A large proportion of dentists who are currently using 1:5 increasing slow speed handpieces seem to be using the handpiece predominantly for removal of zirconia and other crowns and abutment tooth preparation rather than for wisdom teeth extractions. Various types of handpieces were displayed in Kavo stand but only regular high speed handpiece and 1:5 increasing slow speed handpiece were set up for hands-on trial. This again showed 1:5 increasing slow speed handpiece is at its demand.

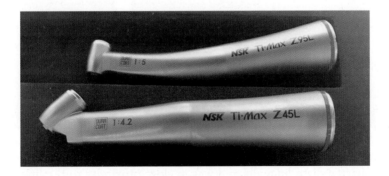

At NSK stand, the same handpiece model as the one author is currently using was displayed. This was also their main advertising product. The handpiece shown on the bottom photo is a 45-degree handpiece which is used worldwide for extractions but is rarely used in Korea. As stated earlier, author normally has a 45-degree handpiece available in the surgery and is currently using this 45-degree slow speed handpiece (1:4.2 increasing). As it is on the market for extraction only purpose it is manufactured so it is easy to turn on/off the air that gets sprayed at the same time with water. For 1:5 handpiece air needs to be turned off from the operating chair. This is dependant on each treatment centre manufacturer. You can watch the video of the handpieces with chip air on/off.

10
Extractions using 45-degree 1:5 slow speed handpiece ★

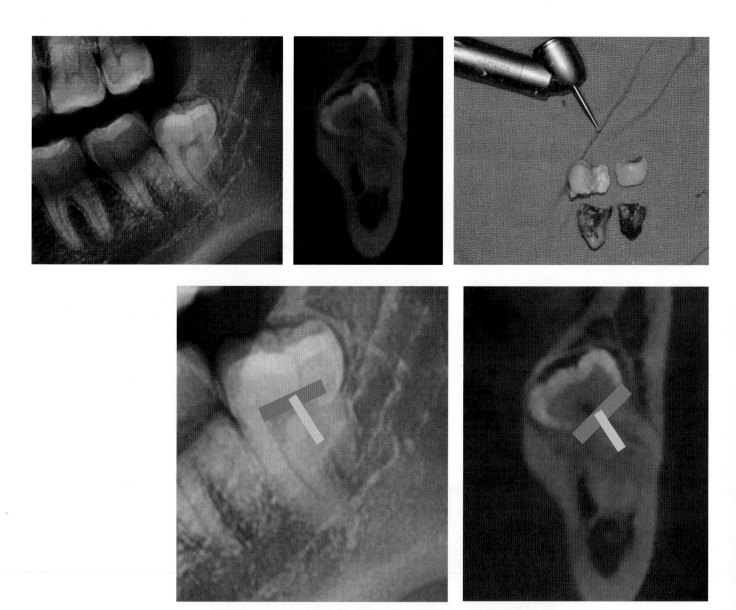

The extraction of lower left wisdom tooth on this 37-year-old female was difficult as the tooth was impacted disto-lingually and was in close proximity to the lingual nerve. As discussed in the crown sectioning technique, 45-degree handpiece was used from the meiso-buccal aspect to make a cut at the cervical region to fracture off the crown. The crown had to be sectioned further at the mesio-distal line for its removal. On the assumption that leaving broken root tip would also be acceptable in case of difficult access or associated discomfort for the patient, the remaining roots were removed by sectioning to mesial and distal root segments.

This is the case where 45-degree handpiece is used appropriately. When you access from buccal to section the crown off and making a slot on the root 45-degree handpiece would be the most suitable.

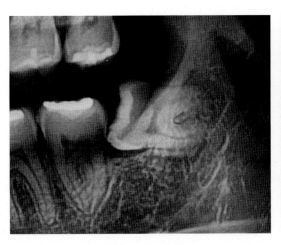
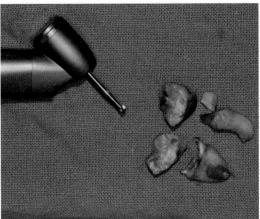

This is an extraction case carried out with the use of 45-degree 1:4.2 increasing handpiece. The tooth was extracted in the same way of using straight handpiece. The wisdom tooth was sectioned to two segments from the lateral aspect for its removal. The crown of the tooth was also sectioned off as the direction of mesial and distal root curvature was different.

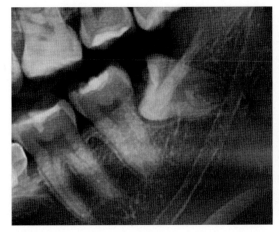
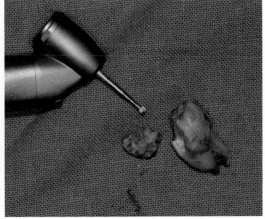

As above, a tooth can still be removed without a division into two segments.

Extraction of a Vertically Impacted Mandibular Third Molar

06
CHAPTER

Chapter 06 translated by

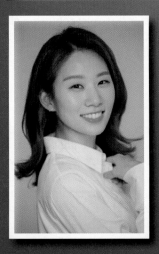

Dr. Addie Yoojung Chang DMD

Private office in Tukwila, Washington
B.A. Chemistry, Carnegie Mellon University, Pittsburgh, PA
D.M.D., Tufts University School of Dental Medicine, Boston, MA

I am honored for the opportunity to review Dr. Kim's world-famous textbook. This textbook is a must read for those who are interested in easy and safe extraction methods.
Like he mentions in this book, please read it more than once! This chapter is originally translated by Drs. Mike Zhou and Somin Kwon.

01
Classification of vertically impacted mandibular third molar ★★

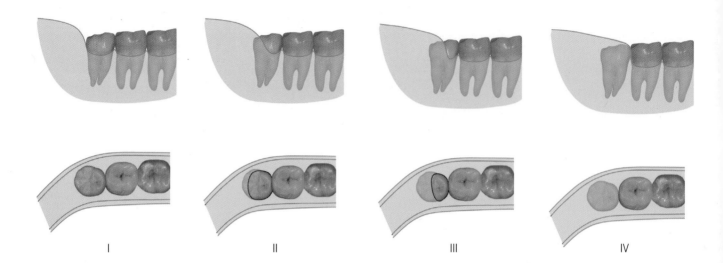

I   II   III   IV

I: Fully erupted (full crown visible)

In many cases where the crown is fully erupted, I mainly use forceps due to the lack of strong cortical bone to serve as a fulcrum point around the crown. If forceps extraction is unsuccessful, then the tooth should be sectioned. Usually the periodontal ligament surrounding functioning teeth are very strong, which makes the extraction more difficult. This is especially true in men with prominent jaws.

II: 2/3 erupted (more than half of crown visible)

Extraction of teeth in this classification is relatively easier than teeth in other classifications. In most cases, extraction can be done with an elevator engaged in distobuccal area without incision.

III: 1/3 erupted (less than half of crown visible)

Extraction of teeth in this classification is also relatively easier but may require a slight buccal incision since it can tear the lingual tissue as the tooth comes out. These teeth also can likely be removed by luxation forces with an elevator engaged in the distobuccal area.

IV: Fully impacted (crown not visible)

First, a full thickness flap is made in the gingiva to expose the crown of the impacted third molar. Then, using an elevator or surgical curette, examine to see if the distal occlusal surface of the crown is covered by the alveolar bone. If the distal area is covered by the bone, I often apply the distal crown sectioning technique (½ to ⅓). Some teeth can be removed without sectioning despite how they appear on radiographs. However, bone removal, in addition to the tooth sectioning, may be needed in cases where the third molar is positioned entirely lower than the occlusal plane of the second molar or where it is angulated distally, buccally or lingually.

02
How to make the incision line for vertically impacted third molars

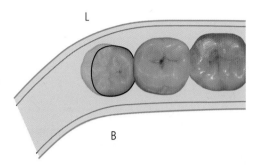
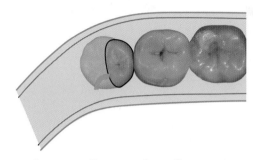

If more than half of the crown is covered by soft tissue, place a small incision buccally to prevent tearing of the tissue during the process of tooth removal. Also, separating the periodontal attachment using an explorer is important. Remember, "It is better to create an incision than get tearing of tissue".

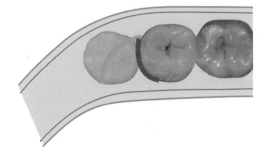

In full soft tissue impaction cases, a semi-lunar shaped incision is recommended. The incision should be performed while the cheek is fully retracted to the buccal, and the incision should end on the lingual side of the distal of the second molar (green line) to prevent tearing during extraction. If necessary, the incision can be extended to the buccal of the second molar (red line).

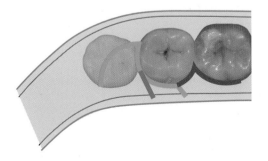

Extending the incision line to the mesial area of the second molar (green line) is only necessary in cases where greater exposure is needed such as when the cervical bulge of the crown is below the cortical bone or when there is significant buccal or lingual tilting.

Extracting fully erupted mandibular 3rd molar

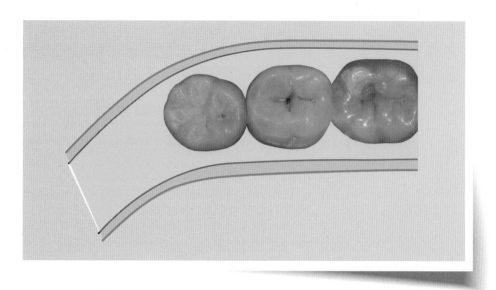

Fortunately (or not), I graduated dental school never having performed an extraction alone because the instructors always helped me. Perhaps this is an indication that dental school education was flawed and inadequate at the time. Not all students graduated never having had a chance to perform extractions on their own – I know this because I was an extraction patient for one of the senior students. One day, senior students gathered lower class men with fully erupted third molars to be used as extraction cases. I was among those who were gathered up. But the pain I experienced during that extraction is the worst pain of my life to date. I could not even count how many students took turns after the first senior student was unsuccessful. In the end, it took over an hour to extract one of my mandibular third molars. I wonder now why both the residents and students alike were trained so poorly, and where were all the attending professors? Anyway, my point here is that extracting fully erupted third molars has the greatest chance to be most difficult.

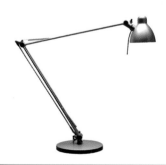

01
Using forceps to extract fully erupted mandibular third molar ★★

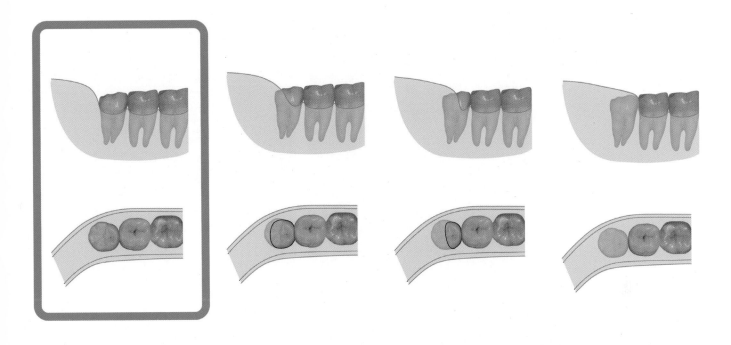

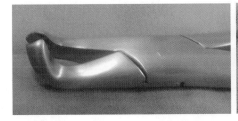
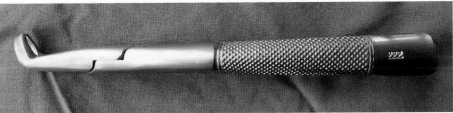

For most fully erupted teeth, extractions can be successfully performed by mainly using the forceps. However, if the disto-buccal area of the tooth is covered by gingiva or by alveolar bone, the tooth can be extracted by luxation forces with an elevator engaged in the disto-buccal area. The indication for forceps extraction is that the cervical bulge of the crown must be above the cortical bone to allow forceps to engage the tooth with maximum grip strength and to avoid slippage. If not, forceps slippage can damage the opposing dentition, surrounding soft tissue, and alveolar bone. Dentists who have less wrist strength must be even more cautious about slippage. In the beginning, I used to teach students to use 60% of their strength to grip the tooth and 40% to actually extract the tooth. However, nowadays, I emphasize allocating 70% of the strength to grip the tooth because I still witnessed too many doctors slipping around when first using forceps. It is important to use far more strength to properly grip the tooth with forceps than to move or luxate the tooth. This way the forceps do not slip, causing iatrogenic damage.

02
Basic forceps positioning for mandibular third molar extraction ★★★

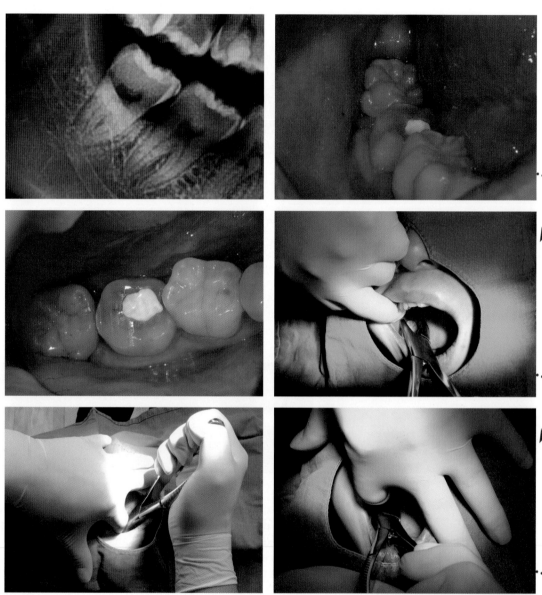

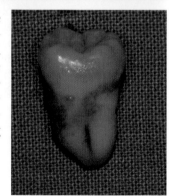

Preventing slippage is the most critical consideration during extraction using forceps. The importance of gripping the tooth tightly and securely with a steady hand cannot be emphasized enough to avoid any damage to the surrounding tissues. Sometimes, the tooth removal can occur unintentionally just from gripping the tooth securely with the forceps. At the same time, the back of the forceps can unexpectedly hit and damage the opposing dentition. To prevent accidental injury of the opposing dentition, gripping the tooth with gradual increase of strength is recommended and just before applying the strong force, you must check once again that the crown of the tooth is securely gripped. When the forceps are properly engaging the crown, I place my left index finger against the opposing maxillary teeth for protection. Some dentists avoid doing 3rd molar extractions because they are afraid of complications, such as cracking or fracturing opposing teeth from forceps.

03
Example of using forceps to extract fully erupted mandibular third molar ★

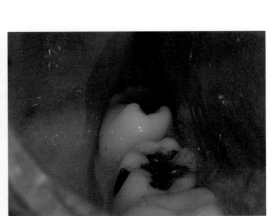

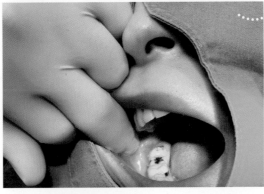
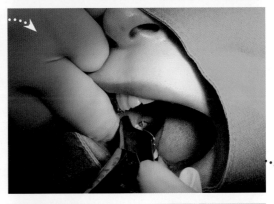

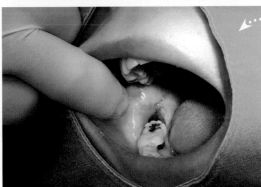
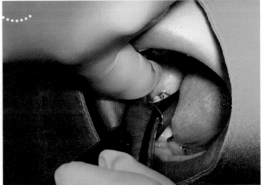

Radiograph and intraoral photographs illustrate that the cervical bulge of the crown is above the gingiva. In order to apply elevators in these cases, the buccal bone must be removed after a full thickness flap to create space to accommodate elevators. Therefore, in such cases, it is best to attempt with the forceps first. Even for someone with a weak wrist strength, such elongated, single rooted wisdom teeth can be extracted easily. Make sure the left index finger is placed on the opposing dentition since just from gripping force of the crown may abruptly luxate the tooth out of the socket. The forceps often 'jump' and damage the maxillary anterior teeth too as this happens, so the left index finger must also cover up to the maxillary anterior teeth as much as possible, as illustrated by the photo.

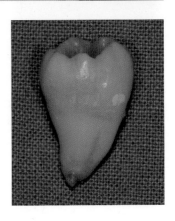

04
Forcep movements for mandibular third molar ★★

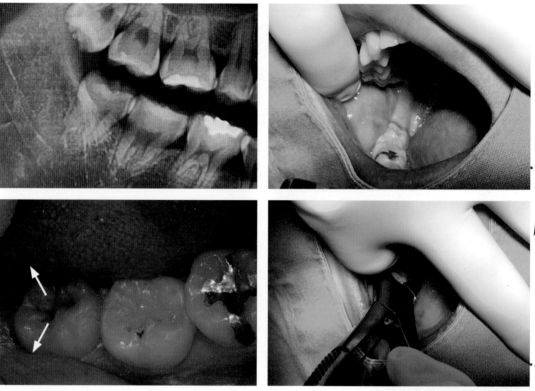

During luxation with the forceps, keep in mind that the mesial of the third molar is contacting the distal of the second molar. The pressure of luxation movement by the forceps can crack the second molar. Please refer back to the section where it explains how to use forceps. From my experience, third molars must be luxated first to feel whether the buccal or the lingual movement of the tooth is easier. More luxation force should be applied toward that direction. Based on my experience, more teeth are extracted with buccal luxation.

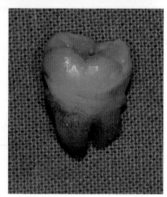

 Additional tips for challenging extractions of fully erupted mandibular third molars using only hand instruments such as forceps or elevators will be covered at the end of this chapter.

05
QR code videos

Fully erupted mandibular third molar extraction using forceps

Fully erupted mandibular third molar extraction using forceps after attempting with elevator

Fully erupted mandibular third molar extraction using forceps after attempting with elevator

Fully erupted mandibular third molar extraction using forceps after attempting with elevator

Fully erupted mandibular third molar extraction using elevator engaging on the distal aspect in an orthodontic patient.

Here are some videos but more to come upon completion of this book. Refer to Youtube on the link below for more videos!

Fully erupted mandibular third molar extraction using 5C elevator due to wider space around the crown

Fully erupted lingually tilted mandibular Third molar and buccally tilted maxillary third molar extraction using forceps

Wait!

I want to be a person who's good at teaching extraction ★★ not who's good at extraction

One's extraction skills cannot be objectively measured or assigned numerical values, but if it was possible, I would not rate my skills high. Especially the wisdom teeth that are on the inferior border of the mandible or ones with cysts or tumors, I have never attempted to remove them nor am I capable of such procedures. As a dentist in South Korea, I admire and appreciate from the bottom of my heart the South Korean oral and maxillofacial surgeons who continue to provide important services of tumor removal, maxillofacial reconstruction, and wisdom teeth removal at very low fees (true in South Korea). Sometimes I am concerned that my book may come across as an arrogant statement or a challenge against the expertise of the oral and maxillofacial surgeons. I do not wish to be someone who is good at extracting wisdom teeth but someone who enjoys it within the scope of general dentistry and exchanges related information with colleagues. While I meet most dentists as their instructor at seminars these days, I am just another dentist who wants to communicate and share with an open mind.

Wait!

How did I end up extracting a lot of third molars? ★★★

Third molar extraction fees are extremely low in South Korea. Since not many people were willing to do them because of low fees, I was able to extract as many wisdom teeth as I wanted. I opened my practice in February of 2002, where the daily foot traffic was over a million young people near the Gangnam station. In those days a posterior resin restoration was around $88 and an implant around $2,650, but a full bony impacted wisdom tooth extraction was around $26 dollars. Because of this ridiculously low fee set by the government (and illegal to charge more), extracting wisdom teeth was something that dentists generally avoided. Thankfully, due to this, someone so lowly such as myself was given a lot of opportunities as a new dentist. From the beginning I have always enjoyed surgical procedures and I was better at extracting teeth than doing restorative procedures. So even if patients had visited my office for some other procedures, I began offering wisdom teeth removals and since then I have been a dentist who enjoys wisdom tooth removals and works hard to be good at them.

Partial Soft Tissue vertically impacted Mandibular Third Molar Extraction

★

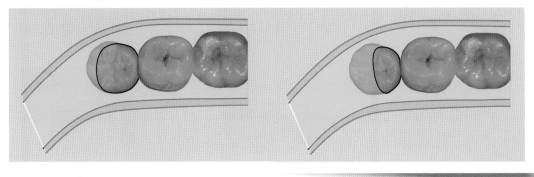

▬Occlusal surface of the wisdom tooth is covered by the gum but not bone.

As mentioned previously, fully erupted wisdom tooth extractions can be the most challenging extractions. Then what about the vertically impacted wisdom teeth that are about half covered by the gingiva? Truth be told, these are the easiest to remove. It may depend on the case but generally these are the easiest, and most can be extracted with just the elevator alone. If dental schools had to teach wisdom tooth removals, I believe these would be ideal to practice using elevators. Of course the training would have to cover proper uses of both the forceps and the elevators, but if I had to place an emphasis on one only, I would recommend removing these partially exposed vertically impacted wisdom teeth with elevators. The elevator applications form the basis of all extractions. When one becomes proficient in extracting these types of wisdom teeth, the horizontally impacted wisdom teeth extraction become easier. Therefore, I recommend that one practices the use of elevators several times on vertically impacted wisdom teeth to improve extraction skills overall.

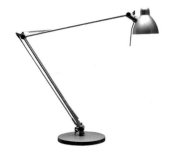

01
Extraction of vertically impacted 3rd molar with elevators ★

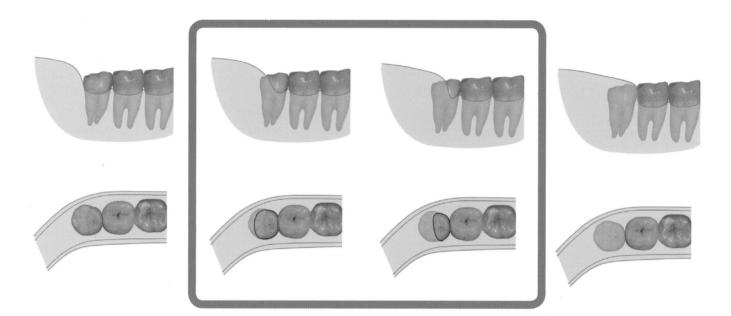

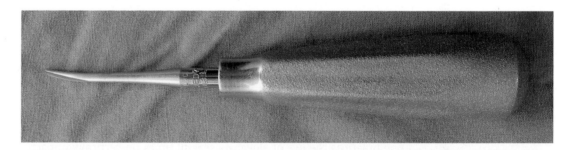

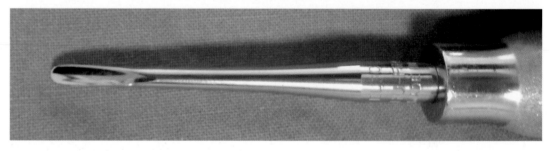

Extraction of wisdom teeth with about half of the crown visible can be the easiest among the different classifications of mandibular third molar extractions. Most of these cases can be extracted with an elevator alone without incisions. These can be extracted within a few seconds once you have mastered the proper technique of engaging the tooth and controlling the elevator.

02
Where to engage the elevator? ★★

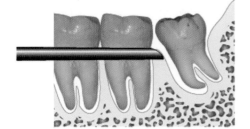 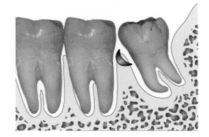 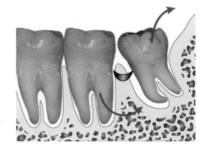

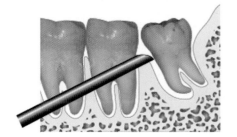 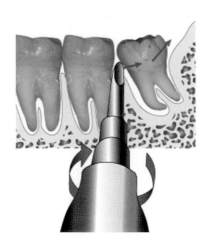 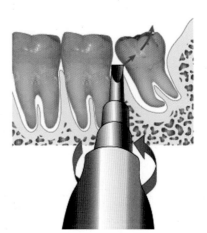

The illustrations above were created in a similar fashion to those found in a typical oral surgery textbook. The thing that I emphasize the most in extractions is to avoid creating anything that makes me sad. As I always emphasize, the general dentists avoid doing third molar extractions because they get stressed out after the procedure is performed, not because they do not know how to.

When you apply the elevator between the second molars and third molars as illustrated above, it is easier to damage the distal of the second molar. Perhaps you never had a problem even after doing a few hundred extractions this way. However, if you extract over a ten thousand like me, a few second molars are sure to have distal root damage on the buccal side. Even on the distal of maxillary second molars, where there is more soft tissue than dense bone, avoid using elevators. Do not place elevator on the mesial of the mandibular 3rd molar - the distal of the 2nd molar will be damaged. I will go over where to put elevator for a safe and easy extraction in the next page.

03
Video clips found on extractions using the elevator between the second ★ and third molars

Here are some general wisdom tooth extraction videos from YouTube when you search for it. I added my personal opinions about other people's techniques, and I will leave it up to you to decide if their techniques are correct or not.

 Watch 1

Start watching from 4:45 min. If you do multiple extractions like this, there will be cases where patients will have micro-cracks in the distal of second molars, and complain that they have sensitivity after the extraction. Sometimes you will see that dentists pushing down the 2nd molar when extracting 3rd molar to ensure the 2nd molar does not move – this shows how dangerous this method is. I would have engaged the elevator in the distobuccal area.

 Watch 2

This is the typical way of engaging an elevator in mesial area of the third molar. If I were in this situation, I would again engage the elevator in the distobuccal area. From my experience, engaging in the distal area of the third molar is easier and gives me more leverage during elevation.

 Watch 3

These videos demonstrate what's called EWF technique (Extraction Without Forceps). In this case, I also suggest engaging the elevator in the distobuccal area. If this fails to extract the tooth, I recommend switching to forcep extraction rather than trying to engage the elevator in the mesial area.

04
For mandibular vertically impacted teeth, apply the elevator right here! ★★

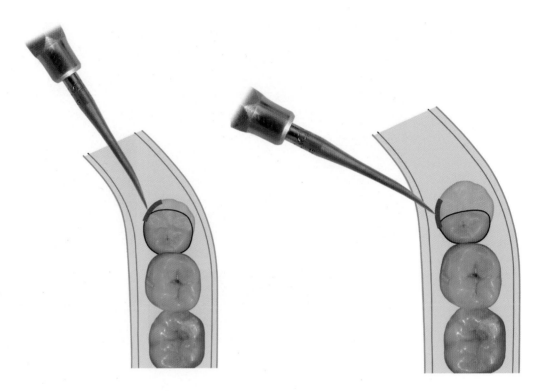

When it comes to vertically impacted wisdom teeth, the easiest way to extract them may be by applying the elevator with the fulcum on the distobuccal bone. Dentists who have trained on a thicker instrument like the EL4S tend to have a difficult time understanding this part. You must have a Hu-Friedy EL3C, which is slightly curved so that it can get around the buccal height of contour of the tooth; and it is narrow and sharp, which allows it to stick in between the alveolar bone and the tooth without removing buccal bone.

Remember! The elevator must engage the disto-buccal of the mandibular third molar.

"Hu-Friedy EL3C & Distobuccal"

05
How to position the elevator on the buccal? ★

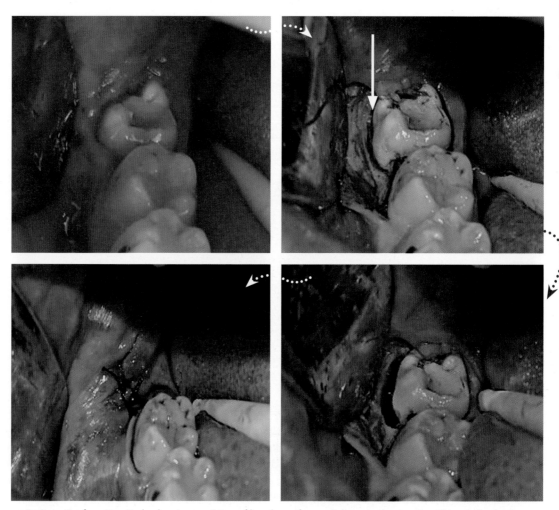

Dr. Peter Kim from New Zealand sent me a picture of how he performs wisdome teeth extractions through Facebook messenger.

The case above demonstrates the most widely used process to extract wisdom teeth. Majority of oral surgeons are trained this way in their graduate programs. This is a typical and textbook way to train and prepare residents for bigger surgeries, probably using a wider and thick elevator like the EL4S. However, by using a narrower and smaller elevator like the EL3C, you can still easily extract these wisdom teeth while avoiding more complicated methods like the one demonstrated above. If I were to perform the procedure on the same case above, I would have applied the elevator in the disto-buccal (white arrow in the second photograph) without making an incision, flapping, and taking away bone. Now, let's take a look at cases using my technique.

06
Extraction of vertically impacted 3rd molar with the elevator <1> ★★★

CASE 1

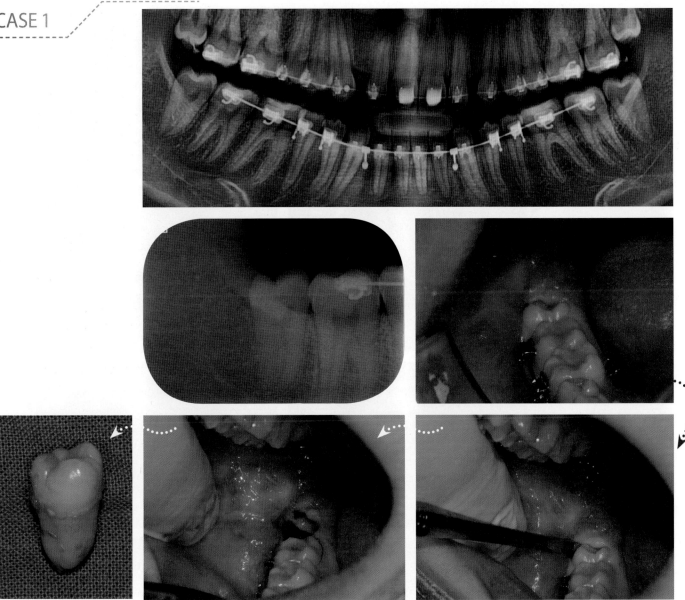

The crowns of both #38 and #48 (#17, 32) pictured above are mostly above the alveolar bone and partially covered by the soft tissue. There would be a high risk of soft tissue damage if I were to use forceps here. In my experience, an elevator creates a greater force than forceps. In many cases, if these teeth were erupted just slightly more or if the bone level on distal was slightly lower, the elevator cannot find a good purchase point. The best case to use the elevator is when just the height of contour of the distal aspect of the crown appears to be slightly encased in the alveolar bone. For #48 (#32), I used the elevator engaging in the disto-buccal bone without incision because the size of the crown was not too big and the root anatomy also allowed for an easy removal.

Extraction of #38 (#17) one month after extracting #48 (#32) ★★★
on the same patient

CASE 2

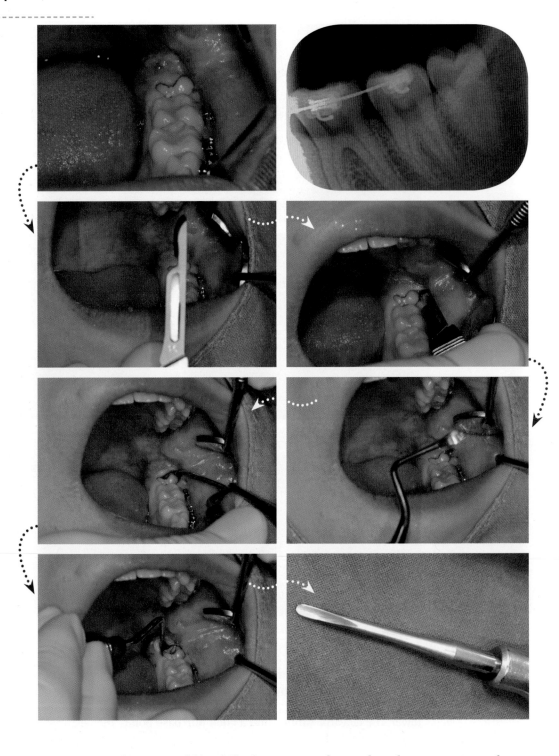

This is a case where it would be difficult to extract the tooth without an incision due to the size of the crown. In such cases, I place a very small buccal incision. The purpose of this small incision is to create space just large enough to insert an elevator on the disto-buccal. The gingiva above the occlusal surface is then released with a surgical curette (concave side down) using the 2nd class lever movement (see Chapter 5-1) while checking for presence of bone on the occlusal surface.

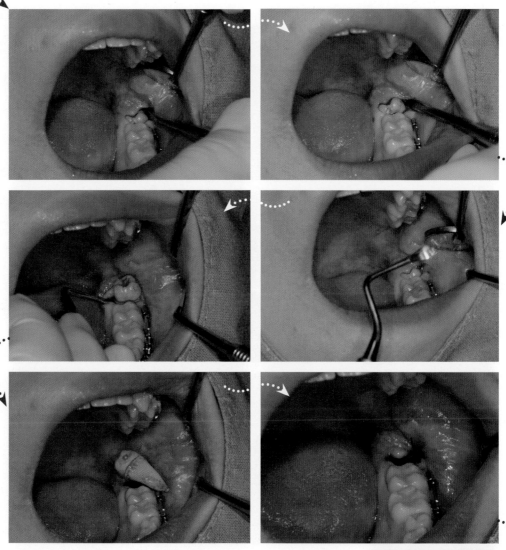

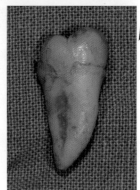

Once the tooth is completely luxated, I apply the surgical curette on the lingual and remove the tooth towards the buccal where the incision line is. A surgical curette is very useful in a variety of ways. And then I just put a small suture on the small incision line. I prefer making small incisions as we should always remember "it is better to create an incision than get tearing of the tissue." If soft tissue is torn during the extraction, this means that the elastic limit of the tissue has been exceeded and there is greater trauma to the area than you might think. In cases such as this, if the elevator was forced from buccal to push the tooth out lingually, disto-lingual gingiva could have been torn.

Extraction of vertically impacted 3rd molar with the elevator <2> ★

CASE 3

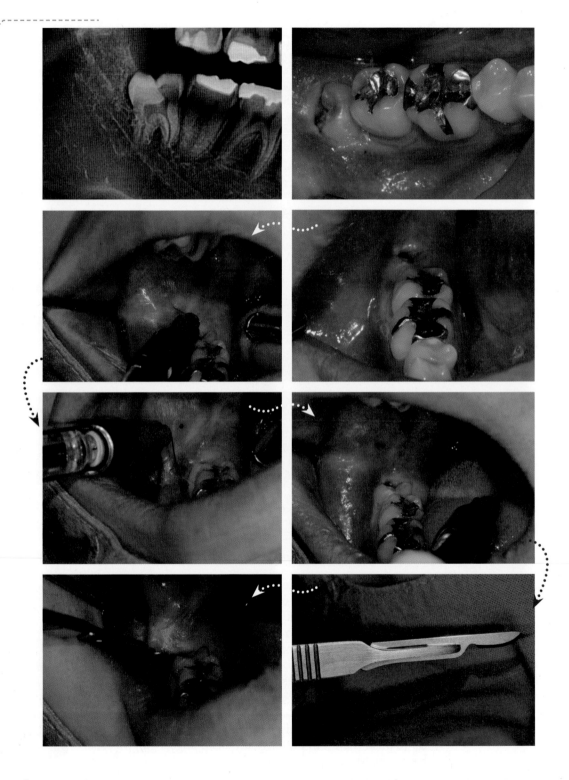

This case above is an extraction of my nephew's mandibular 3rd molar. Local anesthesia was provided to the ramus, the buccal, and the lingual, in that order per usual. The distal portion of the crown may appear to be impacted in alveolar bone based on the images, but most of such cases can be extracted just using an elevator.

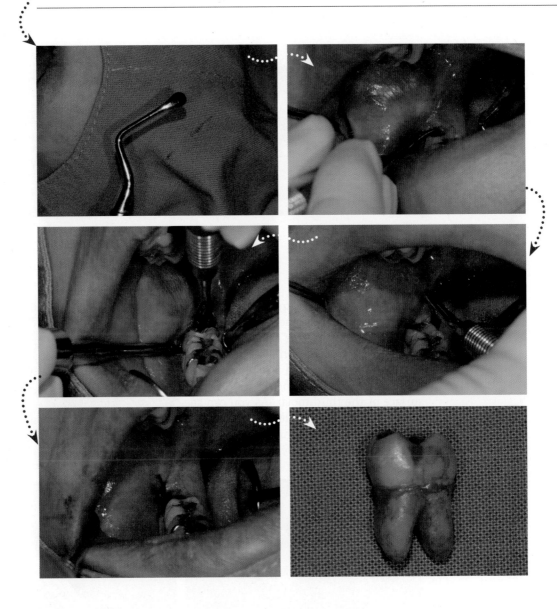

Use the convex surface of a surgical curette to release the distal gingiva and to determine the presence of bone on top of the disto-occlusal surface of the crown. In many cases as this, most of the occlusal surface is covered by soft tissue only. In order to remove the tooth luxated by the disto-buccal application of an elevator, place periosteal elevator on the lingual between the tooth and the lingual soft tissue, preventing lingual tearing of the soft tissue. This is a very useful technique, but you must be very cautious not to use any more force than what is minimally necessary to retract the disto-lingual tissue. This technique is very useful when the crown is very big or tilted lingually. Despite the usefulness of this technique, it is still very important to design an appropriate incision line to minimize tissue trauma.

Extraction of vertically impacted 3rd molar with the elevator <3> ★

CASE 4

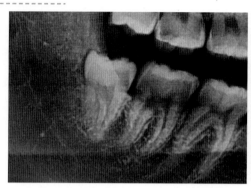
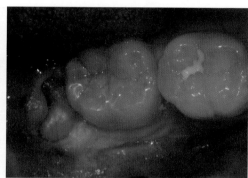

In this case, a buccal incision was made (I never make lingual incision). The most important factor in this case is using the surgical curette, like in the previous case, to retract the tissue and also checking for presence of alveolar bone on the occlusal surface of the third molar. As you can see from the photos, the occlusal surface is visibly covered only by the gingiva.

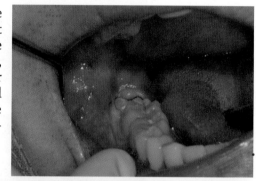

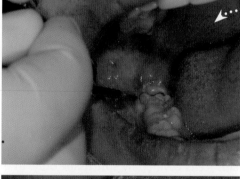
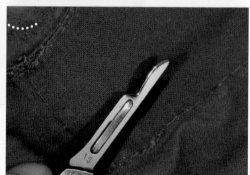

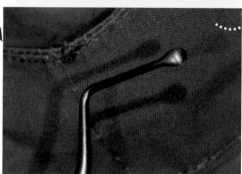
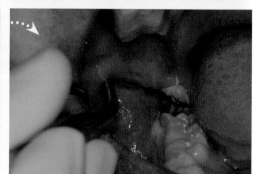

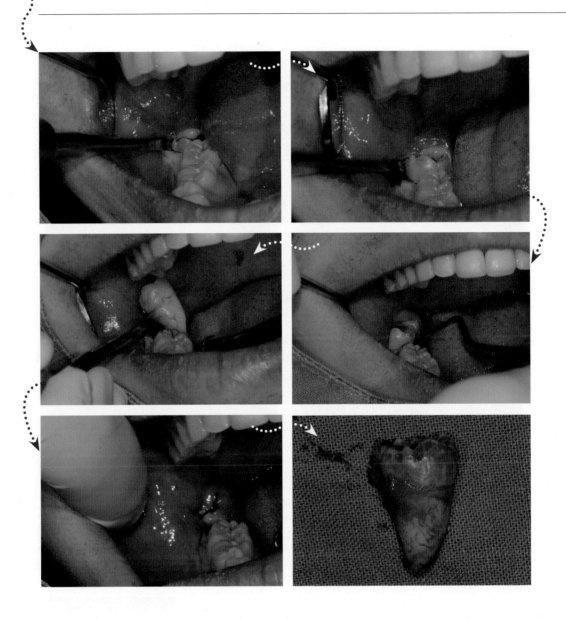

The procedure for this case is very similar to the previous case, except that the lingual gingiva would have been torn if I had tried to remove the tooth only using an elevator from the buccal without lifting the tooth out toward the buccal from the lingual with a surgical curette. When the office is very busy, I am often tempted to skip this step. But this can end up taking more time because I could tear the lingual tissue and take more time to place sutures. Of course, it is highly unlikely that there would be any notable anatomical structures such as the lingual nerve where the tear would be, but because the degree of lingual anatomy variation is too great and unpredictable, we must always be careful on lingual area. If you extract enough teeth this way, tearing lingual tissue, eventually you might run into a big problem.

Extraction of vertically impacted 3rd molar with the elevator <4> ★★

CASE 5

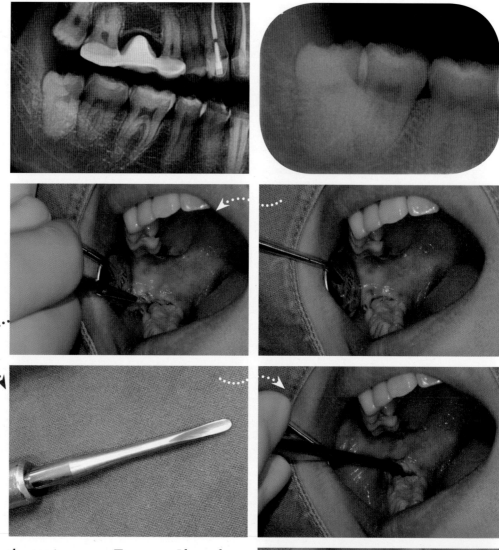

This case is also similar to the previous cases. The reason I keep showing similar cases is because when you master extracting vertically impacted 3rds, all the other cases become easier. You must get used to performing extractions this way. Even horizontally impacted 3rds are extracted basically the same way as the vertically impacted cases once the crown is cut off. If you can, first focus on vertical impaction cases before moving onto mesially tilted 3rds cases.

When I am really busy, I sometimes just use the EL3C elevator to make the incision (because the tip is sharp and narrow), flap, and remove the tooth. In this case, I also used EL3C to check for presence of bone on the distal occlusal surface.

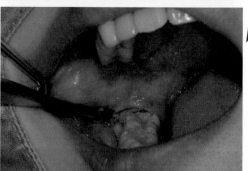

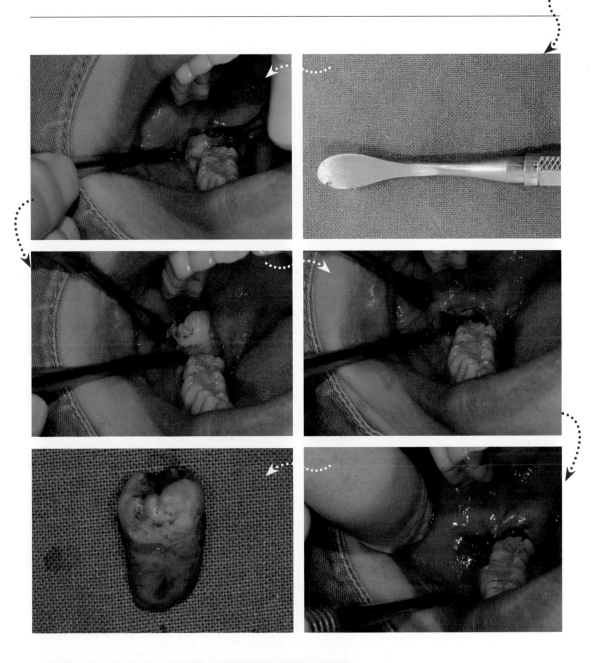

Place periosteal elevator on the lingual so the wisdom tooth does not tear the lingual gingival tissue as it comes out

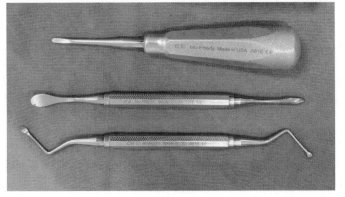

Only these 3 key hand instruments are needed in my surgical armamentarium (in addition to the basic instruments) for mandibular 3rd molar extractions in my clinic. Even though I extract more than a few hundred wisdom teeth per month, I rarely need any other instruments.

Extraction of vertically impacted wisdom teeth with the elevator <5> ★★★

CASE 6

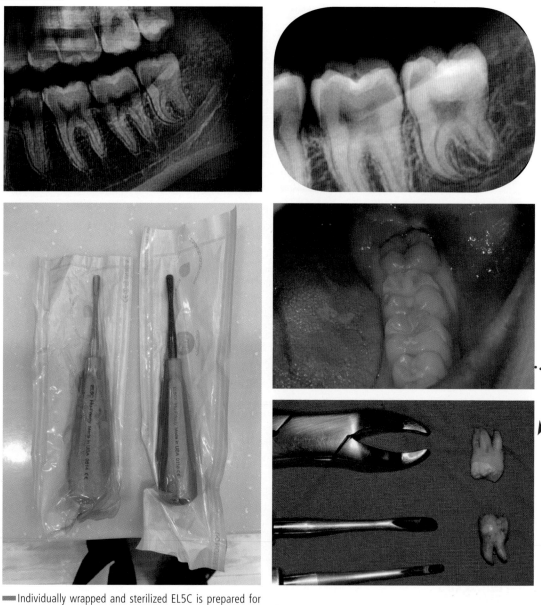

━━Individually wrapped and sterilized EL5C is prepared for extraction in certain situations.

This tooth is fully erupted into the occlusal plane, so the occlusal table is all exposed but the distal appears to be surrounded by bony tissue. I predicted that an elevator extraction would be easier here than with forceps, so I attempted with the elevator. But in such cases, the space between the buccal bone and the tooth is a bit too large for the EL3C and does not engage properly. So I extracted with the EL5C elevator. I stated before that it is a habit of mine to take post-operative photos of teeth with instruments next to them to remember which instruments were used in the process. The lower right photo above illustrates that the left maxillary third molar was extracted by forceps and the left mandibular third molar was first attempted by EL3C but finished with EL5C.

Extraction of vertically impacted wisdom teeth with the elevator <6> ★★★

CASE 7

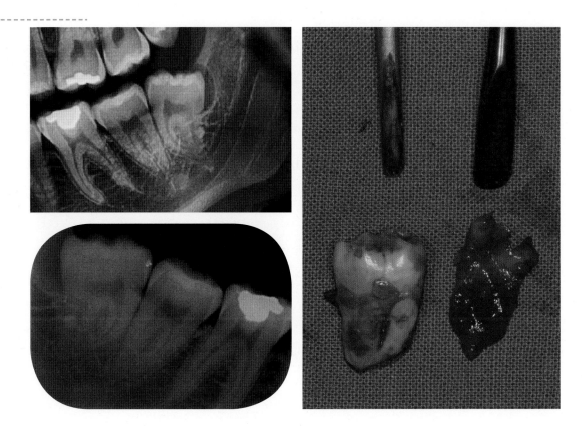

Similar cases like this are commonly seen in the clinic. In this case, the alveolar bone level seen on the radiograph may seem like it would be a quick extraction with the EL3C, but these are often more difficult than you might think. The inflammatory lesion (pericoronal follicle) distal to the mandibular third molar has been present for a long time and has caused bone resorption, which created extra space between the tooth and the buccal bone. The EL5C, which is wider than the EL3C, was used here. The inflammatory tissue was removed along with the tooth.

07
Video clips of extractions with an elevator without incision ★★★

 1/2 of the tooth exposed – elevator with no incision

 1/2 of the tooth exposed – elevator and surgical curette

 2/3 of the tooth exposed – elevator and surgical curette

08
Video clips of extractions with an elevator with incision ★★

Less than 1/3 of the tooth exposed, elevator used after incision

Less than 1/3 of the tooth exposed, elevator and surgical curette used after incision

Less than 1/3 of the tooth exposed, elevator used after incision and suture placed

Less than 1/3 of the tooth exposed, elevator used after incision then surgical curette used from the lingual

Less than 1/3 of the tooth exposed, elevator used after incision

Less than 1/3 of the tooth exposed, elevators (EL4S → EL3C) used after incision

A debate regarding wisdom tooth extractions

Which Tooth (Mandibular or Maxillary) Should be Extracted First?

Oral surgery textbooks recommend to extract maxillary teeth before mandibular teeth (except for teeth with bony impactions). The rationale behind this sequence is: 1) the onset of anesthesia is faster with maxillary teeth and 2) debris may fall into the bony sockets of the mandible if maxillary teeth are extracted after mandibular teeth.

However, in the real world, sequences differ from school to school. To me, it feels a bit awkward to always remove maxillary teeth first just because this is what is taught by textbooks. Most maxillary wisdom teeth are removed within few seconds while most mandibular wisdom teeth take a few minutes to sometimes over 30 minutes. But while working on mandibular teeth, there is continued bleeding from the maxilla and debris from cutting mandibular teeth can wind up in maxillary sockets. It is hard to say which way is the correct way because everyone has their own philosophy that works well for them.

Personally, my rule is to extract mandibular wisdom teeth first because mandibular third molars typically require more time and more often need tooth sectioning. Some say the maxillary teeth should be removed first because they take less time to be anesthetized but if an appropriate injection technique is followed correctly, regardless of whether it is mandibular or maxillary teeth, profound anesthesia can be achieved quickly. Even though it does typically take longer to extract mandibular third molars, it is rare to have anesthesia wearing off in maxillary third molars while working on mandibular teeth (because they are also removed quickly) or have mandibular teeth take longer to become anesthetized. It might be better to say that you should remove ones that will take longer rather than saying you should always remove the mandibular wisdom teeth first. Following the same rule, I believe it would be wise to extract the more time-consuming one first when extracting both wisdom teeth from the same arch; and this is what I do.

Extraction of vertically impacted Mandibular Third Molar with Full Soft Tissue Coverage

The distal occlusal surface is impacted in alveolar bone

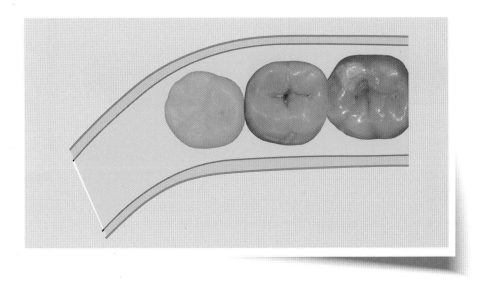

For these cases, despite being fully covered in soft tissue, the protocol for extraction with an elevator is the same as that of other vertically impacted mandibular third molars once the incision and flap are made. However, some cases where the distal occlusal surface is impacted in bone requires either removing the bone or sectioning the tooth. In most cases, I will extract by sectioning the tooth. It is difficult to tell from panoramic radiographs whether the distal occlusal surface is actually impacted in bone regardless of the degree of soft tissue coverage or how much of the crown is visible. In the end, a small incision is needed to examine the distal and buccal of the occlusal surface to see if all of the occlusal surface is above the alveolar bone. It is also useful to examine if the height of contour is above the bone. If the tooth is vertically impacted deep in bone, in addition to sectioning the distal portion of the crown, either remove the buccal bone or section the lingual portion of the crown to create space. I will touch on this again later in the book. In this chapter, we will focus on extracting vertically erupted third molars by distal crown sectioning.

01

Extraction of vertically impacted mandibular third molar with full soft tissue coverage ★★

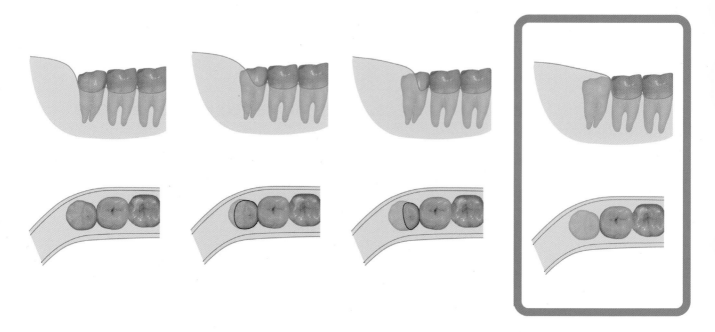

Now we are going to talk about tooth sectioning for extraction. My fundamental philosophy on extracting teeth is minimizing tissue damage around the tooth to be extracted. That is why I prefer sectioning the tooth instead of bone removal.

Dr. Youngsam Kim's Basic Principle of Extracting Impacted Wisdom Teeth

1. Avoid incisions and flaps as much as possible.

2. Avoid removing bone as much as possible.

3. Section the tooth into 100 pieces if necessary.

When the 3rd molar is vertically impacted with full soft tissue coverage, the most important factor to consider is whether the alveolar bone is above or below the occlusal surface or the height of contour of the 3rd molar. When the distal height of contour is below alveolar bone, the key is to section the distal portion of the crown, rather than removing the distal bone. I will call this technique here "distal crown cutting". When sectioning the crown, we need to make purposeful cuts in a straight line, which makes it easier to have clean breaks and leaves adequate tooth structures for better elevator adaptation.

02
Distal Crown Cutting (sectioning distal portion of the crown) ★★★

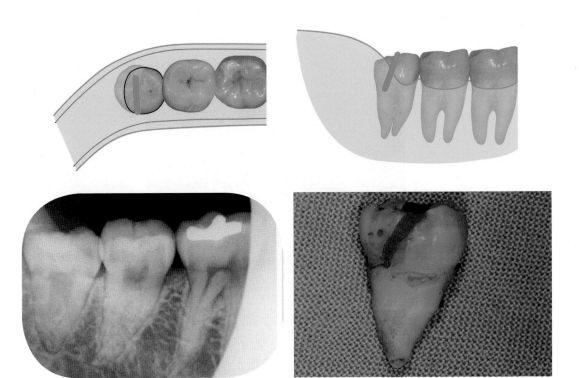

Removing the distal part of the crown is quite simple. First, the cut into the distal crown should be deep and narrow following the blue line in the diagrams above. I prefer using a 1.4 mm diameter No. 4 surgical round bur, which allows enough space for the elevator to engage and fracture the crown. Sometimes I use a No. 6 surgical round bur if a No. 4 is not available – with No. 6 round bur, the depth of cut needs to be deeper. You will see that most of the cases illustrated in this chapter is using No. 4 round bur.

As the photos illustrate, the cut is oblique. Oblique cuts are often made naturally due to the angulation of the handpiece and limitation of interocclusal space in this area. The most important part of this procedure is creating clean cuts, and drilling all the way to the buccal bone in order to create enough space for the elevator to fracture the crown. As you cut toward the lingual, you can stop at the dentin area just before the enamel to avoid lingual tissue damage.

03

Extract wisdom tooth like you are extracting Kudzu off your grandfather's grave ★★

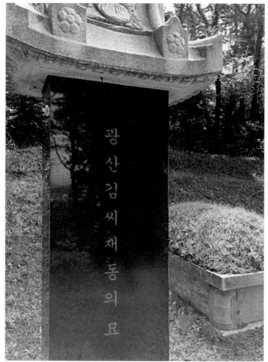

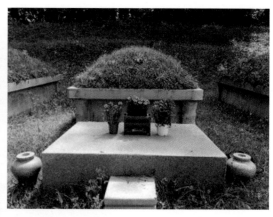

This is the grave of my grandfather. Every year I visit here on Father's day and I can see many kudzu (an herb that looks like wild ginseng) on his tomb.

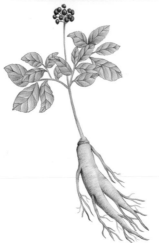

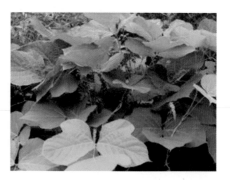

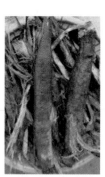

Kudzus are used in herbal medicine and have many health benefits. How do we collect them? The roots are deep inside the soil. If I want to remove them without damaging their roots, then the soil will be disturbed but I cannot disturb my grandfather's grave. This is similar to extracting 3rd molars (think kudzu as 3rd molar and grave as bone). We need to minimize the damage to the soft tissue and alveolar bone around the tooth just like we should not ruin our ancestors'grave in order to collect kudzus. Whenever you are tempted to remove alveolar bone to extract the toot, remember: "do not ruin our ancestors' grave."

04
Important tips for Distal Crown Cutting ★★

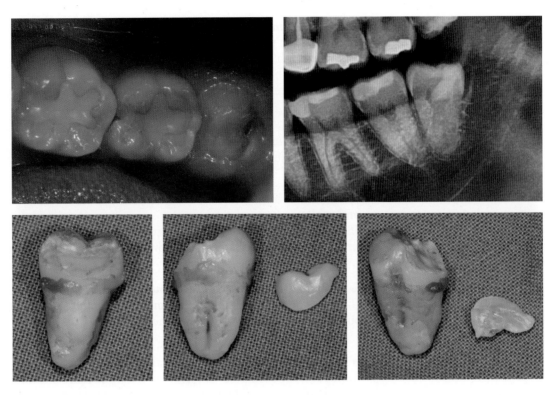

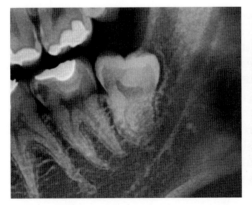

The tooth above was removed using an elevator after distal crown cutting. As you can see from the images, most of the cutting is from the buccal and I do not cut all the way to the lingual. Enamel is easy to break so there is no need to take a risk cutting with a bur all the way to the lingual side.

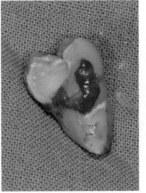

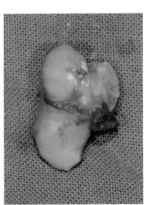

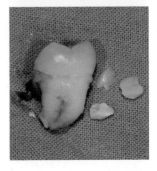

The tooth in this case was also extracted with the same procedure. It is common to have undercuts in the distobuccal area of mandibular third molars due to the ramus. That is why as long as you section the distobuccal portion of the crown completely, the rest of the tooth is easy to remove.

05
Dr. Youngsam Kim's basic rule – section the teeth ★★★

Section into multiple pieces for impacted 3rd molar
This is a basic principle when you extract wisdom teeth. As mentioned with vertically impacted teeth, we need to section teeth, rather than remove bone. If you remove bone, you may have better visibility but you will lose cortical bone that can serve as fulcrum for elevators. Therefore, I section tooth as much as possible, rather than removing bone.

There are rules to sectioning teeth.
We must absolutely avoid sectioning teeth without a clear purpose.

When removing sectioned crown pieces, consider the distal undercut of the second molar.
The extent, shape, and area of undercuts are different for each tooth. There are many cases where the crown is cut again due to different undercut areas ('crown dividing technique').

Rotate out the sectioned pieces buccally or lingually.
The distal of a 2nd molar is convex only in the middle. Sectioned pieces can be removed buccolingually since there is wide space.

If the roots are split, often it is easier to remove.
If the roots are separated, the extraction may be more difficult than the single root. However, it becomes actually easier to remove, because they are now two single rooted teeth after sectioning. The most difficult cases are where the cross-section appears peanut shaped or shaped like a duck's flipper where the roots look separated but are connected in the middle with concavity. Be mindful that radiographs can be misleading.

When there are two roots, remove the more difficult one first.
Because I tend to extract with an elevator without removing bone, when there is inadequate cortical bone, it is harder to extract. When you remove the easier root first, the bone support becomes weaker and it may require more bone removal when removing the more difficult root. But this is just my opinion.

Do not be afraid to leave root tips if necessary.
You should not consider it a failure when you fail to remove all root tips after removal of the crown. As I discussed previously, it is still a successful extraction. Just make sure all of the crown is completely removed.

Various Teeth Cutting Methods for Wisdom Tooth Extraction

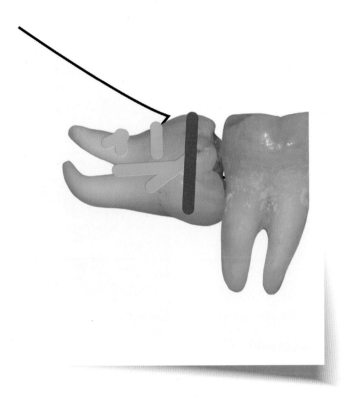

To extract wisdom teeth well, there should be minimal post-operative complications. In order to do this, we need to minimize bone removal and that is why tooth sectioning is so important. However, sectioning the tooth should not to be performed without proper planning. Randomly sectioning the tooth will not increase the ability to extract it. Have a clear purpose and direction when sectioning and name each distinct cut, like 'mesial cutting', 'distal cutting', etc. I almost always use a high speed handpiece for extraction. Before discussing the actual extraction methods, you will first learn how to use the handpiece to section teeth. Let us now look at different sectioning types that I named.

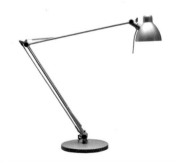

01
Techniques of traditional Korean wrestling

The picture explains techniques of Korean wrestling.

Each movement of Korean wrestling has a distinctive name based on its direction and is easily distinguished from other movements. Just as these techniques, tooth sectioning techniques have distinct names.

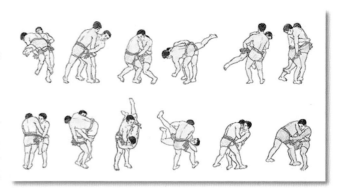

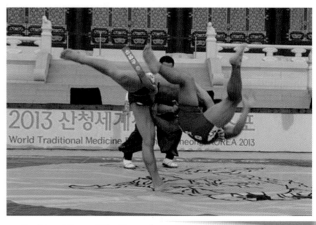

Traditional Korean Wrestling

When you watch traditional Korean wrestling, it may appear like it is a game for boasting one's strength, but every technique has a name and steps to it. There is a great difference between someone who would try brute force only and someone who uses power in strategic movements with purpose and strategy. The same is true for sectioning teeth in wisdom tooth extractions. You must have a clear plan and purpose when cutting.

★★

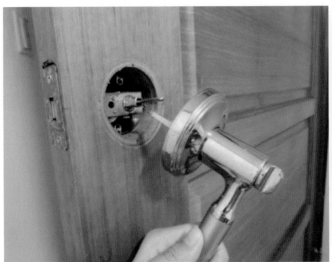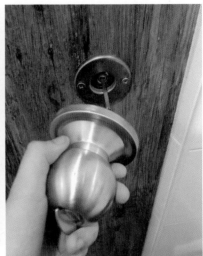

If you section teeth aimlessly and just start cutting away whatever you see, it is equivalent to taking the handle off the door. If you remove the visible part of the crown, just like the door handle, now you have made the extraction harder since you have to take out the pieces of the tooth that you cannot see. Also, it makes it harder to apply the elevator. For beginners, I suggest taking multiple radiographs in between steps to determine the progress and precision of your cuts.

★

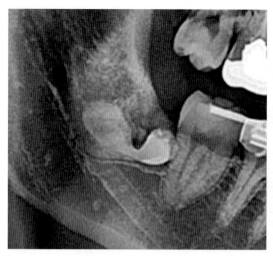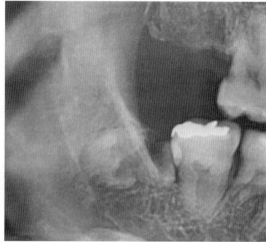

This case on the left was previously discussed in the coronectomy chapter. This is a typical 'door without the handle', where only the visible part was cut and vertical sectioning was not performed completely. The photo on the right is similar.

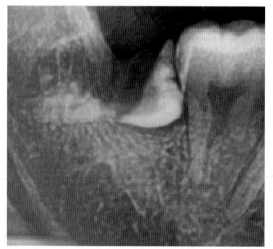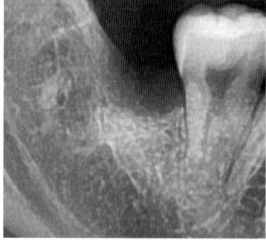

The picture above is a photo uploaded by a friend on Facebook. You can see the 'door knob' missing from the first image. The first vertical sectioning was probably intended to remove the mesial part of the crown, yet it seems that he removed or ground away all the visible parts of the distal root while leaving the mesial portion of the crown left in place. Sometimes we do extract third molars this way when the distal undercut on the second molar is severe, and you see a cut like this especially when using either a low speed handpiece or a 45-degree handpiece. But from now on, let us section teeth with a clear purpose and precision. For this purpose I put a clear name for each sectioning technique. The name is not important, but it must have a clear purpose and direction.

02
Tooth cutting (section) #48 ★★★

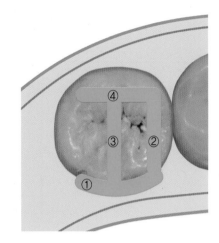

▬▬ Crown cuting

① Buccal bone cutting

② Mesial crown cutting

③ Distal crown cutting

④ Lingual crown cutting

⑤ Cervical cutting

⑥ Disto-cervical cutting (groove creating for elevator adaptation)

⑦ Coronectomy

⑧ Crown division [horizontal division (8-1) & vertical division (8-2)]

▬▬ Root cutting

⑨ Lift & Cutting

⑩ Root separation

⑪ Oblique cutting

⑫ Distal root cutting (creating groove)

⑬ Creating groove between roots

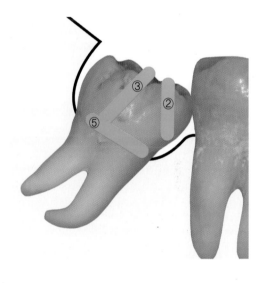

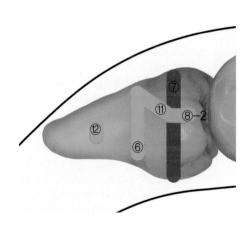

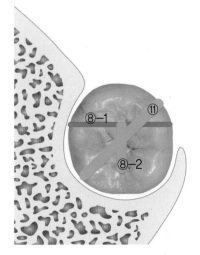

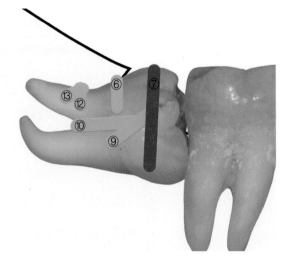

03
Why we should cut 1 mm more on the buccal and 1 mm less on the lingual side? ★★★

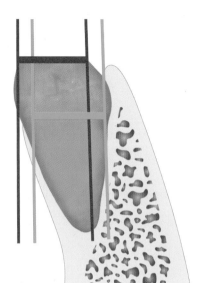 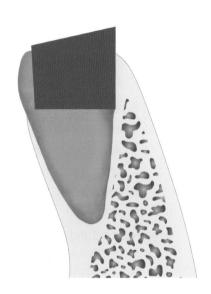

▬ The cross-section of the tooth cut by the bur will be as illustrated above if you cut the buccal 1 mm more and the lingual 1 mm less.

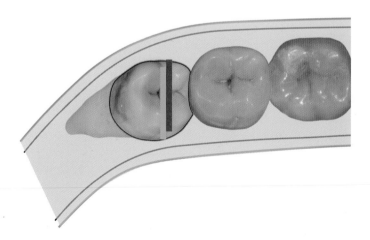

▬ The red line above demonstrates the exposed, visible buccolingual dimension from the occlusal surface. The green line demonstrates where the cut should be made to section the tooth.

The reason why I say we should cut 1 mm more on the buccal side and 1 mm less on the lingual side than what is visible is to prevent damaging the lingual tissue and minimize risk of complications like nerve damage and excessive bleeding. I believe this is why I have never had a nerve injury in my career. Generally the lingual side has a greater undercut the further apically you go, so cutting 1 mm less is safer. Despite not cutting all the way through the lingual portion of the tooth, there is no trouble causing a clean fragment with an intentional fracture because enamel is brittle. Also, because I often use the 'oblique cutting' technique, this is even less likely to cause me trouble. However, we should for sure cut 1 mm more on the buccal because unlike the lingual side, the buccal anatomy of the tooth is very convex, which requires cutting more in that direction than what you see on the occlusal table. Although we generally minimize tooth cutting, the buccal needs to be cut all the way through for the instrument to work well and cause a clean, intentional fracture even when the lingual portion is not cut all the way through. In my live surgery courses, new dentists often are very afraid of extending the cut both lingually and buccally, which makes extractions difficult. On the buccal side, you need a clean, definitive cut for visibility and instrumentation. Let us memorize – 1 mm more on the buccal and 1 mm less on the lingual.

04
These radiographic images explain in detail ★★★

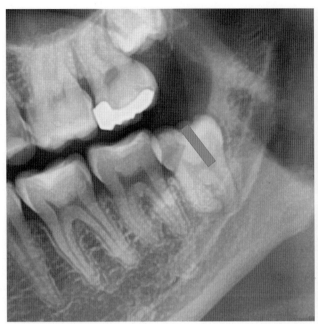 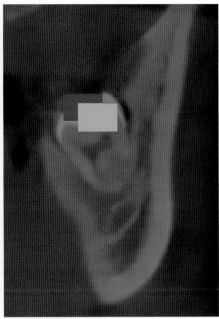

If we plan to extract the third molar here using 'distal crown cutting' technique, the cut made following the visible portion of the occlusal table would be as indicated by the red area, but the cross sectional cut we need to make is indicated by the green area. The green area demonstrates a cut that extends 1 mm more to the buccal and 1 mm less to the lingual, which does not extend to the lingual bone.

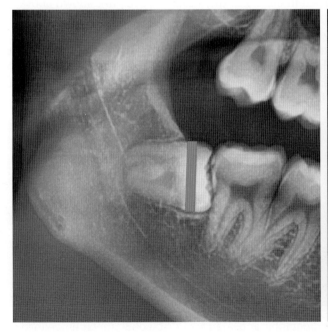 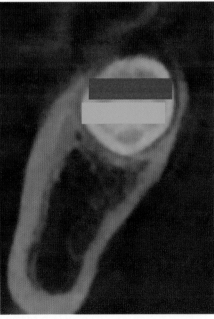

When it comes to cutting the crown of the horizontally impacted tooth, we also can use the same technique as above. Please remember "cut 1 mm more on the buccal side and 1 mm less on the lingual side."

05
Case 1: Sectioning the distal crown (distal crown cutting) ★★★

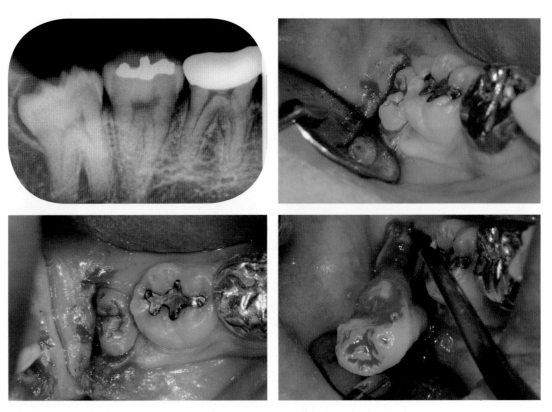

Even when completely covered by gingiva, the mandibular third molars often do not have alveolar bone on top of the occlusal surface. While it is rare to find a case where the distal occlusal surface impacted in bone and the mesial exposed like shown above, I photo-documented it for convenience. Most such cases are performed with a small incision. Normally, I insert a surgical curette between the occlusal table and the covering gingiva to check the distal portion for the bone and section the distal without raising a flap like shown above. It is very useful to perform extractions this way with 'distal cutting.' For this reason, when I teach hands-on seminars, I instruct my mentees to section the distal on a vertically impacted tooth for practice even when it is unnecessary for a successful extraction.

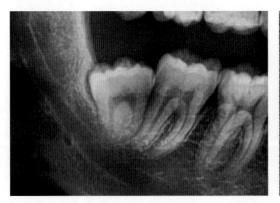
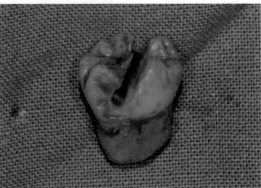

Despite the radiographic appearance of distal of 3rd molar embedded in bone, in most cases, they are not actually covered in bone. The more experience you have, the better you will be at predicting the clinical position of the 3rd molars by looking at the radiographs. Pictured is a case from a hands-on course where one of the mentees practiced 'distal cutting'– the elevator was inserted and turned to create a fracture of the tooth but the tooth came out in one piece.

Case 2: Sectioning the distal crown (distal crown cutting)

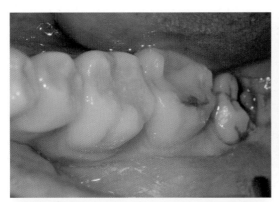

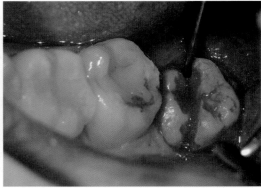

This case is similar to the previous case. In most cases, a small flap would be created but it was intentionally avoided here to take photographs. Even if you do not start the cut on the distal, the bur will naturally go distally, as you cut further down towards the cervical. This is why the distal segment fractures off first when elevator is used and there is enough space created by the thickness of the bur that allows the distal fragment to come out towards the mesial.

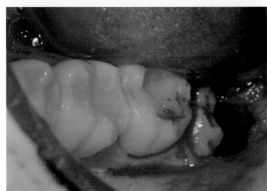

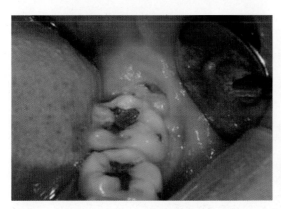

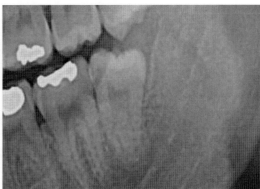

Above is a typical case indicated for applying distal crown cutting. Of course, if you are a beginner, it is necessary to make an incision and check with a surgical curette that the distal occlusal surface is free of bony impaction. Even when radiographic appearances are the same, the clinical findings may be different based on bucco-lingual positioning. If the third molar is buccally tilted, the bone from the ramus could be causing an impaction on distobuccal occlusal surface, which may require distal bone removal. When the tooth is angulated more towards the lingual, I perform a distal crown cutting even when the distal occlusal surface is not covered by bone; the reason is because when the tooth is angulated towards the lingual, you can have an over-stretching or tearing of the gingival tissue as the tooth is being removed. So if you start the extraction by performing the distal crown cutting, the whole process of extraction becomes easier. In most cases of tooth sectioning, I start the cut from the buccal and do not extend all the way to the lingual. This is especially true for teeth tilted lingually because the actual time spent on sectioning the tooth is very short.

06
An examination of extracted teeth using the Distal Crown Cutting ★★ technique

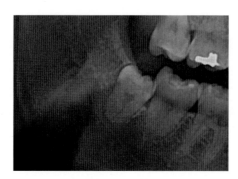

In these photos, extracted tooth fragments using the distal crown cutting technique are reattached by wax. You can see from the images that while the appearance of the occlusal surface may imply that the cut was made through-and-through buccolingually, the bur actually did not cut all the way to the lingual height of contour. All of my extracted teeth look this way upon examining after procedures.

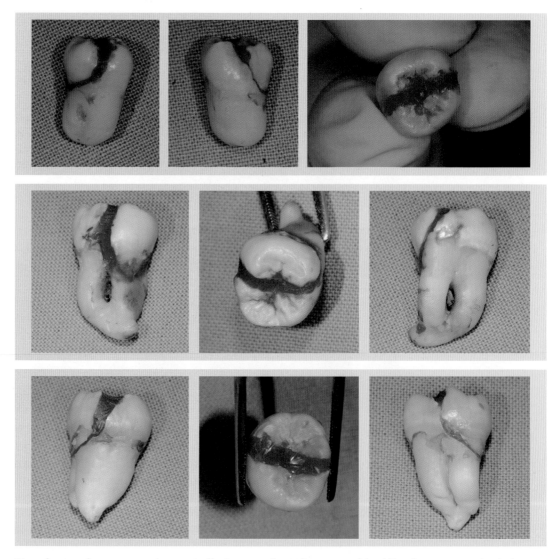

The photos above are again vertically impacted teeth removed by 'distal crown cutting'. As you can see, the buccal was cut all the way while the lingual was fractured. The same goes for horizontally impacted teeth - you do not need to cut all the way past the enamel where you will cause an intentional fracture. The enamel has a very low tensile strength without dentin and is brittle and easy to fracture.

07
'Distal Crown Cutting' cases depending on amount of crown exposure ★

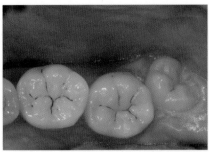 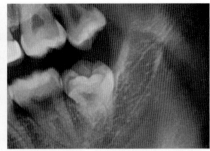 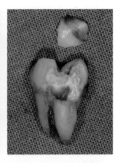

When more than ⅔ of the crown is exposed, the distal crown portion can be sectioned without making an incision. In such cases crown sectioning may be unnecessary and most are sectioned for practice. I will discuss again in the upcoming chapter of horizontally impacted teeth but if you section the crown to create more space even when it is not absolutely necessary, the extraction process becomes easier and safer.

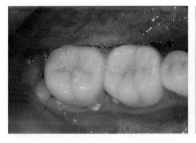 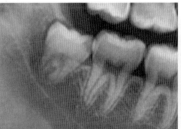 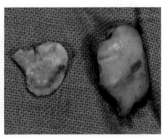

When most of the crown is covered by gingiva, distal crown cutting can be performed after a small incision. In truth, the incision does not even reach the periosteum, so a small incision is adequate.

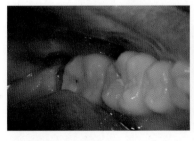 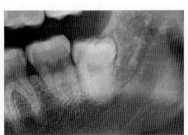 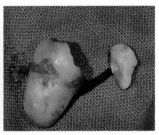

When the third molar is completely covered by gingiva, a full incision is necessary, sometimes even extending mesially with a flap. While the incision and flap design vary greatly among practitioners, the sectioned and extracted teeth should be similar in appearance.

08
More cases depending on the tipping ★★

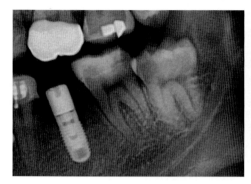
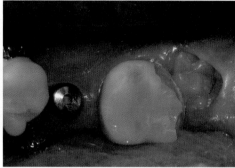
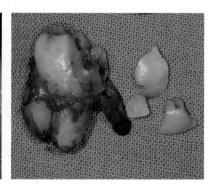

The patient presented to my office after an implant placed at another clinic. In situations like this, there is a key point to remember in performing third molar extractions – do not place elevator on the mesial of the 3rd molar. When the 1st molar is absent and you put force in between the 2nd and 3rd molar, the 2nd molar can be traumatized or even be extracted. 3rd molar is very stable inside the bone and is supported by the hard ramus, unlike the 2nd molar. In this case, the extraction becomes easier if you create space by distal crown cutting.

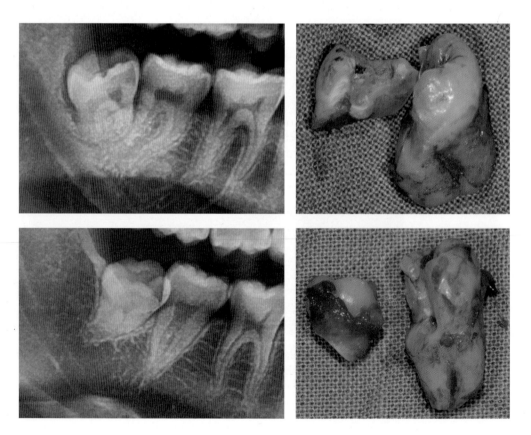

When the tooth is distally tilted, the distal crown cutting is especially useful, but it is also useful in cases where the tooth is mesially tilted. You might contemplate whether to perform a distal crown cutting or mesial crown cutting but the end results are similar. There is no huge difference but a mesial cut is easier to perform while a distal cut tends to allow for an easier extraction.

09
Distal Crown Cutting Case <1> ★

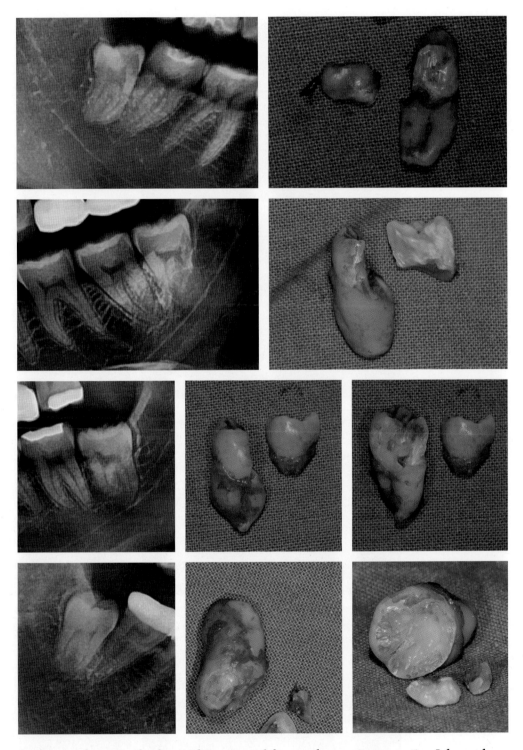

As discussed previously, due to the nature of the very busy private practice, I do not have very many pre-op photos but I have many post-op photos, which do not require complicated patient consent forms. While I do not document most extraction cases that do not require crown sectioning, my staff photographed countless cases where crowns were sectioned.

Distal Crown Cutting Case <2> ★

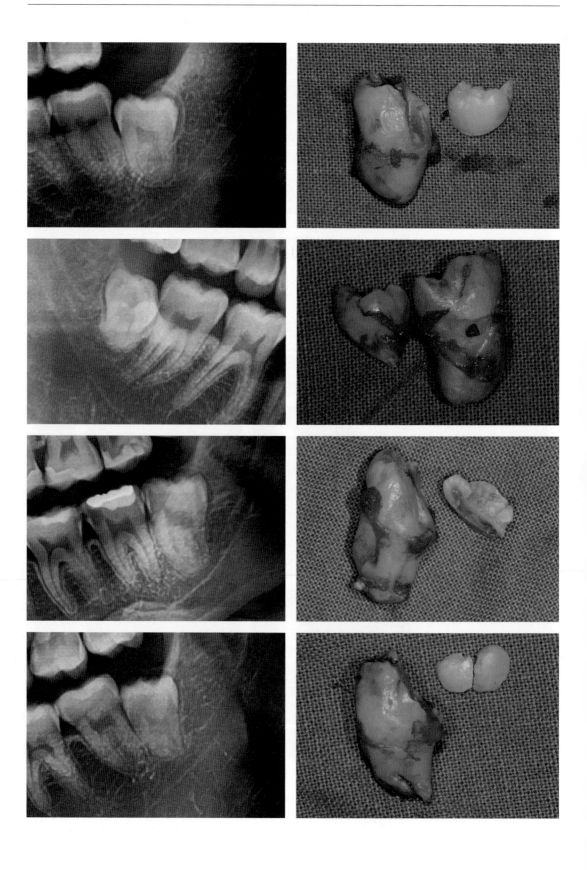

Distal Crown Cutting Case <3> ★

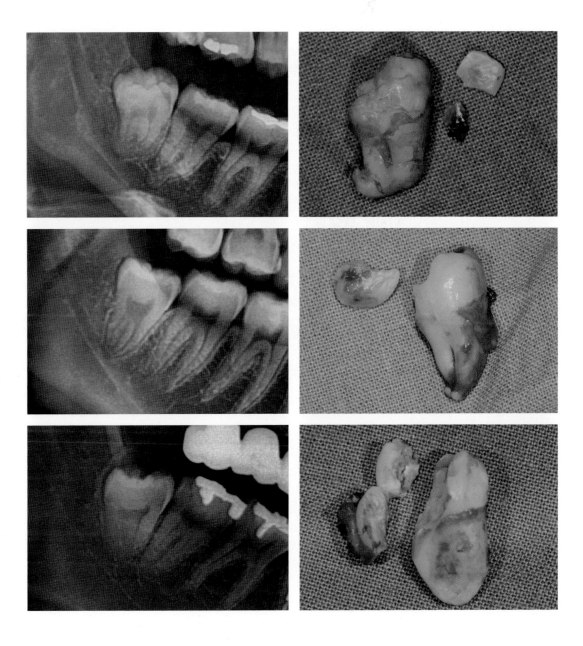

10
QR code videos ★★

 Vertically impacted mandibular 3ʳᵈ molar extraction using an elevator after distal crown cutting

 Vertically impacted mandibular 3ʳᵈ molar extraction using an elevator after distal bone removal

 Vertically impacted mandibular 3ʳᵈ molar extraction using forceps after distal crown cutting

Very Difficult Extraction of Fully Erupted ★★ Mandibular Third Molar

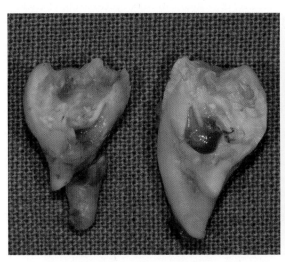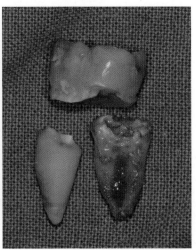

I mentioned earlier that extracting fully erupted, functioning mandibular 3rd molars can be the most difficult cases. In most fully erupted cases, I use forceps, but sometimes you will find that they do not budge at all with forceps. The periodontal ligaments surrounding non-functioning teeth are weak and the residual roots can be easily removed with just an explorer. However, the periodontal ligaments around functioning teeth are strongly developed and the bone around the roots are also harder and denser, making the extraction more difficult. In these cases, I section the tooth vertically into two pieces, removing the root one by one.

Let us discuss separating roots into two segments. There are two ways – one is vertically sectioning the whole tooth from the crown down, and the other is sectioning the roots after first removing the crown. Let us now take a look at the pros and cons of the two methods.

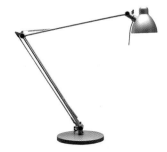

01

Very difficult extraction of a vertically impacted (very strong attachment) ★ mandibular third molar

If you have some experience with third molar extractions, you already know that the fully erupted, functioning third molars are the hardest teeth to extract. I also find that the most difficult third molars to remove are the vertically fully erupted and functioning third molars of middle aged or older men. In the past I preferred splitting the tooth vertically in halves but it is not applicable in single rooted teeth and it takes too much time. It is also more difficult to achieve profound anesthesia in these cases, which can make you struggle. These days, I do not waste a lot of time and I remove the crown first. Let us take a look at both methods.

Extraction with vertical hemisection

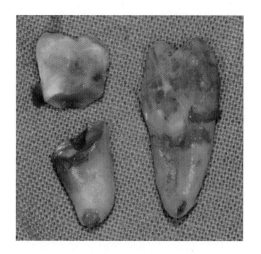

Extraction with crown sectioning first and vertical hemisection

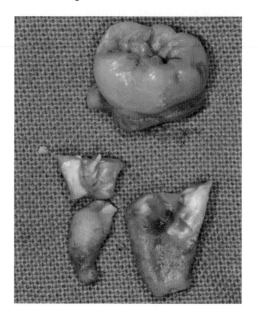

02
Referral for extraction

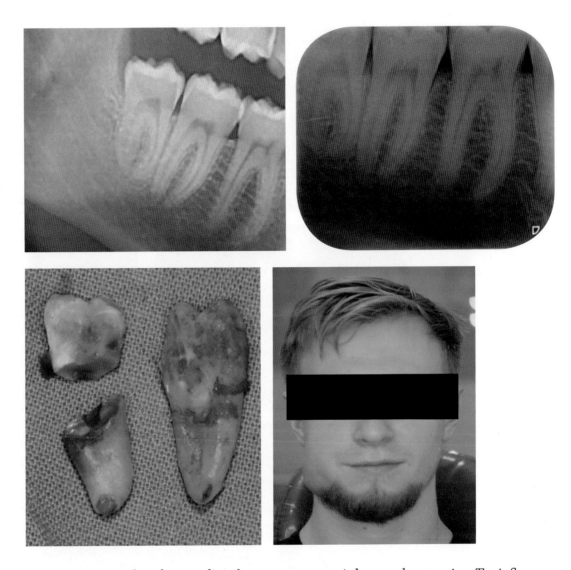

This patient was referred to my clinic for an emergency wisdom tooth extraction. The inflammation seemed unrelated to the third molar and looking back, it seems like a case of an acute bacterial infection in the area. Anyway, I was asked to extract the third molar only by the referring dentist and I performed the extraction.

My clinic is located at Gangnam Station, which has many language schools, so I frequently treat foreign patients, especially many Arabic and Turkish patients (because only one Turkish restaurant is nearby). The patient in this case is a Caucasian male with a well-developed jaw, which would make extractions more difficult. The 3rd molar did not budge to elevator or forceps. I then immediately performed a vertical hemisection and extracted the tooth. Despite the vertical sectioning down the middle, it is common to have a separation of the crown and the root, especially the distal root and the crown. It is unnecessary to place too much emphasis on cutting exactly down the middle.

03
Extracting vertically erupted mandibular third molars with vertical ★★ sectioning <1>

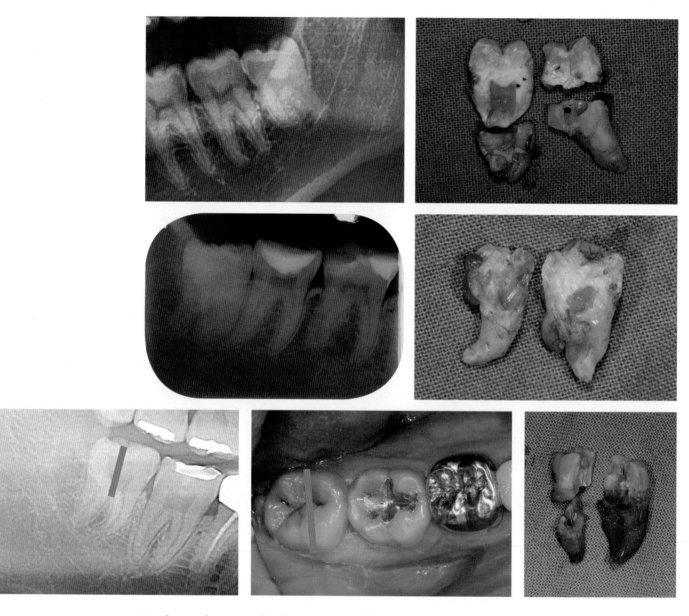

I only use this type of technique when the tooth does not budge at all with forceps and the buccal application of an elevator is not feasible - usually because most of these cases are multirooted teeth. Most single-rooted teeth respond well to forceps. Even when performing a vertical hemisection, it is better to initiate the cut more mesially (60/40 ratio) and another key point is that the cut should be made a lot deeper than you think. Because of the depth of the cut, the No.4 bur's shank will get stuck, so I sometimes section off the distal crown and then go deeper to cut in between the roots. The surgical fissure bur can be used here too.

Extracting vertically erupted mandibular third molars with crown division ★ (vertical sectioning) <2>

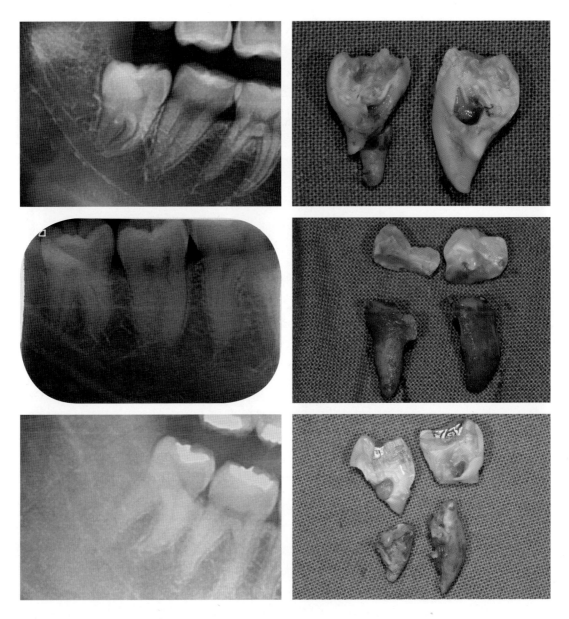

One negative aspect of the vertical hemisection is that you may have difficulty achieving profound anesthesia just like what you sometimes encounter during second molar root canal treatments. Most root apices of impacted mandibular third molars are close to the lingual plate because of the inadequate space, so the local infiltration of anesthetics on the lingual side works very well. However, roots of fully erupted wisdom teeth are positioned in the middle of the dense cortical bone, similar to mandibular second molars, which can cause difficulty with profound anesthesia. In these situations, instead of attempting to cut from the occlusal table, I recommend cutting vertically from the CEJ. It is easy to approach from the CEJ to pulp. Intrapulpal anesthesia can be performed at this time if patients are complaining of pain. This method can also be used similarly in extracting horizontally impacted mandibular third molars.

Extracting vertically erupted mandibular third molars by hemisection <3> ★★

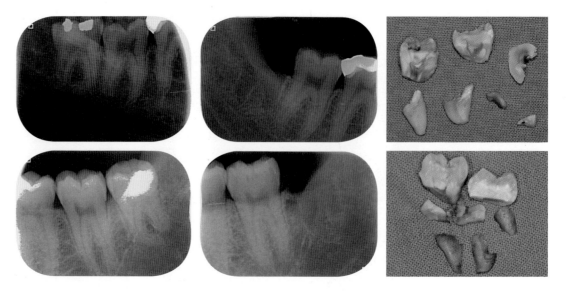

It may appear in this case that it would be easy to section the tooth vertically and remove the curved roots, but that is just in theory and I do not believe it to be that simple. It may be better to intentionally leave the curved root tips.

I am more embarrassed now looking back to when I used to try to remove every single root tip thinking leaving root tips behind is something to be embarrassed about. Now I think that it might be better to just use forceps to break off the roots to begin with. When I use forceps to extract, I often first break the roots on purpose because that is easy and safe.

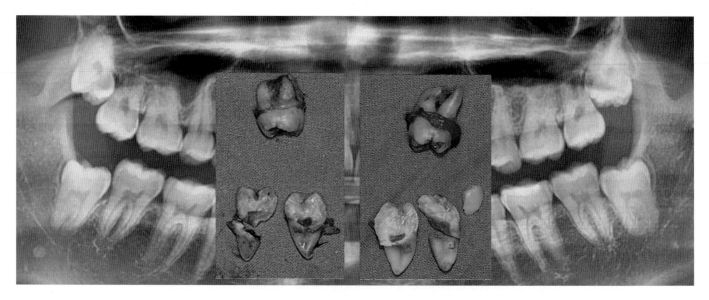

The above case is of a 28-year-old male, whose third molars were very hard to remove due to full impaction in the alveolar bone. Often, when one side is difficult, the other side is also difficult. Contrary to what the images suggest, none of them were easy to remove.

04
Attempted vertical hemisection to separate the roots ★

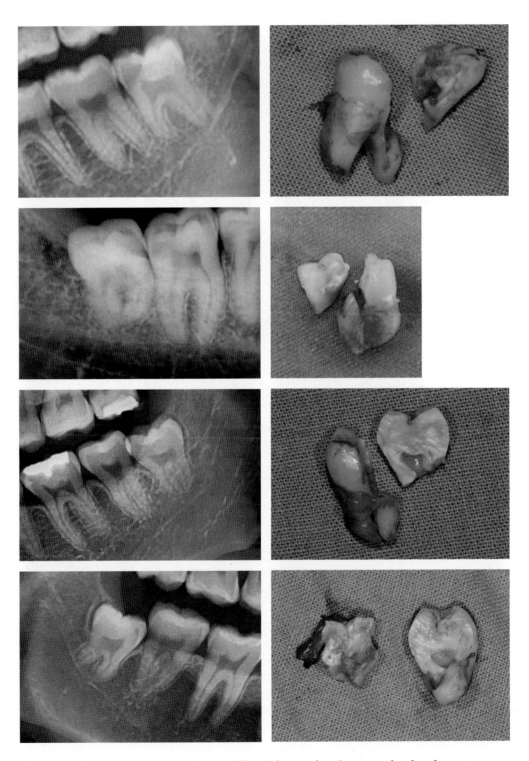

When we think we are cutting the middle of the tooth, often just the distal portion gets cut. Even in cases where we attempt a hemisection of a multi-rooted tooth, more often the tooth does not split in halves but end up sectioning off the distal portion. Still, the extractions were successful.

05
Extracting vertically erupted mandibular third molars with ★★★
'cervical sectioning' (horizontal sectioning) <1>

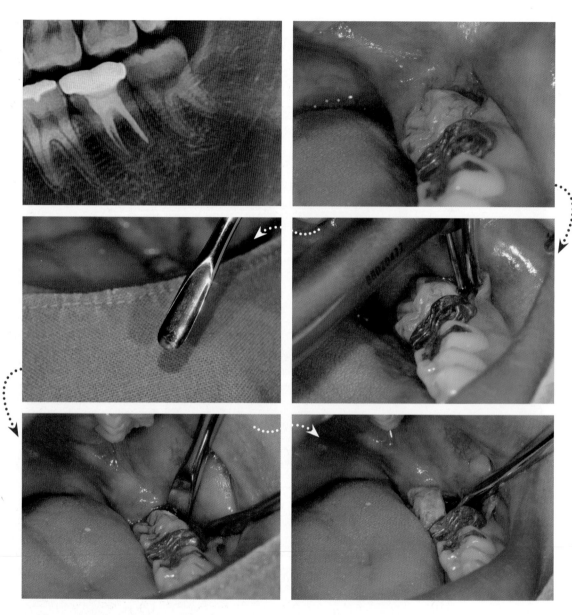

When a tooth is not easily extracted using forceps or elevators, it is good to cut off the crown and remove the residual roots. I also believe that a coronectomy is a good option as well. If the objective from the beginning is to perform a coronectomy, a flap should be made and the sectioning should be performed as close to the crestal bone as possible. However, if the objective is to remove the roots after cutting off the crown, the roots may be more difficult to remove if the crown was sectioned too close to the roots. But perhaps the most important thing in this case is trying to educate patients that a third molar like this does not have to be extracted.

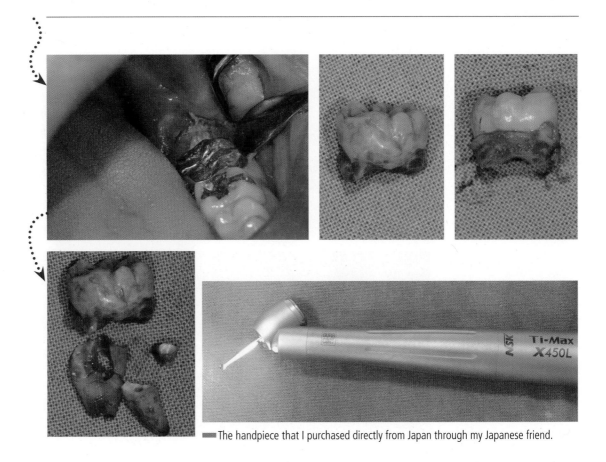

The handpiece that I purchased directly from Japan through my Japanese friend.

All parts of the tooth was removed by crown being removed first after cervical sectioning. With a conventional contra-angle high speed handpiece, only the fully erupted teeth are approachable from the buccal. Sometimes I come across practitioners who section from the lingual but I do not believe this is safe. For this reason I have been using a 45-degree handpiece for sectioning and removing the crown. This type of surgical handpiece was not officially available in Korea until about 2 years ago. I obtained this handpiece through a Japanese friend who shipped it to me after I made a direct purchase from the NSK headquarters in Japan. I met this friend at UCLA dental school 10 years ago, who is now faculty member at a dental school in Japan. I am very satisfied with the 45-degree handpiece. Now NSK Korea has been established and the handpieces are available for purchase through them. Let us remember that a dentist cannot be a good dentist without good instruments. I believe you just need one in your office.

Extracting vertically erupted mandibular third molars with ★★ 'cervical sectioning'(horizontal sectioning) <2>

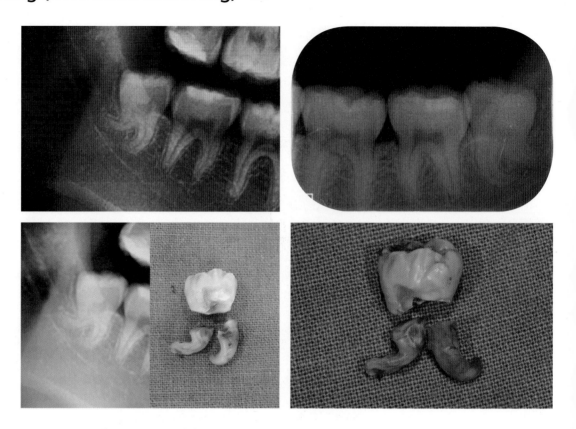

This is a case where I removed the crown for the purpose of removing the root tips as well. Generally when you use forceps or an elevator to extract a third molar with curved roots like this, the apical portions tend to break off. When the roots are superimposed with the nerve and you see a warning sign like the dark band around the roots, it is best to leave them alone. However, in this case, I first sectioned the crown off and removed the roots with an elevator near the CEJ with the intention of uploading the photos on social media. The picture on the left was taken on my phone by me to upload onto Facebook and the picture on the right was taken by my staff, which broke my heart when I saw it later. Over the years I have had to throw out many photographs because of misorientation of fragments or losing pieces post-operatively. The indentation of the inferior alveolar nerve canal can be seen on the inferior aspect of the distal root.

Cervical sectioning case <1> ★★★

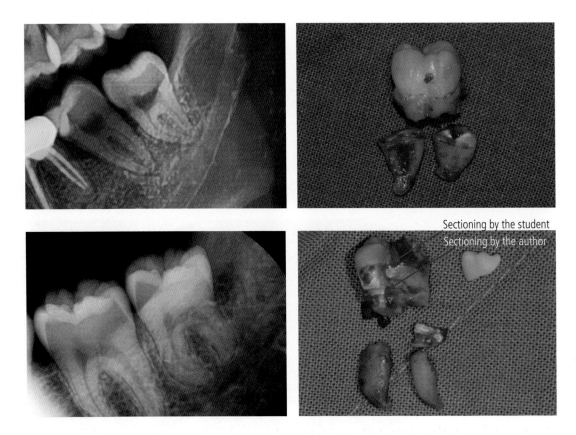

Sectioning by the student
Sectioning by the author

This tooth was extracted during my live surgery course. I was going to perform the extraction in a normal fashion here but one of them asked me to show them how to use the 45° angled surgical handpiece. A mentee at my course started to section the tooth too high (the upper arrow in the picture). I sectioned the cervical area again 3 mm lower than where the crown was originally cut (the lower arrow in the picture) and removed the crown. In most cases when a tooth is cut with just enough depth and width to insert an elevator, the crown will fracture easily and be removed. Sometimes the 5C elevator, which has a wider tip, can be useful.

 The QR code video for this case above.

06
Cervical sectioning case <2> ★

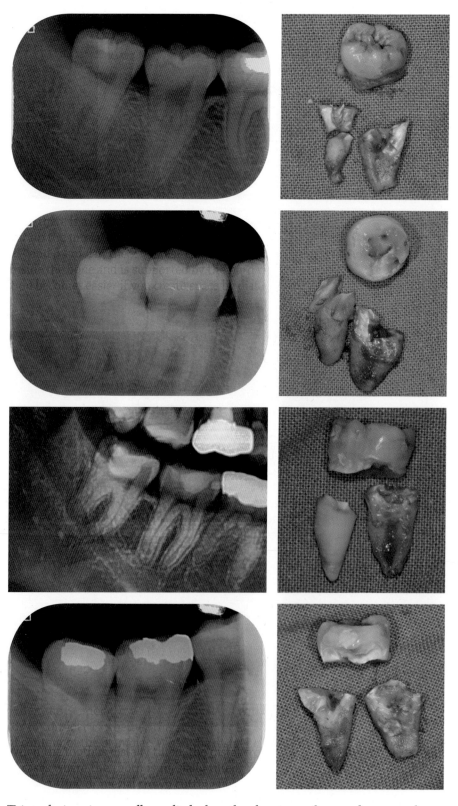

This technique is generally applied when the elevator or forceps do not work.

Wait!

The more wisdom tooth extractions you perform, the better you will become at other surgical procedures

A quote by Kyung-Ju Choi, the PGA golfer

The reason why Tiger Woods is a better golfer than I am is because he practices much harder than I do. Once you've set a goal of hitting 1000 balls today, you have to hit 1000 balls today. The moment you start to think you will hit 999 today and hit 1001 tomorrow, you might as well not even think about being successful.

You cannot improve your golfing skills because you just play a lot. In order to improve your overall golfing skills, you have to practice driver, putting, and bunker shots separately. The same philosophy is also applied to wisdom tooth extractions. Practice how to raise a flap, section the tooth, and learn how to properly use the instruments, which will all come together and you will be a better surgeon.

To become noticeably better at something, you have to practice until you're nearly sick of doing it. – Youngsam Kim –

Like everything else in this world, merely just observing how to perform a task or performing it only once or twice does not make you become proficient at that task. You have to observe and repeat the the task yourself over and over to truly improve your skills. For this reason I recommend that rather than thoroughly reading this book once, you read this book at least twice even if you skim through it both times. I hope you watch the video clips multiple times as well. A skill is only mastered by training your body to be used to the process.

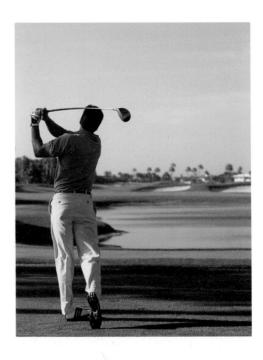

Mesioangular Impacted Wisdom Teeth Extraction

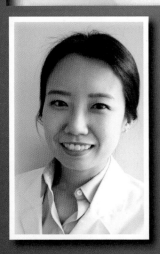

Chapter 07 translated by

Dr. YouRee Lim DDS

Dr. YouRee Lim obtained her Bachelor of Science with Honours from York University and Doctor of Dental Surgery degree from the University of Toronto. She practices general dentistry in Toronto, Canada.

01
Difficulty of mandibular third molar extraction ★★

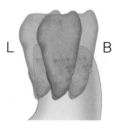 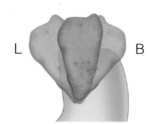 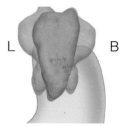

These figures show the various bucco-lingual position of vertically erupted mandibular third molars. In general, it is more difficult to extract if the crown of a third molar is located towards the lingual side.

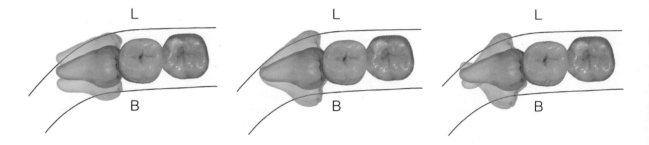

These figures show the various bucco-lingual position of horizontally erupted mandibular third molars. If the crown portion is positioned more lingually, it is more challenging to extract. The same rule applies for mesially impacted mandibular third molars.

The most important aspect of mastering extraction of third molars is to determine the difficulty level of each case. Once you are comfortable with that you can start training with simple cases. However, in many cases, there are unexpected variations so it is important to pay attention to details to reduce those variables.

As mentioned before, any lingually positioned mandibular third molar is challenging to extract. If a third molar is lingually tipped, the lingual plate is usually thinner which can fracture easily. Also, there is an increased chance of damaging the floor of the mouth and lingual nerve. This also applies to mesioangular and horizontally impacted mandibular third molar cases.

Difficulty of wisdom teeth extraction ★★★

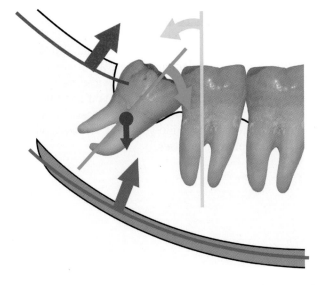

This figure shows the degree of difficulty of third molar extraction. Difficulty increases in the direction of the arrow.

▬ Violet arrow:
If the mandibular third molar is positioned more apically relative to the second molar, it is more difficult to extract.

▬ Green Arrow:
If the mandibular third molar is more mesially inclined, it is more difficult to extract because more coronal tooth structure must be removed prior to removing its root. Also, visibility is compromised.

▬ Yellow Arrow:
If the mandibular second molar is distally inclined, it is more difficult to extract the third molar due to compromised visiblity from the undercut. Also, a larger coronal portion should be removed first.

▬ Blue arrow:
When the inferior alveolar nerve is located higher than normal, it is more difficult to extract a mandibular third molar. Sometimes, the third molar itself is not much impacted, but the inferior alveolar nerve is positioned high.

▬ Red arrow:
The more the alveolar bone covers the mandibular third molar, the more difficult the extraction is. It is important to assess alveolar bone level because we cannot avoid bone removal in this case. Minimal bone removal is best, but if more bone must be removed, remove up to the CEJ or the buccal height of contour.

Wait!

What are the other variables of difficulty? ★

In general, if the patient is older and/or if the patient is male, extractions tend to be more difficult. From my own experience, I don't feel a big difference. However, most of the difficult and time consuming mandibular third molar extraction cases were for older or male patients.

★★

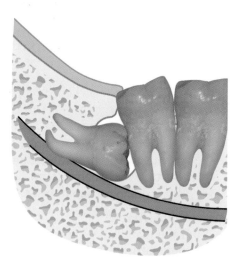

Based on difficulty level assessment as mentioned above, horizontally impacted mandibular third molars are the most challenging. There are many factors to consider for this case. An experienced dentist will extract using their own approach. If you are not experienced, it is best not to attempt these cases because it is more important to build your skill from successful extractions of simpler cases.

It is hard to predict the time it takes to extract mandibular third molars. About 95% of the cases that you expect to be challenging turn out to be easy. On the other hand, about 5% of the cases that you expect to be easy turn out to be challenging.

For any challenging cases, I try to use the similar technique keeping things simple but sometimes I use other techniques.

You can learn how to assess the difficulty level of extraction from your own extraction experiences. If you are a beginner, you must rely on examining the basic factors affecting difficulty level.

02
If other conditions are same, an important distance in wisdom teeth extraction ★★★

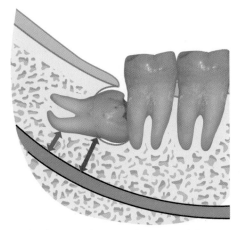

■The distances between the IAN and the root (blue) and the CEJ (red). The latter (red) is important to consider.

Most inexperienced dentists focus on the distance or relationship between the mandibular canal and roots (blue arrow) on a panoramic radiograph. There is no reason to be too concerned about this because it is okay to leave the roots in the bone if there is no associated pathology. If necessary, you can do a coronectomy and leave the roots remaining in the bone.

The most important aspect of horizontally impacted mandibular third molar extractions is the distance from the CEJ to the mandibular canal (red arrow), not the distance between the root and mandibular canal (blue arrow). The key to this extraction is the complete removal of the crown.

Nowadays, a CBCT is widely available and it makes the assessment of 3D relationship between the mandibular canal and root possible, but there is not a significant difference in difficulty of mandibular third molar extractions. After all, complete removal of the crown is the most important part of mandibular third molar extractions (especially in horizontally impacted cases).

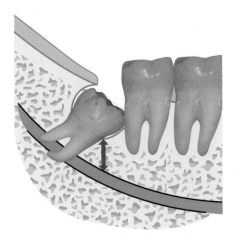

This figure shows that the root is superimposed on the inferior alveolar nerve (IAN) but there is sufficient distance between the nerve and mesiocervical area of the crown so it is possible to do a safe extraction with more caution on root removal.

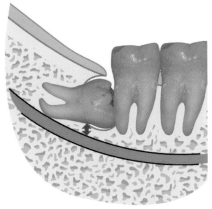

This figure shows when the root is not superimposed on the IAN but the distance between the nerve and crown is very close. In this case, more attention is required when sectioning the coronal portion of the tooth. This case can be considered a difficult case for inexperienced dentists.

03
Mesial impacted third molar extraction (complicated case) ★★

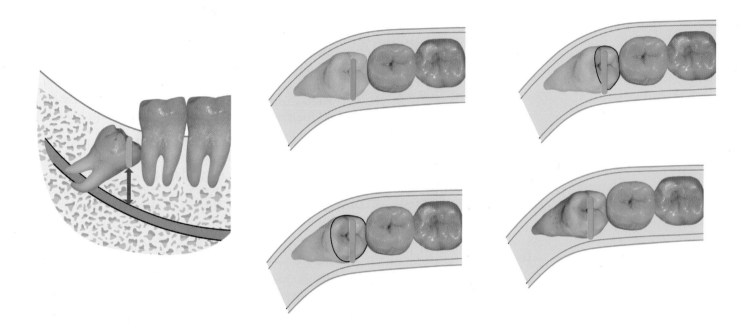

For the extraction of mesially impacted mandibular third molars, the most important step is the removal of the coronal portion caught under the distal portion of the second molar. Once you remove the undercut area, there is not much different from vertically impacted cases. I tend to eliminate or minimize an incision and a flap raising and section the mesial part of the crown as shown above (blue line) - which is the key. When I section the mesial portion, I use a #4 round bur to section enough to split it. After removing the mesial portion, the rest of the extraction is almost similar to a vertically impacted case.

04
Typical oral surgeon style extraction examples ★★

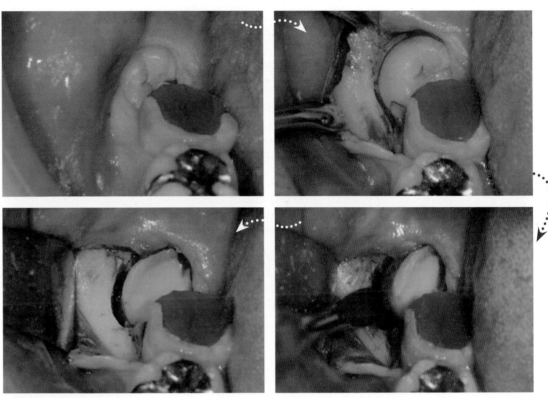

■ This is the case of Dr. Min-kyo Seo, who had seen in the flap part.

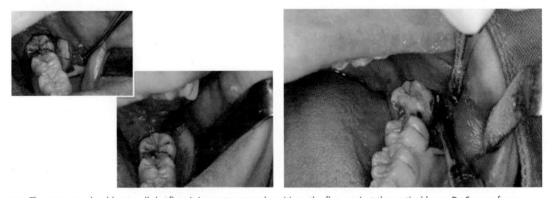

■ The retractor should not pull the flap, it just retracts and positions the flap against the cortical bone. Dr. Seo performs wisdom tooth seminar with the author.

This is a typical extraction style of an oral surgeon. If I were to do this case, I would section the mesial portion and extract the rest without raising a flap. For inexperienced dentists, it is important to raise a flap to achieve a better visiblity. Dr. Seo is a faculty member of my wisdom tooth extraction course.

The above figures show the typical extraction style of an oral surgeon. The mucoperiosteal flap have been extended slightly more than usual to take photos, but this is a textbook style extraction. However, this amount of flap and bone removal can lead to more postoperative bleeding and swelling. If the extraction is done properly, postoperative bleeding and swelling can be less than expected, but if you don't raise a flap or remove bone, it won't happen at all.

My goal for any tooth extraction is minimal incision, minimal flap, and minimal bone removal. The incision and flap can cause postoperative pain and swelling. By performing an incision and raising a flap, the surgery takes a longer total time and also involves more suturing. However, if you are inexperienced, you should raise a flap to practice and improve the visibility during the surgery.

If you have good visibility by raising a flap, you can reduce the time for the extraction portion of the surgery. As mentioned earlier, this is why I teach inexperienced dentists to raise a flap when extracting third molars when learning at the start of your career.

I also would like to highlight the minimal amount of bone removed in this case. The main reason is to use my favorite EL3C elevator for the extraction. Extensive buccal cortical bone removal not only causes postoperative bleeding, pain, and swelling but it also makes it harder to elevate off the buccal bone.

What if you go to the past with a time machine?

In the movies, the main character takes a time machine to go back to the past and adventures. Let's imagine that we go back to 500 years ago. As in the movie, we can reveal our identity and save the hero from the crisis and so on. If the King asks me what I do for living in the future, I have to say that I am a dentist. However, if you don't have any instruments, there is nothing I can do.

So what would you do if you go back to 500 years ago and the King lets you do anything you want? First of all, I would go to the blacksmith and make scalers. If I can invest more time, I would make mirrors and simple air or suction system. After that, I would make Gracey curettes. Dr. Gracey invented curettes less than a hundred years ago, so you could have named those curettes after your name or my name such as Youngsam curette.

Why do I talk about us going back to the past? If we do not have proper instruments, we cannot do anything. If you still do not have proper extraction instruments and tools that I recommended in the beginning, get them and practice my extraction technique. For example, you cannot learn how to play golf without having a golf club. You can learn from the book but you also need to practice physicially with proper instruments.

05
Third molar extraction seminar, live surgery case comparisons ★

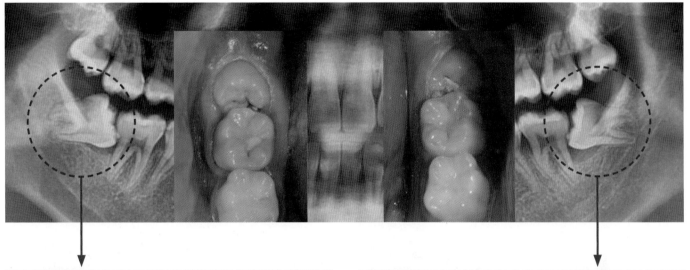

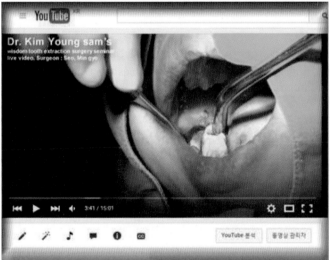

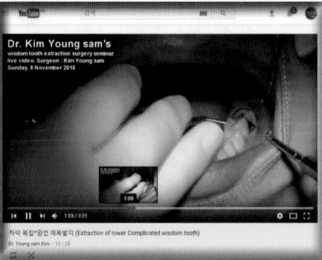

Sep 20, 2015
Nov. 8th 2015 Seminar

Dr. Seo, Oral Surgeon case Video
Author's case(Dr. Kim) Video

These two surgeries were performed for two mandibular third molars which are in similar positions. The lower right third molar #48 (#32 in universal system) was extracted neatly by Dr. Minkyo Seo using his oral surgeon technique. The patient suffered from post operative swelling and pain. The patient declined to extract the lower left third molar #38 (#17 in universal system). I persuaded the patient to do #38 extraction promising no postoperative pain and swelling. I sectioned a mesial portion of the crown only and completed the extraction, without raising a flap. As expected, postoperative swelling and pain was minimal. There are advantages and disadvantages to each extraction style, but the postoperative swelling and pain is definitely less in my extraction style.

06
The way of cutting mesioangular impacted third molars ★

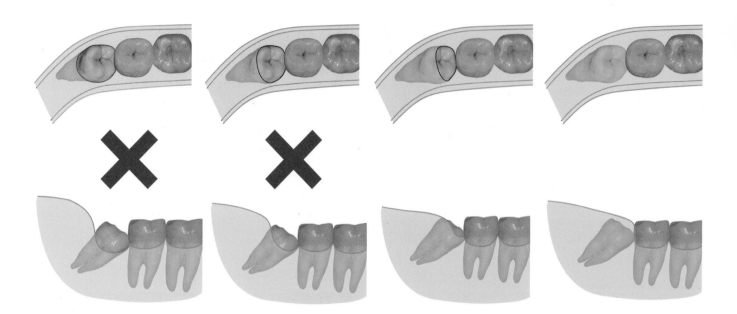

For the sake of simplicity, cases are classified into four. The first two cases are treated the same as vertical impaction cases - extraction can be done without raising a flap and bone removal. The frequency of incision for mesioangular cases is slightly higher than that of vertical impactions, however, the extent of incision is smaller.

The incidence of incision is higher for mesioangular cases because you must section a tooth and you need to have better visibility from the buccal side. However, it is not necessary to extend the incision line extensively because once the mesial portion of the crown is already removed, the rest can be delivered by elevating mesially.

If 1/3 of the coronal portion is impacted, an incision can be made toward the buccal side to prevent the gingiva from tearing during the extraction. Since the mesial portion of the crown is removed anyways, it does not improve visibility a lot.

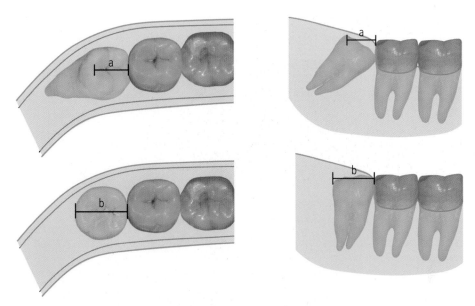

As shown in the figure below, if it is completely covered by gingiva, the incision line is in a half-moon shape. The distal portion of the third molar crown is closer to the second molar than in the vertical impacted case, so the amount of incision is slightly smaller.

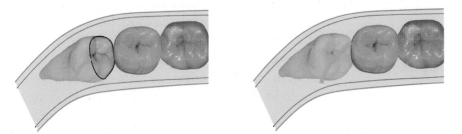

The end of the incision should be on the lingual side of the contact points between the second and third molar as shown by the green line. The purpose is to get better visibility, but also to minimize the damage on the lingual gingiva. The lingual gingiva around the crown is usually damaged by a bur during sectioning. Therefore, it is better to extend the incision to expose the area where the bur would pass.

It is also important to release the periodontal ligament with an explorer like a vertical impaction. As mentioned in the previous chapter, if the wisdom tooth is properly erupted, the periodontal ligament tends to be strongly attached to the distal surface of the crown.

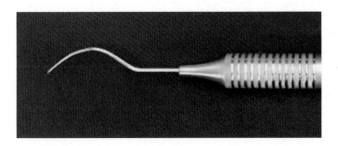

Crown Cutting ★★

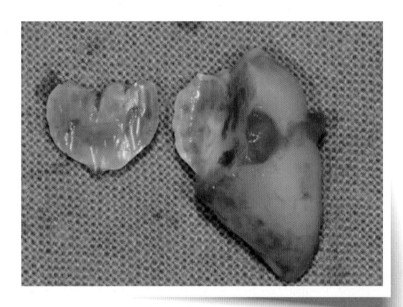

In my case, 'Mesial Crown Cutting' only is enough to extract most mesioangular impacted third molars. Removing the tooth portion impacted under of the distal of second molar is the key. After that, the remaining part is removed using the same technique as in the horizontal impaction case. When the mesial portion of the crown has been removed, an elevator is placed against the disto-buccal side and push the tooth forward and expand the periodontal ligament space. Based on the degree of impaction or root shape, the remaining part of the tooth is removed using various methods used in the vertical impaction.

'Mesial Crown Cutting' is the most important part of the mesioangular impacted wisdom teeth extraction.

Let's take a look at the case which 'Mesial Crown Cutting' can be used for mesioangular impaction.

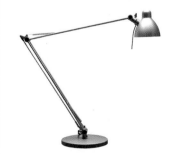

01
Mesioangular impaction ★★★

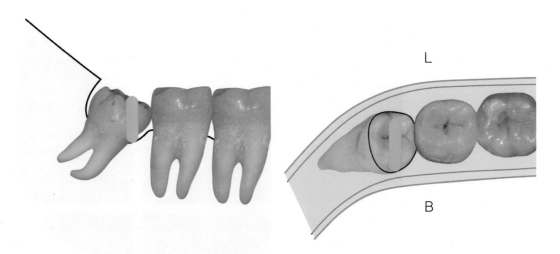

The most ideal sectioning surface of 'Mesial Crown Cutting' is shown from the occlusal and buccal view. The line is thicker in the figure because I use the #6 burs more these days. In the past, I used a thin fissure bur or a needle bur that was used for crown or inlay preparation. However, recently I have been using only #6 or #4 round burs because it creates more space for the sectioned portion to be removed easily.

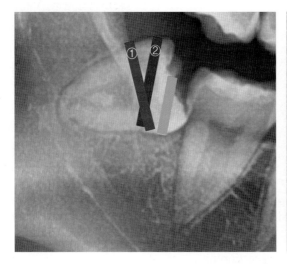

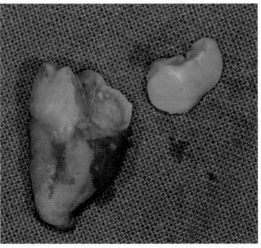

Most dentists try to section like red line ①, but due to the wrong angulation of the handpiece, it ends up like ② red line. I would rather section the tooth following the blue line as close as possible to the second molar. If you aim to section the tooth more coronally, it is easier to section because the crown is likely to be surrounded by a follicle. Also, a sectioned fragment can be easily fractured and removed because it is mostly enamel.

02
Mesioangular impaction Cases ★★★

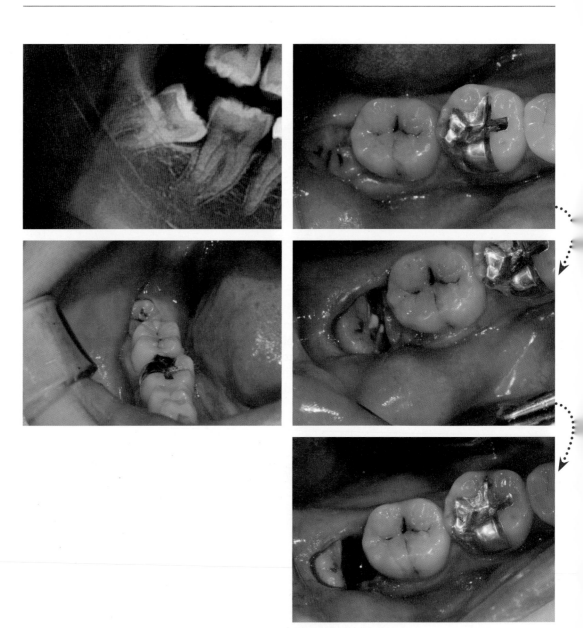

For the cases like the above, the third molar can be extracted by sectioning without a gingival incision. As you can see in the figure, this can be easily cut in a few seconds.

In most cases, even if there is an undercut, the mesial portion can be removed due to the space created by the bur during sectioning.

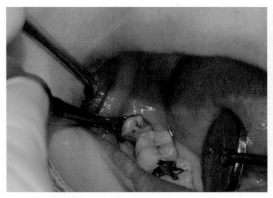 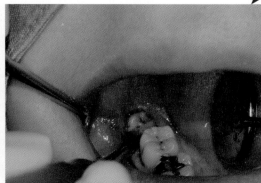

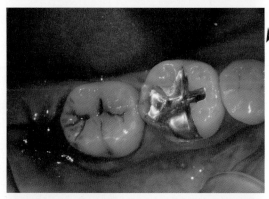

Once the mesial crown portion is removed, the elevator is applied to the distobuccal side as in vertical impaction cases.

However, unlike vertical impaction cases, you can use an elevator from the mesial side but you need to be careful not to damage the distal of the second molar.

At this stage, if the elevator is not working from the distobuccal side as in a vertical impaction case, various extraction methods can be used to extract the remaining part. On the radiograph, if the alveolar bone level is below the CEJ of the third molar, forceps can be used.

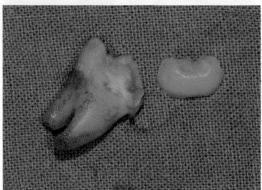

03
It is easy to remove the mesial part of a crown even if the visible part is small ★★

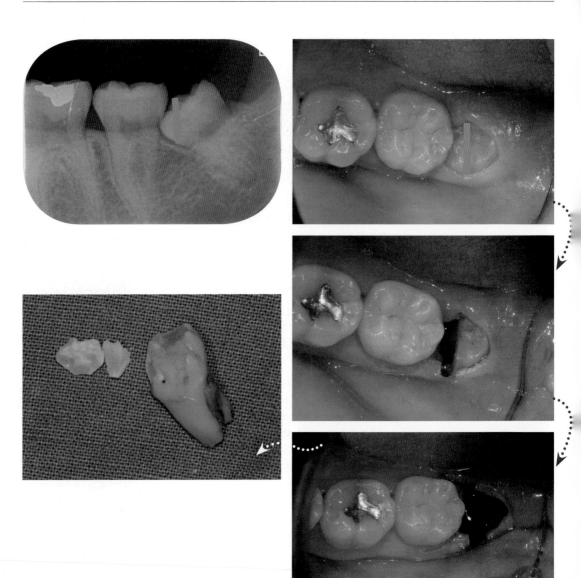

The shape of the tooth can be easily guessed even though there is a small portion of the third molar that is visible. In this case, the tooth was sectioned and extracted. The key point here is deep sectioning of the buccal part of the crown. It is difficult to section all the way to the lingual side of the crown, so it is important to be sure that the buccal side is sectioned completely.

For beginners, there is a tendency to not section the buccal side deep enough. However, with practice, you can improve your sectioning skill.

04
Similar case ★

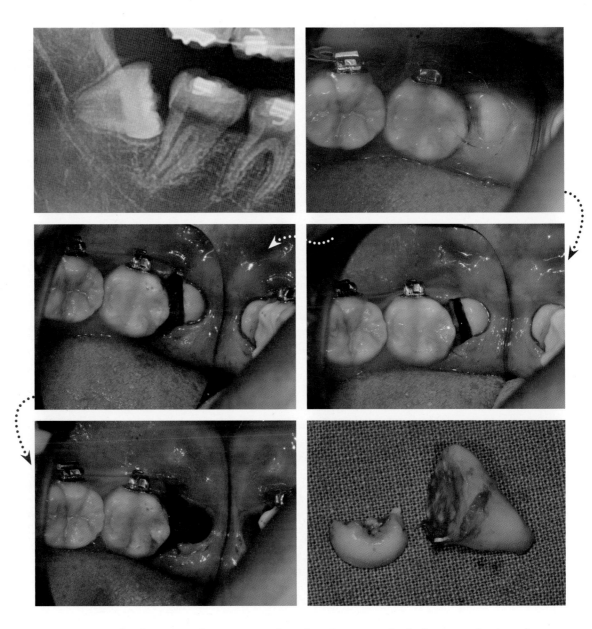

In most cases, the duration of extraction is less than 3 minutes (excluding anesthesia and suturing) and there is usually minimal postoperative bleeding, swelling and pain. If you are familiar with my extraction technique, most beginners can complete this extraction within 10 minutes.

05
Even if you do not see wisdom teeth at all ★★

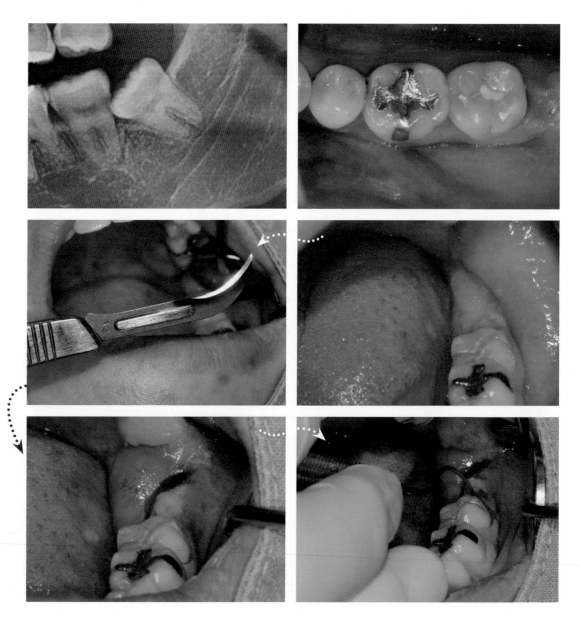

If the gingiva completely covers the third molar, use a No. 12 scalpel to cut the gingiva all the way to the distal of the second molar. Unless the height of contour of the third molar is deeply impacted in the bone, the flap is not extended to the mesial of the second molar. With a modified explorer, it is good to release the periodontal ligament off the distal and buccal of the second molar and the distal of the third molar if accessible.

If a third molar is not in function, the distal periodontal ligament is usually weak.

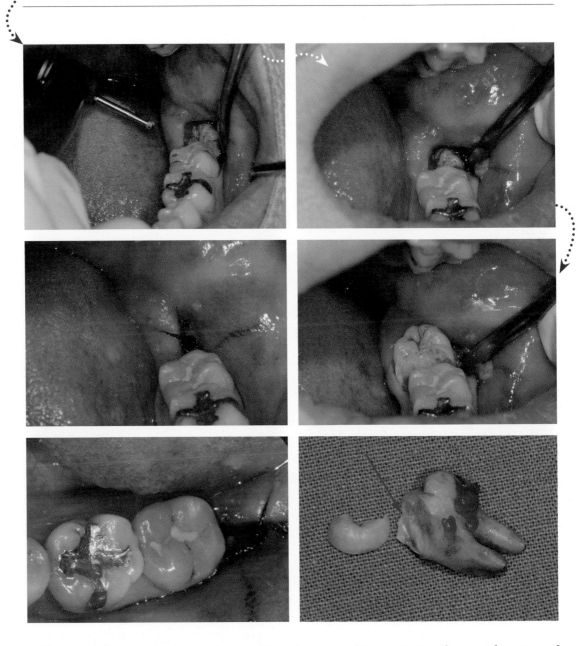

Fully impacted mesioangular wisdom teeth can be removed by sectioning the mesial portion of the crown as in the vertical impaction case. It is not different from the vertical impaction case if you raise a flap and remove the mesial portion of the crown. The elevator can push the third molar forward by pressing against the distobuccal side. The red arrow shows the incomplete sectioning of the lingual part - this is acceptable because complete sectioning of the lingual part is not necessary.

06
It is common that the lingual side is cut less ★★

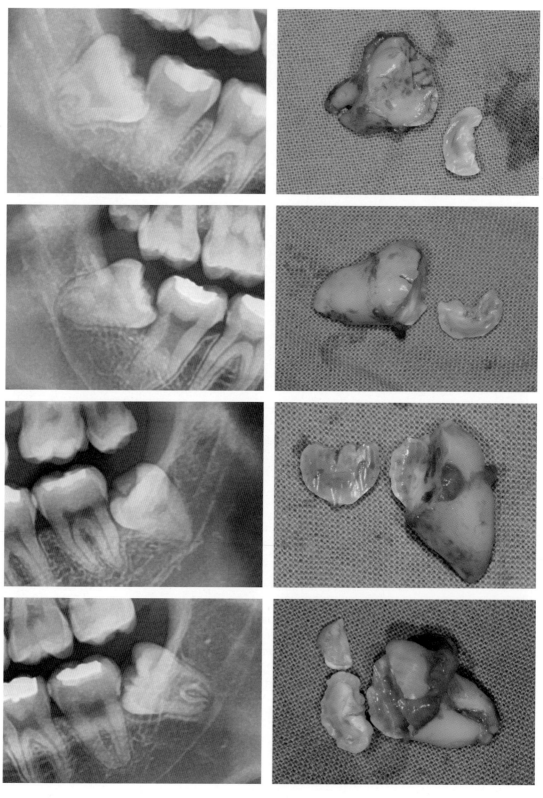

It is necessary to remove the portion under the undercut. A slightly incomplete sectioning of lingual part is not a big concern.

07
Mesially impacted case - mesial crown cutting <1> ★★

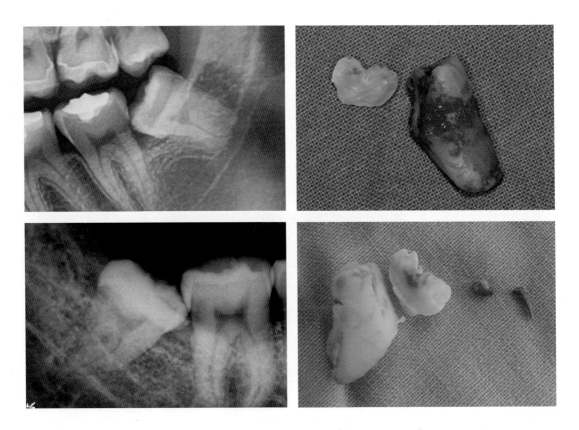

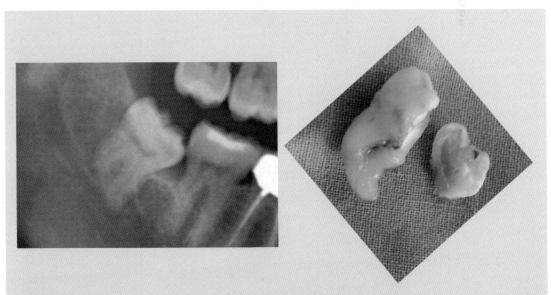

In the case above, considering the direction of the roots, this third molar needs to be elevated forward. We should keep in mind that it is important to push the distal surface forward in other cases.

Mesially impacted case - mesial crown cutting <2> ★

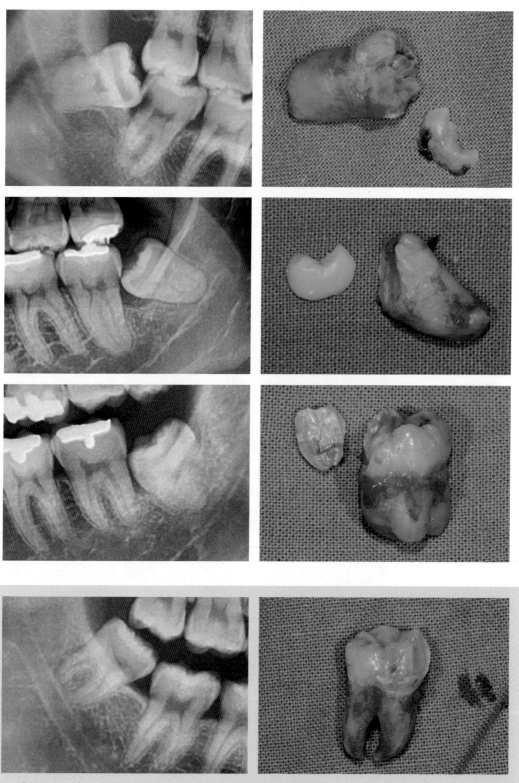

In this case, the sectioned mesial portion was not photographed because it was cut very thinly and sucked into the suction.

Vertical Division of Mesial Crown Portion ★★★

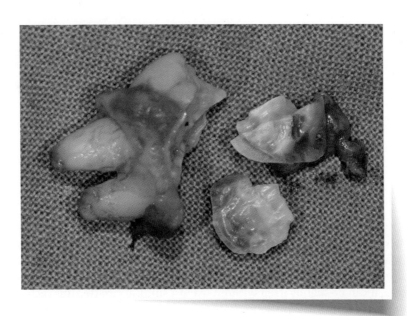

Even though the mesial portion of the crown is sectioned already, it may not be easy to remove the fractured portion if the undercut of the distal portion of the second molar is very deep. This can happen often when you use a small-sized bur, such as #4 round surgical bur. This is a case in which the mesial portion of the third molar crown is caught under the distal of the second molar or surrounding tissues. In this case, rather than pushing the piece out forcefully, I vertically section the fractured mesial portion again. And I use the surgical curette to rotate the piece out or deliberately break the piece into two. I named the vertical cutting method of mesially sectioned crown portion as <Vertical Division of 'Mesial Crown Cutting' Portion>

It is not commonly done in the mesial impaction case, but it is used all the time in the horizontal impaction cases. I will just mention it briefly here, and further teach this technique in the horizontal impaction section.

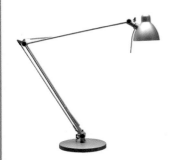

01

\<Vertical division of mesial crown cutting portion\> if the 2nd molar has severe undercut ★★★

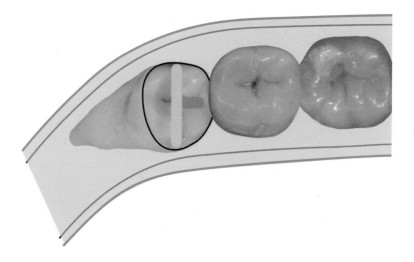

As shown in above picture, after cutting the mesial portion of the crown, section it again vertically along the central groove without damaging the distal of the second molar. Then, a surgical curette can be placed in the cut space to split and remove the pieces. In a mild mesial impaction case, it can be split by itself without using a surgical curette. This technique is not very important in the mesioangular impaction cases but it is very important in a complete horizontal impaction case.

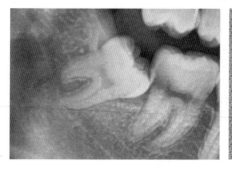
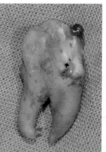
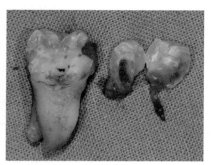

Since the wisdom tooth was deeply impacted and the undercut was severe, the sectioned mesial portion could not be removed. Additional vertical sectioning was done to split the mesial portion into two pieces and then removed.

02
Vertical division of mesial crown cutting portion ★★

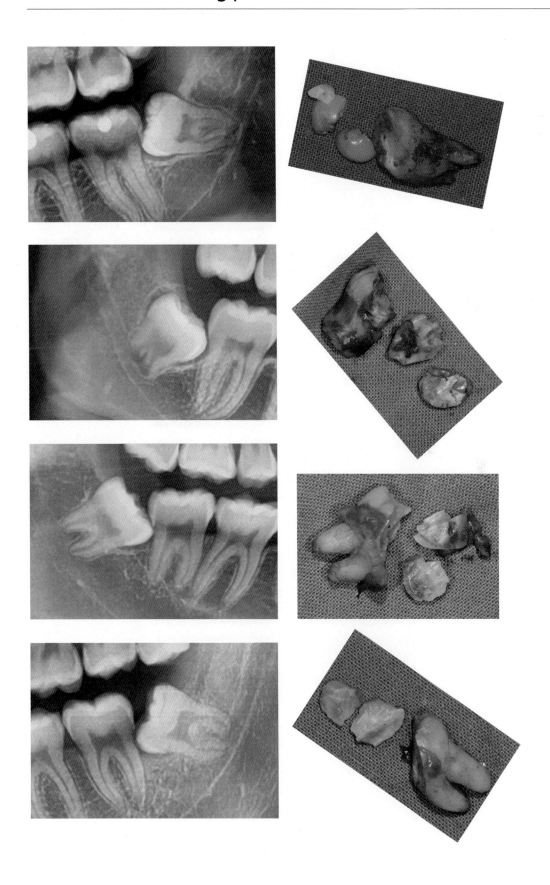

03
Intentional split or split by itself… ★

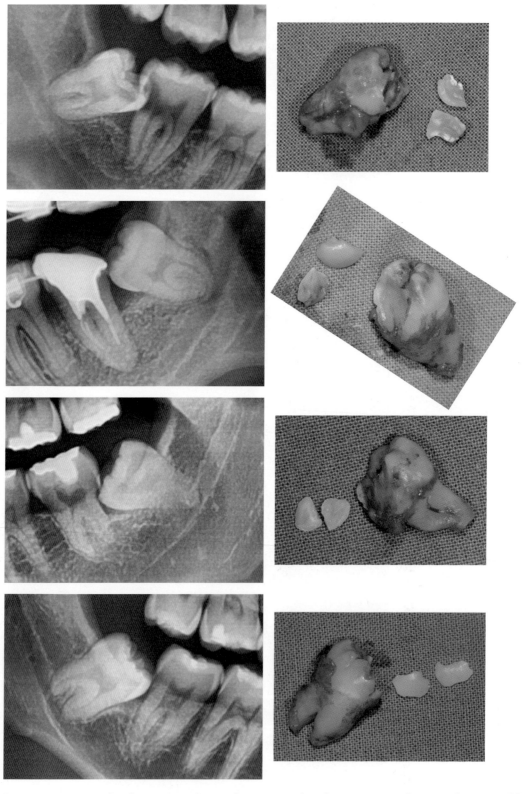

It is very common for the sectioned mesial portion to break spontaneously since the enamel has a very low tensile strength. Again, this technique can be used to extract horizontally impacted third molars.

04
Easiest extraction exercises for beginners ★

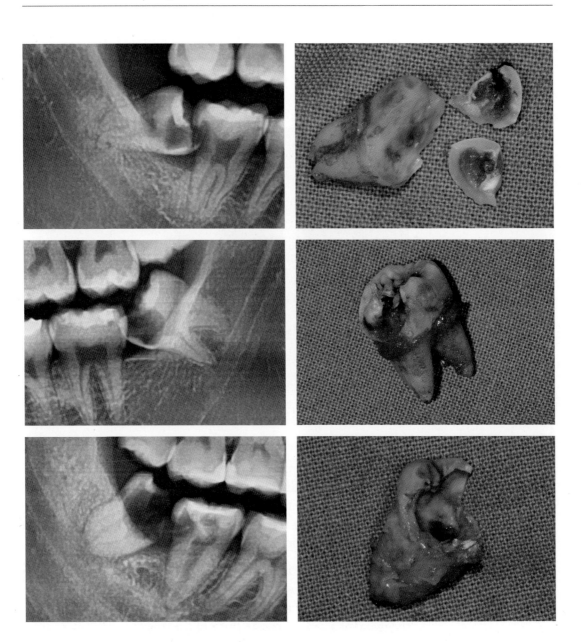

I often make inexperienced dentists to practice sectioning a mesial portion of the crown in the cases like the above. The removal of a mesial portion is the key here so practicing in these cases will lead to more successful and complete extraction of third molars. The last case is an extreme case of a grossly decayed third molar, but it is a great case to practice sectioning although a very thin layer of crown is remained.

Mesially Impacted Third Molar Extraction ★ with Forceps

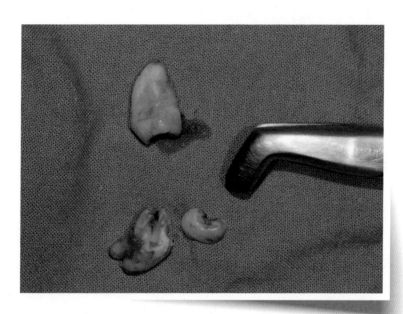

I chose the title of this chapter as a mesioangular third molar extraction with forceps. Most dentists will proceed by sectioning a mesial portion of the third molar that is caught under the distal portion of the second molar. However, it is more difficult to remove the remaining crown and root if the crown is not covered by the alveolar bone. Many dentists may not know that forceps can be very useful in this case. If a wisdom tooth is erupted more, it is much easier to remove it with forceps.

After removing the mesial portion of a mesioangular wisdom tooth, it is easy to extract the remaining part with forceps than a vertically erupted wisdom tooth. When you hold a vertically erupted tooth with forceps and luxate, you have to be careful not to damage the distal of a second molar, but not for this case. However, you need to be careful not to slip with the forceps since the crown is smaller.

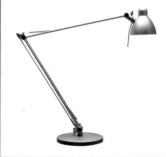

01
Mesially impacted third molar extraction with forceps <1> ★★

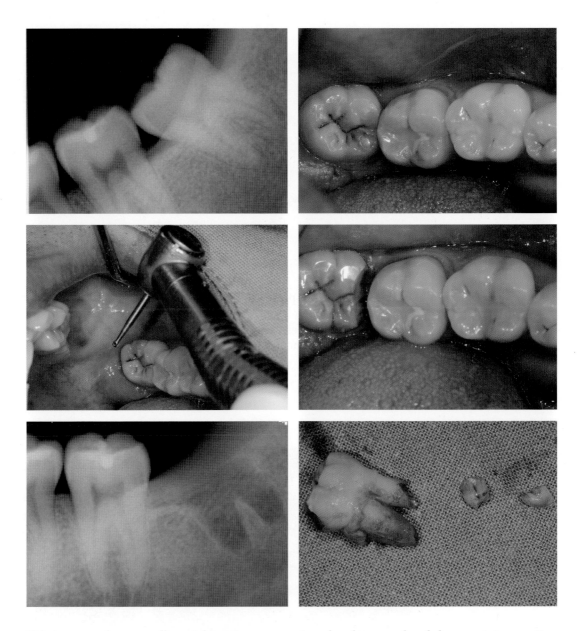

This is a case that a small mesial portion was sectioned and removed and the remaining portion was removed with forceps. You can still extract this tooth without sectioning, but if you remove the mesial portion first, it is much easier to luxate and the path of extraction becomes less limited.

We can often observe a distal crack on the second molar that was caused by forcep luxation if the mesial portion is not removed prior to the removal of the third molar. In Korea, the fee for extraction becomes more when you section the tooth because it becomes a complex impaction case.

Mesially impacted third molar extraction with forceps <2> ★★

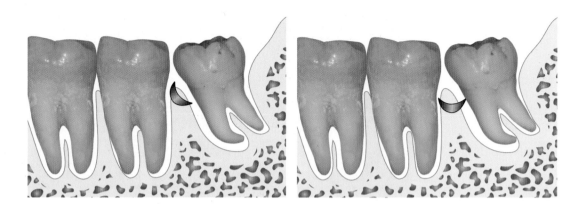

In this case, you can press the occlusal surface of the second molar with one finger and lift the third molar with an elevator because you may extract the second molar accidentally instead. I prefer not to use an elevator against the mesial of the wisdom tooth because you may damage the distal of second molar.

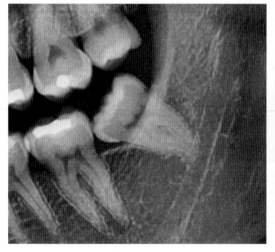 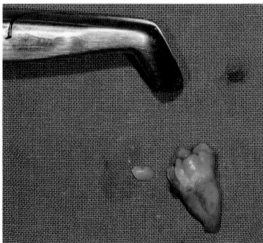

If you section and remove the mesial portion first, you can often use forceps to extract the third molar as in the vertical impaction case. Forcep delivery in this case is much easier than in a vertical impaction case. Since there is a free space between the second molar and the mesial of the third molar, it is easy to move the tooth. In order to remember the instruments that I used, I usually take a picture of the third molar and the instrument together.

02
Habit of taking pictures with used tools ★

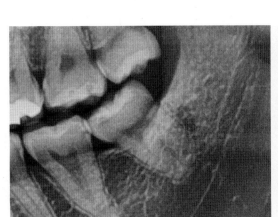 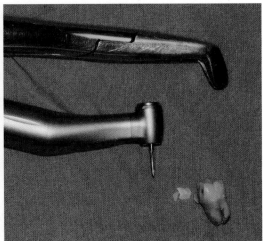

If the third molar is slightly tilted mesially and in function, it can be very difficult to extract. In cases like this, if you use forceps, you may need to luxate the tooth aggressively side to side and back and forth many times and this can lead to the damage of the second molar. However, if you perform 'Mesial Crown Cutting', you can create a free space, so you can extract the wisdom tooth easier and prevent damaging the second molar. In the past, 'Mesial Crown Cutting' was done with a thin diamond bur that was used for crown preparation. You can use any cavity preparation bur – either round bur, diamond bur or fissure bur.

You may have already seen pictures of the third molar and instruments taken together in this book. I do not always do that, but when I have a chance, I ask my staff to take pictures. The above figures show that a NSK 5x Contra Angle low speed handpiece and a 25 mm MANI fissure bur were used to remove a mesial portion of the crown, and the rest was removed with a Hu-Friedy 222 forceps.

03
The habit is older than I thought ★

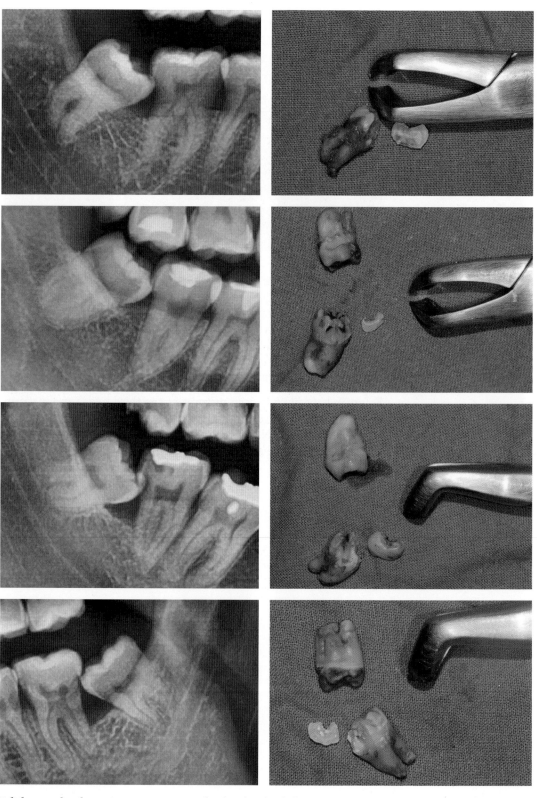

I did not take these pictures to write this book. I had the courage to write this book because I had so many post op pictures that I have collected over many years.

04
Third molar extraction with forceps after a slight removal of mesial portion ★

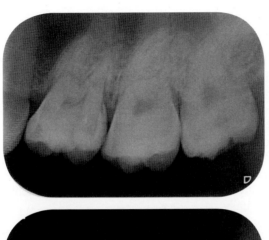

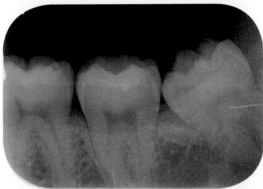

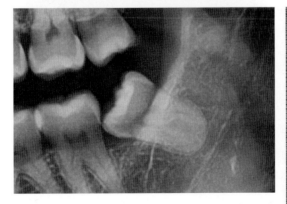

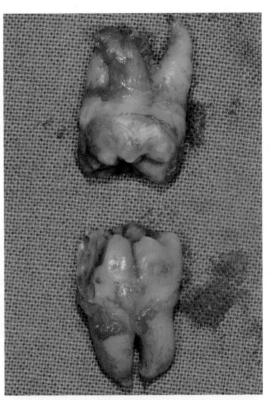

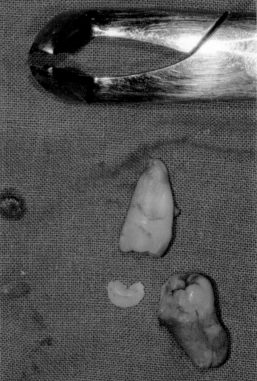

Often, I use mandibular forceps to extract a maxillary third molar when my assistant brings the wrong forceps or when the maxillary extraction is very simple after the mandibular extraction.

It is difficult to get enough strength with the wrong forceps so do not attempt this.

Wait!

American and British not love and war, but wisdom teeth war ??

In In the late 1990s, the United Kingdom announced that wisdom tooth extraction is not necessary in "the Guidance on the extraction of the wisdom teeth". In summary, wisdom tooth should not be removed if possible. It says that less than one in ten people experience any wisdom tooth problem if there is no caries or periodontal disease. They listed numerous side effects of prophylactic wisdom tooth extraction such as nerve damage...etc. On the other hand, the United States announced why wisdom tooth should be removed because many people are already suffering from cavities or periodontal disease. The longer the wisdom tooth is retained, the greater the damage caused by the wisdom tooth, thus the longer the postoperative effect. If the wisdom tooth is kept longer, more people experience problems and they end up extracting them eventually.

These days, the United States' claim is more accepted than the United Kingdom's claim. However, we do not have to follow either of these articles because these research results can be biased. As we all know, the U.K. has a socialized healthcare system. Anyone can get free medical and dental benefits. Of course, extraction of a wisdom tooth is free. If you are a dentist in the U.K., would you like to extract wisdom tooth? What about the U.S.? Wisdom tooth extraction fee is the highest in the world. Advanced impacted case can be charged up to several hundred dollars. I cannot find the exact reference of this article that I read a few years ago but I just wanted to share it with you. Of course, the ratio of wisdom teeth extraction in the United States, which earns a lot of money, is higher than in the U.K. In Korea, fee for a wisdom tooth extraction is much lower than the U.S. According to that article, the ratio in Korea was just halfway between Britain and the United States. Anyways, I am grateful for the U.S.'s claim is getting accepted more and more because I am a snob, after all, who extracts wisdom teeth for a living ^^.

Various Types of Wisdom Teeth Extraction ★ in Mesial Impaction

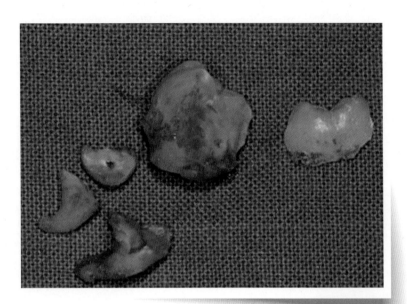

After the mesial portion of the crown is sectioned and removed, it becomes very similar to a vertical impaction case so you can use the same method to extract the rest of the tooth as in a vertical impaction case. After removing the mesial portion, the elevator can be used. However, if the elevator is not effective, forceps can be used immediately. You can also section the tooth again or section the whole crown off and remove the roots separately. Those cases will be discussed here.

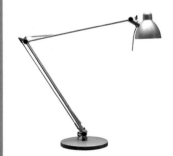

01
What if an elevator or forceps cannot remove a tooth after sectioning a mesial portion of the crown? ★★★

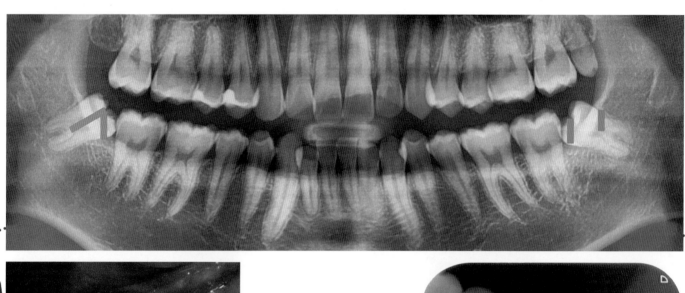

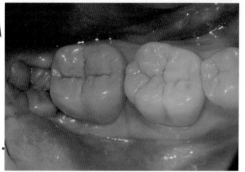

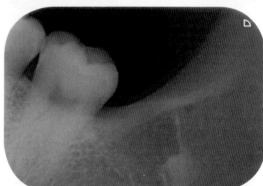

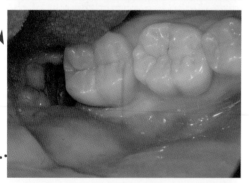

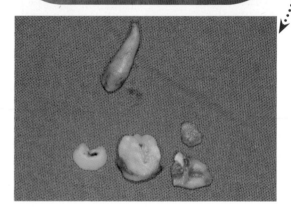

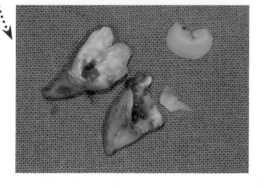

This case should be treated the same as a vertical impaction case. You can section the root into two halves to deliver them separately or section and deliver the crown first and deliver the rest. For #38, it was a challenging case and the distal root apex was left behind.

02
Hemisection approach of a mesially inclined tooth ★★

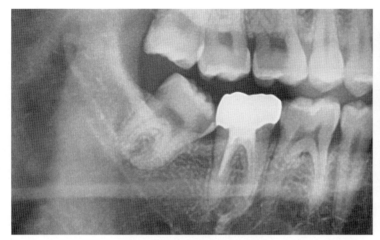

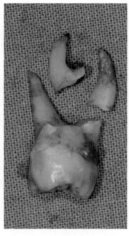

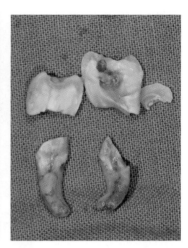

A mesially inclined wisdom tooth in a muscular young male patient can be more challening to extract than a typical horizontally impacted wisdom tooth. In the above case, both maxillary and mandibular wisdom tooth extractions were very difficult. In particular, I do not recommend removing broken roots of maxillary wisdom teeth if you are inexperienced.

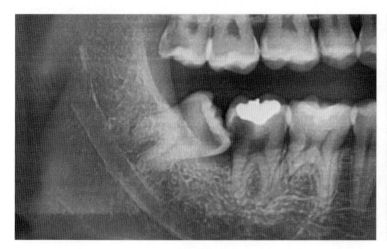

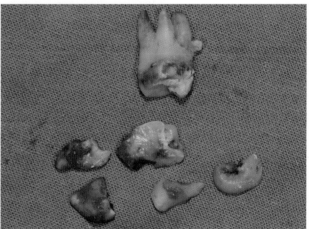

This is also one of the most difficult cases. In addition, Youngsam's sign is visible in the apex of the distal root. If a wisdom tooth is grossly decayed, when the forceps are used aggressively, the crown can be fractured off. In this case, you may want to consider doing Distocervical cutting or L-extraction instead.

03
Root delivery after the crown removal in a mesial impaction case

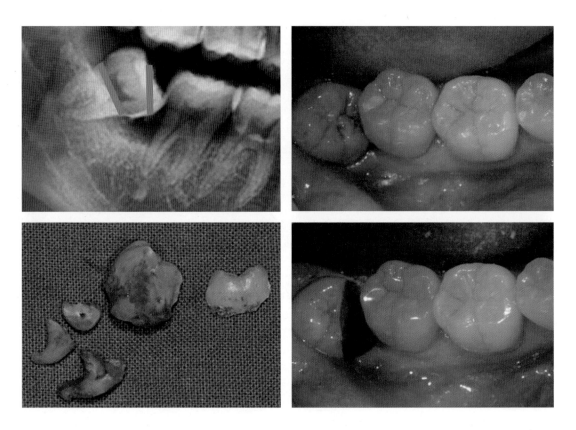

The extraction was attempted with 'Mesial Crown Cutting' as usual, but due to the excessive root curvature, the root portion was difficult to extract. Thus, Crown Cutting method was used.

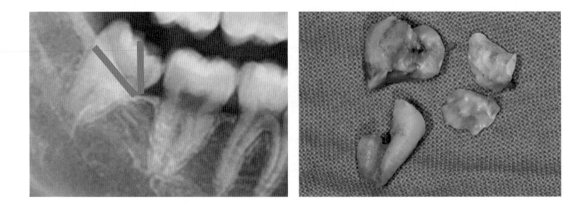

It seemed like a simple case from the panoramic radiograph, but after performing 'Crown Cutting', I attempted to section the center of the root as you can see in the right side. When the roots are fused, it is more difficult to extract (I call these roots that are fused by a thin piece, a "flipper"). Among them, it gets more challenging if the shape of the overall root is round and thick (I call this round and thick fused root, a "bum").

04
If the occlusal surface is higher than the occlusal surface of a second molar ★★

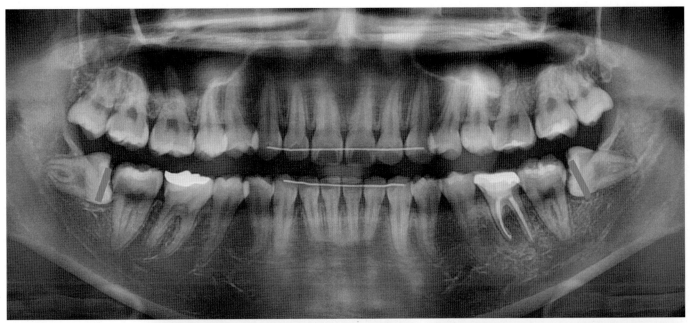

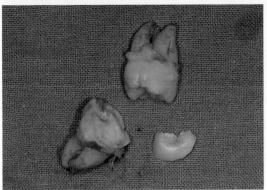 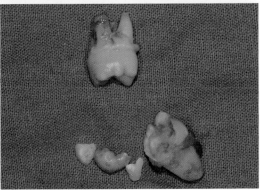

Many dentists divide the entire portion of the crown into half and extract them. I consider the remaining crown as a handle, so I do not remove an unnecessary portion of a crown. I only remove the portion that is caught under the second molar as shown above. In this case, the angle of the handpiece should be adjusted to prevent damage to the distal of a second molar. In most cases, it is unlikely to damage the adjacent tooth if you section from the buccal side and there is usually enough room from the distal of second molar. Using fissure burs is not recommended to section the crown.

Lift & Cutting ★

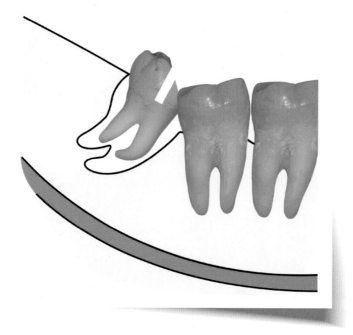

If you try to lift a mesially impacted wisdom tooth, it can get caught under the distal of a second molar if only the enamel of the undercut is removed. For the most part, you can lift the wisdom tooth by elevating towards either lingual or buccal side using the elasticity of the tooth or the alveolar bone.

When a third molar is caught under the undercut as it comes out, I would cut the part that is caught under the undercut while it is lifted. I named this technique 'Lift & Cutting'. In general, when removing a piece of tooth by sectioning and breaking it off, I use a #4 round bur in most cases. I strongly encourage inexperienced dentists to use a #4 round bur.

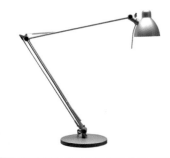

01
Lift & Cutting ★★★

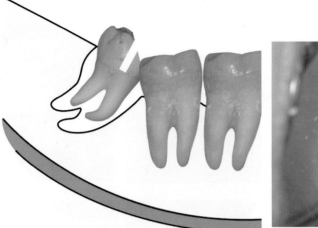 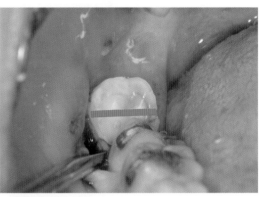

When the mesio-distal distance of the third molar is larger than the distance between the distal surface of the second molar to the distal alveolar ridge of a third molar, the third molar will be caught under the distal side of a second molar as above. In this case, you can remove the distal alveolar bone. However, if you remove a portion of the third molar that is caught under, you can easily extract the rest.

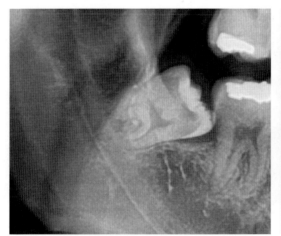 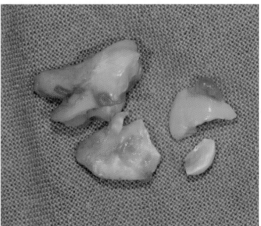

This case is s a typical example of 'Lift & Cutting'. I tried to extract after removing a small mesial portion, but the tooth itself was too big to pass through the space. So, I tried 'Lift & Cutting'. In this case, there are many different approaches such as removing the distal alveolar bone, bisecting the root with a slow speed handpiece, or dividing the tooth with a surgical high speed handpiece. However, I would like to minimize the use of different tools, so I removed only the parts that are caught under the undercuts by using the same handpiece.

02
Lift & Cutting process ★★

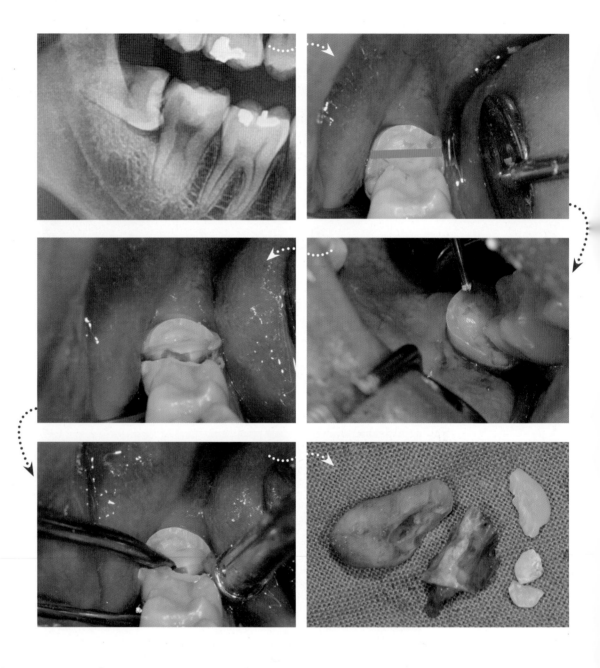

03
Lift & Cutting is necessary in this case ★★

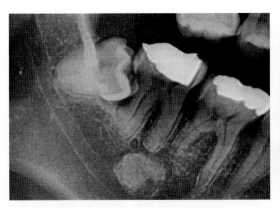
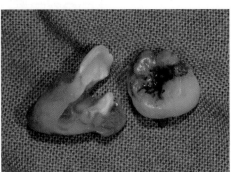

In most cases that need 'Lift & Cutting', the distance between the distal surface of the second molar to the distal alveolar ridge is narrower than the width of the third molar. In that case, most of them are caught under the distal part of the second molar as shown above. In this case, I used the elevator to break the sectioned part, but instead the whole tooth came out. It might have been misaligned, or caught within the elastic limits of the alveolar bone. Sometimes you can extract the tooth during the process of 'Lift & Cutting' because the third molar may have moved in the direction of least resistance in the process of cutting with a handpiece.

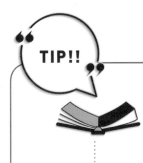

TIP!!

In the figure above, the notch on the distal surface of the extracted third molar was created to make room for the elevator. In this case, I intended to drill into the tooth, not the alveolar bone. As mentioned earlier in the panoramic radiograph part, when the inflammation of the crown is severe, the root gets stuck to the posterior alveolar bone by the coronal pressure, so the elevator cannot be inserted. Therefore, a notch is made into the disto-cervical portion of the wisdom tooth to pull out remained part with an elevator (Disto-Cervical Cutting). This is covered later in this chapter.

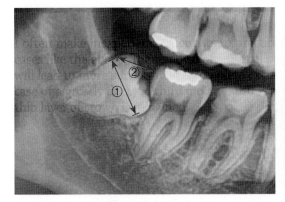
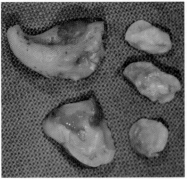

In this case, the distance between the distal surface of the second molar and the distal alveolar bone ② is smaller than that of the mesio-distal width of the crown of the third molar ①. I always try to minimize alveolar bone removal, thus I performed 'Lift & Cutting'.

04
Lift & Cutting video ★

45 degree impaction: During extraction it was caught so "Lift & Cutting" was done.

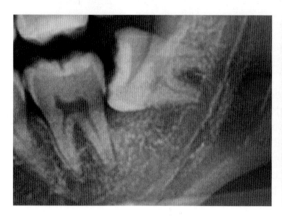

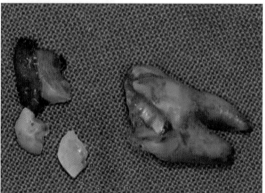

In comparison to Dr. Seo Min-kyo's video, you can see that as the tooth comes out after the "Mesial Crown Cutting", it was caught under the undercut so "Lift and Cutting" was performed.

Even though "Oblique Cutting" method was used, the tooth can be caught. (After Oblique Cutting, it was caught so an explorer was used to lift and the roots were sectioned)

05
Different angle view after Lift & Cutting

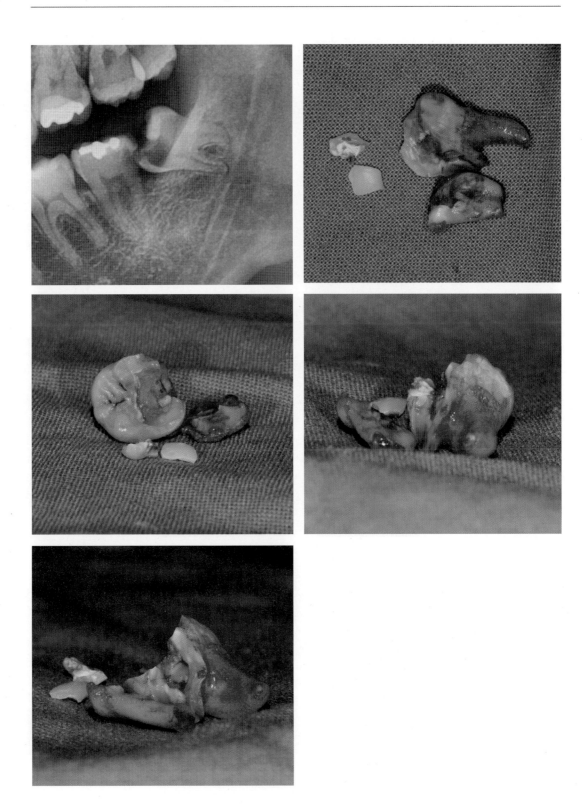

06
Lift & Cutting case <1> ★

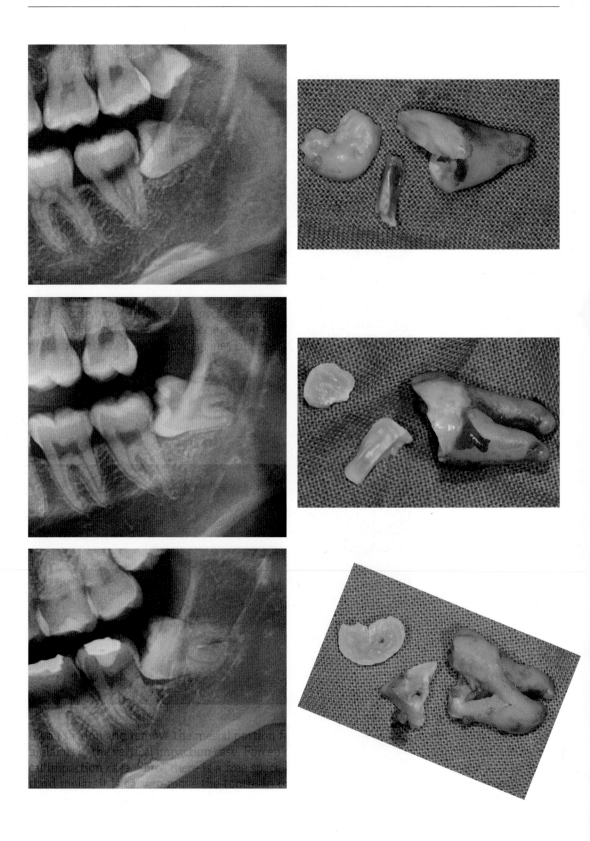

Lift & Cutting case <2> ★★

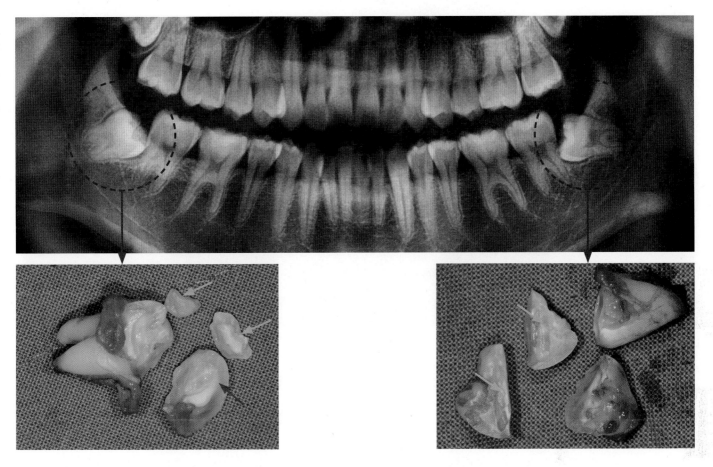

The yellow arrow shows 'Mesial Crown Cutting', and the red arrow shows 'Lift & Cutting'.

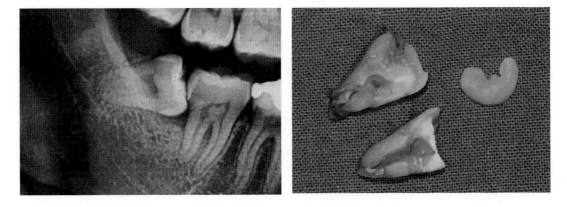

During 'Lift & Cutting', the root of the tooth is almost cut in half, and this can happen commonly in multi-rooted teeth. Even though I do not intend to divide the root, but it can be sectioned because it is probably the weakest part. If the furcation is close to the crown, it is the weakest part of the tooth.

Lift & Root Cutting ★★

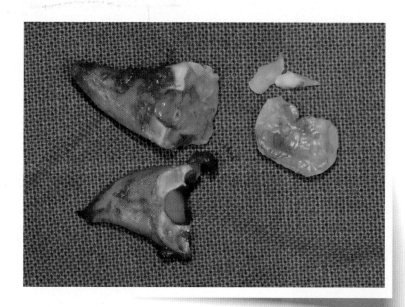

When the space is too small, we usually do the 'Lift & Cutting' method. If the third molar is multi-rooted and the furcation is high, roots will be sectioned then the extraction becomes very easy. Repeating this process will naturally lead 'Lift & Cutting' to 'Root Sectioning'.

The difference from the 'Crown Division' method is that the third molar is already being dislodged from the alveolar bone and loose inside the socket. With more experiences, 'Lift & Cutting' and 'Crown Division' is proceeded very similarly to each other, but I have classified these techniques separately because inexperienced dentists must section and remove the portion of a tooth with a clear purpose.

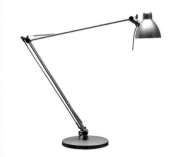

01
From 'Lift & Cutting' to 'Root Separation' ★

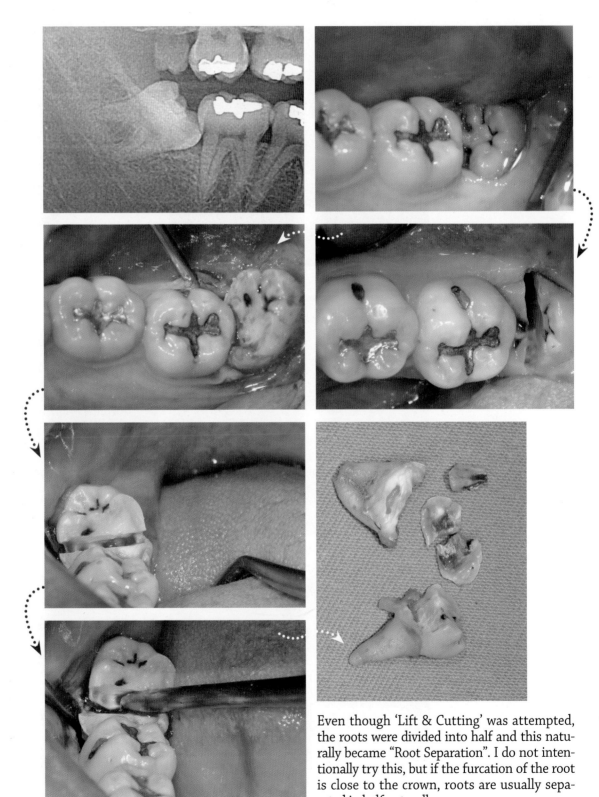

Even though 'Lift & Cutting' was attempted, the roots were divided into half and this naturally became "Root Separation". I do not intentionally try this, but if the furcation of the root is close to the crown, roots are usually separated in half naturally.

02
Lift and Root separation case <1> ★

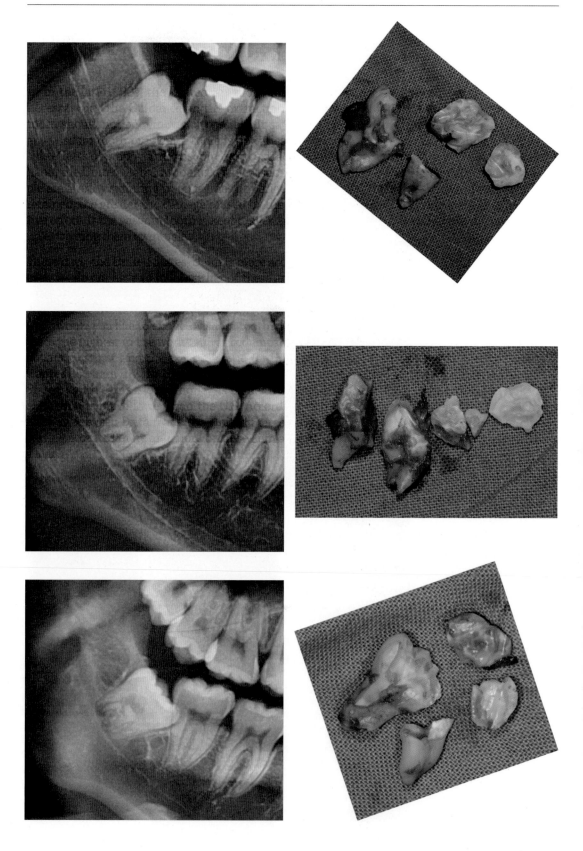

Lift and Root separation case <2> ★

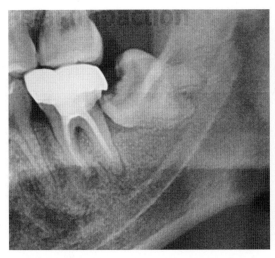 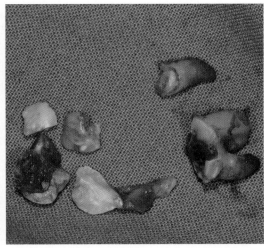

It does not appear as a 'Lift & Root Separation' case, but it divides one of the roots because there are three roots.

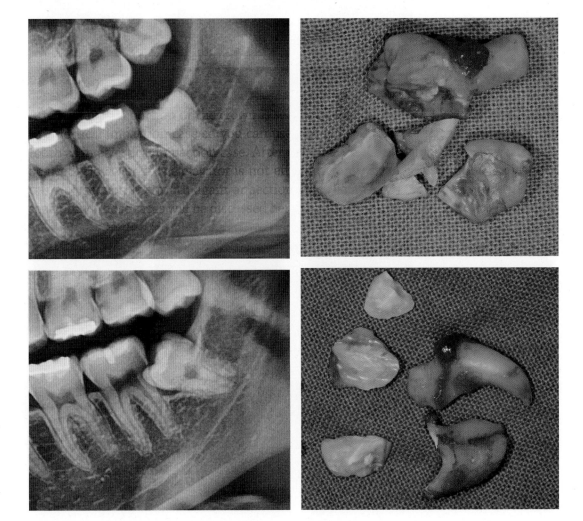

Lift and Root separation case <3> ★

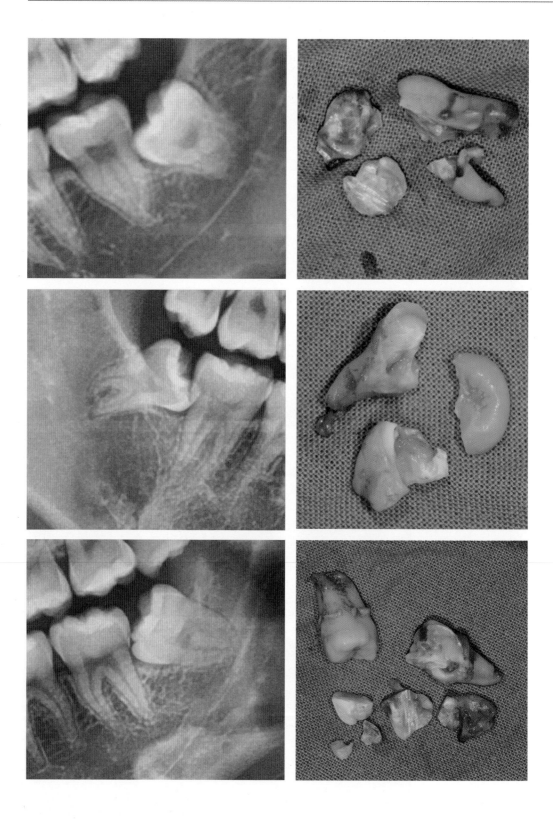

03
If root division is clear ★★

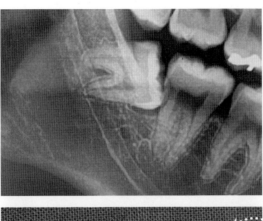
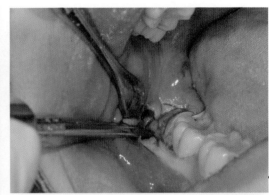
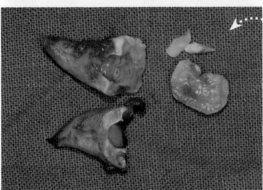
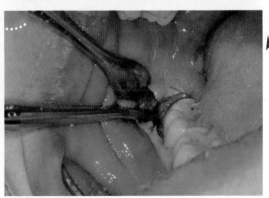

When a third molar is caught under the second molar, if the furcation is high and the roots are sectioned clearly, the elevator can be inserted between two roots to separate them completely. This is the technique that I use most often. Even though the root is fractured like the figure on your right, the root can be easily removed.

I try not to use a high speed handpiece too much after the third molar is already dislodged. This is to prevent the extraction socket from being filled with distilled water and tooth pieces. However, in order to shorten the surgery duration, we sometimes need to use a high speed handpiece after dislodging.

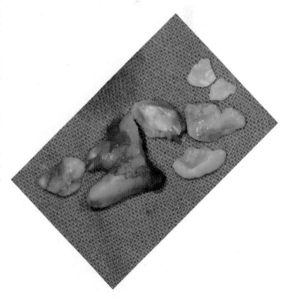

04
Root separation with elevators ★

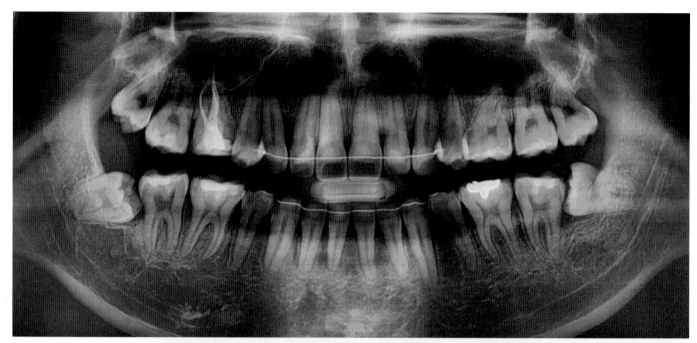

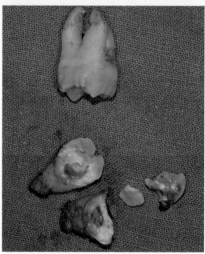
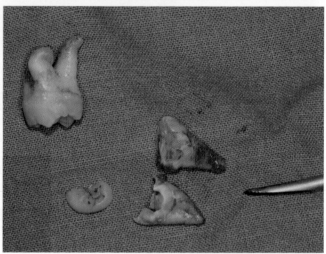

Both wisdom teeth were extracted in the same way. I have already mentioned that I have a habit of taking a photo of third molar that I extracted and the instrument that I used. Perhaps this picture can be inferred. For tooth # 48, when you look between the roots, there is no evidence of handpiece use. After the removal of the mesial portion of the crown, the remaining part of the third molar is dislodged with the EL3C elevator. During this process, if the remaining portion is caught, I insert the elevator between two roots and fracture it. I do not have too many clinical photos of this method because it is usually done in a few seconds. However, if the elevator does not fit well between the two roots, 'Disto-Cervical Cutting' or 'Lift & Cutting' methods should be done immediately.

Oblique Cutting ★★★

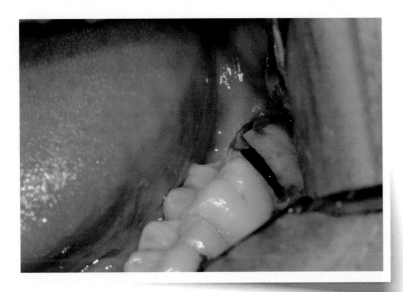

'Oblique Cutting' is the technique that after removing the mesial portion of the crown, you remove another fragment by sectioning it in an oblique line as shown above.

This is my favorite approach to an easy and safe extraction. I do not use this method every time, however if there is any challenging case, I return to the basics and proceed to 'Oblique Cutting'.

This method is also consistent with my basic rule of extraction - minimal bone removal but sectioning a tooth instead. 'Oblique Cutting' is one of the most popular techniques that many participants of my extraction seminar learn and use after the seminar. Let's learn why 'Oblique Cutting' is important and efficient.

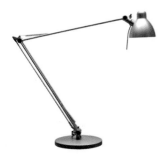

01
Oblique Cutting ★★★

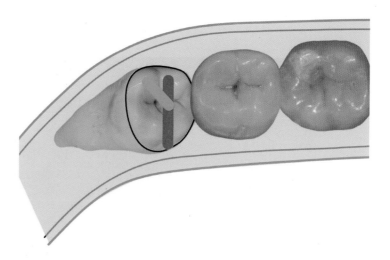

'Oblique Cutting' is the technique that after removing the mesial portion of the crown, you remove another fragment by sectioning it in an oblique line (blue line) as shown above.

It is similar to 'Lingual Crown Cutting' (discussed later) in a vertical impaction case. However, it is called 'Oblique Cutting' because the cutting line looks oblique not only from the occlusal plane, but also from the coronal plane.

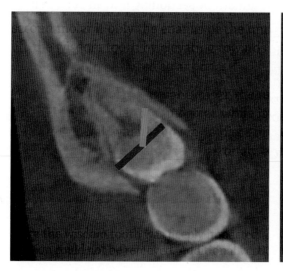 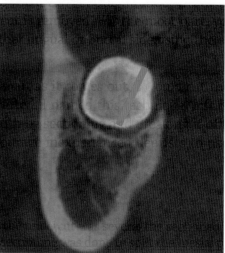

This CT image shows the cross section and coronal plane. As you can see in these images, the cutting line is oblique (Blue line) and this is why it is called 'Oblique Cutting'. For this method, you need to remove the sectioned fragment thus I strongly recommend inexperienced dentists to use a #4 round bur so it is easier to break the sectioned part.

Oblique Cutting ★★

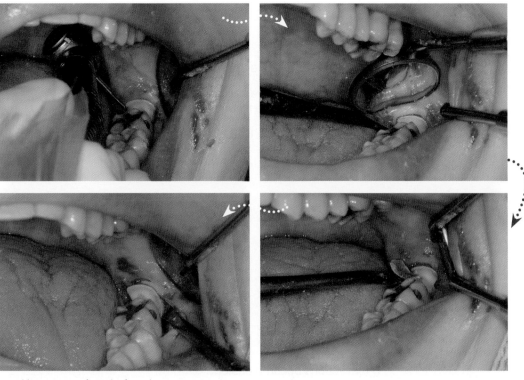

Oblique Cutting from the frontal view

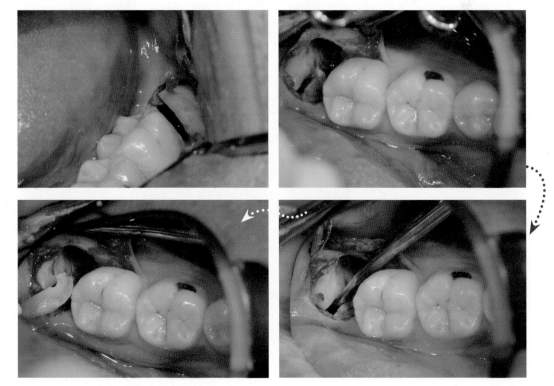

It is easy to visualize from the occlusal view.

02
Advantages of Oblique Cutting ★★★

There are many advantages to Oblique Cutting.

1) Extraction becomes easier.

2) It can prevent the fracture of lingual cortex.

3) It is easy to remove the mesio-lingual portion of the crown which can be troublesome.

4) There is a pre 'Lift & Cutting' effect.

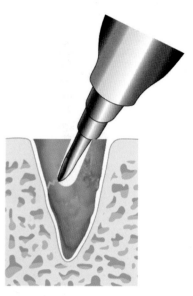

▬ "Oblique Cutting" is performed by sectioning some of the remained parts after the removal.

First advantage of 'Oblique Cutting'

1) Extractions become easier.

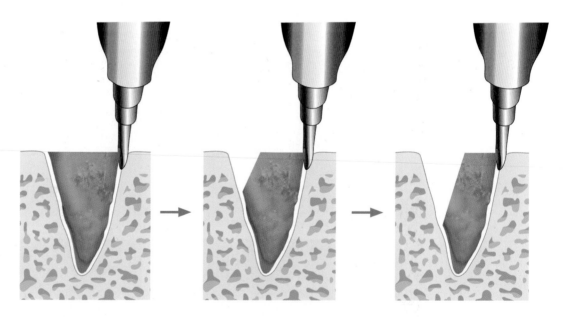

First, extractions become easier. Let's look at the figure above. As we proceed to the right, the extraction will become easier. In general, I apply the elevator in the disto-buccal side of the third molar. If you remove the mesio-lingual portion of the crown first and apply the elevator to the disto-buccal side (which is the opposite side), the extraction will be much easier.

The second advantage of 'Oblique Cutting'

2) Lingual cortical bone fracture can be prevented

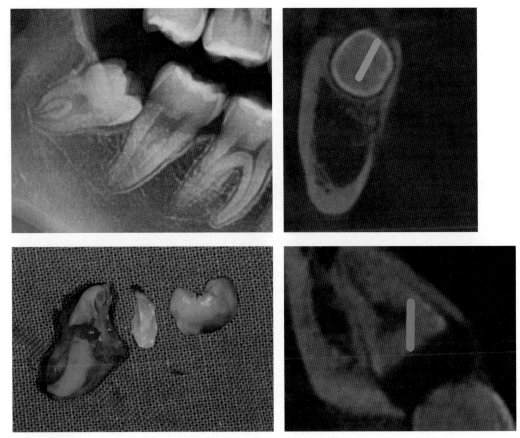

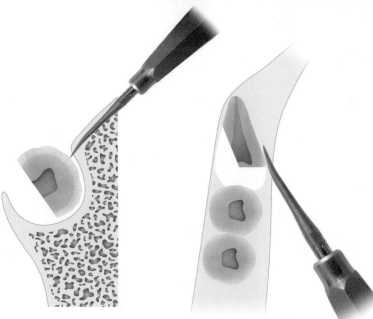

In the above case, you can see that the wisdom tooth is deeply impacted. The CBCT image shows that the lingual bone is very thin. In this case, 'Oblique Cutting' can prevent the fracture of the lingual cortical bone. I definitely see less lingual bone fractures when I do 'Oblique Cutting'.

After 'Oblique Cutting', the rest can be extracted by applying some force from the buccal side and in turn, less force is applied to the lingual cortical bone.

'Oblique Cutting' is a useful technique in removing a deeply impacted or lingually tipped third molar.

The third advantage of 'Oblique Cutting'

3) It is easy to remove the troublesome lingual portion of crown.

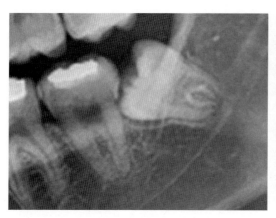 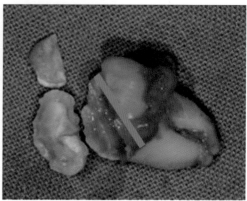

When 'Mesial Crown Cutting' is done, the lingual side is usually not sectioned completely, and this lingual part can get caught under the distal of the second molar or under the soft tissue. It is good to remove this troublesome mesio-lingual portion of the crown first. The yellow arrow in the figures below shows that the mesio-lingual portion of the crown that is sectioned and removed.

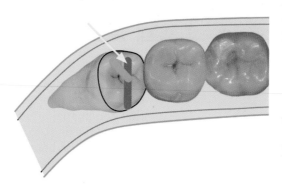 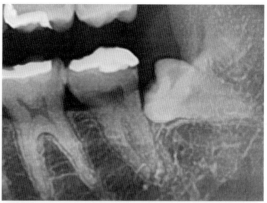

The figure above will make it easier to understand. Especially, in the case of wisdom teeth that are impacted deeply, even though 'Mesial Crown Cutting' is done, it is very likely that the third molar is caught under the distal of the second molar. The 'Oblique Cutting' is done in almost all horizontally impacted cases. The yellow arrow is the fragment that is removed from 'Oblique Cutting'.

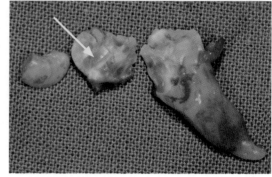

The fourth advantage of 'Oblique Cutting'

4) There is a pre-'Lift&Cutting' effect.

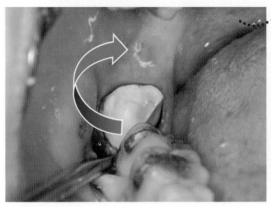 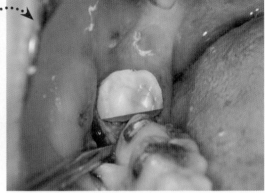

■ Even though the third molar is dislodged, it can get caught under the distal of the second molar. In such cases, you can do "Oblique Cutting" in advance and turn the wisdom tooth clockwise.

■ If you rotate clockwise (counterclockwise if you are on the left side of the mandible), it will end up in the same position as in the 'Lift & Cutting' method.

I mentioned earlier that you can do 'Lift & Cutting' when a third molar gets caught under the distal of the second molar as it comes out of the socket. If you do 'Oblique Cutting' first, even though it is caught under, you can rotate the tooth in the direction of the arrow (either clockwise for #48 or counterclockwise for #38). Once the third molar is released from the undercut, the extraction becomes easy. If you practice this technique several times, you can see how the extraction can get easier.

03
Oblique Cutting video ★★

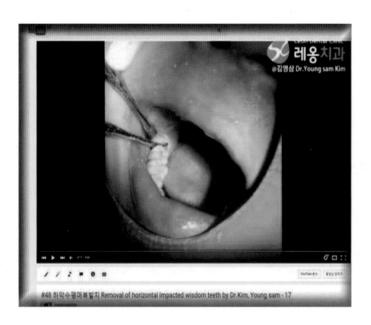

 "Oblique Cutting" for a 45-degree horizontal impaction

 "Oblique Cutting" for a horizontal impaction

 An 80-degree horizontally impacted tooth extracted by forceps after sectioning

04
A comparison of the buccal and lingual surface of wisdom tooth extracted ★★
with 'Oblique Cutting'

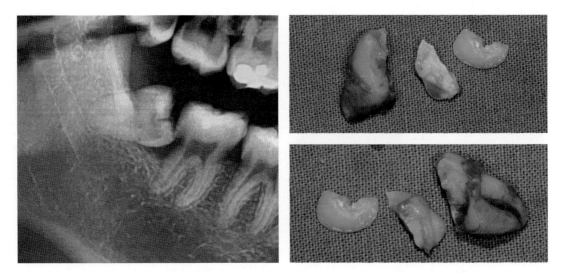

The images above shows a lower third molar that was extracted by 'Oblique Cutting'. If it is hard to visualize by looking at the buccal view (top right), you can see the sectioned surface from the lingual side (bottom right). This cut surface looks similar to the 'Lift & Cutting' because they are done similarly but the cut is made at a different angle.

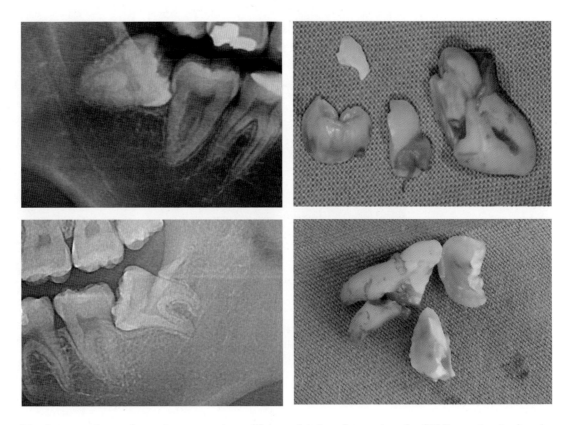

The images above show the extraction of lower third molars using the 'Oblique Cutting' technique (lingual side view) . You can see the sectioned pieces and surfaces where the cut was made.

05
'Oblique Cutting' cross-section view from a different angle ★★

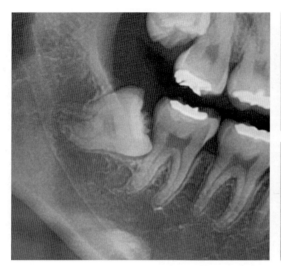
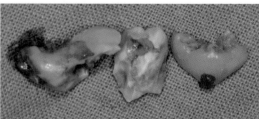
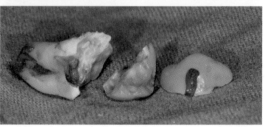

If you observe the wisdom tooth from the bottom, you can see two surfaces where the cut was made.

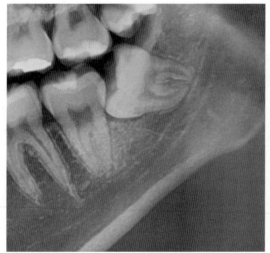
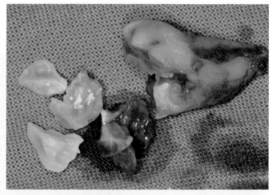
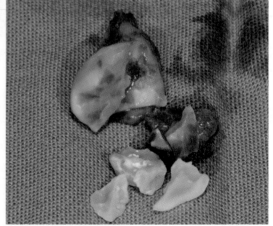

06
Oblique Cutting Case <1> ★

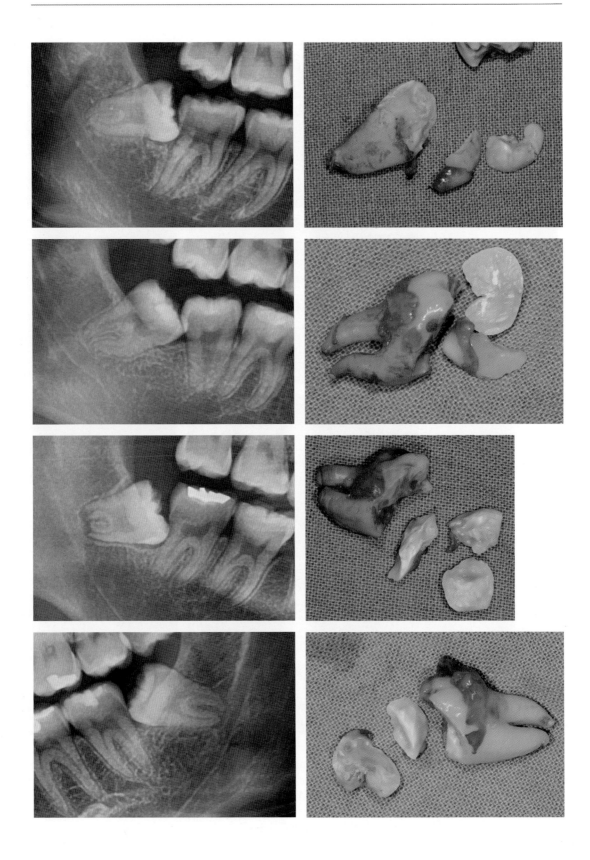

Oblique Cutting Case <2> ★

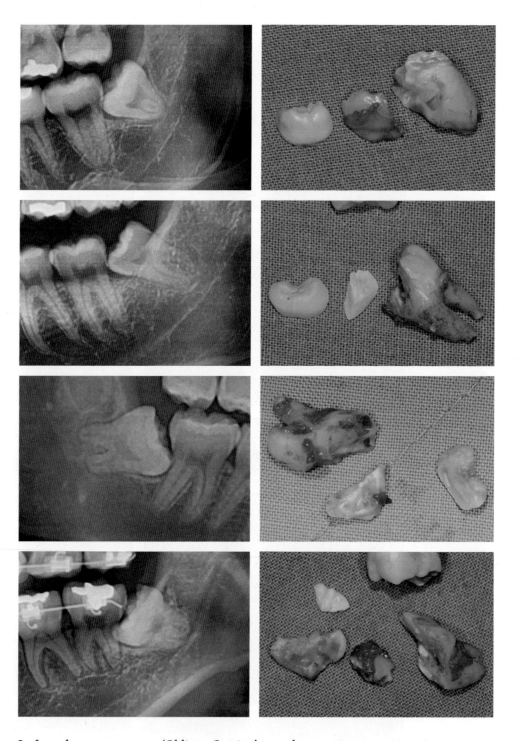

In fact, there are so many 'Oblique Cutting' cases because in most extraction cases, some extent of 'Oblique Cutting' is done. This technique certainly helps inexperienced dentists to do an easy and safe extraction. Whenever I face any challenging cases or couldn't remove a third molar by only doing 'Mesial Crown Cutting' (taking shortcut when I am busy), I always go back to my basics and do the 'Oblique Cutting'.

07
Vertically deep impacted and mesially inclined third molars ★

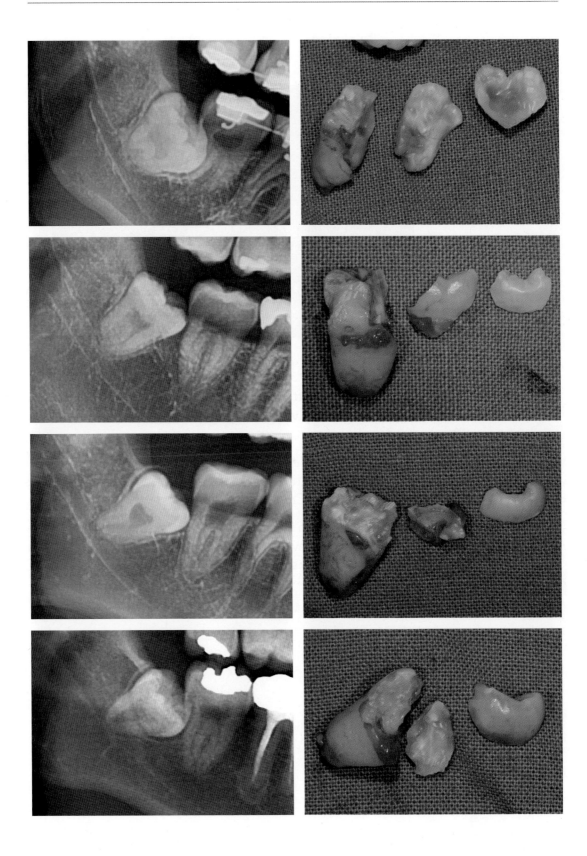

Lingual Crown Cutting ★★

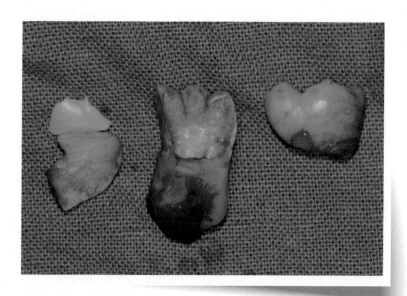

'Lingual Crown Cutting' is used mainly when a mandibular third molar is less mesially tipped or in a deep vertical impaction case when the height of contour is covered by the bone.

In this case, most dentists will remove the alveolar bone around the crown to expose the tooth before extraction, however I tend to section the tooth into smaller pieces instead. The key is 'Lingual Crown Cutting'.

It can be seen as an 'Oblique cutting' for a deep impaction case or in a slight mesial impaction case. However, since this technique is very useful for a deep impaction case, I named it separately as 'Lingual Crown Cutting'.

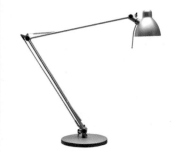

01
Vertically deep impacted wisdom teeth cutting method ★★★

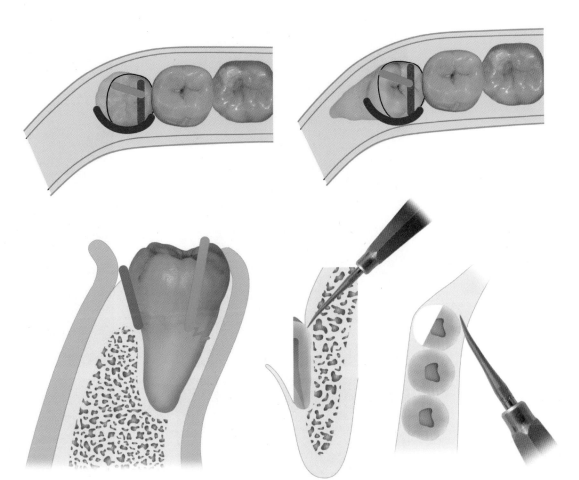

In the case of a deep vertical impaction, I approach the extraction similar to any other cases unless it is a complete horizontal impaction case. I was planning to discuss this case within the 'Vertical Impaction' chapter, but I decided to discuss in this chapter with other mesial impaction cases. As a result, I treat them in the same way as above, whether it is vertically or mesially impacted.

Since the alveolar bone is positioned above the height of contour of the third molar, it is difficult to remove. In this case, most dentists tend to remove buccal and distal alveolar bone and extract the wisdom tooth (as shown by the purple line). However, as I try to minimize alveolar bone removal, I section and remove the mesio-lingual portion of the tooth first as described above ('Lingual Crown Cutting') and elevate the rest forward by placing an elevator at the disto-buccal corner.

'Lingual Crown Cutting' is almost the same angle as 'Oblique Cutting', depending on the degree of impaction. I believe that this method is very efficient and results in less postoperative bleeding and swelling. In addition, damage to the lingual cortical bone can be minimized.

02
Vertically deep impacted wisdom teeth extraction ★★

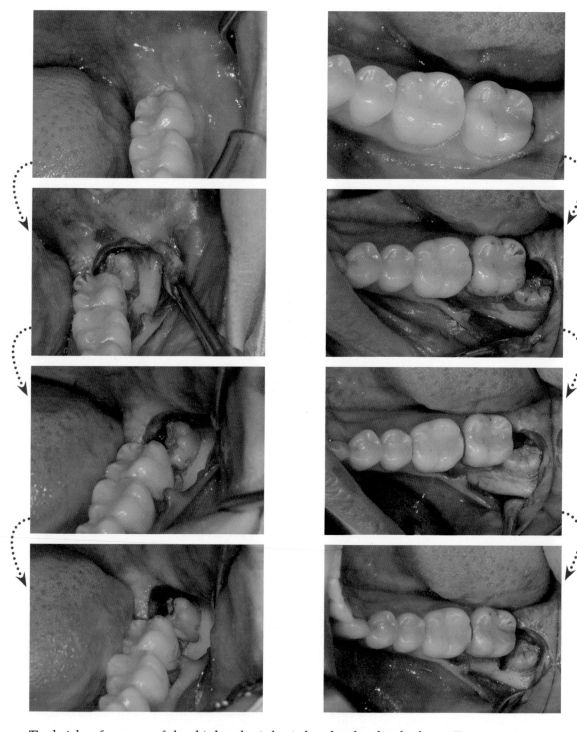

The height of contour of the third molar is buried under the alveolar bone. The extraction was carried out by raising a flap. Instead of removing the disto-buccal alveolar bone, I removed the lingual portion of the crown using the 'Lingual Crown Cutting' technique first(similar to 'Oblique Cutting'). In a deep vertical impaction case, it is important to remove a sufficient amount of the mesial portion of the crown extending to the buccal bone, similarly to 'Mesial Crown Cutting'.

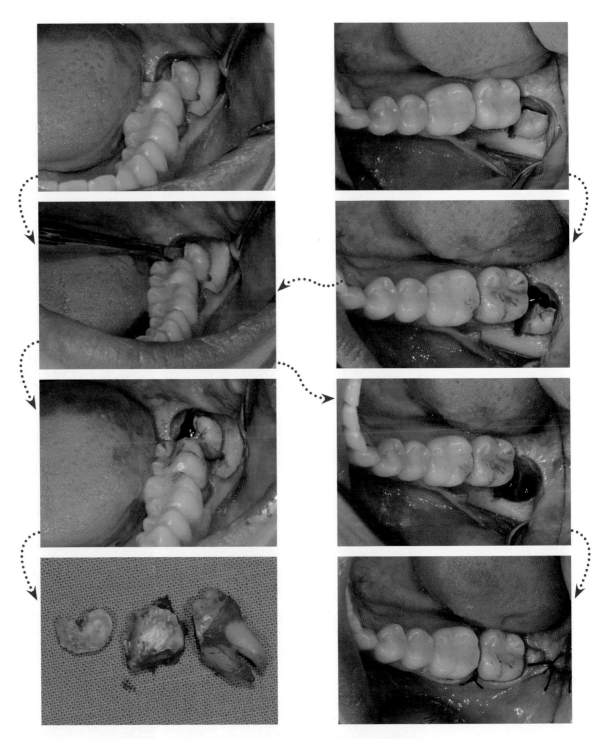

After sectioning the third molar with 'Mesial Crown Cutting' and 'Lingual Crown Cutting', you remove the fragments using an elevator and surgical curette. The 'Lingual Crown Cutting' technique not only makes the extraction easier but also reduces postoperative complications. This case had a large open flap to allow for taking photographs. Routine extractions usually do not require to have such wide incisions and flaps.

03
Lingual Crown Cutting case slightly different from Oblique Cutting <1> ★

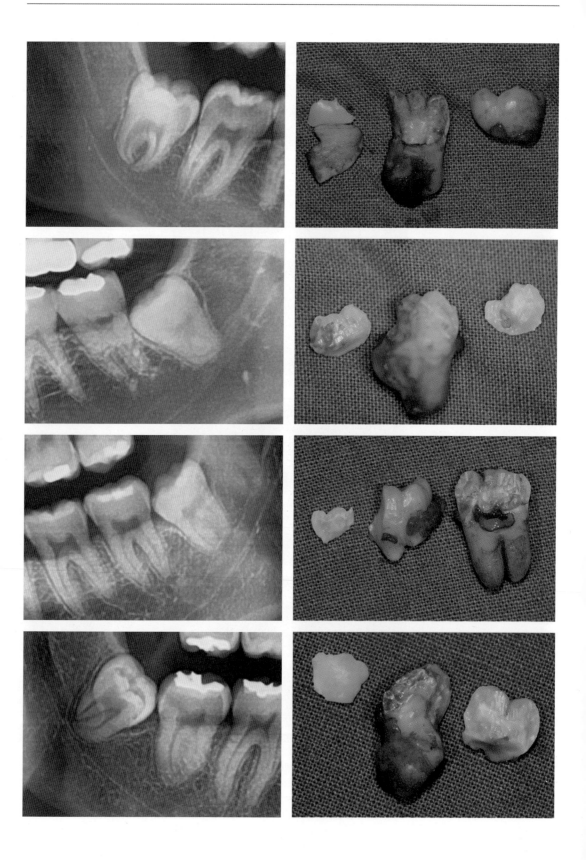

Lingual Crown Cutting case slightly different from Oblique Cutting <2>

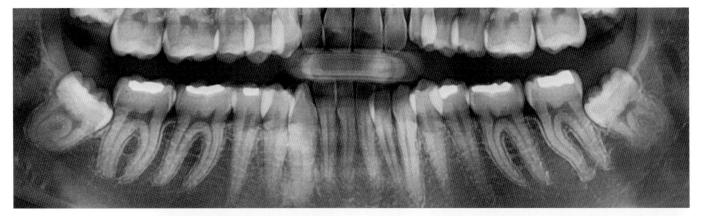

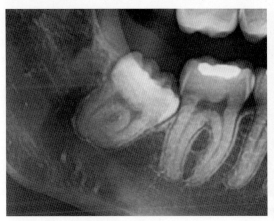

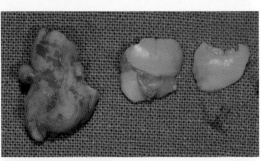

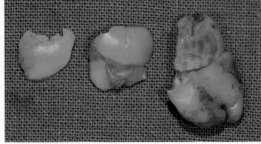

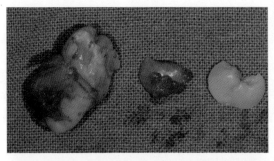

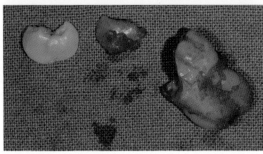

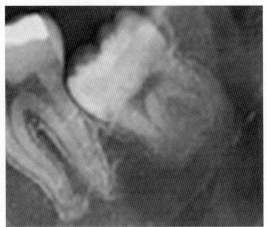

04
As a Crown Cutting method ★

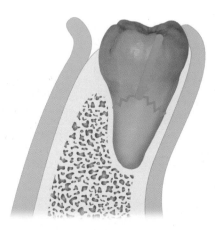

In the case of limited opening, the handpiece can be tilted too much, and the buccal portion of a crown may be fractured instead. In this case, the extraction may be continued or can be terminated with a coronectomy if necessary. Sometimes, coronectomy is planned and performed like the above approach.

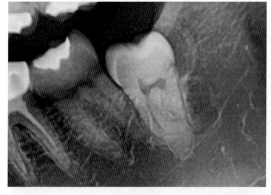
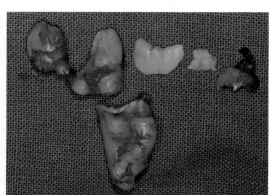
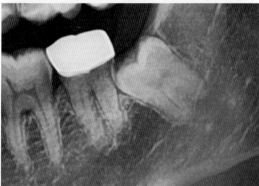
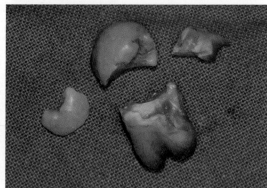

Wait!

Look at this book twice

If you read this book again, you will see cases that were extracted in the same way as above in the radiograph and coronectomy sections. This is the reason why I recommend you to read this book twice. You can read once to get the basic flow of this book and you can review each case when you read again. You can also learn more as you do extractions in your practice.

Disto-Cervical Cutting ★★★

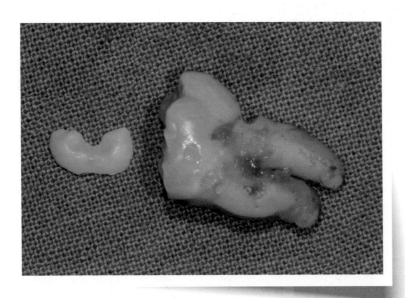

'Disto-Cervical Cutting' is a technique to use if you still cannot extract the third molar even after 'Mesial Crown Cutting' and/or 'Oblique Cutting'.

'Disto-Cervical Cutting' leads to a faster extraction and less post-operative edema and pain compared to doing an extraction with buccal alveolar bone removal.

It is not necessary to try this technique if you can remove a third molar with elevators or forceps before 'Disto-Cervical Cutting'. When you do 'Disto-Cervical Cutting', I recommend a small bur, like a #4 round bur. I often use the same No. 6 round bur that was used to remove the mesial portion of the crown because it is often inconvenient to change the bur. I would recommend using a #4 round bur for beginners.

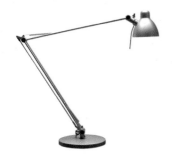

01
Disto-Cervical Cutting ★★★

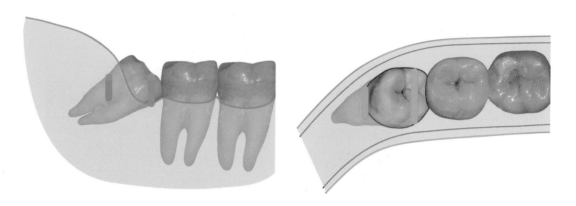

These figures show the position, direction, and degree of 'Disto-Cervical Cutting' which is performed in the case of mesially impacted third molars. Just as the patient's mouth condition is not always the same, it can appear in various forms.

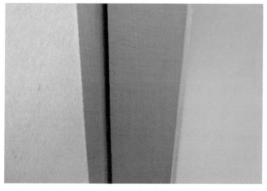 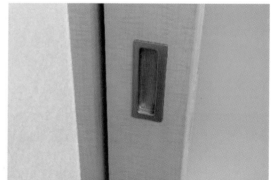

It may not be the right example, but it may be good to think of it as the case. If there is a door like the picture on the left above, it will be hard to open. It is easy to open and close the door if you make a groove. I originally called it 'Notch Creation' but I decided to call it 'Disto-Cervical Cutting' while writing this book.

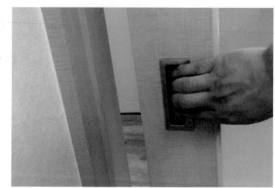

02
Disto-Cervical Cutting process <1> ★★

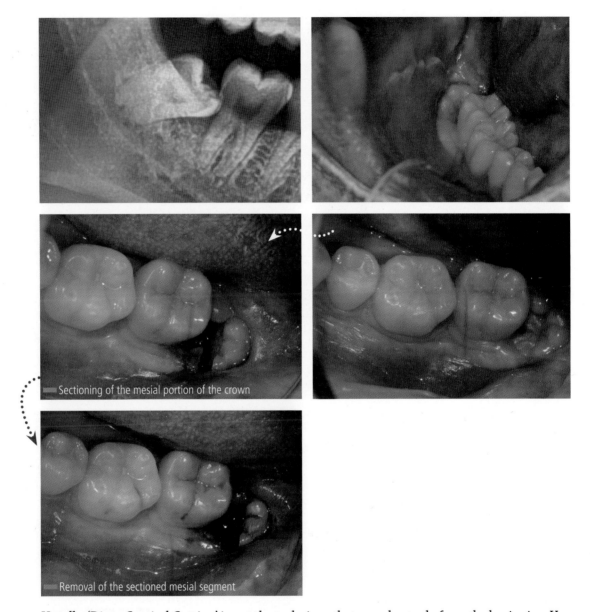

Sectioning of the mesial portion of the crown

Removal of the sectioned mesial segment

Usually, 'Disto-Cervical Cutting' is not the technique that you plan to do from the beginning. You can proceed with 'Disto-cervical Cutting' if the third molar does not come out even though the usual methods such as 'Mesial Crown Cutting', 'Oblique Cutting' and 'Lingual Crown Cutting' are done already.

As mentioned in the radiograph section, 'Disto-Cervical Cutting' is mainly used when an elevator cannot be used, for example, when the crown is completely exposed or when the root is pressed tightly against the alveolar bone due to severe inflammation around the crown. In these cases, I strongly recommend the use of forceps, but it is hard to use forceps if the third molar is impacted.

I have recently seen cases where forceps can be used for an impaction, however I was not interested in them because my goal is perform extractions while using a minimum number of instruments.

It is good to do 'Oblique Cutting' beforehand, but if the elevator cannot move a tooth from the buccal side, I tend to do the 'Disto-Cervical Cutting'. This is a very useful method.

Disto-Cervical Cutting process <2> ★★

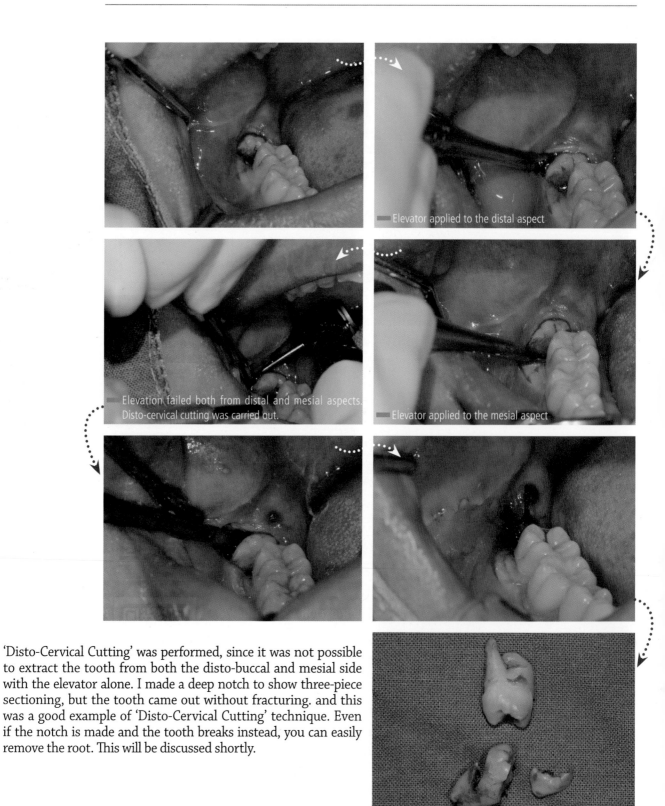

Elevator applied to the distal aspect

Elevation failed both from distal and mesial aspects. Disto-cervical cutting was carried out.

Elevator applied to the mesial aspect

'Disto-Cervical Cutting' was performed, since it was not possible to extract the tooth from both the disto-buccal and mesial side with the elevator alone. I made a deep notch to show three-piece sectioning, but the tooth came out without fracturing. and this was a good example of 'Disto-Cervical Cutting' technique. Even if the notch is made and the tooth breaks instead, you can easily remove the root. This will be discussed shortly.

03
The No. 4 round surgical bur is the most useful in 'Disto-Cervical Cutting' ★★★

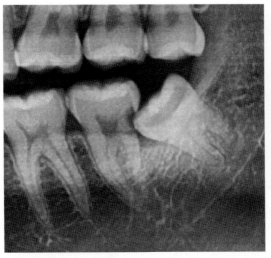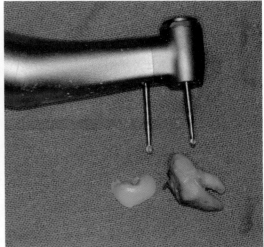

The picture on the right shows you what I did to extract the lower left molar. I used a NSK 5x contra-angle low speed handpiece and a #6 round bur for the 'Mesial Crown Cutting', and a #4 round bur for 'Disto-Cervical Cutting'. In hindsight, for this mesial impaction case, using a #4 round bur would be ideal for both 'Mesial Crown Cutting' and 'Disto-Cervical Cutting'. This photo was taken to record that I used a 5x low speed contra angle handpiece, not to emphasize that the 'Mesial Crown Cuting' was done with a #6 round bur and the 'Disto- Cervical Cutting' was done with a #4 round bur.

In any case, I recommend you to use a #4 surgical round bur (diameter of 1.4 mm) for 'Disto-Cervical Cutting'. These days, I do the first 'Crown Cutting' with a #6 round bur and proceed with the 'Disto-Cervical Cutting' with a #6 round bur (diameter of 1.8 mm) as well to avoid changing burs. However, if you use a #6 round bur for the 'Disto-Cervical Cutting', you need to make a deeper groove or notch to place an elevator, then it is easy to fracture the tooth unfavourably. In turn, it may not be easy to pull the rest of the tooth out. This is why I strongly recommend to use a #4 round bur to do the 'Disto-Cervical Cutting' if you are a beginner.

If you have any surgical fissure burs in your dental clinic, those are recommended as well. Commonly used surgical fissure burs are 1.6 mm in maximum diameter and the cutting head is about 0.8 - 1.0 mm in diameter. If you have a fissure bur with a short cutting head, you can use it. However, most of the fissure burs available in Korea have a long cutting head (at least 9 mm) and they damage the gingiva easily. So nowadays, I recommend using a #4 round bur again. Otherwise, as described in the 'Disto-Cervical Cutting' section, you can use a #6 round bur but you need to make a deeper notch or groove.

04
Disto-Cervical Cutting cases ★★

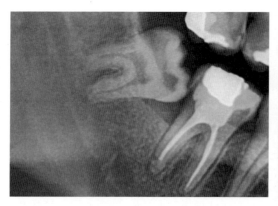

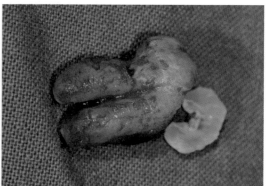

In this case, the lower right third molar was mesially impacted, and it would be ideal to extract using a dental elevator but there is no alveolar bone around the crown. In this case, if you make a notch or groove in the disto-cervical part with a high speed handpiece, the elevator can be placed into the groove and pull the third molar forward.

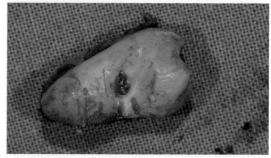

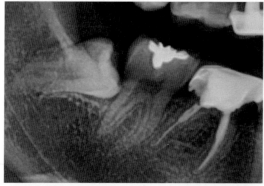

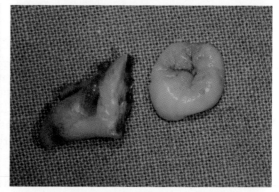

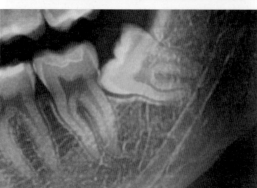

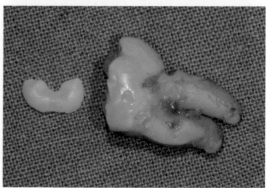

In fact, you won't need to do 'Disto-Cervical Cutting' in most mesial impaction cases because most cases will be extracted before you do the 'Disto-Cervical Cutting'. However, if the mesial inclination is more than 45 degrees, it is difficult to use the forceps so 'Disto-Cervical Cutting' can be very useful. 'Disto-Cervical Cutting' is the basis to the 'L-Extraction' or the 'Three Sectioning' techniques which will be discussed later.

Disto-Cervical Cutting and L-Extraction ★★★

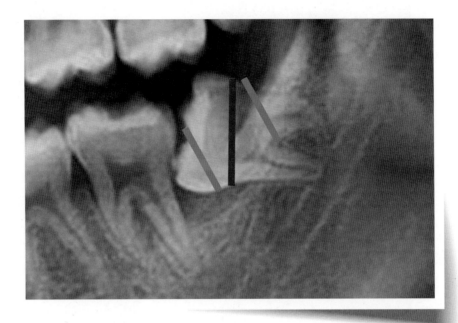

If the wisdom tooth does not come out easily with the elevator after removing the mesial portion, it is good to section off the distal root with the 'Disto-Cervical Cutting' technique. When you separate one of the roots of the third molar, the force required for the extraction will be reduced by half. In addition, the 'Disto-Cervical Cutting' technique also creates a groove (notch) where the elevator can act on. This is particularly advantageous when the upper root is bent downward, opposite to the direction of the extraction.

I call this technique 'L-Extraction' because one of the segments of the tooth after extraction looks like the capital letter "L". In this case, there are many dentists who want to section the tooth like the red line. As I have mentioned before, I personally think it is unwise in this case. It is necessary to section and remove the tooth fragment with a clear purpose such as 'Mesial Crown Cutting' and 'Distal Crown Cutting'. The sum of cutting surface made with the two blue lines is much less than the cutting surface of the red line.

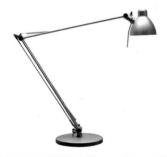

01
L-Extraction ★★★

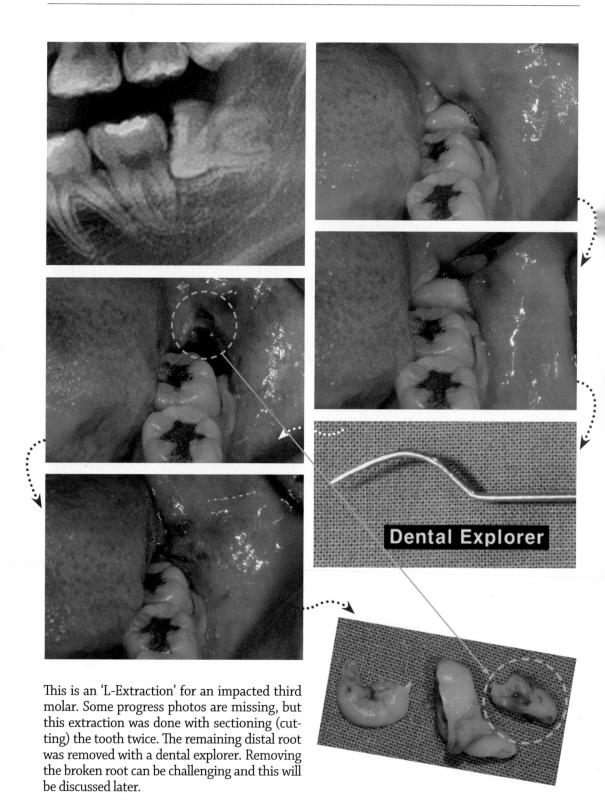

This is an 'L-Extraction' for an impacted third molar. Some progress photos are missing, but this extraction was done with sectioning (cutting) the tooth twice. The remaining distal root was removed with a dental explorer. Removing the broken root can be challenging and this will be discussed later.

Dental Explorer

02
Radiographic examples of L-Extraction process <1>

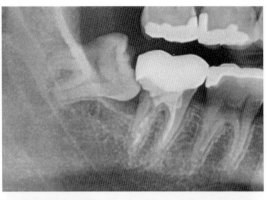

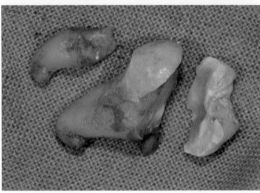

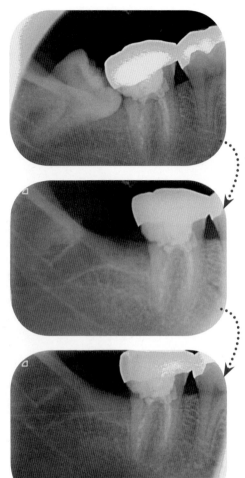

This is a standard shot of the 'L-Extraction' procedure. If you are a beginner, it would be good to take x-rays during and after the extraction.

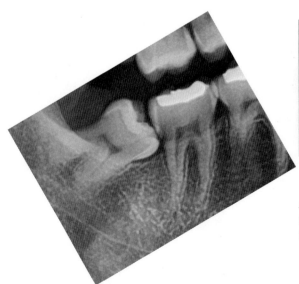

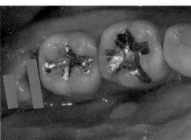

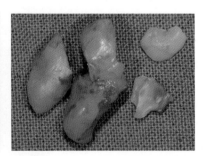

An impacted wisdom tooth like this case can be easily removed by sectioning the tooth twice without raising a flap using the 'L-Extraction' technique.

Radiographic examples of L-Extraction process <2> ★

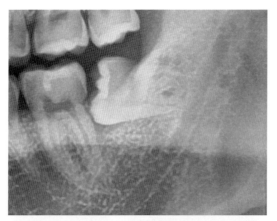

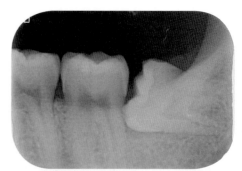

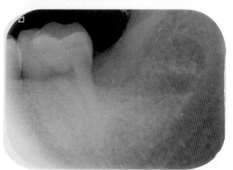

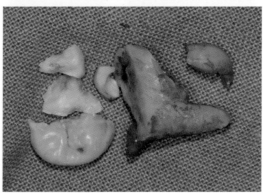

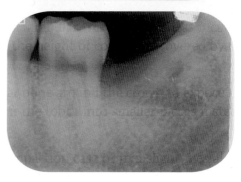

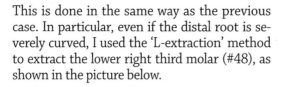

This is done in the same way as the previous case. In particular, even if the distal root is severely curved, I used the 'L-extraction' method to extract the lower right third molar (#48), as shown in the picture below.

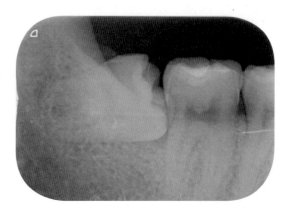

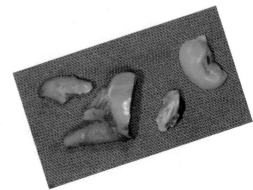

03
L-Extraction case: Both side same case ★

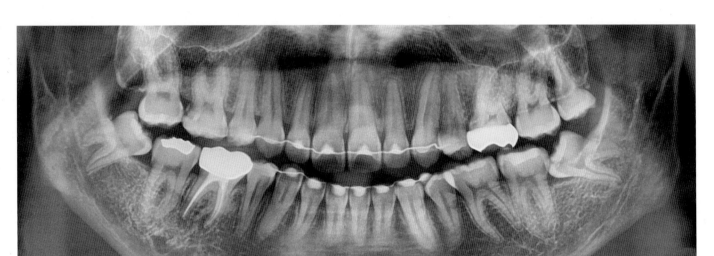

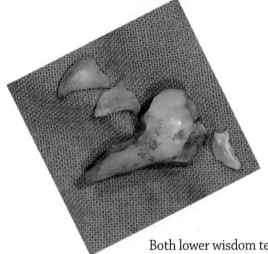

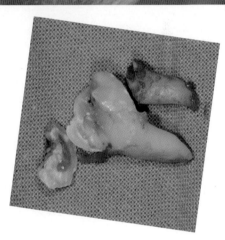

Both lower wisdom teeth were extracted using the 'L-Extraction' technique. 'L-Extraction' is beneficial because you can extract with a minimal incision and no alveolar bone removal. It is very fast and simple because you just need to section twice. It is much easier, faster, and safer than removing alveolar bone and cutting the center of the crown.

Typical L-Extraction cases

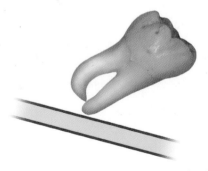

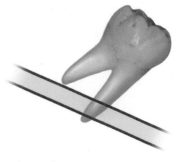

Mesial root is overlapped with IAN or distal root is severely curved.

04
L-Extraction case <1> ★

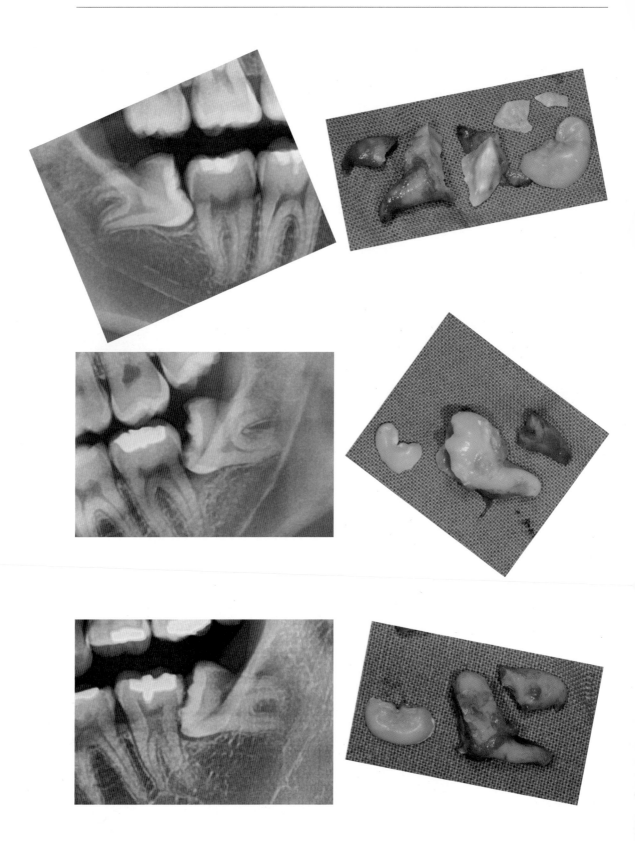

L-Extraction case <2> ★

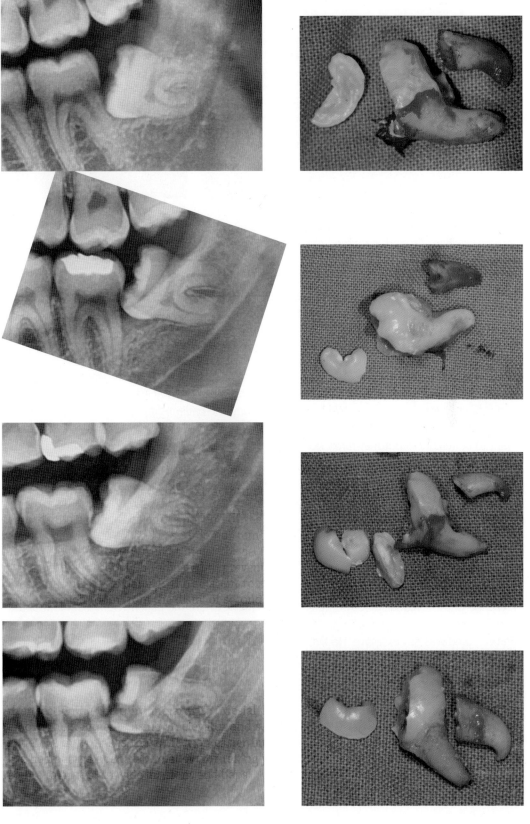

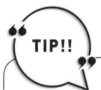

TIP!!

Post Operative Bleeding ★★★

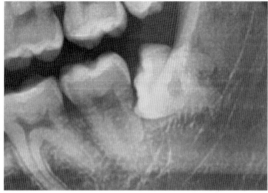 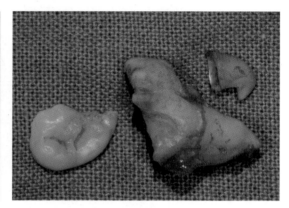

This patient was a young male in his mid twenties and his mother was a dentist who referred her son to me for wisdom tooth extraction. Around that time, three more patients whose mothers were dentists also came to see me. I was honored that other dentists are recognizing me for my extraction skill. This extraction took less than 3 minutes. The patient's mother, who is a dentist, asked me not to take a CBCT scan (in this case, I did not think it was necessary), and asked me not to use any hemostatic agent. I did not see any excessive bleeding and the patient did not report any pain during and right after the extraction. However, I got a call from the mother of the patient the next day reporting that excessive bleeding suddenly started at night so the mother tried to achieve hemostasis by compressing with gauze but bleeding did not stop. They ended up going to the hospital emergency where bleeding was controlled.

The patient's mother asked me if there was any complications during the surgery and she seemed quite concerned. I usually do 300 to 400 third molar extractions per month and a few patients end up going to the emergency department at night due to excessive bleeding. We always mention to the patient during their post operative instructions that post operative bleeding is possible, and if necessary, they can go to the emergency. Most patients go to the emergency because they want to be reassured but they rarely need to receive any special treatment. As a matter of fact, most emergency clinics are busy and they may not have a dentist who can manage dental emergencies. When the mother of the patient asked me what could be the cause of it, I sent the above images and explained it.

My explanation was "In my opinion, Youngsam's sign appears at the root apex. The distal root might have been embedded in the lingual cortical bone and the lingual cortical bone might have been fractured or punctured during the extraction. It seems that the distal root was curved significantly towards the lingual cortical bone. Since there was no incision and flap made on the buccal side, I believe that the bleeding is not from the buccal side." She did not seem to be convinced by my response.

I reached out the acquaintance in the emergency room where the patient went last night and asked him what happened and the answer was very interesting. Only a new resident was present to manage the patient in the emergency department and bleeding was not excessive. He first tried to remove the sutures and place surgicel into the socket, but it would not go in. Also, he mentioned that bleeding was mild so he had the patient bite down on gauze. Even a dentist who has sufficient knowledge on post-operative bleeding can panic in this situation.

05
Seminar student's case ★

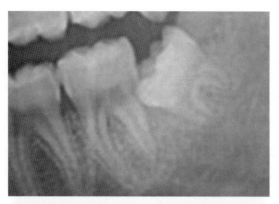

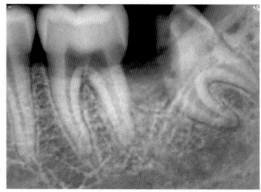

This is the case of my extraction seminar attendee. He shared this case in our group chat. If it was my case, I would have sectioned the mesial portion closer to the distal of the second molar.

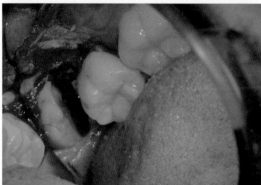

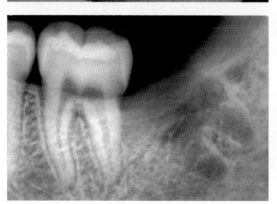

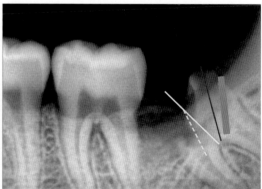

Many different opinions were presented. I can see that he has already done more sectioning after removing the mesial portion of the crown. I recommend you not to do any sectioning without a clear purpose because that can complicate your situation more.

In this case, I would try elevating the tooth out after 'Mesial Crown Cutting' and if it does not come out, I would have done 'Disto-Cervical Cutting'. It could progress to the 'L-Extraction' so I could remove the mesial root and body. Especially when the root is close to IAN, this method is very useful. Most oral surgeons would suggest separating the two roots with a slow speed handpiece. After training, you will find my method easier, faster and safer.

06
What if it breaks during extraction? 'Three Part Sectioning' ★★★

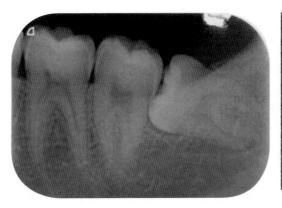 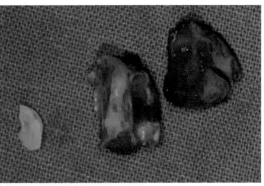

It is a principle to remove the residual root if it is broken, but it is not necessary to take the time and effort to remove the remaining root if you follow my extraction technique. This is because you already did enough for the coronectomy. However, if possible, I always try my best to remove the residual roots. The method to remove the residual roots will be discussed when we discuss complete horizontal impaction.

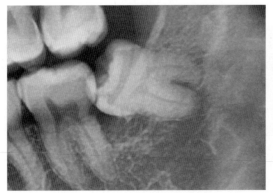 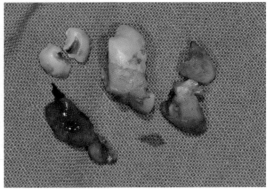

As mentioned in the radiograph section, if the inflammation is severe around the crown, the roots are pushed apically and they can be almost attached to the alveolar bone. Therefore, the apical portion can break when the tooth is elevated after the 'Disto-Cervical Cutting' technique is used. I ended up removing the broken root.

07
Extraction with 'Three Parts Sectioning' after 'Disto-Cervical Cutting' ★★

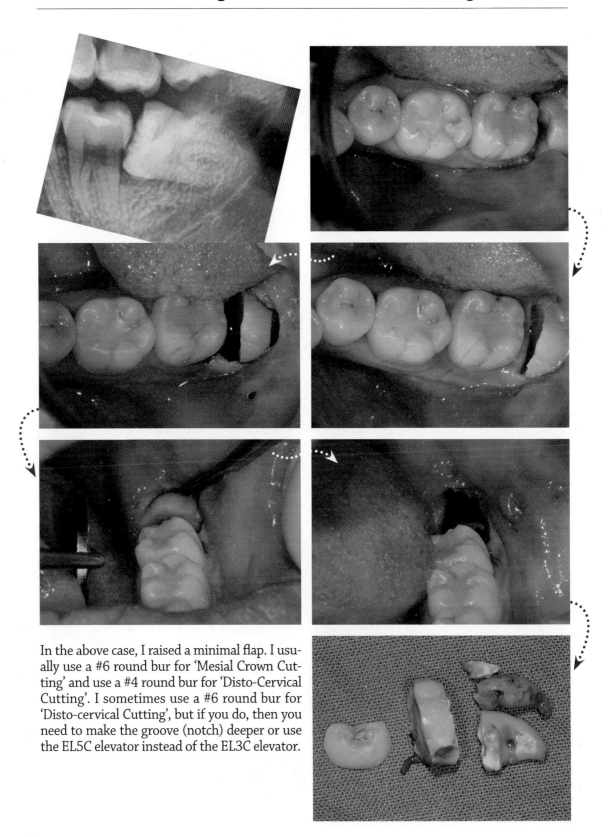

In the above case, I raised a minimal flap. I usually use a #6 round bur for 'Mesial Crown Cutting' and use a #4 round bur for 'Disto-Cervical Cutting'. I sometimes use a #6 round bur for 'Disto-cervical Cutting', but if you do, then you need to make the groove (notch) deeper or use the EL5C elevator instead of the EL3C elevator.

08
Three parts crown division case ★

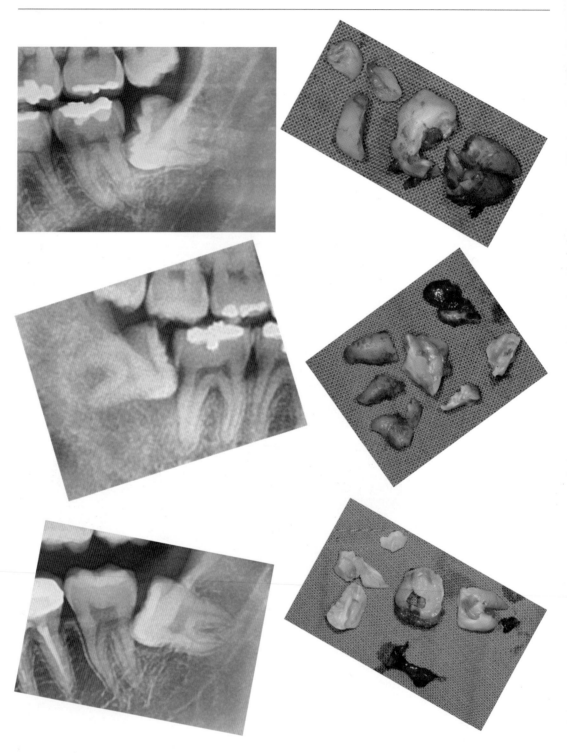

Although the tooth is not sectioned into exactly three parts, I decided to call this technique the 'Three Part Extraction' technique - a mesial crown portion, mesial root and body portion, and distal root portion. There are many ways to remove the remaining root. I will discuss it in the 'Horizontal Impaction' chapter.

Horizontally Impacted Wisdom Tooth

Chapter 08 translated by

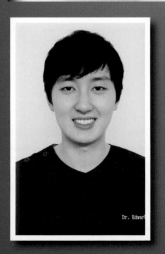

Dr. Edward Jh Lee
Bdent. Mdent. MSc. FICOI. DICOI.

The Bachelor of Health Sciences in Dentistry / Master of Dentistry
(La Trobe University)

The Master of Science (MSc.) in Oral Implantology
(Goethe-University Frankfurt)

Diplomate of International Congress of Oral Implantologists (DICOI)
Principal dentist at With U Dental

It is my great pleasure to participate in this project. As much as this knowledge has been very informative to myself I have no doubt that this book will be of great help to you.

01
Incision methods for horizontally impacted tooth ★★

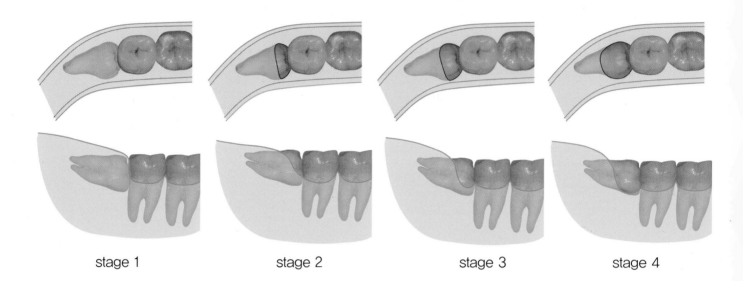

stage 1   stage 2   stage 3   stage 4

For convenience, let's divide the amount of gingivally submerged wisdom teeth into four stages. The tooth will be extracted without any gingival incision when most of the crown is exposed in the oral cavity (stage 4). This means that no flap or bone reduction will be required during the extraction. Comparably, an incision made on horizontally impacted wisdom teeth will be larger than the incision made on a mesially impacted wisdom tooth. A small buccal incision needs to be made for stage 2 horizontally impacted wisdom tooth in order to obtain visibility of the extraction site.

It is critical to have a consistent length and shape of the incision line from the occlusal surface to the distal surface of the tooth regardless of the visibility. That line should always be in mind when making an incision. Usually, I extend the incision line mesial to the 7 if the tooth is fully impacted and not visible (stage 1), or slightly visible with a portion of the crown showing in the oral cavity (stage 2).

TIP!!

An incision line must be extended longer if you are using a fissure bur instead of a round bur. You must have a gingival separation along the lingual, raise full-thickness mucoperiosteal flap, and also create a mesio-buccal flap in order to prevent gingival damages if you decide to utilize a fissure bur.

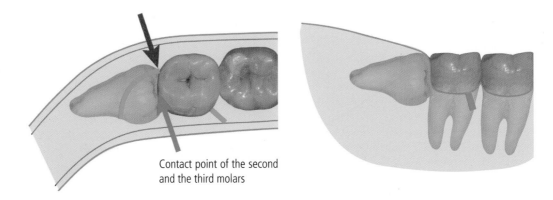

Contact point of the second
and the third molars

As I have mentioned before, the incision line should end lingually to the contact point of 7th and 8th teeth. Such incision provides visibility as well as minimises gingival damages near the lingual contact points of the 7th and 8th teeth during sectioning of the crown. Therefore, it is highly recommended to create the incision line up to the pathway of the bur.

Generally, the vertical incision line on the mesial of the 7th tooth and raising the full-thickness mucoperiosteal flap allows sufficient space to implement the procedure. However, the flap can be extended beyond the interdental papillae under special circumstances without a vertical incision. On a very rare occasion, a vertical incision can be made on the distal of the 7th tooth depending on the surgeon's need.

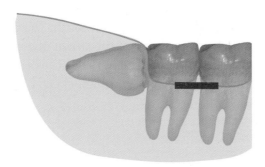

The incision line is made below the papillae of the 7th and 6th teeth and full-thickness mucoperiosteal flap is raised, but I personally do not prefer this type of incision.

Crown Cutting of the Wisdom Teeth

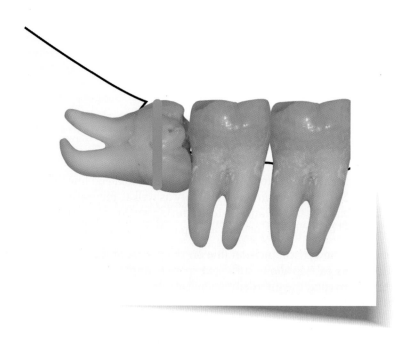

Typically, sectioning a crown of a horizontally impacted wisdom tooth is not so much different from cutting a mesially impacted wisdom tooth. There are several more different sectioning methods through a mesial side of the crown of a horizontally impacted tooth. I have used many different instruments and burs but the best way of cutting and removing the crown is with a surgical round bur on a high-speed handpiece.

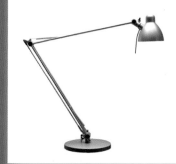

01
Crown Cutting of the wisdom teeth ★★

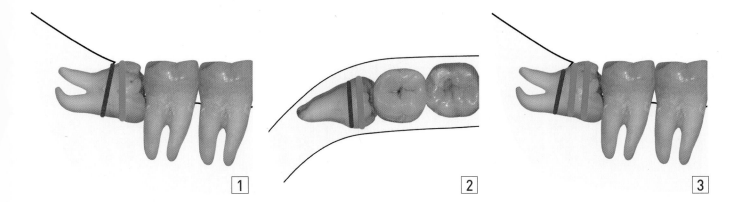

I have named it 'Crown Cutting' for cutting a crown portion of the wisdom tooth. As I have mentioned before, I have been contacted by numerous dentists all over the world related to the wisdom tooth extraction techniques. Thus, I have tried to simplify the terms for any dentist around the world to easily understand. I also created the names of different sectioning techniques for dentists to easily remember, and to think outside the box.

Image 1 shows the complete cutting of the crown with a single cut. As I have mentioned in the 'Mesioangular Impacted Wisdom Teeth Extraction' chapter, I always cut as close to the distal contact of the 7th tooth as possible. Usually, most dentists cut as per red line indicated in the images.

Sectioning through the red line will be easy compared to the recommended blue lines but this will make it even harder for the sectioned crown to be removed.

Extraction time can be unnecessarily increased especially when you do not know what to do in the middle of the procedure. Methodical crown sectioning of once or twice more is more predictable than sectioning a large chunk at once. Moreover, a Crown Cutting does not consume much time. Consequently, I prefer to cut the crown several times during extraction.

As shown in image 3, I tend to cut the crown twice when severe undercut is noted on the distal of the 7th tooth.

02
Sectional view of the Crown Cutting according to the size and shape of the burs

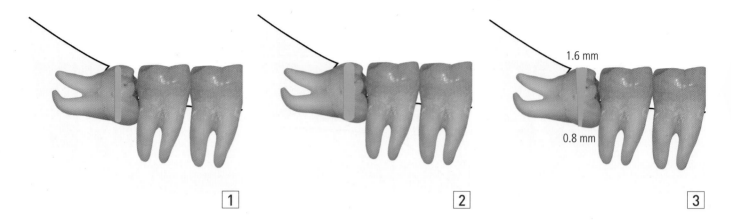

| 1 | 2 | 3 |

These pictures convey sectioning of the horizontally impacted tooth according to the size and shape of the different burs. Image 3 demonstrates sectioning of the crown using the fissure burs. This is the reason why I personally do not like using the fissure bur during Crown Cutting. The fissure burs have a narrow bur diameter towards the tip of the bur (1.6mm near the shank, and 0.8mm at the tip). This creates the difficulty in removing the mesial piece of the crown and also has a high chance of damaging the gingiva during sectioning. Furthermore, under-experienced dentists may potentially damage the distal surface of the 7th crown during sectioning.

Whereas, a round bur is uniform in its shape which allows the initial cutting point to be the same as the final cutting point of the crown. Some dentists like to use the No. 8 surgical round bur (2.3mm in diameter) which creates higher stress on the handpiece than No. 6 surgical round bur (1.8mm in diameter). I prefer to use the No. 6 surgical round bur which has a slightly smaller shank diameter of 1.6mm than its bur size. It is much easier to remove the mesial portion of the crown when the cutting is uniform all the way down to the inferior portion of the crown.

03
Crown Cutting: Cut completely with a single movement ★★

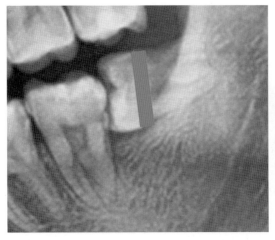
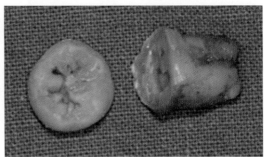

The image illustrates a horizontally impacted tooth that was cut in a single movement since the undercut on the distal of 7th tooth was minimal and the alveolar bone was below the height of the contour. As the inferior alveolar nerve (IAN) is away from the site it is important to cut completely down to the alveolar bone to easily remove the sectioned crown. It is also critical to never cut completely on the lingual side and stop near the enamel portion to prevent damages to gingival tissues and the lingual nerve. Once the tooth is cut near the lingual enamel, it can be easily fractured and removed. It can be visualized on the image above that the tooth was not cut completely through to the lingual side.

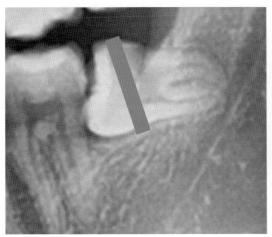
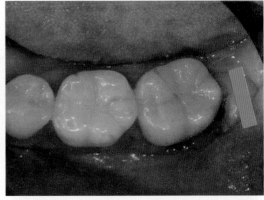
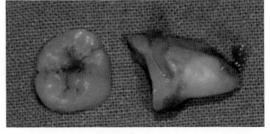

The case above also demonstrates minimal undercut and the alveolar bone is located below the height of the contour of the crown. I usually cut the crown then remove the remainder of the tooth without creating an incision line and raising the full-thickness mucoperiosteal flap when the tooth is well exposed and visible.

The remaining root portion of the tooth is elevated towards the distal of the 7th tooth after the portion of the crown has been removed. The No. 6 surgical round bur of 1.8mm in diameter provides sufficient reduction of the tooth during sectioning hence the separated root portion of the tooth is easily removed even with some undercuts on the distal of the 7th tooth.

04
Crown Cutting: Clinical cases of a single cutting of the crown

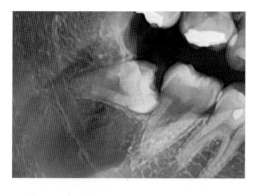

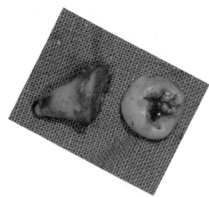

A single cutting case due to a small size of the crown

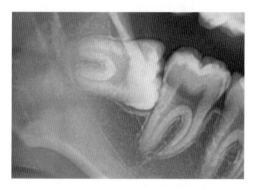

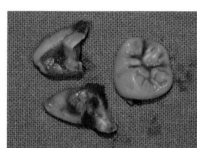

A single cutting case due to a small undercut on the adjacent tooth.

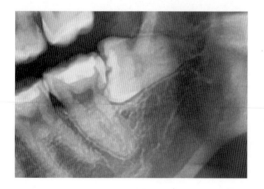

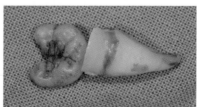

Sometimes, the crown's enamel portion can chip off due to the vibration of the handpiece whilst the crown is being cut close to the 7th tooth.

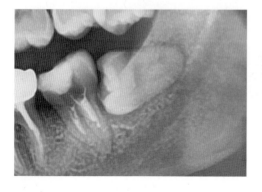

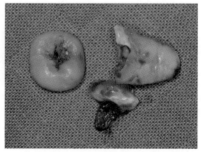

A resorption of the alveolar bone near the crown of the wisdom tooth occurred due to the chronic inflammation around the crown as I have mentioned in the 'Radiology' chapter. This leads to an increase in the inferior alveolar bony space and I would recommend removing the tooth by sectioning the crown with a single cut.

05
Instruments used to fracture a crown after Crown Cutting ★★

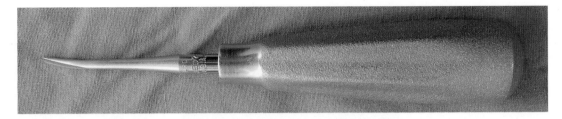

I usually use a slightly backward bent elevator, EL3C, since I would like to minimize the number of instruments used during a procedure. All you need is a light force since the tensile strength of the sectioned tooth is very low. Due to its backward bent tip, it also permits a buccal approach when you do not have many angles to work with.

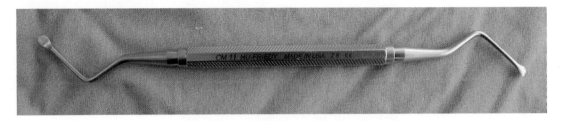

A surgical curette is often used to fracture the sectioned crowns or to remove fractured crowns by rotating the separated crown out.

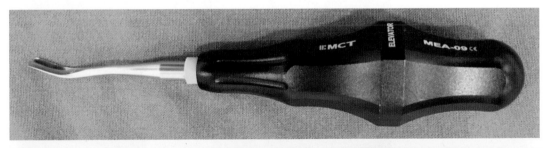

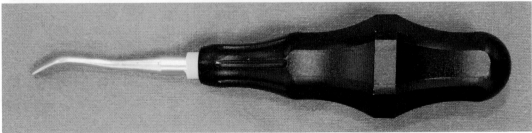

Sometimes, I do recommend special elevators that have steeper angulation towards the end of the instruments to less experienced dentists. The typical elevator is used to fracture the crown by approaching buccally and pulling forward by expanding the bur reduced space. In contrast, the angled elevators can easily engage the lingual and inferior portion of the bur reduced space hence fracturing the crown by pushing the crown towards the distal of the adjacent tooth can be much easier. This instrument is from MCT (Mr. Curette www.2875mart.co.kr). Most companies have similar instruments available. It would be a good idea to have one in each office as an option. It is also a useful tool to have during the Disto-Cervical Cutting and L-Extraction.

06
Removal of wisdom teeth on a patient undergoing orthodontic treatment

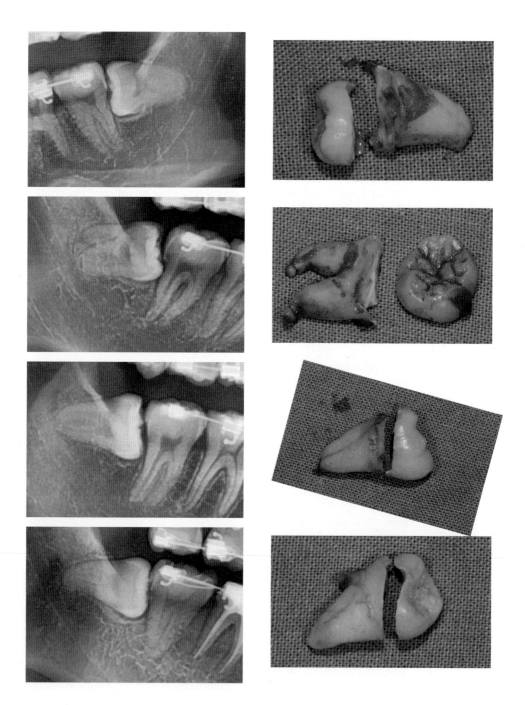

Many dentists do not like to remove lower wisdom teeth on a patient undergoing orthodontic treatment due to the bracket being located on the buccal of the 7th crown of the tooth. However, I prefer to remove these even more. Generally, there are more spaces around the crown due to the movement of the 7th crown resulting in an easier cutting and removal of the fractured crown of the wisdom tooth. Of course, every case is different as the patient may be in different stages of orthodontic treatment, have different treatment plans of where and how the teeth will be moved, etc. All the removed crowns on the photos indicate that the teeth were not fully cut into the lingual portion of the teeth.

07
Limitations of the handpiece angulation during wisdom teeth extraction

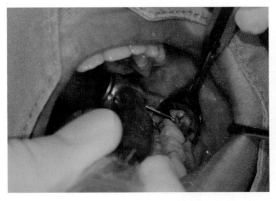 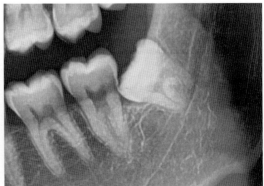

The picture shows a close-up of the handpiece during sectioning of the mesially impacted tooth. Usually, you will picture how the handpiece can be angled to be perpendicular to the tooth, but it cannot be done due to the interferences with the opposing teeth. There are some cases where the handpiece can be perpendicular to the impacted tooth due to a large jaw opening and wisdom tooth being positioned more mesially. Most of the time, the handpiece has to be tilted hence I am more used to cutting in this angle. It is very difficult to cut deeply into the lingual portion of the crown because of the angulation of the handpiece. Also, this is another reason why I do not prefer to use the fissure burs. The most important factor in wisdom teeth extraction is how to approach effectively and cut the lingual lower portion of the crown safely without complications.

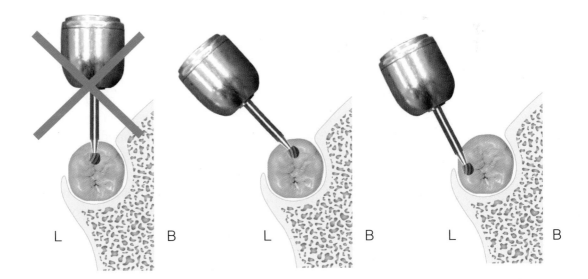

Most of the time, dentists will assume that a handpiece will be positioned as shown in the image above.

In reality, the handpiece is angled lingually due to the interference with the opposing teeth. As you cut the crown and section more deeply, you can angle the handpiece more perpendicularly. The rule of thumb is to utilize round burs as the fissure burs can damage the tissues when accessed lingually.

Crown Cutting: Horizontal Division ★★★

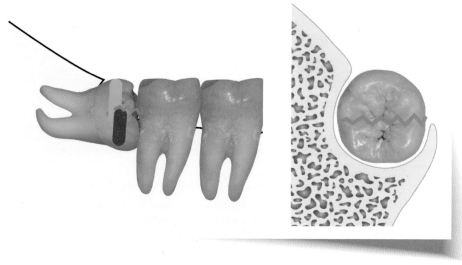

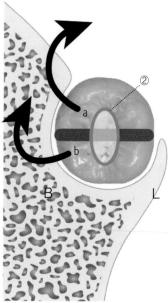

This is a method implemented to cut and fracture a more superiorly located portion of the crown first. Followed by cutting the lower remaining crown. I usually perform this on the following:

- A large crown limiting the access of the bur to the lower end of the crown
- Not able to achieve visibility of the crown after cutting
- Lower end of the crown is very close to the alveolar nerve where accurate crown reduction is required.
- Severe caries limiting the crown removal with a single cut.
- Require performing vertical division on the lower crown portion.

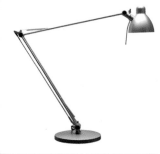

Blue circle indicated as ② on the above image is where the point of the wisdom tooth crown contacts the distal of the 7th tooth shown in the cross-sectional view. Commonly, the concave surface of the wisdom tooth wraps around the distal of the 7th tooth. Therefore, the remaining lower half of the crown can be easily removed without interfering with the undercut of the 7th tooth when turned or rotated to buccal or lingual directions.

01
Step by step Horizontal Division of the crown ★★★

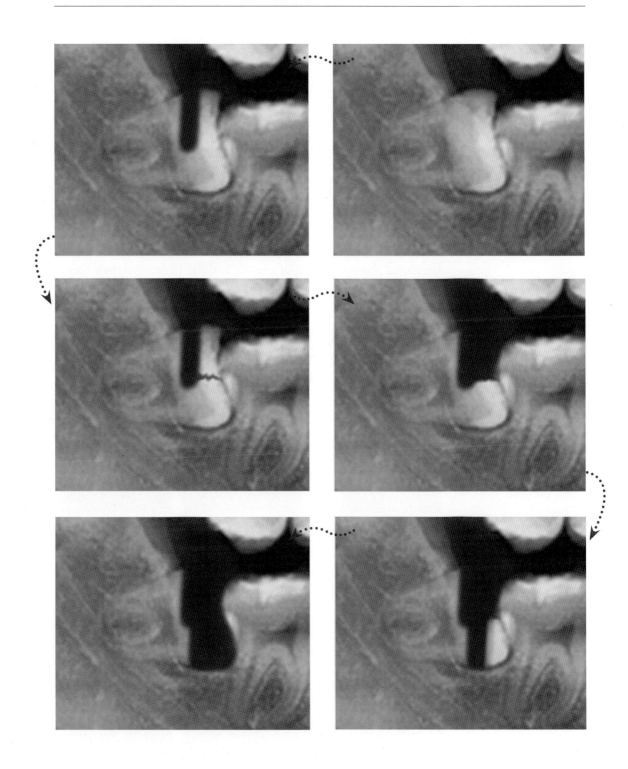

02
Clinical cases: Horizontal Division of the wisdom teeth ★★

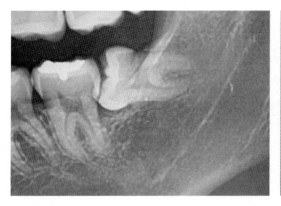 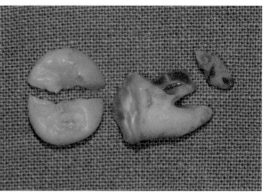

A No. 4 round bur has a diameter (1.4mm) with a larger shank size (1.6mm) is often used to cut the crown above the point of contact in order to remove the upper half of the crown. Then the lower half of the crown is removed.

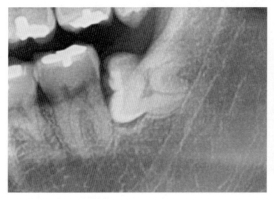 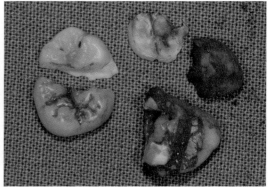

The upper half of the crown was removed initially to obtain visual and physical access to the deeper portion of the crown as the crown is positioned lower than the point of contact of the 7th tooth.

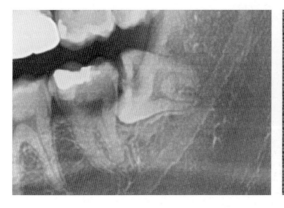 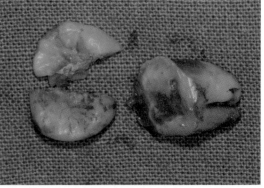

The upper half was removed first due to the carious activity in the wisdom tooth. If the upper portion of the crown was not removed first then the crown may have fractured in an undesirable manner. Sometimes, a crown is cut deliberately in multiple pieces to desirably fracture and plan the pieces.

03
Horizontal Division of the crown for better visibility ★★

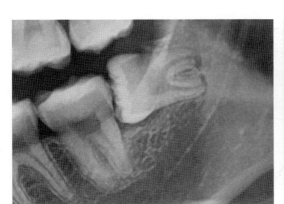
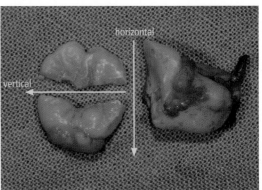

I have a habit of removing the upper portion of the crown because I used to use a No.4 surgical round bur (1.4mm diameter bur with 1.6mm diameter shank) which is difficult to cut completely to depth. Therefore, I am more used to separating crowns in pieces. As I get older I have a difficulty cutting precisely with smaller sized burs, hence I started using No.6 surgical round bur (1.8mm diameter bur with 1.6mm diameter shank) to cut deeper and at once when it is safe. Nowadays, the dental handpiece contains fiber-optic to provide better visibility of the surgical sites so I do not need to cut the crown for visibility anymore. I still recommend horizontal division to less experienced dentists because obtaining visibility is critical.

There are several key points to cutting the crown. Do NOT cut too deep. It will separate the whole crown which can result in more difficult extraction. Do NOT cut too deep (cut less than 2/3 of the crown). I recommend cutting a smaller upper portion than the lower portion for better visibility. In many cases, crown shatters, and is sucked into the suction unit unlike the case above. I usually remove the upper portion of the crown with a horizontal division then remove the remaining crown with a vertical division to further separate and remove the crown.

A clean horizontal division is rare because of the enamel fracture and tends to shatter. A vertical division is usually followed by the initial horizontal division. You will see more details later in this chapter.

04
Vertical Division of the crown ★★★

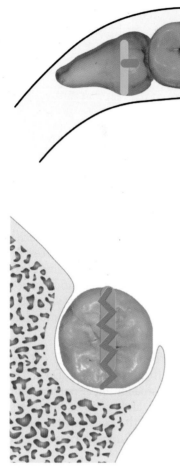

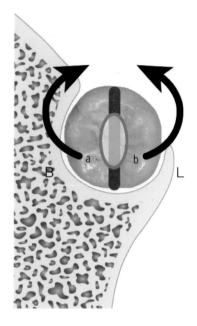

It is critical to not cut through the crown completely but to fracture the remaining crown off in order to prevent the damage on the distal of the 7th tooth when the vertical division is performed. Since the enamel is brittle, the crown often gets shattered into multiple pieces to be suctioned into the evacuation system.

As shown on the upper left diagram, the wisdom tooth is impacted underneath the distal height of the contour of the 7th tooth. Most of the time, a wisdom tooth is impacted underneath the height of the contour of the adjacent tooth. This is when the vertical division comes in handy. The vertical sectioning begins from the separated portion of the crown towards the 7th tooth as demonstrated as the dark blue line on the diagram. Then fracture the tooth vertically with a surgical curette. If the vertical cutting completely passes through the dentine then the brittle enamel will fracture easily. I recommend using the No.4 round bur to those under-experienced dentists.

When the crown is fully separated from the root but persists to be removed, the vertical division is performed to section the separated crown and then removed by rotating the pieces out as indicated by the arrows on the upper right diagram. Remove the 'a' piece first then 'b.' The 'b' piece can be easily rotated clockwise and slid into where the 'a' piece occupied.

05
Review of a vertically divided crown surface <1>

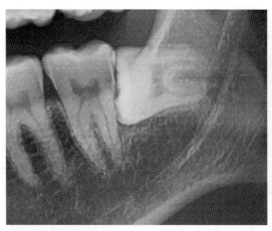

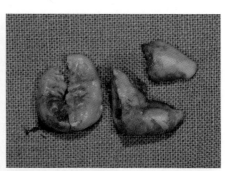

The above image demonstrates a typical case of Vertical Division of the crown. Then the remaining roots were removed using the L-extraction technique. Let's focus on the Vertical Division as the L-extraction will be discussed in detail in the later chapter.

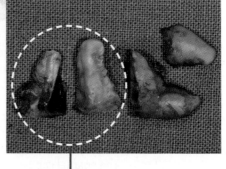

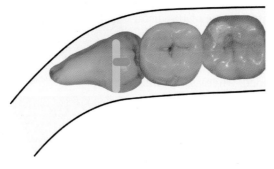

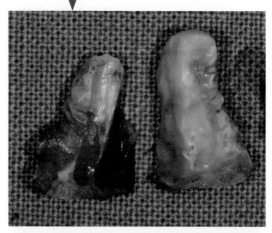

Typically, two divisions are required to completely remove the crown. The first section is performed at the sky blue line. The partially sectioned crown is then fractured; separating the crown from the roots. The vertical division follows the dark blue line and the crown is fractured into two pieces and rotated out with a surgical curette. The important key point here is to not cut through the crown completely and fracture the remaining portion.

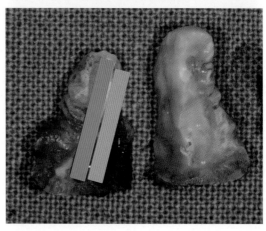

06
Review of a vertically divided crown surface <2> ★

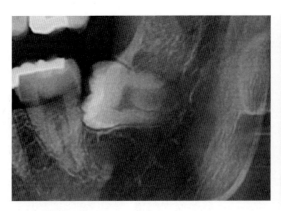

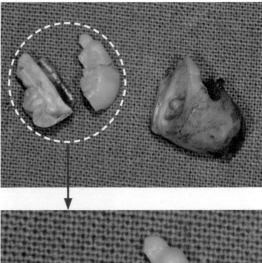

The extraction process is very similar to the previous case. The only difference being the splayed wisdom tooth roots are now joined together. Similar to the previous case, please visualise the crown that is not fully sectioned through on the lingual portion of the crown. Usually I do not cut through the lingual at all as the enamel can be easily fractured with curette. When the crown is vertically cut and divided again then the crown can be easily rotated and removed without the interference of the distal height of the contour of the 7th crown. The lingual and inferior surfaces do not need to be fully reduced with the bur. The lingual surface needs to be always avoided, whereas, the inferior surface does not need to be fully sectioned to fracture off the crown despite the IAN is located far away from the tooth. Even in the case where the IAN is located just below the tooth, the usual method of Crown Cutting can be completed without the nerve damage.

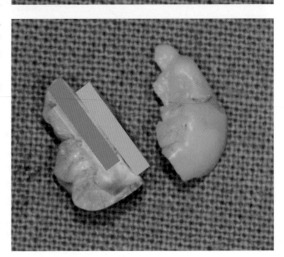

07
Clinical cases of Vertical Division ★

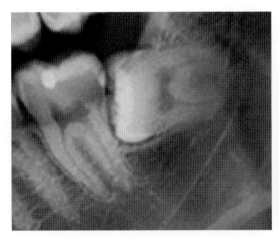

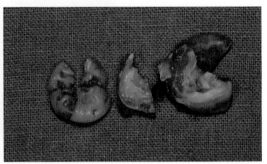

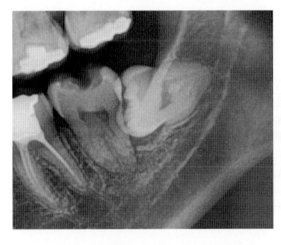

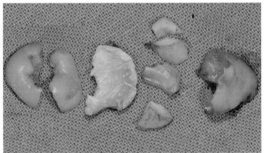

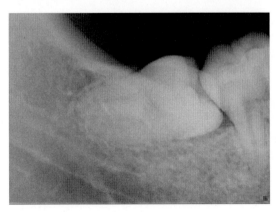

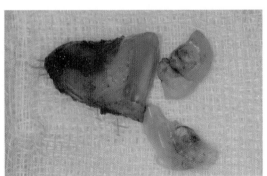

★

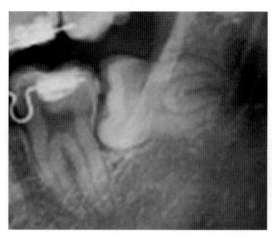 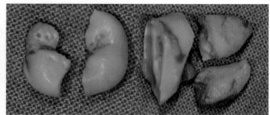

A Vertical Division is a very useful technique when the crown of the wisdom tooth is impacted below the undercut of the 7th tooth. Preventing any damages on the distal of the 7th tooth is critical. You do not have to cut so close to the distal of the 7th tooth. The tensile strength of enamel is very weak, so once the dentine portion of the crown is cut the unsupported enamel can be easily fractured off. In most cases, a surgical curette would do the work.

A No.4 surgical round bur is very good for these vertical divisions. Lately, I have been just working with a No.6 surgical round bur for all of my Crown Cutting. But I insist that beginners start with a No.6 surgical round bur to section the crown horizontally and a No.4 surgical round bur to divide vertically.

For beginners, it is often difficult to cut the crown from the center. Therefore, when they attempt to vertically cut the crown, they enter the crown perpendicularly, and often the crown is cut and separated erratically. If this process is repeated then the crown can be fractured into three or four pieces.

Crown Cutting: Horizontal - Vertical Division ★★★

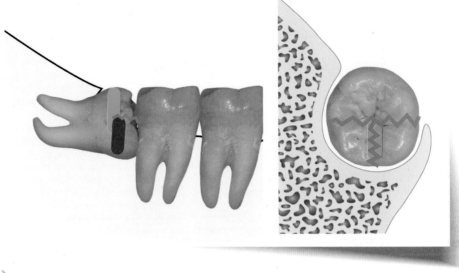

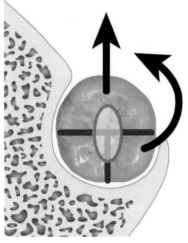

A combination of Horizontal and Vertical Division is often performed together. There are cases that require each procedure to be implemented separately, however, it is more difficult to perform each division separately. In most cases, each method is delivered one after another.

By planning the precise cutting of the internal surfaces of the tooth, separating, and removing the sectioned pieces of the crown, we are able to minimise the surrounding bone removal and complete the Easy, Simple, Safe, and Efficient extraction.

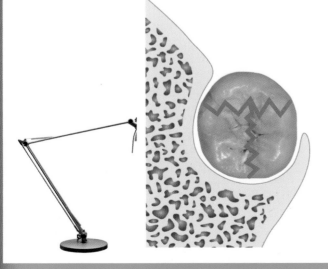

It is important not to section the upper portion of the crown more than ⅓ of its size. If the crown is sectioned larger than ⅓ then the crown may be fractured in wrong directions providing inadequate visibility. When you perform the procedure and section less than upper ⅓ of the crown then the visual access would be enhanced and ease the Vertical Division process as we begin the removal of dentin from the flatter surface of the crown.

01
Why do we require rotational movement? ★★

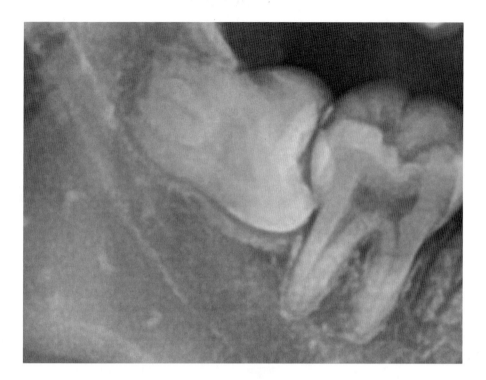

The most crucial point that we need to consider is that wisdom teeth are often positioned below the height of the contour of the 7th tooth. The distal of the 7th tooth is usually convex and contacts the concave occlusal surface of the 8th crown resulting in severe undercut interference. If the surgical bur is able to reach and completely cut the crown vertically and lingually then the space created from detaching the crown may allow the easy removal of the remaining roots. This is theoretically feasible, however, clinically it is not easy to do in most cases. Even if it was possible we do not completely cut the crown through and through in order to prevent damage to the surrounding structures.

Therefore, it is highly recommended to cut and assess the neighbouring lingual and inferior structures in each step of the crown sectioning. This method often leads to separation of the crown of the horizontally impacted wisdom teeth into 3 or 4 pieces.

02
Sectional view of the Horizontal-Vertical Division ★★★

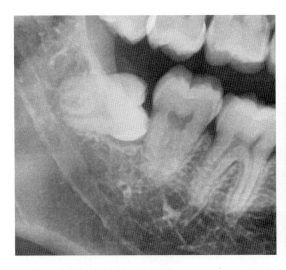
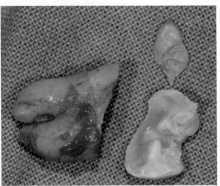

This case demonstrates where a Horizontal Division leads to removal of a small coronal portion of the crown then a Vertical Division is performed to separate the remaining inferior portion of the crown, but the remaining crown was removed in one piece instead. The remaining crown came out from the site during rotation of the surgical curette to fracture the crown as there was minimal undercut.

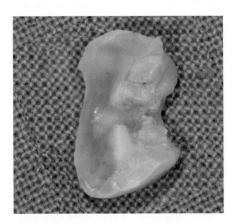
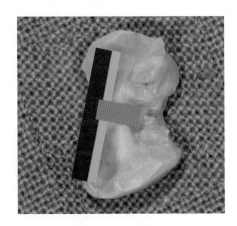

Please review the three cutting lines on the sectional view of the crown in this case. The lingual and inferior portion of the crown is not completely cut through. On the other hand, the buccal portion must be completely sectioned especially for the under-experienced dentists. Frequently, there are cases where the buccal portion of the crown is not completely sectioned as the operator cannot fully visualise the crown underneath the undercut of the adjacent 7th crown. I noticed during the supervision of other fellow dentists that they often miss something this simple more than complex techniques I teach. I would like to emphasise again that the buccal side must be cut completely.

03
Clinical cases of Horizontal-Vertical Division of the crown ★

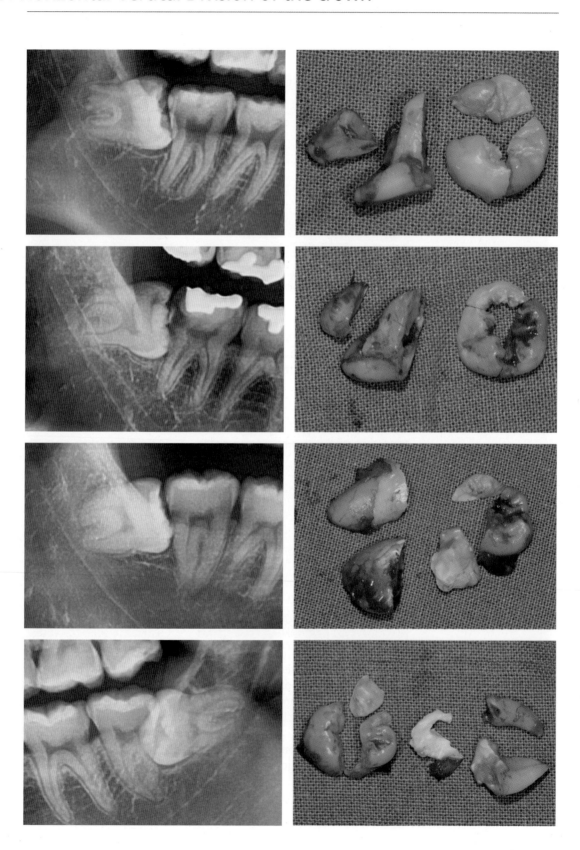

04
Separating a crown into multiple pieces ★★

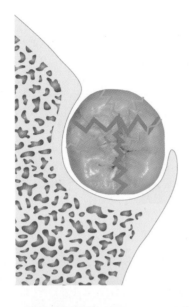

When performed clinically, a crown often does not fracture as intended. The enamels are very fragile and thin on the upper portion of the crown hence they can fracture into small pieces like sand grains and be sucked into a high-speed suction.

You will see numerous clinical cases like this in the next pages. I always follow the same steps not just sometimes. It is easy to get confused and lost when you do not know what you are doing, but when you have a specific goal in mind then cutting and fracturing of the crown is easy to do.

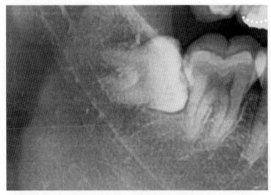
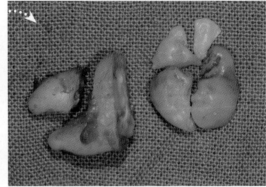
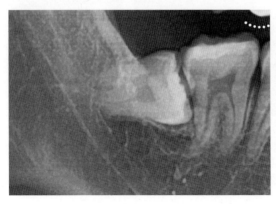
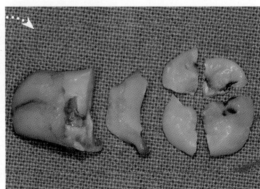

05
Clinical cases of separating a crown into multiple pieces (1) ★

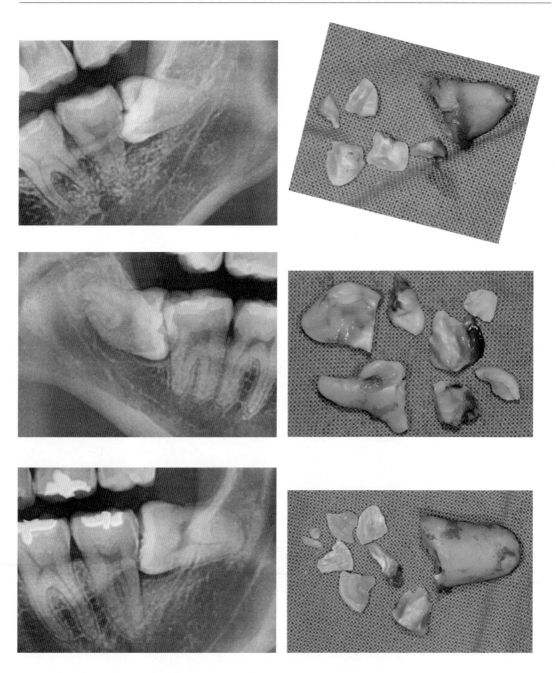

I do not have many good clinical photographs of separating a crown into multiple pieces. It is because most of the pieces are sucked into a high-speed vacuum and my assistants have a hard time putting them together.

Clinical cases of separating a crown into multiple pieces (2) ★

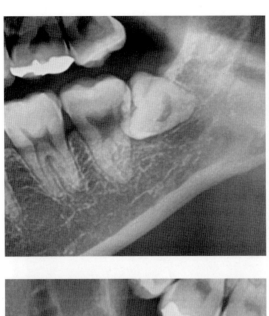
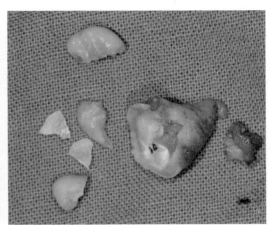
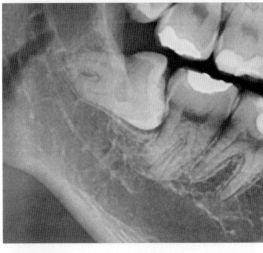
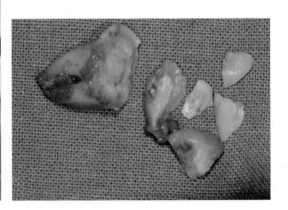
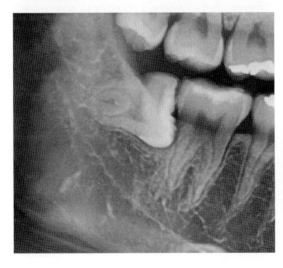
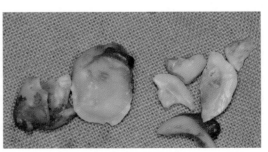

Oblique Cutting ★★★

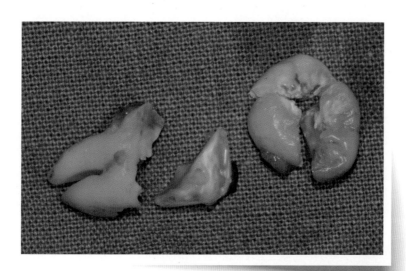

We have discussed the advantages of Oblique Cutting in the chapter 'mesially impacted wisdom tooth.' Let's go through the advantages again.

1. Makes extraction easy and simple
2. Decreases the chance of fracturing a lingual alveolar bone
3. Makes it easy to remove the often troublesome mesio-lingual portion of the crown
4. It can provide Lift and Cutting effect.

Please go back and read over the Oblique Cutting again as it is one of the most valuable techniques in this book. The technique performed in a horizontally impacted wisdom teeth can be slightly different hence we will go over it one more time.

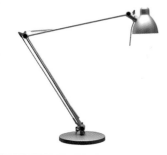

01
Zigzag division of a crown ★★

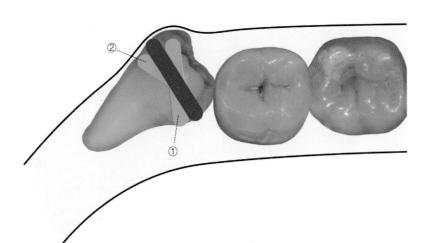

When a crown is located more lingually, the crown is cut more commonly following the line ① which is parallel to the distal of the 7th tooth rather than the red line. Then section the crown one more time following the line ② to remove the crown because it is difficult to remove the lingual portion of the crown with the division of the line ① only. If we apply the same principle to cutting a non-lingually positioned tooth, then it will be shown as below.

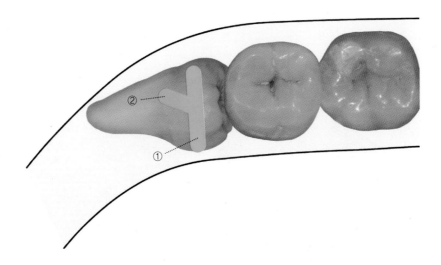

Don't you think the picture is a déjàvu? It is the same Oblique Cutting diagram shown on the mesially angulated wisdom tooth. The Oblique Cutting promotes easier extraction by inducing elevating movement on the tooth and prevents possible interferences during the removal of the crown. However, it is also used when the lingual portion of the crown is not cleanly and completely cut during the procedure.

02
Oblique Cutting to remove a crown including mesio-lingual contact point ★★

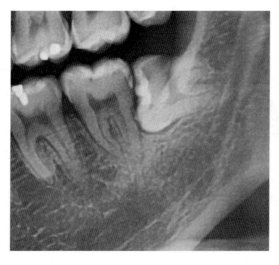

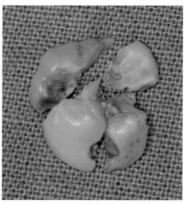

A crown was removed in pieces then reassembled. It may look like the crown was cut into proper pieces but in fact this represents a crown that was separated and removed in an erratic manner. I still make these mistakes where I believe that the crown is completely removed, firmly engage an elevator to elevate from the buccal surface of the tooth, and the tooth is not budging. In such cases, when I look into a mirror there is an inadequate cutting and removal of the lingual inferior portion of the crown. Utilising the Oblique Cutting technique has other advantages but will also enable the removal of the insufficiently sectioned and removed portion of the crown.

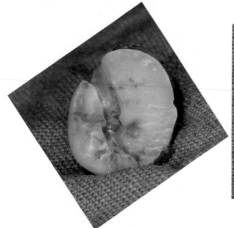

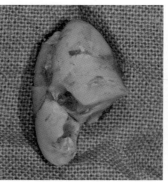

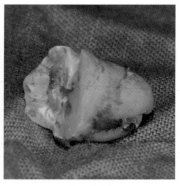

An Oblique Cutting was performed to remove the lingual inferior portion of the tooth then the root portion was extracted and reassembled together. Now this demonstrates how useful Oblique Cutting is in the procedure. Please go back to the 'mesially angulated wisdom tooth' chapter and re-read about the Oblique Cutting technique.

03
Clinical cases of an Oblique Cutting (1) ★

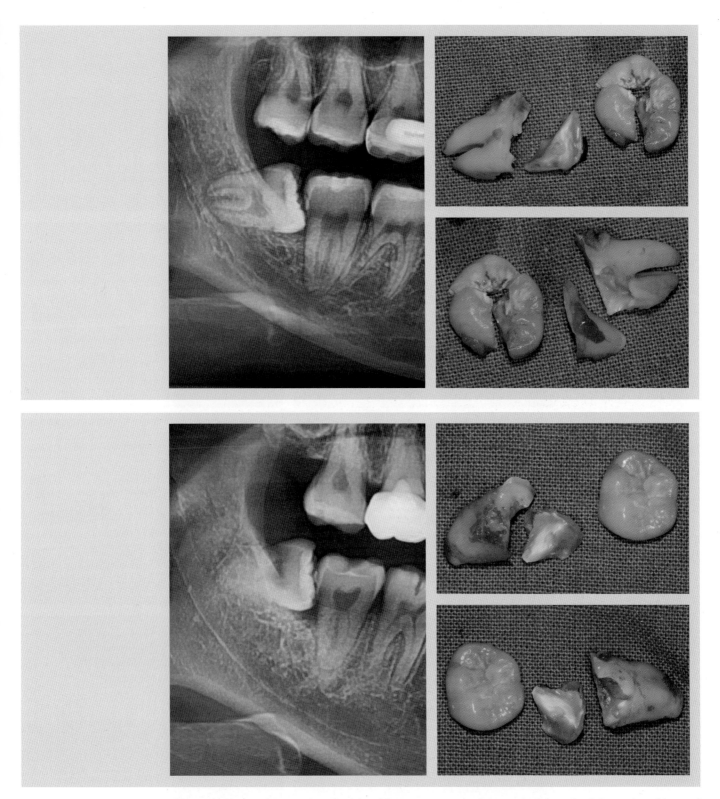

These are the cases completed with Oblique Cutting and examined from both buccal and lingual sectional views. Please review how the crown was removed from the previous pages and compare that information to how an Oblique Cutting was performed.

Clinical cases of an Oblique Cutting (2) ★

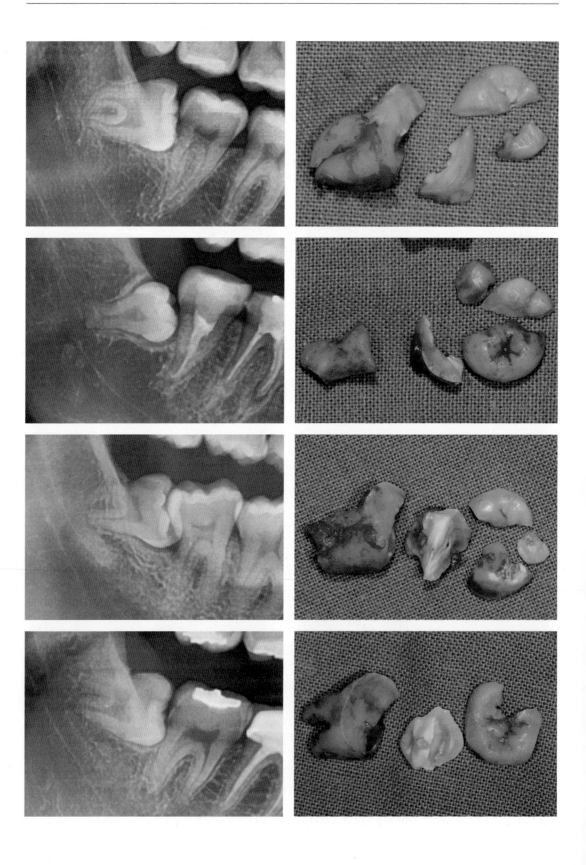

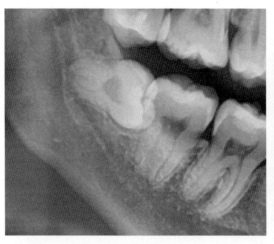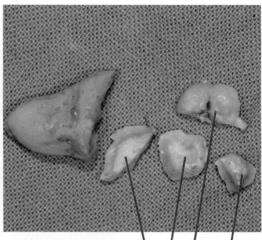

This is a clinical case that involves all the cutting methods we have learnt previously. Now we can predict how the tooth was sectioned and removed by reviewing the images.

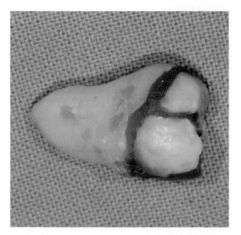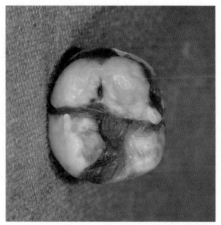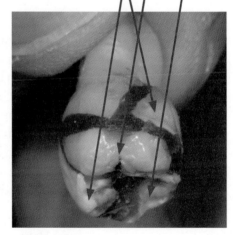

The sectioned pieces of the tooth were put together with red wax. We can safely assume how the tooth was sectioned and removed. It is important to understand that removing a tooth employing a combination of different sectional techniques is not rare and utilised in most of the wisdom teeth extractions.

Lift and Cutting ★★

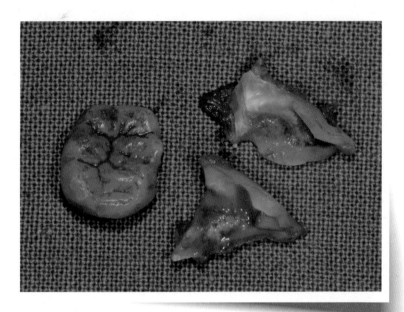

This technique is the same as the previously discussed method in 'mesially angulated impacted wisdom tooth' cases. There is a higher chance of performing Lift and Cutting technique in horizontally impacted teeth than in mesially angulated impacted teeth. This seems to occur more often as I tend to cut the crown close to the 7th tooth and limit the alveolar bone removal. Since the tooth will be removed anyway there is no harm sectioning the tooth into more pieces. In most cases, an Oblique Cutting can sufficiently provide a space for the extraction of the remaining tooth, but there are cases where an Oblique Cutting will still have some interferences during extraction. This is when you perform Lift and Cutting along with the Oblique Cutting.

The Disto-Cervical Cutting that will be discussed in the later pages can be utilised in this case. However, if the remaining tooth is still interfered by the bone and the distal portion of the 7th tooth, the tooth is sectioned again. The dislocated wisdom tooth from its socket is like a tooth that is already extracted. The last process is to remove the interferences. Do not cut all the roots and interferences before dislocating the wisdom tooth out of its socket. The loss of the purchase points will make the job much harder.

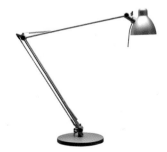

01
Method of Lift and Cutting ★★

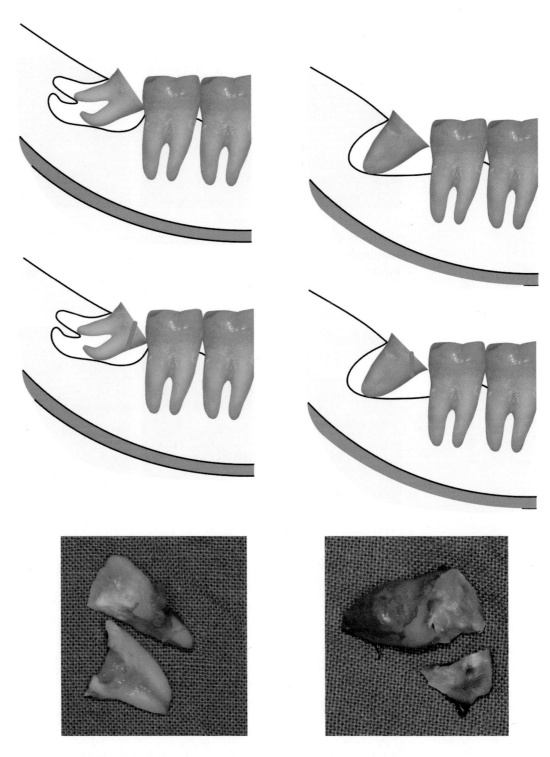

The method does not change whether a tooth is single-rooted or multi-rooted. The way that the tooth is lifted and angulated will result in different shapes of cut pieces. It is easier to remove a multi-rooted tooth when the roots are separated. Consequently, consider separating the splayed roots before executing this method.

02
Clinical cases of Lift and Cutting of the horizontally impacted wisdom tooth <1> ★★

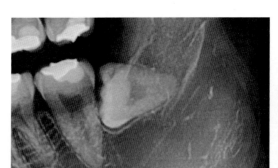 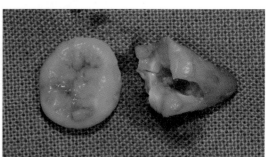

The tooth that underwent the Lift and Cutting was reassembled together. Please visualise the angulation of the cut on the lingual surface of the root. I recommend No. 4 surgical round bur for cutting, but I mostly use No. 6 surgical round bur because I feel lazy to change the bur. This means that I must cut deeper.

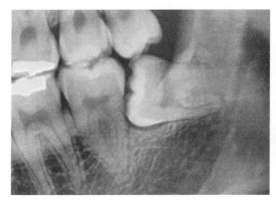 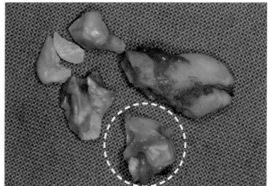

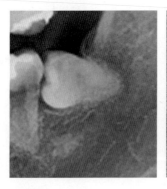 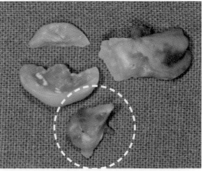 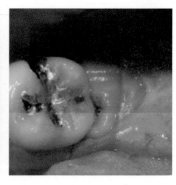

In this case, the tooth was removed without making an incision and flap of the gingiva through the process of Crown Cutting and Lift and Cutting of the interfering portion of the root. In order to enhance visual access and prevent injuries to the gingival tissue, the crown was further cut horizontally during the sectioning of the crown of the tooth.

Clinical cases of Lift and Cutting of the horizontally impacted wisdom tooth <2> ★

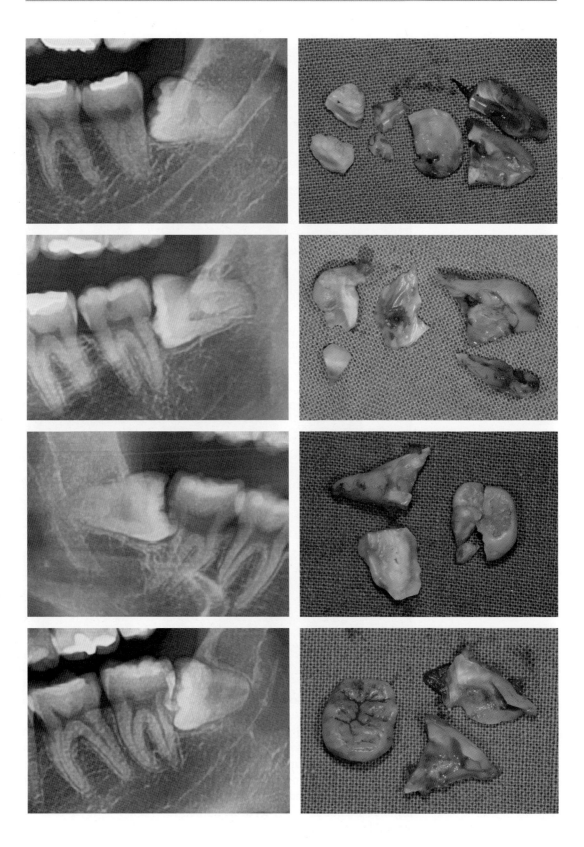

Clinical cases of lift and cutting of the horizontally impacted wisdom tooth <3> ★

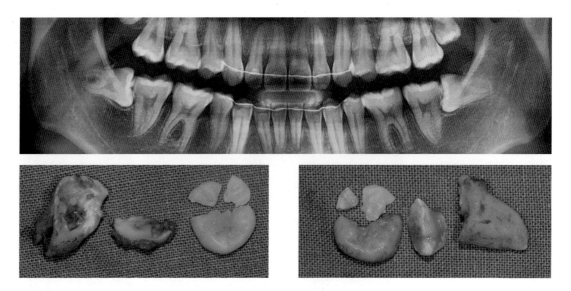

The Lift and Cutting was performed on the tooth 48 while the Oblique Cutting was executed on the tooth 38 to fracture and remove the lower lingual portion of the crown. Please compare the differences between the fractured fragments of these different procedures in the pictures above.

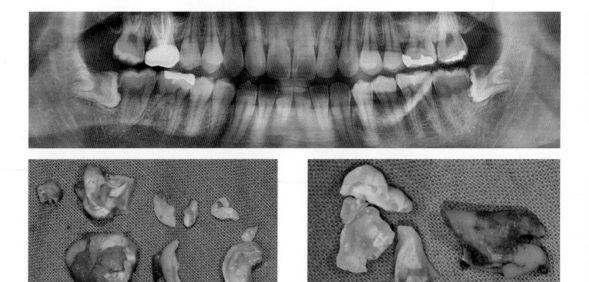

The teeth above are positioned incorrectly on the photo. The root fragments are upside down. I sometimes find out about this positioning error once my staff have taken the photo of the extracted tooth. It appears that my staff are not as enthusiastic as I am in reassembling the tooth.

This case also demonstrates the tooth 48 being extracted using the Lift and Cutting technique and the tooth 38 employing the Oblique Cutting technique as per the previous case.

Separation of the Roots ★★★

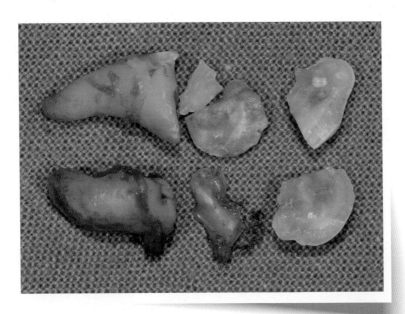

Separating the splayed roots of the tooth is usually completed naturally when the Lift and Cutting technique is utilised. Conversely, after removing the crown of the tooth and the splayed roots are difficult to mobilise then the roots should be separated. In this chapter I do not tend to separate these clinical situations with such details because my average surgery time is very short, and the method carried out is not recorded in every case. Thus it can become quite difficult to distinguish what methods have been performed by looking back at the fractured tooth pieces. Since I rarely use a surgical low-speed handpiece and tend to avoid raising the flap, there is limited access using only the high-speed handpiece hence most of the removal is performed using Lift and Cutting technique. Therefore, it is often seen as the Lift and Cutting of multi-rooted teeth or separation of the roots on multi-rooted teeth.

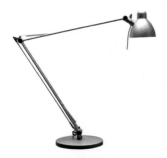

01
Separation of the roots ★★

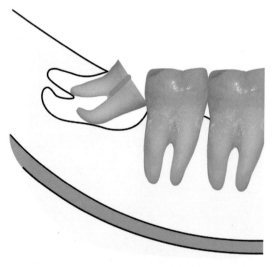

The technique is not specifically cutting between the roots. When the tooth is lifted it naturally cuts between the roots and the splayed roots can be removed separately. However, if a tooth is not dislocated from its socket, it is often difficult to separate the roots with a high-speed handpiece. The Disto-Cervical Cutting technique is performed which will be addressed in the later chapter. If the tooth still does not budge, then there is another method to separate the roots to dislocate the roots from its socket. This will also be discussed in the next chapter.

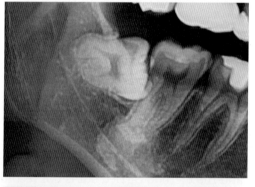
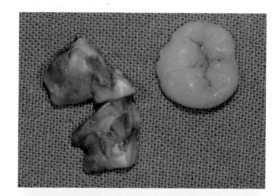
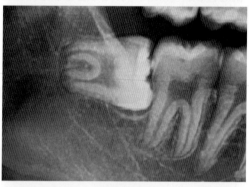
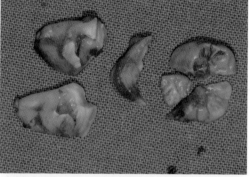
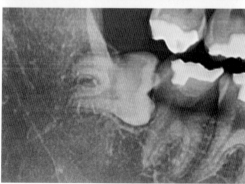
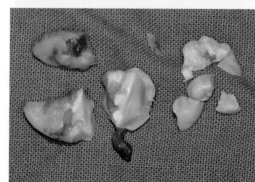

02
Clinical cases of separation of the roots <1> ★

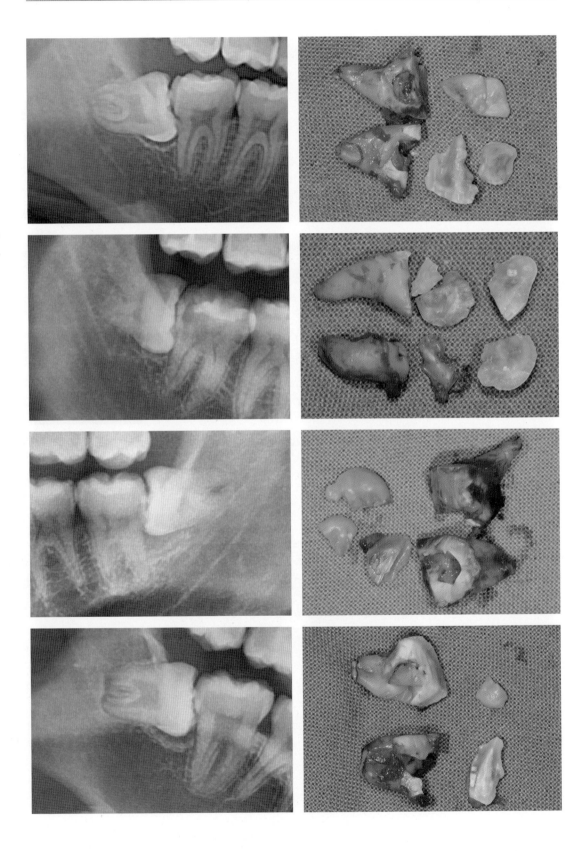

Clinical cases of separation of the roots <2> ★

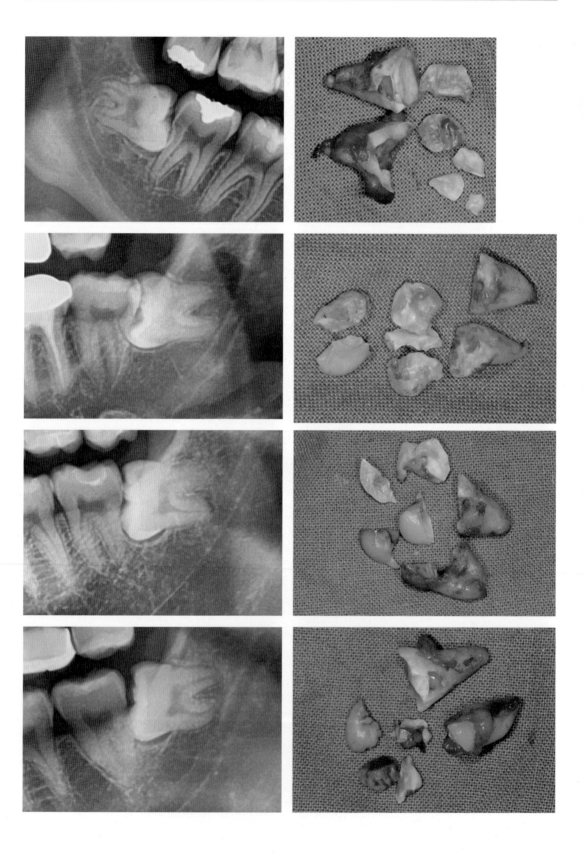

Clinical cases of separation of the roots <3> ★

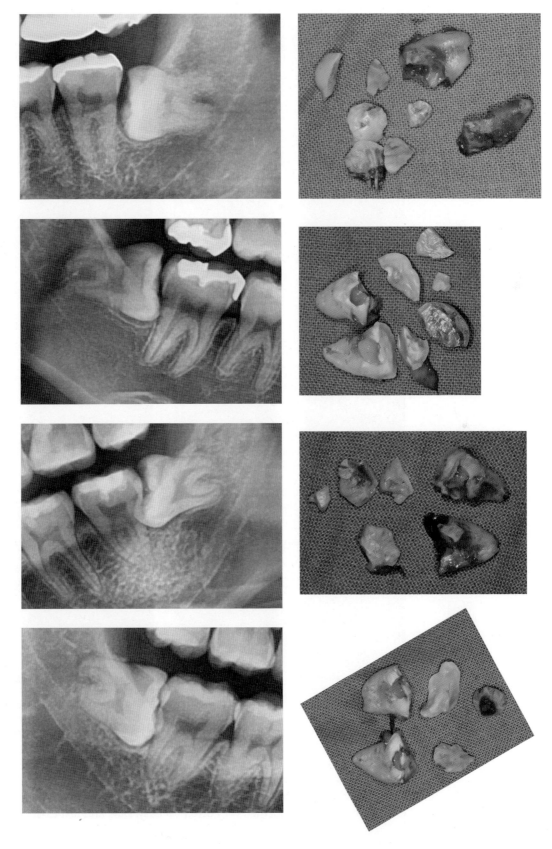

03
Dislocating a tooth with an elevator then separating the roots ★★

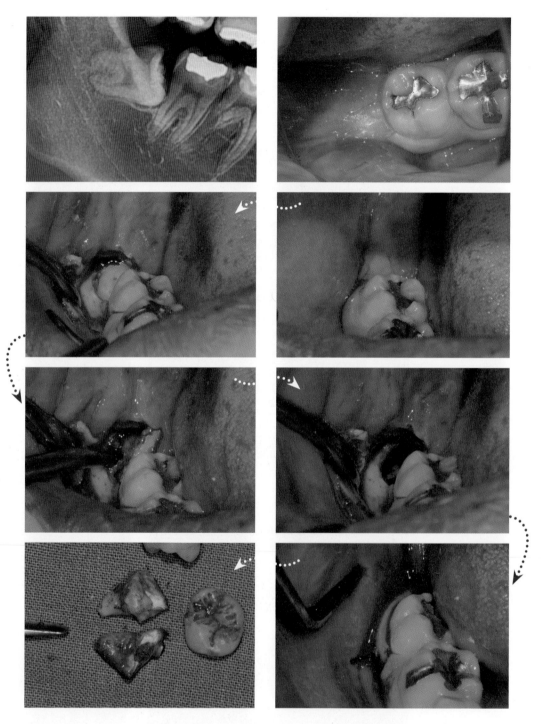

There are too many patients scheduled for wisdom teeth extractions every day hence I have to reduce my surgical time in every way. For this type of multi-rooted wisdom tooth, the crown of the tooth is sectioned off then the remaining tooth is dislocated from its socket. Then an elevator is placed between the roots to fracture and remove each root separately. Air, water and other debris may enter the socket when you use a high-speed handpiece on a dislocated tooth. Therefore, this elevator method is performed very often for easy, safe, and fast extractions.

04
Clinical cases of separation of the roots <4> ★

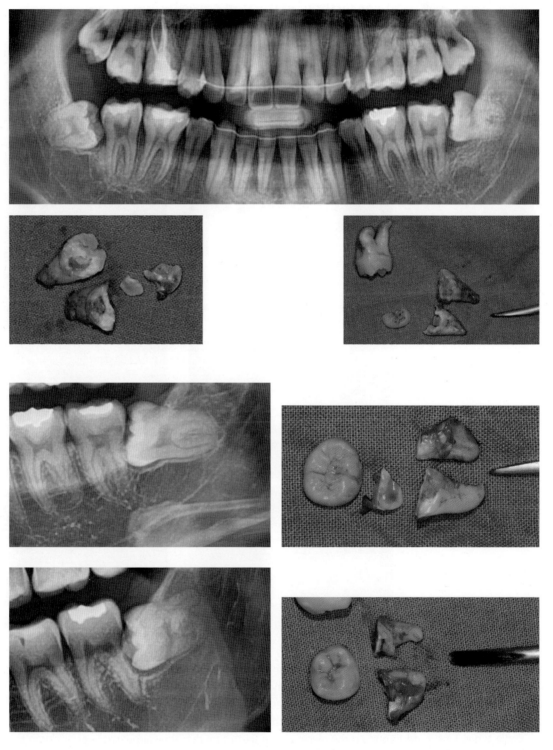

When an elevator is placed between the separated roots as shown in the photos, it indicates that the roots are separated using an elevator. Sometimes, radiographs reveal that a tooth has splayed roots however it may not be the case. Then you can implement the Lift and Cutting technique as usual.

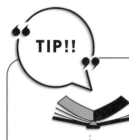

TIP!!

4 consecutive extraction cases within an hour ★ (excluding maxillary wisdom teeth)

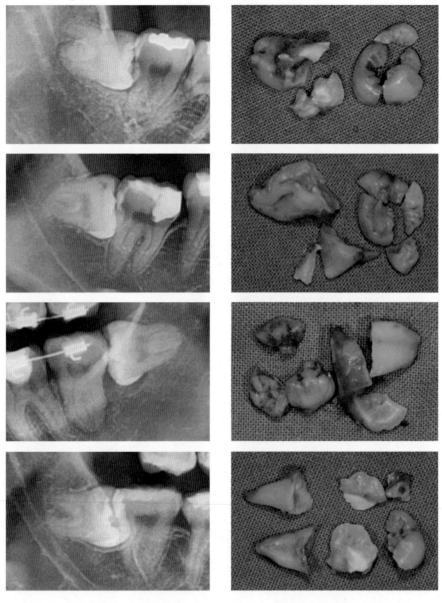

These cases are shared not to brag about how quickly they are extracted but because all these four teeth were extracted exactly the same way. Wisdom teeth extraction cases are randomly scheduled every 15 minutes by my staff and I do not know what kind of case will arrive until I see the patient. Some days, treatments are scheduled with all vertically impacted wisdom teeth where extraction can be executed quickly and still be relaxed. On the other days, all maxillary wisdom teeth are severely impacted in bone. But somehow, this day was scheduled with all horizontally impacted wisdom teeth. Interestingly, when I returned to putting the pieces of the teeth together they appeared very similar in shape hence I have decided to share these four cases. It was one Saturday afternoon in 2015, a day before the wisdom teeth extraction seminar. I presented these four cases the next day so I remember them well. I also wanted the readers to know that every case that I present and discuss in this book is not only shared for presentations but they are my daily routine procedures.

Disto-Cervical Cutting ★★

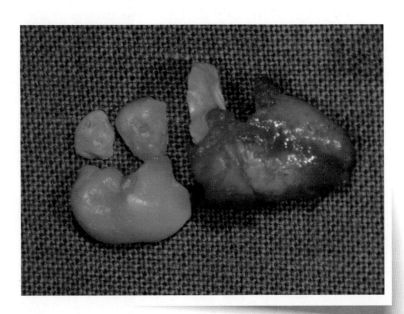

An elevator is used to remove the remaining horizontally impacted wisdom tooth after the crown is sectioned off. If the tooth is able to be dislocated from its socket and there is interference then the Lift and Cutting method can be utilised. However, if the tooth is difficult to dislocate from its socket then the Disto-Cervical Cutting technique is implemented without any hesitation. Mostly, it is when the periodontal ligament space is too narrow for an elevator to engage without any bone removal. I tend to use the Disto-Cervical Cutting technique and place an elevator in the purchase point to extract the tooth.

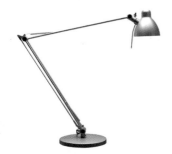

01
Disto-Cervical Cutting ★★★

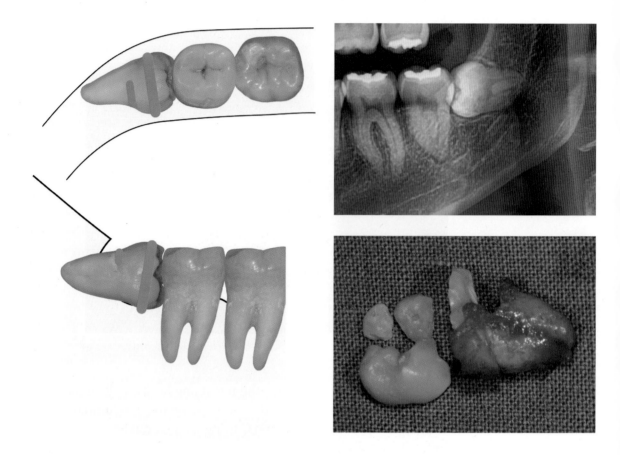

Usually, the crown sectioning is completed with a No.6 surgical round bur and I was too lazy to change the bur so I completed Disto-Cervical Cutting with a No. 6 surgical round bur (diameter 1.8mm). When you use a No.6 surgical round bur, you must cut deeper, otherwise, a crown may fracture in an unplanned direction and an elevator may be difficult to engage leading to a more difficult extraction. For under-experienced dentists, I strongly recommend to use No.4 surgical round bur for the Disto-Cervical Cutting. This method is very useful especially for those teeth that have inflammation near the crown resulting in the tooth being pushed back and is almost adhered to the alveolar bone.

02
Clinical cases presented in the radiology chapter ★★

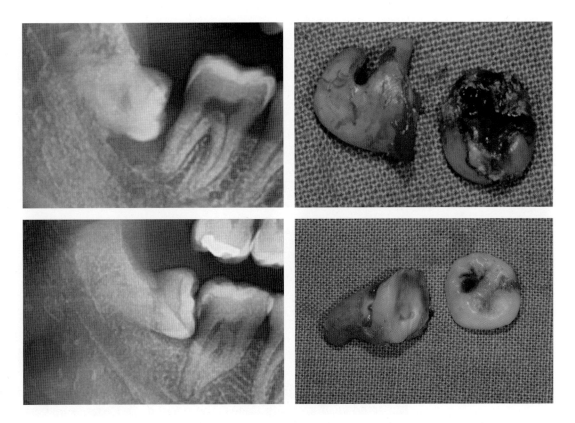

Due to an inflammation of the soft tissues around the crown, the tooth was pushed back distally resulting in a narrower periodontal ligament space. It appears on the radiograph that the teeth have nearly adhered to the bone. There is no space for an elevator to engage. Therefore, a Disto-Cervical Cutting technique is implemented to pull out the tooth.

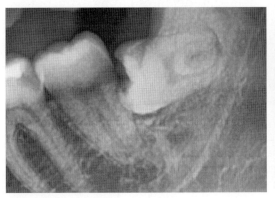
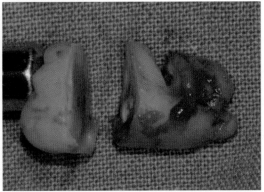

This is a case with severe inflammation around the mesial of the crown. You can see a small portion of the enamel left on the photo after Crown Cutting. If there is severe inflammation surrounding the crown the space created between the 7th and the remaining tooth allows the crown to fracture off easily despite inadequate cutting of the lingual enamel. But sometimes the root is embedded into an alveolar bone resisting its removal. The above case was completed with Disto-Cervical Cutting to remove the remaining roots.

03
Clinical cases of Disto-Cervical Cutting ★

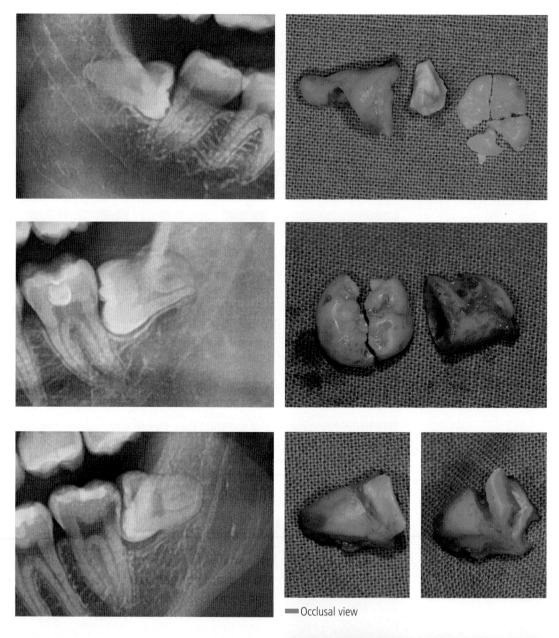

■ Occlusal view

This is a case using a Disto-Cervical Cutting technique. The extracted tooth was flipped to show the lingual surface of the tooth. The photo on the right is showing the lingual surfaces. When looking from the above, the bur mark from the Disto-Cervical Cutting can be visualised, On the other hand, when the tooth is placed to show the lingual surface the cut is barely visible. In fact, the tooth reduction mostly involves the buccal and superior surfaces of the horizontally impacted tooth. The lingual surface of the tooth is rarely touched.

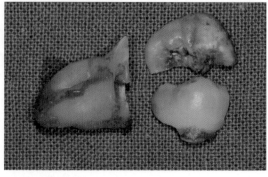

■ Lingual view

04
Three consecutive cases of #48 extraction using a Disto-Cervical Cutting technique ★

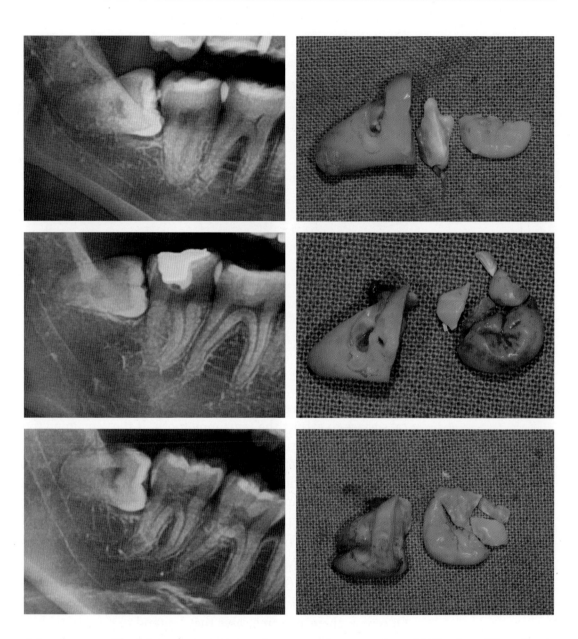

A few days ago, I had three consecutive patients requiring extraction of #48 using a Disto-Cervical Cutting technique. As I have mentioned before, I follow my own strict protocol for each and every extraction. A Crown Cutting is performed to remove the crown then an elevator is placed on the buccal surface to extract the remaining tooth. Nevertheless, the tooth was unable to be dislocated with the elevator and I decided to conduct a Disto-Cervical Cutting instead of removing the buccal bone. To reiterate, the methods and procedures discussed in this book are executed following my daily routine protocol.

Disto-Cervical Cutting and L-Extraction ★★★

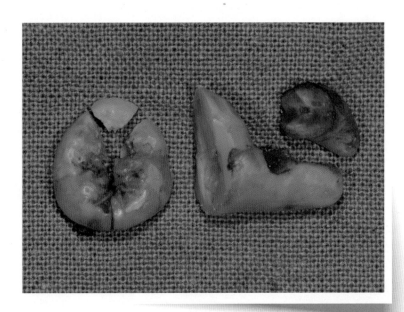

A Crown Cutting is performed to remove the crown then an elevator is used on the buccal surface to extract the remaining tooth. If the remaining tooth is dislocated from its socket, then extraction is almost completed. If the neighbouring tooth is interfering with its removal, then proceed to perform a Lift and Cutting technique. Most often, when the tooth is not easily dislocated from its socket by engaging the buccal surface of the tooth, more buccal alveolar bone is reduced in order to increase the engagement of the elevator. However, I usually proceed with Disto-Cervical Cutting instead of removing the buccal bone.

If the remaining tooth is removed in whole with Disto-Cervical Cutting, then it is extracted using the Disto-Cervical Cutting technique. If the root is separated and removed during the Disto-Cervical Cutting in a multi-rooted tooth, then L-Extraction is performed. Of course, there are some cases that I intend to proceed with L-Extraction from the beginning. Usually, a No.6 surgical round bur is used for a Crown Cutting on a horizontally impacted tooth then uses a No.4 surgical round bur when executing the Disto-Cervical Cutting technique. But lately I became lazy to change the bur in between the procedures, where I end up using the No.6 surgical round bur requiring a deeper cut. Have a look at the sectioned surface of the L-Extraction anticipated root segment and the bur marks on the more inferiorly situated root portion due to a deeper cut.

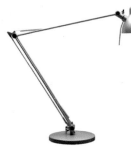

01
Disto-Cervical Cutting and L-Extraction ★★

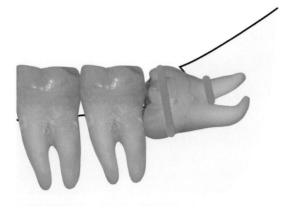

As briefly mentioned on the previous page, the L-Extraction technique performed on the mesially angulated wisdom tooth is the same principle as the one performed here. The impacted wisdom tooth that has multiple roots can be more difficult to extract hence it is often used in extracting multi-rooted wisdom teeth. Have a look at how Disto-Cervical Cutting is performed as shown in the diagram. In most cases, Disto-Cervical Cutting naturally becomes L-Extraction.

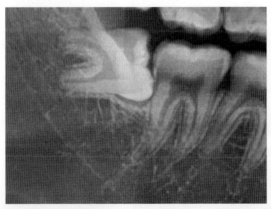
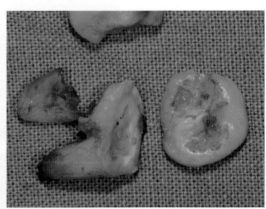

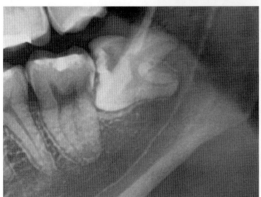
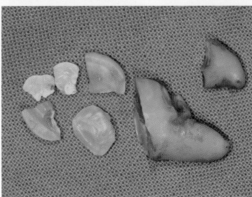
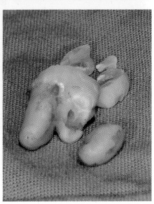

The case above illustrates a wisdom tooth that has large splayed roots thus extraction can be very difficult. In this circumstance, separating the two roots and extracting them one by one can simplify the situation.

02
The process of L-Extraction using Disto-Cervical Cutting ★★

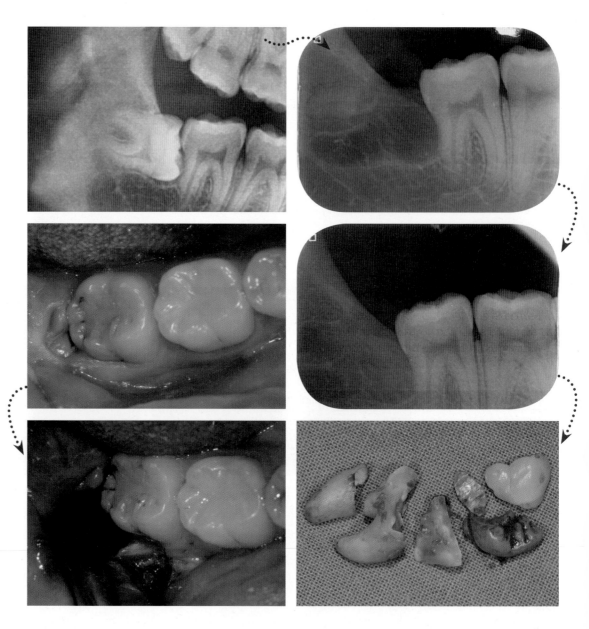

This case demonstrates the process of L-Extraction using a Disto-Cervical Cutting technique. When you have a look at the fractured crown pieces, I have performed a Crown Cutting with a Horizontal Division. Then I executed the Oblique Cutting technique. Despite the further oblique sectioning, the remaining tooth would not budge hence a Disto-Cervical Cutting was exercised which naturally became the L-Extraction. The fractured crown does not exactly exhibit L-shape and it may look like 3 different pieces after separating the lingual portion through the Oblique Cutting. Clinically, the piece that was separated via the Oblique Cutting method does not impact on completing the Disto-Cervical Cutting thus the extraction as a whole. I always remove the more inferiorly located root first. I have completed countless number of L-Extraction cases, but I can count the number of cases where I have left the distal root in its socket with my five fingers. The remaining distal root is mostly removed using an explorer. Sometimes, I may need to perform the Disto-Cervical Cutting and L-Extraction on those tiny remaining roots for complete extraction. But as you can see on the radiograph, it does not seem like a big deal to leave the distal root in the extraction site.

03
Clinical cases of the process of L-Extraction using Disto-Cervical Cutting ★★

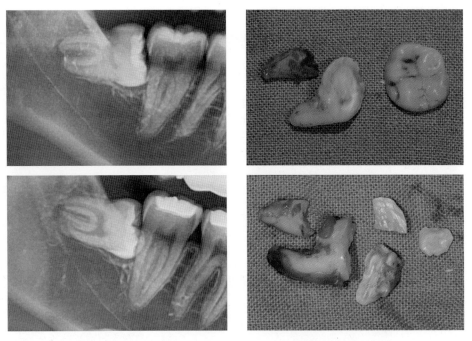

This is one of the most common cases that involve Disto-Cervical Cutting that becomes L-Extraction. In spite of the radiographic multi-rooted tooth anatomy, the tooth may in fact be a single-rooted tooth. In this situation, we should expect that the tooth will end up in 3 pieces.

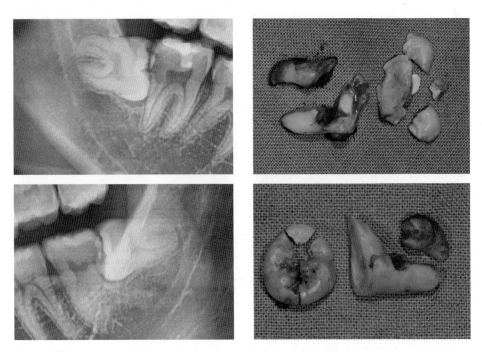

Most of the Disto-Cervical Cutting is completed with a No.4 surgical round bur but due to my laziness, I have cut the tooth with a No.6 surgical round bur that has a larger diameter. When this happens I have to create a deeper purchase point for the narrow elevator (EL3C) to engage the site. Because of this deeper cutting is required and the L-Extraction is performed naturally.

04
Clinical cases of Disto-Cervical Cutting with Oblique Cutting ★★

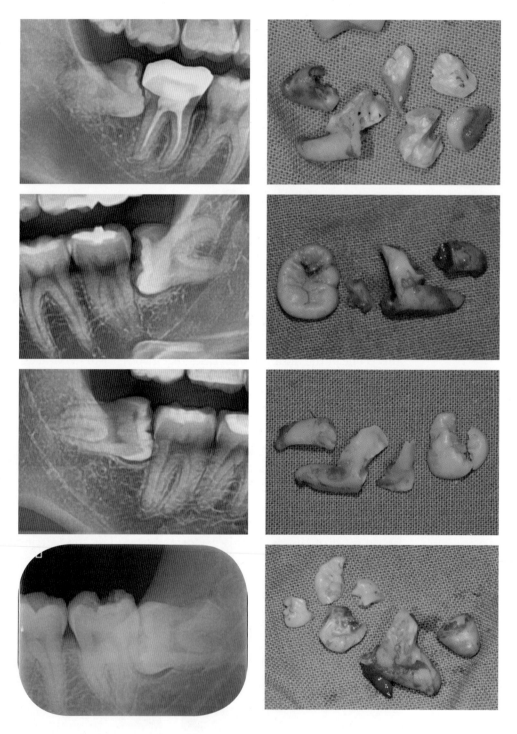

As we know, performing Disto-Cervical Cutting means that an extraction is extremely difficult hence most often Oblique Cutting is completed even prior to engaging an elevator on the tooth. Therefore, it follows a similar pattern of these fractured pieces of the tooth after an L-Extraction.

05
Clinical case of L-Extractions on both sides of the mouth ★

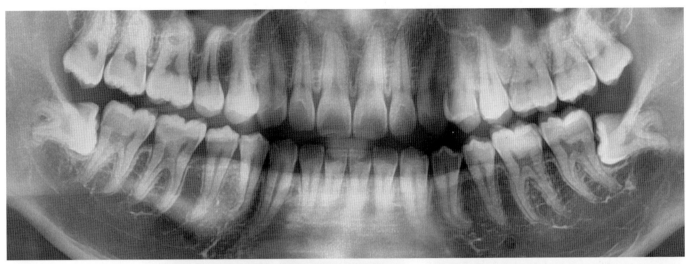

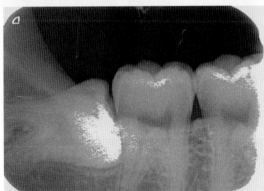

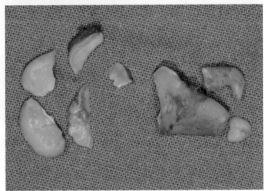

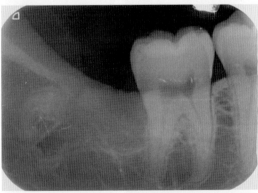

This case demonstrates where both of the lower horizontally impacted wisdom teeth were extracted using the L-Extraction technique. Here the roots are dilacerated inferiorly which is the opposite direction to the direction of the tooth that is extracted. In this case, I prefer to use the L-Extraction technique where the mesial root is removed first then the curved distal root is able to be pushed into the space of the mesial root without breaking the distal root tip. Fortunately, most of the time mesial root is relatively straight thus removing a mesial root is implemented without any complications. Sometimes, a mesial root can be curved like the distal root and positioned close to the inferior alveolar canal (IAC). In this situation, the root tip is often fractured during removal and I must implement its removal very cautiously.

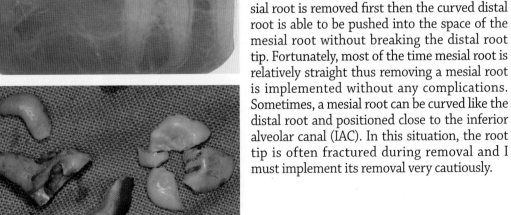

06
Clinical cases of L-Extractions with the inferiorly dilacerated distal root <1> ★

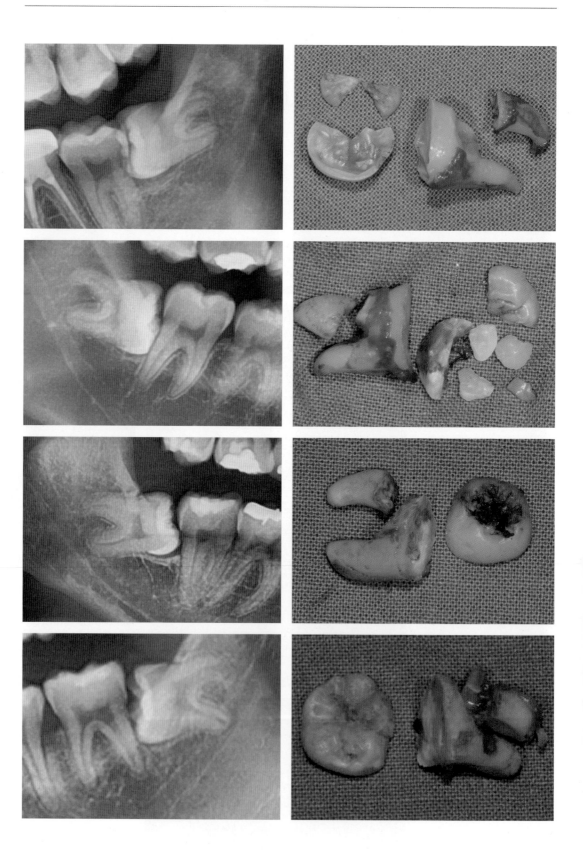

Clinical cases of L-Extractions with the inferiorly dilacerated distal root <2> ★

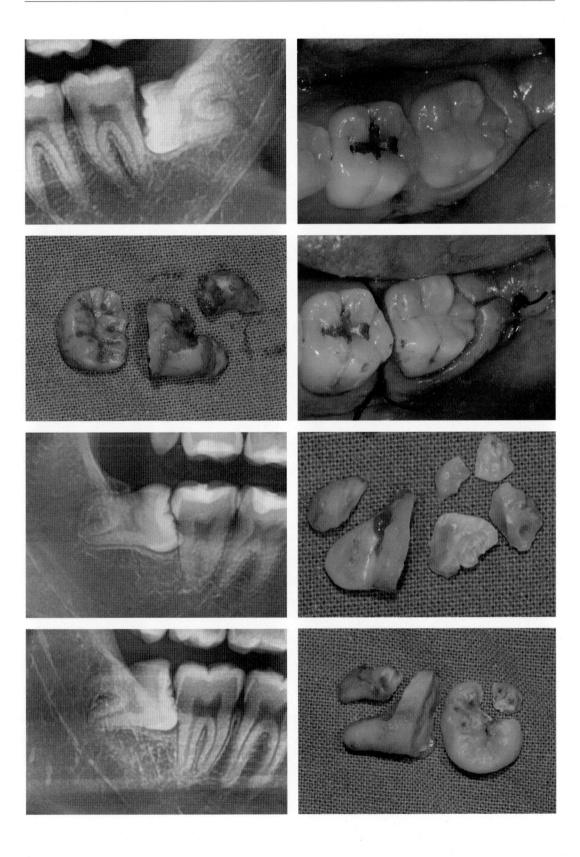

Clinical cases of L-Extractions with the inferiorly dilacerated distal root <3> ★

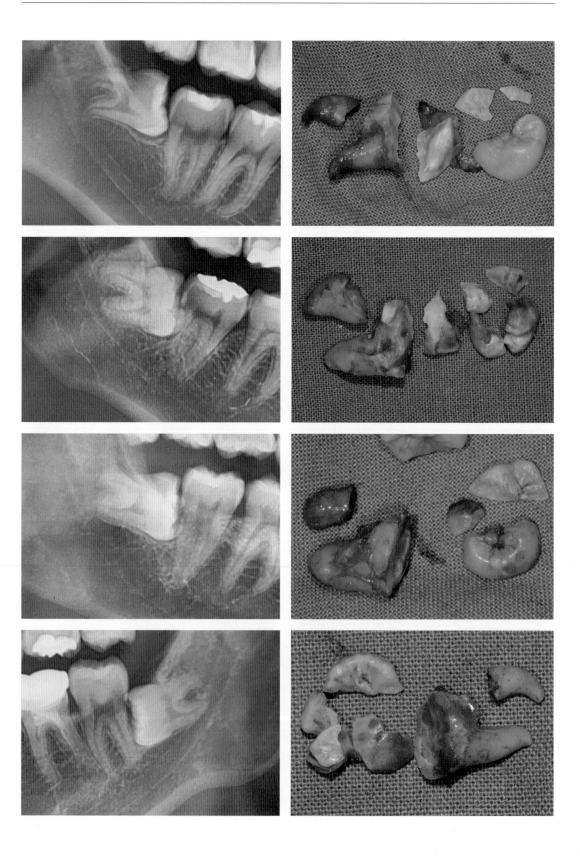

07
Failed cases of Disto-Cervical Cutting and L-Extractions on both horizontally ★ impacted wisdom teeth

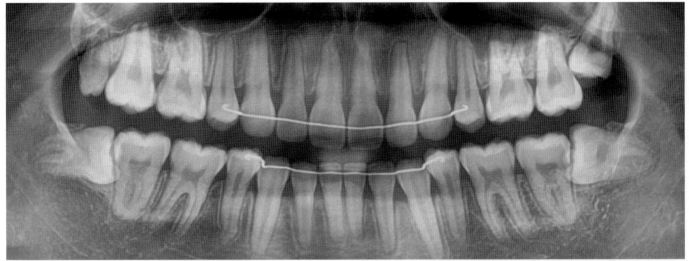

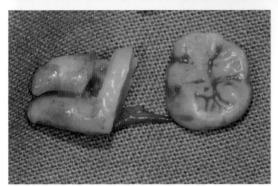

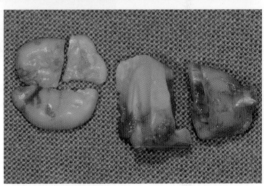

L-Extractions were performed on both mandibular wisdom teeth but failed to execute it completely. Tooth 48 was extracted successfully but failed to complete the L-Extraction technique as the tooth came out before the distal root was fractured off. Disto-Cervical Cutting technique was utilised to remove the remaining root of the tooth 38 but the entire root fractured off. The remaining fractured root was removed with the usual extraction method. I call this kind of case a removal in 3 pieces or trisection extraction. If you leave the remaining root and stop the extraction, it can be called a successful Intentional Coronectomy. Let's discuss a little bit more about the removal in 3 pieces on the next page.

Removal in 3 Pieces ★★

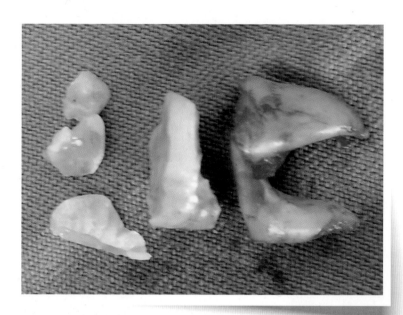

■ The photograph is out of focus but I decided to use this photo as I got accustomed to presenting with this old case of mine.

As the wording suggests, you may intentionally perform the removal in 3 pieces. However, it occurs mostly in the process of implementing Disto-Cervical Cutting or L-Extraction techniques and fracture occurs near the furcation area. The remaining roots are removed with a usual method of extraction. Since the root fracture has occurred deep within the bone, you can leave the remaining roots and consider it a successful Intentional Coronectomy. There is no need to name this type of extraction, but this occurs reasonably frequently and is not considered as a failed extraction. Therefore, I named this kind of extractions as a removal in 3 pieces to signify that this type of extraction is never a failed extraction.

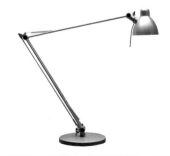

01
Removal in 3 pieces ★★

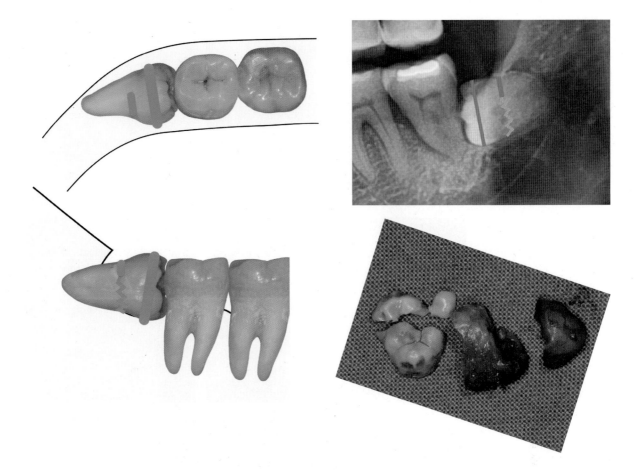

During the removal of the anterior ⅓ of the Crown, the Crown Cutting must be performed to cut through the inferior portion of the crown completely. When removing the mid ⅓ of the crown, the bur should enter only ⅓ to ½ of the crown creating a purchase point as discussed in the Disto-Cervical Cutting method. Therefore, when the extracted pieces are examined, the upper portion of the tooth reveals the complete bur reduction whereas the mid-portion indicates partial reduction with a fracture. The method of removing the remaining root(s) will be discussed later.

02
Clinical cases of removal in 3 pieces <1> ★★

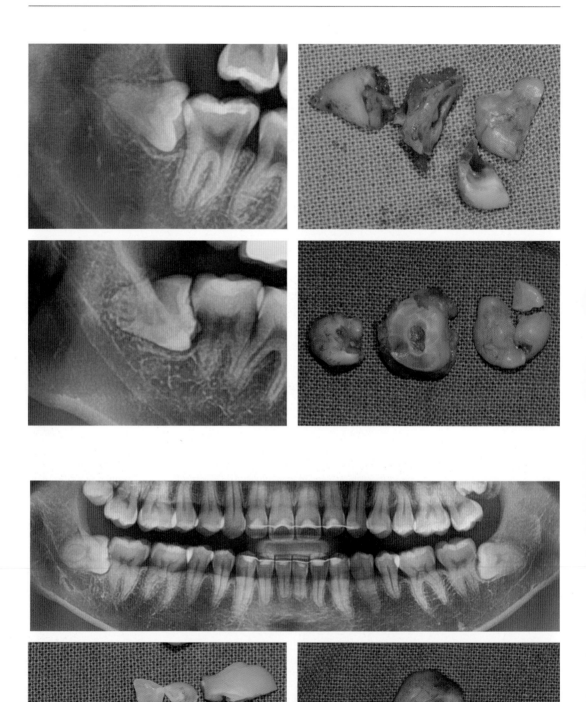

Clinical cases of removal in 3 pieces <2> ★

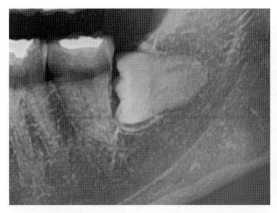
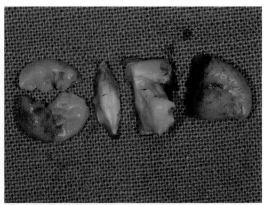

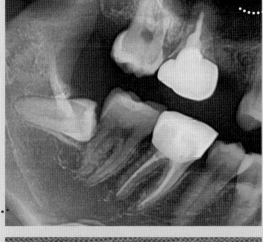
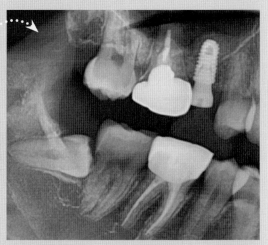

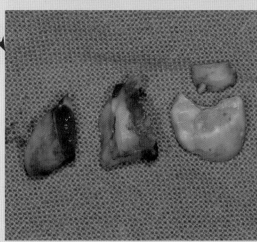
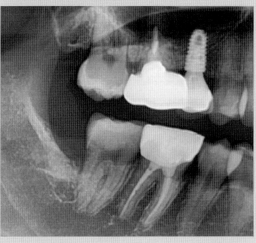

A patient came in to extract a wisdom tooth and decided to place an implant too on that day hence I have placed the implant, took a new panoramic radiograph then extracted the wisdom tooth. I am sharing this case because I wanted to point out that when I extract a wisdom tooth for a patient that patient is most likely to get an implant placed with myself. The panoramic radiograph may show that the implant is placed more towards the distal, however, it is in fact more in the centre of the adjacent teeth.

03
Single rooted tooth that resembles multi-rooted tooth ★★

As conveyed in the title, these are single-rooted teeth that resemble multi-rooted teeth. The removal in 3 pieces occurs mostly in these circumstances because they are the most difficult extraction when performing wisdom teeth extraction.

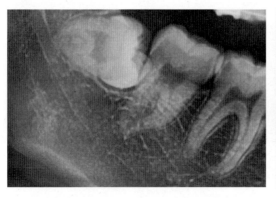 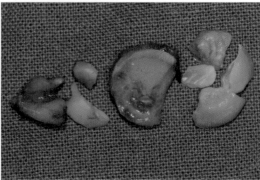

The extraction is the most difficult when the root resembles that shape of a swim fin. As I believe the wisdom teeth extractions are all generally simple to do, when I face difficult extractions and put the teeth together for examination, the roots are connected with a swim fin structure.

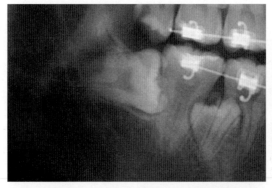 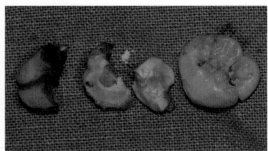

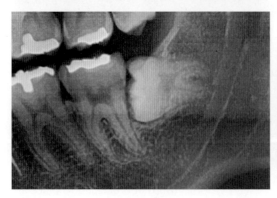 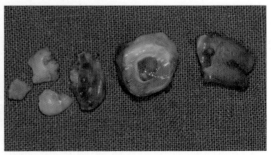

The two cases above are also as difficult as the swim fin shaped roots. The cases above are not as severe as the one I am trying to describe but it serves the purpose for my description. It is when the roots are shaped like a fat person's buttocks. In such cases, the last ⅓ of the root portion is extremely difficult to dislocate from its socket.

04
A severe inflammation resulting in root adherence to the bone ★

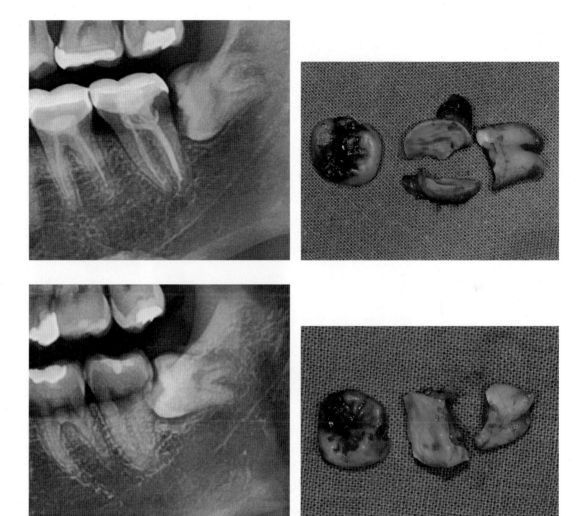

The shapes of the wisdom teeth above indicate straightforward extractions. However, the amount of calculus buildup on the crowns demonstrates how much inflammation there was around the extracted wisdom teeth. In these cases, the inflammatory lesions surrounding the crowns push the tooth into the bone rendering extractions extremely difficult. When this happens, the periodontal ligament space becomes too narrow for an elevator engagement hence the Disto-Cervical Cutting is performed. If the tooth does not budge and break then an extraction will be completed through removal in 3 pieces.

05
Removal in 3 pieces of multi-rooted teeth ★

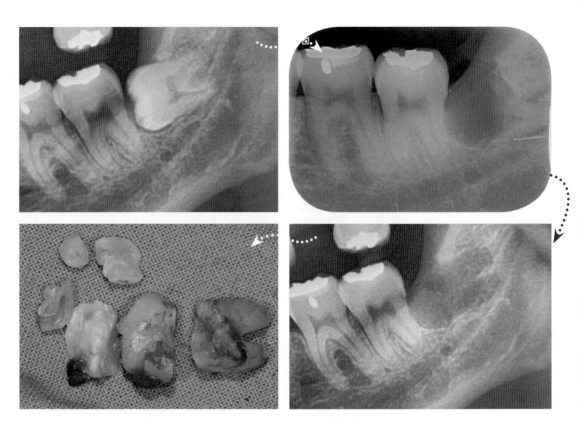

After performing the Disto-Cervical Cutting I have tried to execute the L-Extraction but that mid ⅓ of the tooth fractured. This is more prevalent in a situation where the root furcation is closer to the root apex, however, if the roots can be easily removed then it is not much different to correctly performing the L-Extraction.

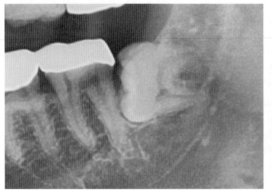

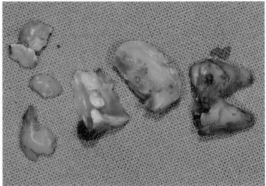

In regards to the above case, as I tried to remove the mesial ⅓ of the tooth as close to the 7th tooth as possible, the mid ⅓ also was sectioned more mesially and fractured in this manner. As mentioned before, it occurs more readily because the root furcation is located close to the root apex but if the root ⅓ can be easily removed then it should be no different to removing any other impacted roots. However, if the remaining ⅓ of the root portion is splayed and multi-rooted then the remaining roots may be difficult to extract.

Disto-Cervical Cutting then Root Separation ★★★ at the Roots

Root separation at the third piece

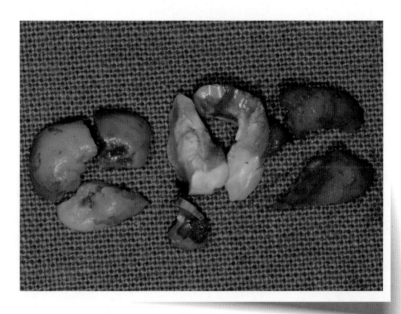

Separating the roots during removal of horizontally impacted wisdom teeth for most dentists is a very common routine procedure. Why would I mention this towards the end of the chapter? It is because I rarely use a low-speed straight surgical handpiece for extractions. You may misunderstand that I use the straight handpiece in this circumstance but I still do not use it during this step of the extraction. I tend to use a high-speed handpiece by creating the best possible angulations to separate the roots and place an elevator between the roots to fracture and complete the extraction. As mentioned before, I hardly used a low-speed handpiece until 2014. However, when utilising high-speed handpiece and accessing from the above it can lead to more severe bone reduction hence I sometimes do use a low-speed handpiece these days. As I need to extract wisdom teeth very quickly, I tend to become a bit impatient to change the handpieces hence most of the cases are still completed with the high-speed handpiece.

01
Separation of multi-rooted teeth in 3 pieces ★★

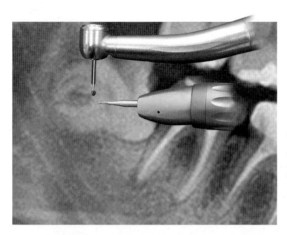

Usually, a low-speed surgical handpiece is used to separate the roots, but I use a high-speed handpiece most of the time.

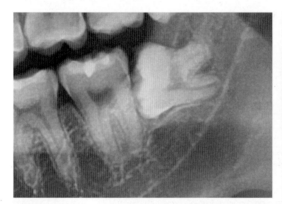
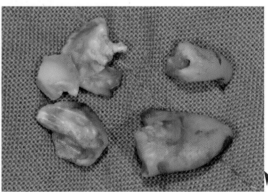

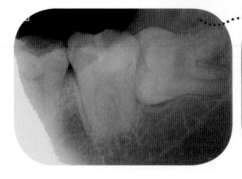
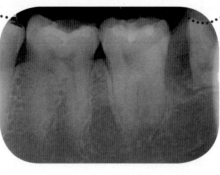
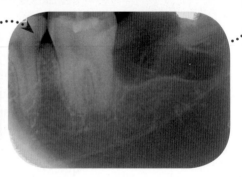

When separating the roots using the high-speed handpiece, the area is approached from the top and the distal root may appear shorter than the mesial root due to bur reduction. It is very critical to minimise reduction of the mesial root for an elevator engagement hence care must be taken.

02
Remove inferiorly located root first ★

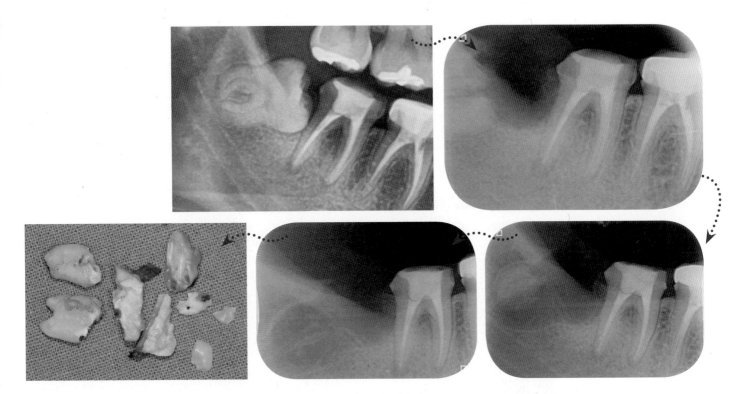

This was a difficult case as the roots were curved and diverged. The teeth that are curved and diverged often fractures in multiple pieces when performing L-Extraction.

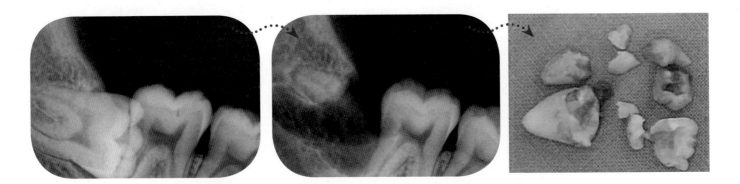

The photo is out of focus, and it is one of my old cases so I am presenting it here. The remaining distal root appears very short as the high-speed handpiece was accessed from the top and reduced a large portion of the distal root.

03
Removing the inferiorly located root first (Dr. Kim's recommended style)

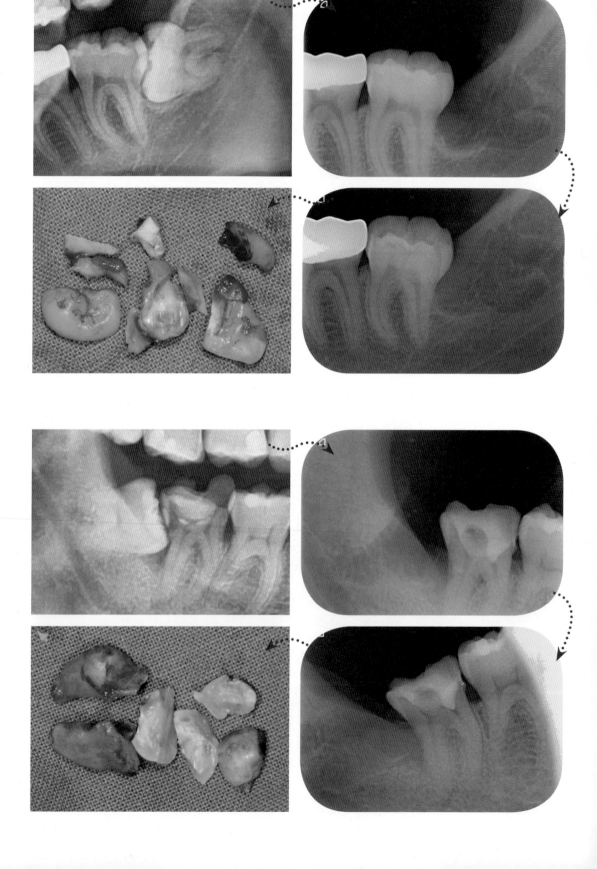

04
Clinical cases of root separation at the roots <1> ★

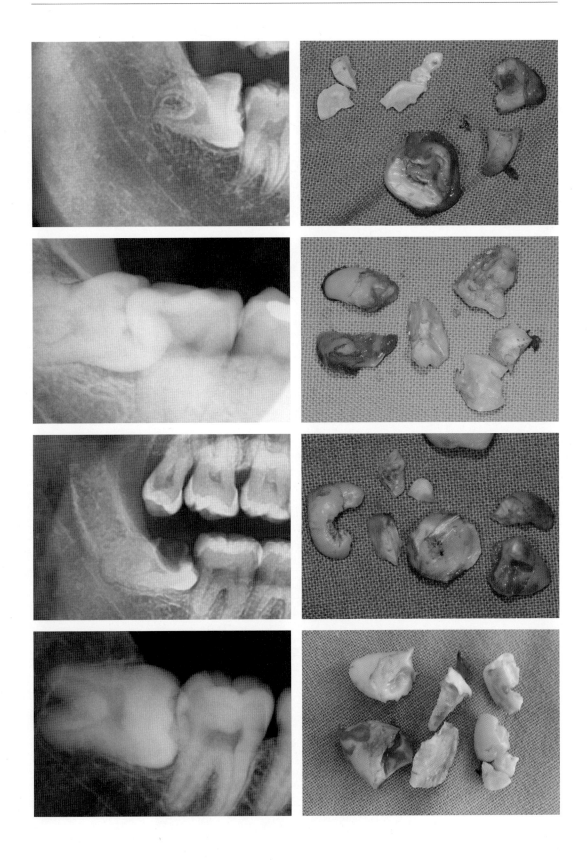

Clinical cases of root separation at the roots <2> ★

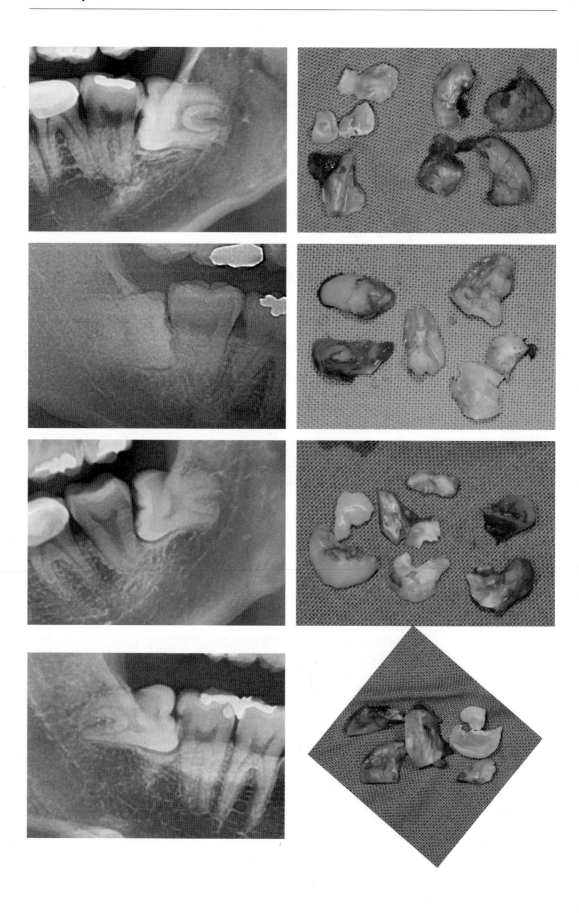

Clinical cases of root separation at the roots <3> ★

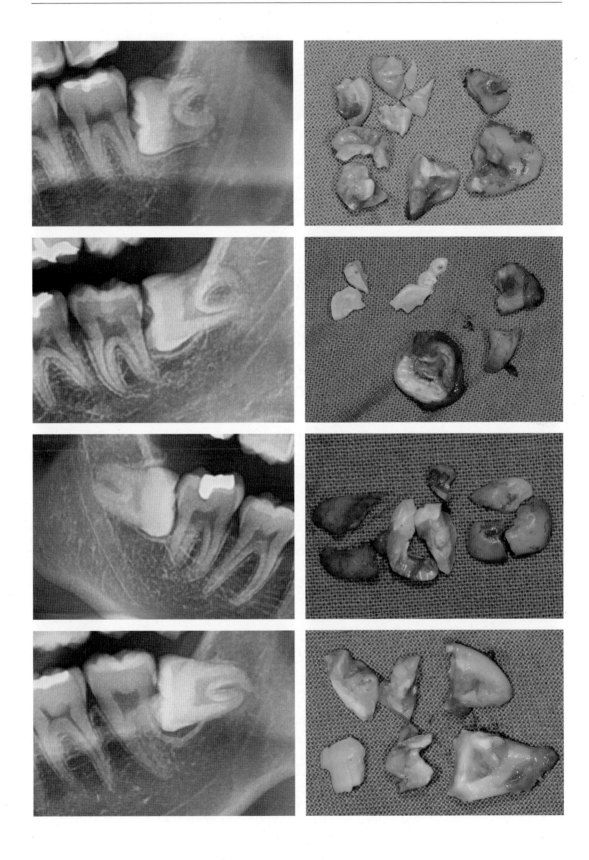

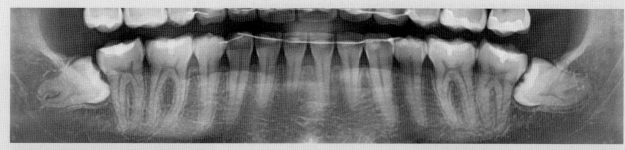

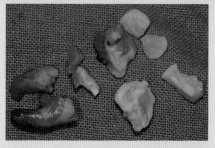

This is a typical case for root separation

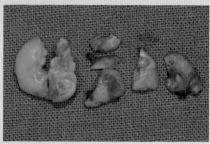

The remaining ⅓ of the root was difficult to remove and the notched area ended up fracturing into four pieces.

Clinical cases of root separation at the roots <4> - when the remaining root is difficult to remove (swim fin and buttocks)

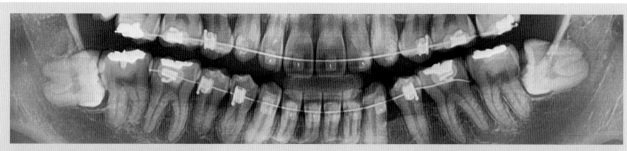

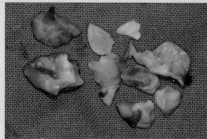

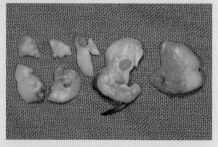

This is a typical case for root separation. The separated pieces that are shown above are erratically placed and I ask for your understanding. When you have a look at the mesial root, there is a notch created with a high-speed handpiece. The remaining ⅓ of the root is also removed by creating a purchase point with a high-speed handpiece as if we are removing the remaining tooth after Crown Cutting in the Disto-Cervical Cutting technique. As expected, the root is shaped like a swim fin.

I do not remember whether I did not, or could not separate the roots near the root apexes. But you can see that the removed root resembles a fat person's buttocks which indicates that the extraction was not easy.

Clinical cases of root separation at the roots <5> ★★

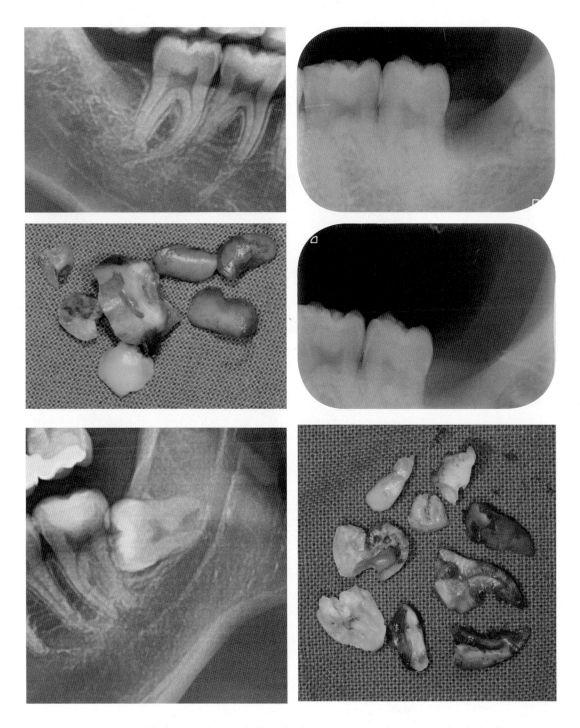

Extraction of a mandibular wisdom tooth with three roots can be extremely difficult. Most of the time, the mesio-lingual third root is so thin and tiny that the surgeon may not realise its existence until the root is outside the mouth. However, if the third root is a similar size as the original two roots then the level of extraction is quickly heightened. Furthermore, the mesial root can be connected with the distal root resembling peanut or swim fin shape will induce a much more complex situation.

Disto-Cervical Cutting at the Roots ★★

Creating a purchase point on the upper portion of the root

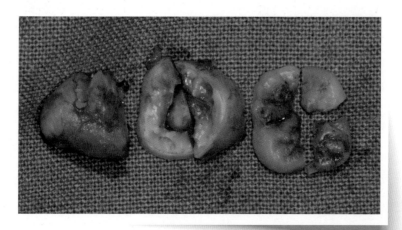

The technique is similar to the Disto-Cervical Cutting method performed on a horizontally impacted wisdom tooth. It is crucial to use a smaller surgical round bur because the thickness of cementum is thinner as you approach closer to the apex of the root. The angulation and access of high-speed handpieces become much more difficult when the position of the wisdom tooth is located more inferiorly. This method is very effective only when the root is positioned more superiorly and closer to the surface.

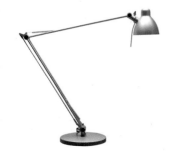

01
Disto-Cervical Cutting at the roots ★★

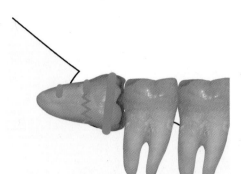

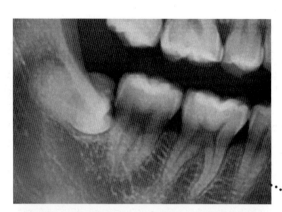

Typically, we may think that three perpendicular cutting is implemented, however, only the first Crown Cutting is sectioned to the end of the crown, and the ones completed afterward are executed by creating a notch and fracturing.

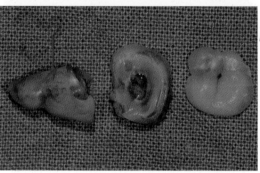

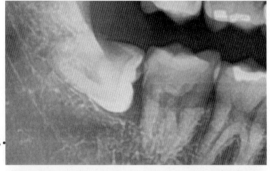

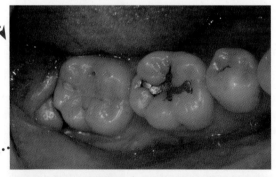

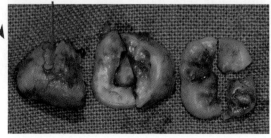

When I tackle a case like this I contemplate on where I should initiate the cutting of the tooth. As usual I was planning to cut the cervical area of the tooth, then I changed my mind and cut more anteriorly. As mentioned in the previous cases, the case like this is when the tooth is pushed back and the periodontal ligament space becomes much narrower thus an elevator is unable to be engaged a lot of times. Consequently, I have performed the Disto-Cervical Cutting but the root ended up fracturing without dislocating the remaining root from its socket. Thus, I have implemented Disto-Cervical Cutting technique on the remaining root and extracted it. In this circumstance, I could have used a low-speed handpiece but I was feeling tired and lazy to change the handpiece. More importantly, the wisdom tooth was positioned more superiorly for me to use the high-speed to create a purchase point to extract the remaining root.

02
Disto-Cervical Cutting at the roots of multi-rooted teeth ★★

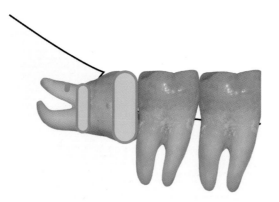

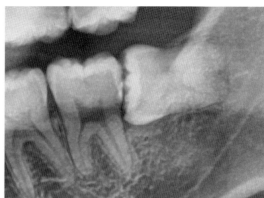

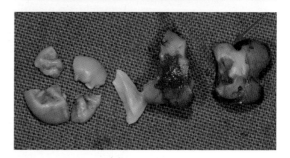

Performing Disto-Cervical Cutting on a multi-rooted tooth at the root portion is not so much different from a single-rooted tooth. To be precise, the cut is already beyond the cervical line thus the name should be something like 'creating a purchase point on the upper root.' But the actual methodology is the same as the Disto-Cervical Cutting, thus I would like to just keep it as Disto-Cervical Cutting at the roots. This technique can only be executed when the vertical level of the roots of the tooth is closer to the crest of the bone.

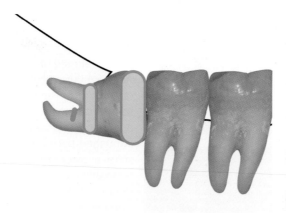

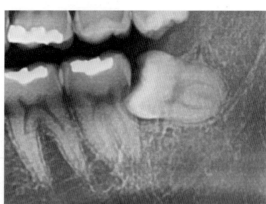

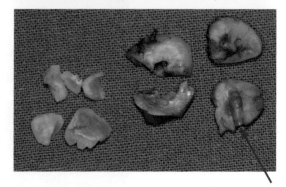

This technique is utilised when a mesial root is difficult to extract, especially when an IAC is located just below the mesial root of the tooth. In such a case, a notch is created to use as a handle to remove the root and avoid damaging the nerve. It is safe to think that this technique has been used in most of the root separation cases. When I am separating the two roots I use a high-speed handpiece to access the roots from the superior portion of the tooth. The bur travels inferiorly to remove the distal root's anterior portion, separates the two roots, and creates a purchase point on the mesial root at the same time.

03
Clinical cases of Disto-Cervical Cutting at the roots <1> ★

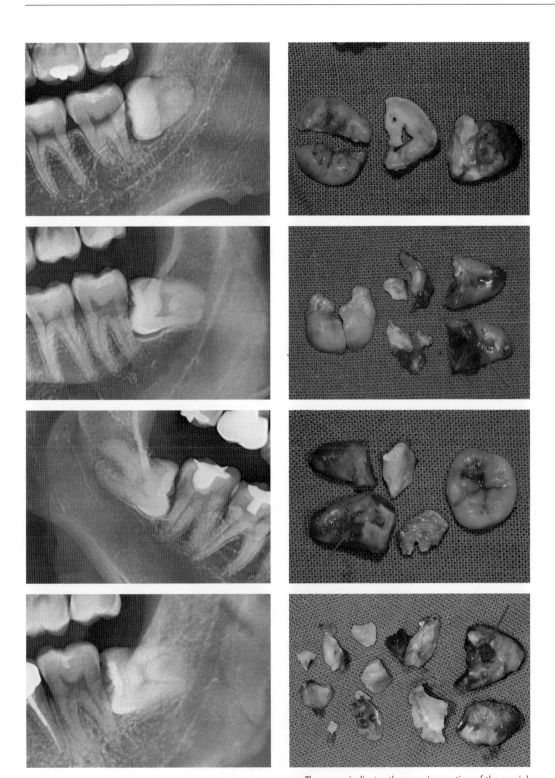

■ The arrow indicates the superior portion of the mesial root

The depth of the created purchase points can vary but when I create a notch on the superior portion of the root, it is used to 'pull out' the remaining root of the tooth.

Clinical cases of Disto-Cervical Cutting at the roots <2> ★

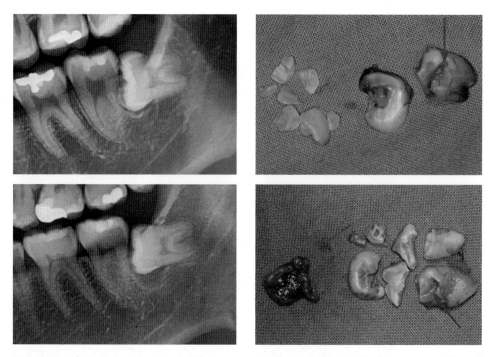

Sometimes, I have to create an oblique or vertical notch due to the limitation of handpiece angulation to create a horizontal purchase point. Since the elevator is engaged from the mesio-buccal surface of the root if the elevator does not slip then the root can be removed successfully.

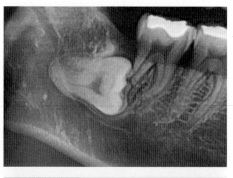

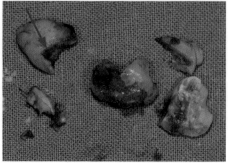

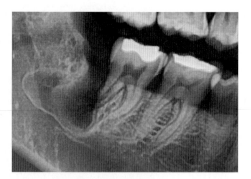

The root of the wisdom tooth is lingually positioned to the IAC. We can clearly visualise the dark band around the root which indicates that the root is closely located to the IAC. Therefore, the tooth was approached buccally and superiorly rather than lingually and inferiorly. As the book is written for the general dentists, most of the extremely difficult extractions for the specialists are excluded in this book. However, this case is presented here as the patient came in due to severe pain and inflammation around the wisdom tooth.

Clinical cases of Disto-Cervical Cutting at the roots <3> ★

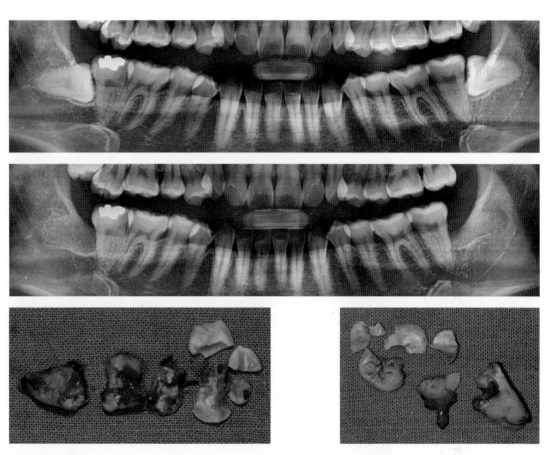

We can visualise that purchase points were created from several different angulations.

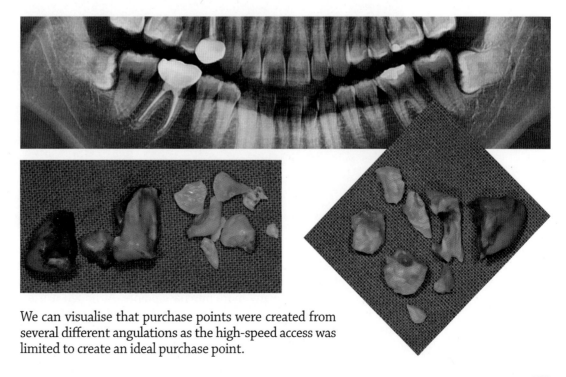

We can visualise that purchase points were created from several different angulations as the high-speed access was limited to create an ideal purchase point.

Clinical cases of Disto-Cervical Cutting at the roots <4> ★

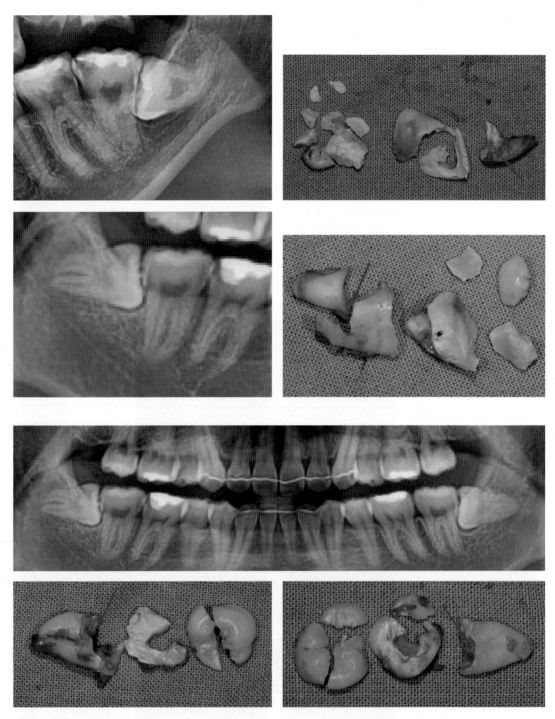

Being able to create a purchase point at the roots does not mean that the remaining root can be easily extracted. As the root structures continuously fracture, the purchase point can be made in the centre of the root rather than the external surfaces of the root, the highspeed handpiece may reach its limit to create any more purchase points. Although it is extremely rare that I have to use a low-speed handpiece, let's have a look at using it to create a purchase point as it will be the most common way of removing the root fragment in this situation.

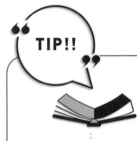

TIP!!

Creating a groove between the roots ★★★
(Flathead Screwdriver Extraction)

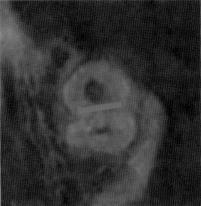

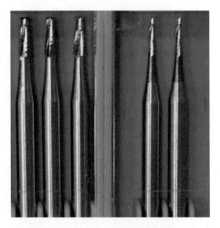

This is a size comparison between the commonly used 016 fissure burs and the 010 used in removing the buccal bones and creating a groove on the root.

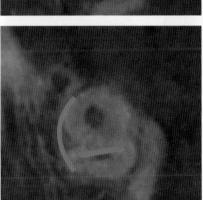

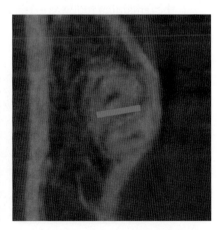

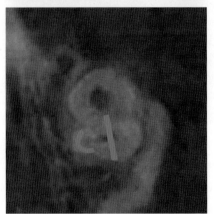

The images above demonstrate how a low speed handpiece can be utilised to remove buccal bones or create a groove depending on the root shapes or locations in the mouth.

Commonly, 010 surgical fissure bur or No.4 surgical round bur can be used. Usually, the surgical burs are expensive hence I tend to use inexpensive generic fissure burs. It is also because I use it for the surfaces where minimal reduction is required. Moreover, due to the fact that the surgical burs with a long shank is not readily imported and accessible in our country, I use it by slightly taking out the regular bur and engaging it in the handpiece.

04
Creating a groove between the roots (Flathead Screwdriver Extraction) ★★

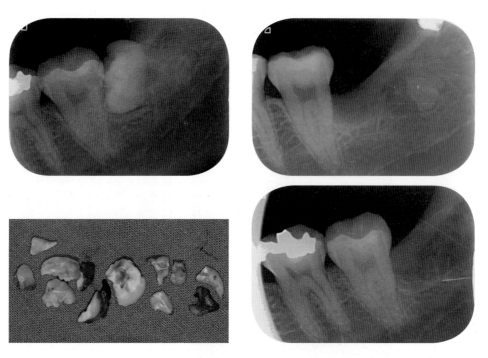

The position of the root was deep so that the access with a high-speed handpiece was difficult. Most of the division was completed using the high-speed handpiece and the remaining root was extracted by creating a groove in between the roots using the straight low-speed handpiece.

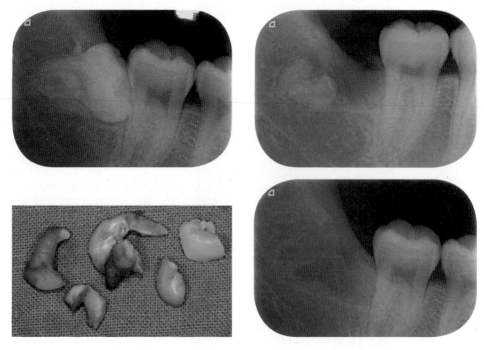

As I do not have many documentations using a low-speed handpiece, I hope you understand that I have to present an image of the pieces of the tooth that is not well arranged.

05
Clinical cases using a Flathead Screwdriver Extraction technique

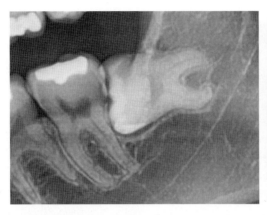

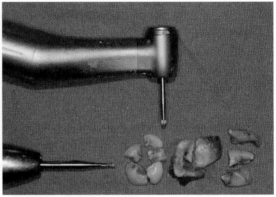

A late 20's Japanese female patient came in for a wisdom tooth extraction that appeared like a common wisdom tooth extraction. Even though I have executed the Disto-Cervical Cutting technique the tooth fractured instead of dislocating the tooth from its socket due to severe root dilaceration. There are two separate roots but the mesial root is shaped like a wide peanut or swim fin. Therefore, they were divided using a straight low-speed handpiece, and then the mesial root was cut vertically to create a Flathead Screwdriver groove to separate and remove the root.

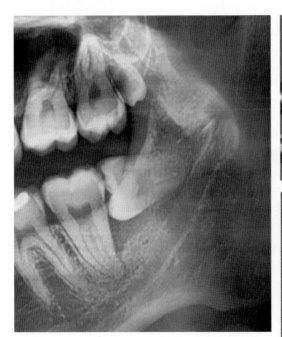

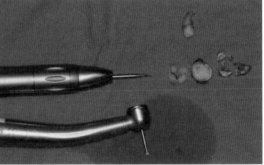

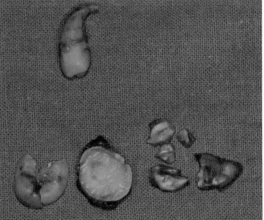

This case is a male patient that appears to have a typically extracted wisdom tooth but as mentioned in the radiology chapter the inflammations around the crown of the tooth lead to roots intruding and adhering to the bone. I can suspect a slight YoungSam's Sign on the upper portion of the root. After creating multiple Flathead Screwdriver grooves in the root, the root fractured into pieces without being extracted. Only after continuous trials, I was able to remove the root. This is a case where the high speed and low-speed handpieces were used interchangeably to section and extract the root. I have just named it as Mix and Match Cutting.

06
Removing the root that can be left as Intentional Coronectomy ★

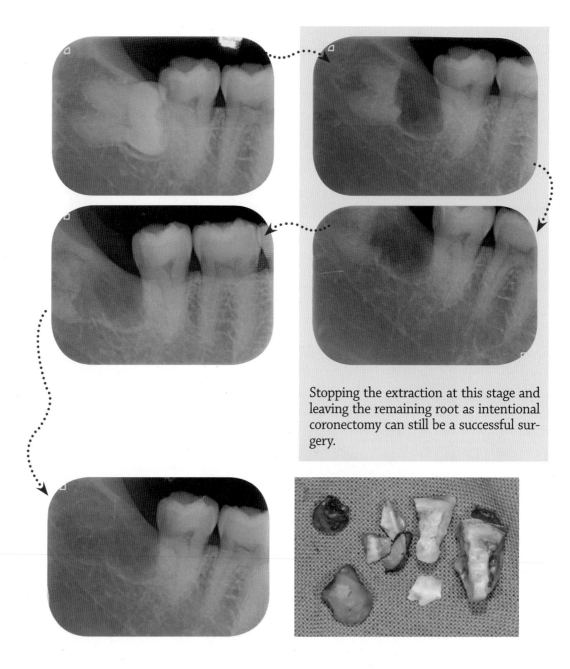

Stopping the extraction at this stage and leaving the remaining root as intentional coronectomy can still be a successful surgery.

07
Mix and Match Cutting ★

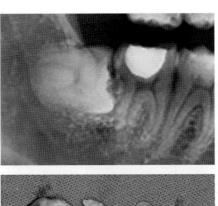

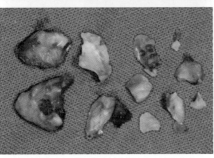

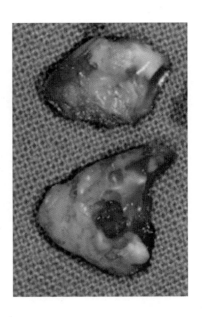

Looking at the pieces of the root it definitely appears like a difficult extraction. I have separated the two roots, and then utilised a high-speed handpiece to create grooves in each root to remove the roots.

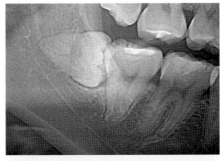

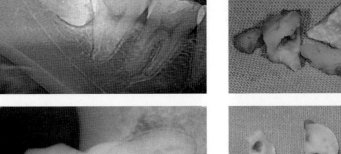

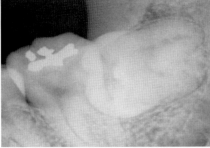

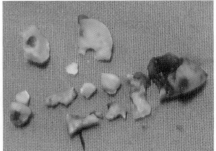

These cases have not been completed recently. It seems that my extraction technique is still improving. There is a reduction in the number of cases where extraction of wisdom teeth becomes severely divided in this manner. In fact, you can also say that there is an increase in the number of cases where I perform Intentional Coronectomy or leave some roots in the bone.

08
Extraction of rotated wisdom teeth ★★

Extraction of vertically impacted wisdom teeth where buccal surface is rotated distally

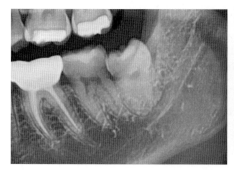
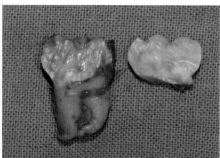

This is a vertically impacted wisdom tooth that is rotated 90-degrees distally. The Distal-Crown Cutting technique was performed then the tooth was extracted regardless of the current tooth position. In this situation, despite the distal crown removal the extraction of the remaining tooth was not easy. It is because a rotated tooth makes it difficult for placement of the elevator where it has to engage on the mesio-buccal surface instead of a usual disto-buccal surface. You may feel somewhat confused to face a rotated tooth just like a right-handed boxer facing a southpaw stance boxer.

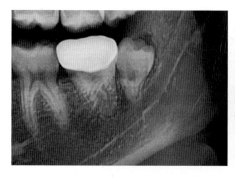
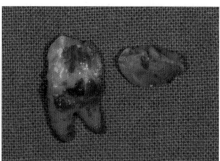

I assumed that this vertically impacted wisdom tooth was an easy typical single-rooted tooth extraction. Surprisingly, the tooth extraction was quite difficult as the wisdom tooth was rotated 90 degrees distally. Same as the previous case, I have performed the Distal-Crown Cutting then extracted the tooth with a little struggle.

Extraction of vertically impacted wisdom tooth where the buccal surface is rotated to the mesial

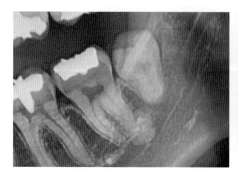
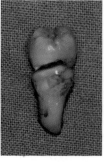
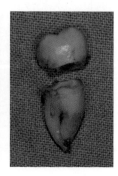

The tooth is lingually tilted with the buccal surface of the tooth rotated 90-degrees and facing the mesial direction. This also is not a common tooth position raising the difficulty of the extraction. A 45-degrees handpiece was used to perform the Cervical Cutting to remove the crown because of the lingualisation of the crown of the tooth.

09
Extractions of rotated horizontally impacted wisdom teeth <1>

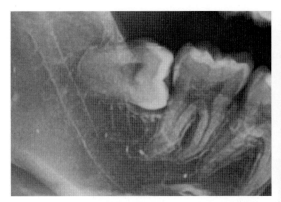
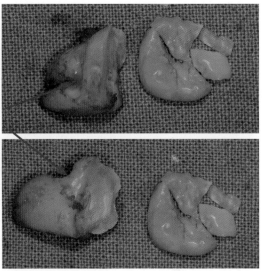

The images above illustrate a horizontally impacted wisdom tooth where the buccal surface of the tooth is rotated 90-degrees to face the occlusal surface. We proceed with the surgery just like extracting a typical horizontally impacted wisdom tooth but I can feel the awkwardness during extraction. The Crown Cutting feels uncommon and the removal of the remaining tooth was not easy. Eventually, I had to implement Disto-Cervical Cutting technique to create a purchase point to extract the tooth with a pulling motion. You can see the buccal and mesial surfaces of the bur marked portion of the tooth. We need to be able to tackle the case with a variety of different methods other than typically engaging an elevator to extract the tooth. In this kind of cases, I often access the middle of the tooth from the occlusal by raising the full-thickness flap then separating the individual roots to be extracted.

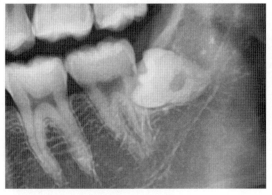
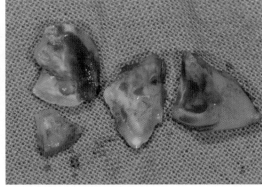

The horizontally impacted wisdom tooth above seems like a single-rooted tooth on the radiograph. When the crown was removed, I realised that the tooth was rotated 90-degrees. Due to the unfamiliarity of extracting the rotated tooth it was more difficult to remove the crown of the tooth than the typically positioned wisdom tooth. I have removed the tooth that clearly shows two splayed roots but a well-trained staff that follows the protocol of taking the photograph as similar to the radiograph as possible has successfully achieved doing it. It would have been nice to present the case with the two diverged roots properly showing. From my experience, the rotated wisdom tooth is much more difficult to section the crown and remove the remaining roots than the unrotated tooth. You may get lucky but most cases will be difficult. Have this in mind when planning to remove the rotated tooth on the radiograph.

Extractions of rotated horizontally impacted wisdom teeth <2> ★★

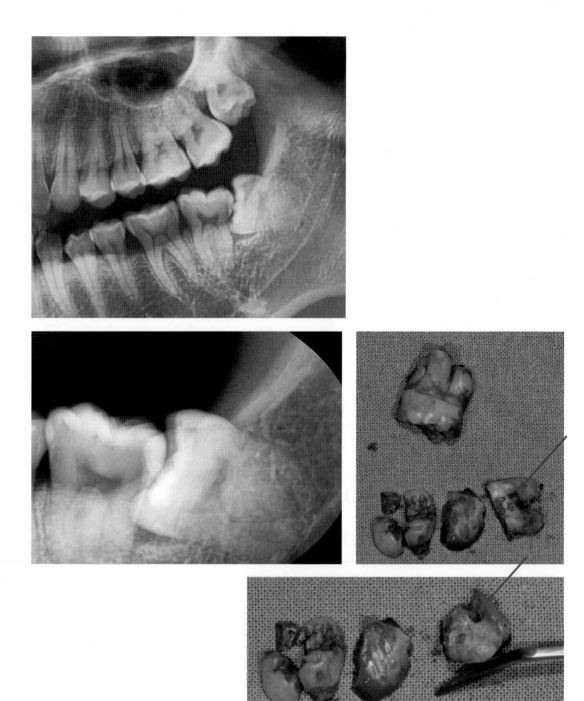

A 30-year-old male patient presented for extraction of his wisdom teeth. The tooth 38 was rotated 90-degrees unlike his tooth 48. The radiograph shows that the rotated buccal surface of the tooth is almost in occlusion. The tooth was not able to be extracted even after the crown was sectioned off hence the Disto-Cervical Cutting was implemented but the tooth broke along the purchase point. The Disto-Cervical Cutting at the roots was further completed to extract the remaining roots. The grooves where the arrows are indicating demonstrate that the two roots were visible from the occlusal view.

10
Extraction of lingually tilted wisdom tooth ★★

Before we discuss the extraction of a lingually tilted wisdom tooth please go back to Chapter 5-2 and revise how I utilized the 5x low-speed handpiece with 45-degrees angle.

The extraction of buccally tilted wisdom tooth is not much different from any other extractions except the amount of bone reduction required according to the position of the wisdom tooth. On the other hand, the lingually tilted wisdom tooth needs to be dealt extremely carefully due to the limitations of access with the handpiece and instruments. I often use the straight low-speed handpiece for the procedure but lately I have started using a 45-degrees high-speed handpiece to complete the Cervical Cutting and remove the remaining root.

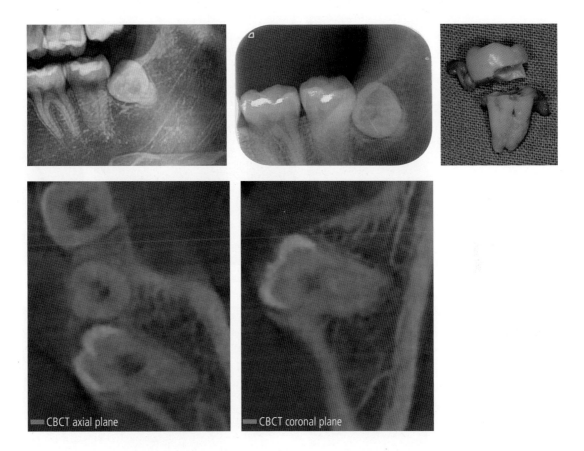

CBCT axial plane

CBCT coronal plane

When you have a look at the panoramic and CBCT radiographic slice of the images the tooth is lingually tilted and the buccal surface is rotated and facing the distal surface. If we proceed with the extraction of this wisdom tooth, it would need to be extracted lingually and the lingual structure will be compromised. We must take the utmost care when the lingual side is involved. I usually use a 45-degrees handpiece to complete the Cervical Cutting from the mesio-buccal surface and remove the crown occlusally then the remaining roots should be extracted.

You can think that the horizontally impacted wisdom tooth that is tilted lingually is approximately 4x harder to extract. On the panoramic views the buccally tilted wisdom tooth may appear similar but it only requires a small amount of buccal bone reduction, and mostly safe and easy to extract.

11
Extraction of severely lingually tilted wisdom tooth ★★

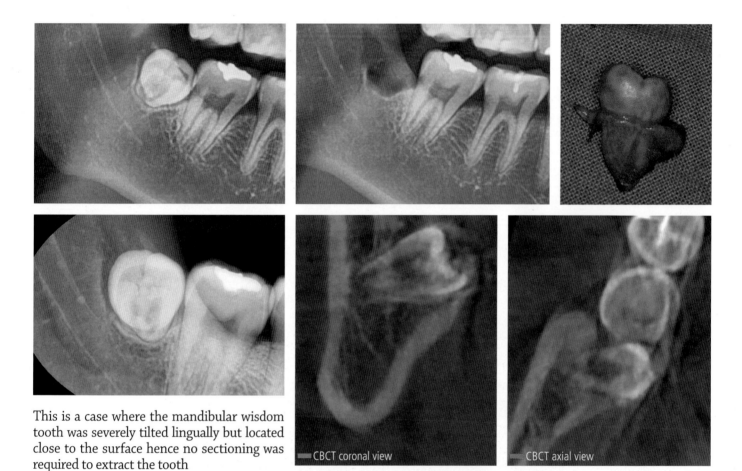

This is a case where the mandibular wisdom tooth was severely tilted lingually but located close to the surface hence no sectioning was required to extract the tooth

CBCT coronal view

CBCT axial view

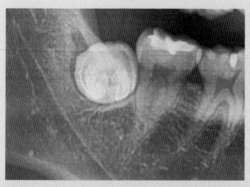

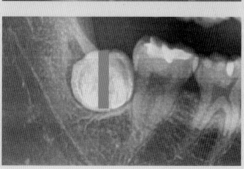

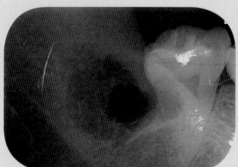

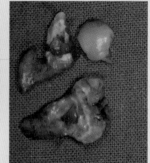

This patient was referred to me from the other clinician due to the severely lingually tilted wisdom tooth. I contemplated on the best possible approach for this case and decided to section the tooth vertically then remove the separated pieces of the tooth. It is very important to plan and tackle the case according to the surrounding alveolar bone conditions. Also, consider the extra time it will take to complete extracting an unusually impacted wisdom tooth.

12
Extraction of incompletely developed wisdom tooth ★★

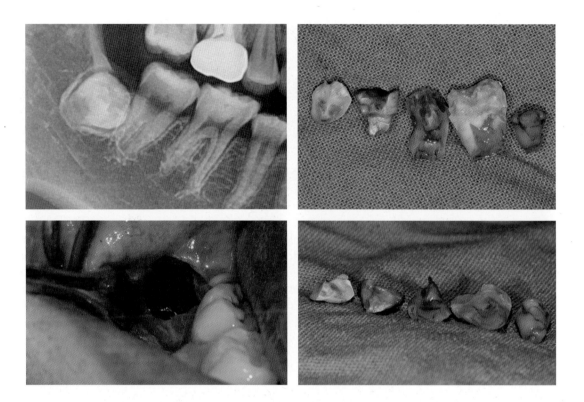

A 20-year-old female patient required an extraction of the wisdom tooth in order to proceed with the orthodontic treatment. The development of the roots of the wisdom tooth varies significantly person-to-person. You may find incomplete root development in some mid 20-year-old patients and also find almost fully developed roots in the late teenage patients. The most important point in the extraction of these wisdom teeth is to section them into multiple pieces and remove them rather than removing a large amount of alveolar bone. I utilized my typical methods of Crown Cutting, Oblique Cutting, and Lift & Cutting to complete the case.

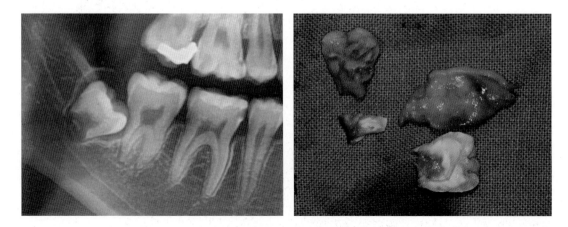

A 17-year-old female patient had an extraction completed by dividing the tooth in half using the straight low-speed handpiece. In order to use a straight handpiece, some of the buccal bones were removed but the distal alveolar bone was hardly reduced at all.

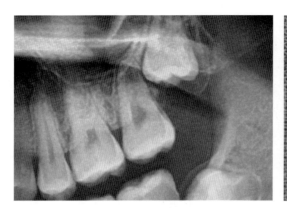 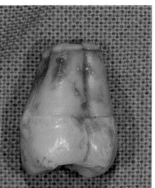

The maxillary incompletely developed wisdom teeth are not prophylactically extracted unless the patient is preparing for the orthodontic treatment. The patient requested its removal for that purpose. The extraction follows typical extraction steps. As the roots are incompletely developed if you remove the bone covering the crown of the tooth then the next step of extracting the tooth is very easy to do. With a proper incision and flap then a slight elevating movement can remove the tooth.

Chapter 09 translated by

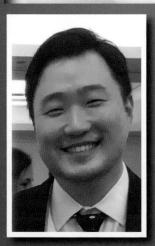

Dr. Leandro Choe DMD

Tufts University School of Dental Medicine 2018
University of California, Santa Barbara 2009
University of California, Davis BS 2010

I am currently practicing as a general dentist after graduating from dental school in 2018. I first began practicing in Los Angeles, CA, as many know it to be a competitive place, especially for new graduates. After starting, one of the first courses I took was Dr. Kim's Third Molar Extraction seminar. Meeting him early in my career truly has set higher standards for my practice—both for implant placements and surgical extractions. He is one of my few mentors that has shaped me into a more competent dentist and I hope the readers also find themselves more clinically competent after reading this book.

Forceps Extraction ★★

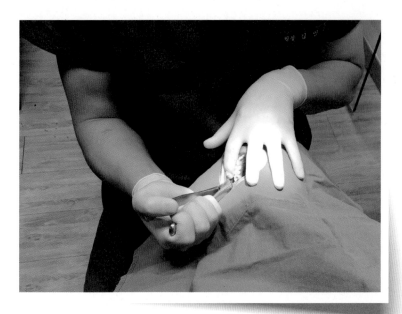

Forceps are the first instrument to consider in upper third molar extraction. Some dentists often think that forceps extraction is for novices and it looks cool when you can take a tooth with an elevator. That's a novice mind set. If you learn and know how to use forceps well, extraction can be a lot safer and faster. I try to keep the cubicle set up simple, but I always request to prepare the upper forceps along with the elevator. It sometimes takes more time to set up when there is an extra instrument. However, forceps allow safer and faster extraction. Elevator assists the extraction when it's not feasible to extract the tooth with forceps. If you use an elevator mainly for upper third molar, I hope you try to be more familiar with forceps extraction.

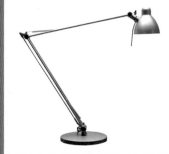

01
How to grasp the Hu-Friedy 10S forceps <1> ★★★

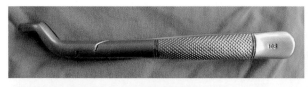

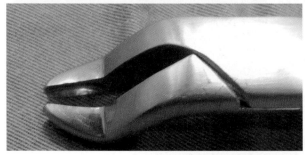

I use Hu-Friedy 10S forceps for the most of upper third molars. It's safer to use an instrument you are the most familiar with. If you are to going to participate a deadly drag race, will you drive a new car? I would get a good universal car, practice with the car every day and will bring that car to the race. Do your best on every procedure even if it's routine for you, it could be the destiny for the patient. Focus not to make a simple iatrogenic complication that will make you sad and discouraged. I extracted a lot of third molars with these forceps and understood the use of it in many different sizes and locations of the tooth.

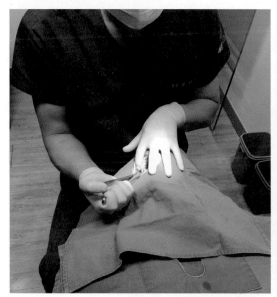

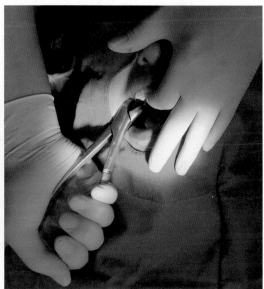

▬ Position for the left upper third molar. Due to my spinal problem, most procedure is done in 9 o'clock position. If the tooth is stubborn, I sometimes move to 12 o'clock position to put strong and stable force. I often confirm the grasp and location of forceps at 9 o'clock position first, and then move to 12 o'clock position.

Due to my spinal problem, most procedure is done in 9 o'clock position. If the tooth is not mobile at all, I sometimes move to 12 o'clock position to put stronger and stable force. I often confirm the grasp and location of forceps at 9 o'clock position first, and then move to 12 o'clock position. When grasping the forceps, my palm faces to upside and the index finger locates the end of forceps.

Dr. Jaewook Lee's comment

If you think about it the other way, the posture and the technique suggested in this book could be less straining to the spine.

How to grasp the Hu-Friedy 10S forceps <2> ★★★

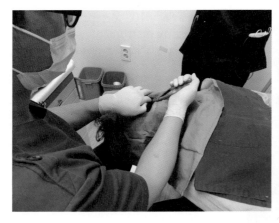 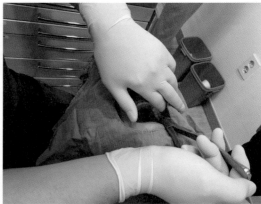

Extraction on #28 (US#16) is performed at 9 o'clock. Extraction is performed as if you push your wrist toward the buccal side. I sometimes place my left index finger on the second molar to feel the movement. More often I place the finger on buccal side to retract the cheek.

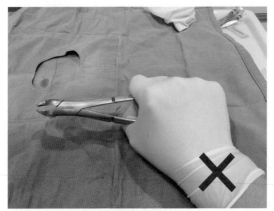

Movie clip for forceps movement

A short clip showing how to open and close forceps properly. Most dentists do it this way, but I sometimes see otherwise.

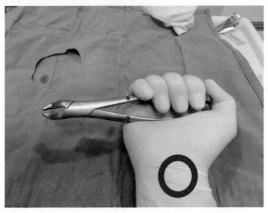 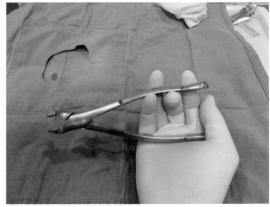

Grasp the forceps in a way that palm faces to upside. This is same for upper and lower wisdom teeth extraction. Use finger to position your forceps.

02
Forceps need to be grasped firmly. Over 60% of force for extraction ★★ is used for the grasp of forceps

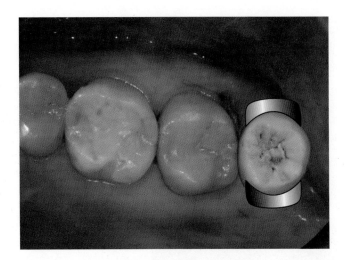

You need to grasp the forceps firmly. If you use 100% of force for extraction, over 60% should be used to grasp the forceps firmly. It is important to avoid any slip of the forceps on the tooth during the extraction. After grasping the tooth tightly, try a slight movement first to confirm the proper location of forceps beaks on to the tooth and see if there is any slip. The adjacent tooth can be easily damaged if the forceps slip and hit it. Remember to confirm the proper location of the beaks of the forceps. One of the reasons many dentists do not want to perform third molar extractions is due to fear of post-op sensitivity of adjacent teeth. Remember, the first rule: focus on avoiding any damage to the adjacent and opposing teeth.

03
Precaution to the adjacent tooth damage ★★

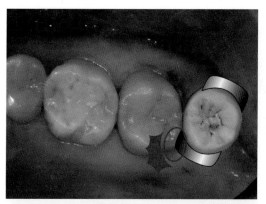

Forceps can push and damage the clinical crown of an adjacent tooth while extracting a third molar even if forceps do not slip. When a third molar is small or rotated, small movements from forceps can damage the adjacent tooth. Remember to not focus on the cases that will please you, rather, focus on the one that will leave no regrets.

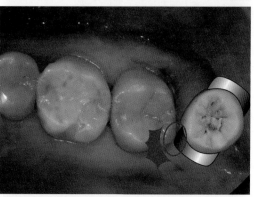

Also, even without direct damage from forceps, pressure from the wisdom tooth to the adjacent tooth can cause cracks. It is important to avoid unnecessary movements of the forceps in random directions. To prevent crack from the pressure to the adjacent tooth, most of the force should be directed toward the distal direction. One of the important concepts in forceps extraction is the direction of the forceps movement.

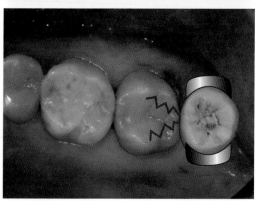

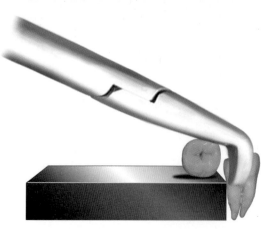

Let's look at the picture. What will happen if you push the tooth while holding the other? It will probably smash the tooth. Beaks of forceps are located close to the adjacent tooth in reality. It can easily damage to the adjacent tooth.

04
Direction of forceps' movement

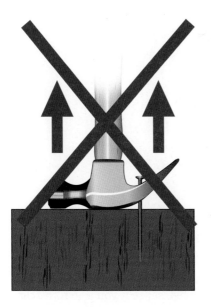
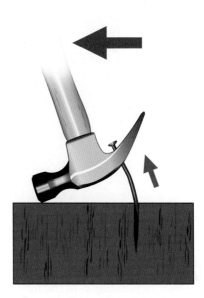

This is an analogy of a wisdom tooth extraction to the removal of a nail as previously shown in the extraction instrument chapter. You twist (or wring) the forceps instead of pulling them. It took time to train students to get used to this twisting motion. Some of them had a difficult time abandoning the bad habit of pulling the tooth.

Precisely speaking, wisdom teeth extraction is more similar to pulling a magnet from a steel wall. When you are trying to remove a magnet from a steel wall, like a fridge, you lift one side of the magnet instead of pulling it flat. While removing a nail from wood takes continuous pulling, you need an instantaneous force to twist forceps. Instantaneous force is more important than continuous force in the forceps extraction.

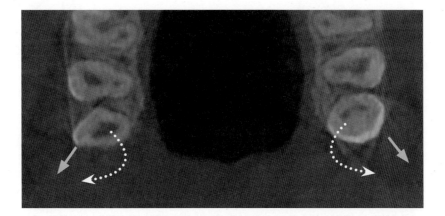

For the most upper wisdom teeth extraction, you rotate the palatal surface of the wisdom tooth to the outside and twist the tooth toward the yellow arrow. It is precise to say you rotate and wring at the same time. You could try to luxate the tooth with forceps, but it is not necessary for most of the upper wisdom teeth.

05
Direction of forceps' action ★★★

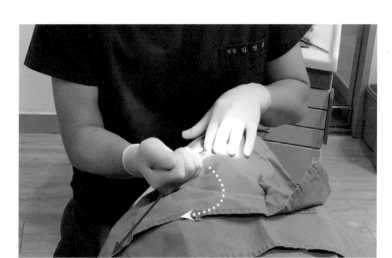

Move forceps towards the outside as you wring them. The direction of forceps movement is demonstrated in the movie clips. It will make sense if you watch the clips. Watch and practice many times just like you watch a golf lesson online and practice to get used to the motion.

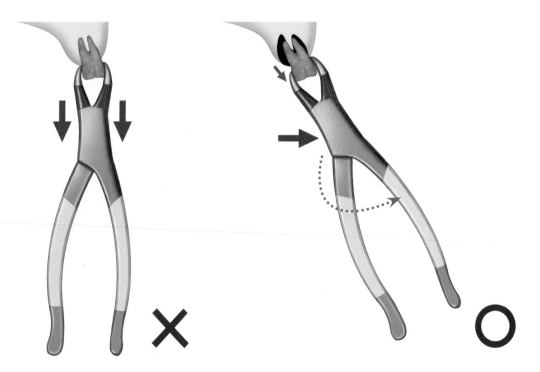

I have changed the previous picture of the clam hammer and nail into forceps and a tooth. Pulling the tooth will damage the opposing teeth or surrounding tissue, which makes extraction more challenging. The correct motion is shown on the right by twisting the tooth. This motion will prevent damaging the alveolar bone.

06
Caution of the distal of second molar when upper wisdom teeth erupted buccally or palatally ★★

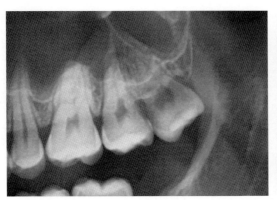

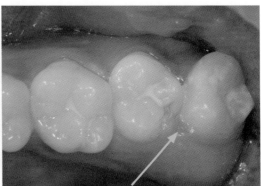

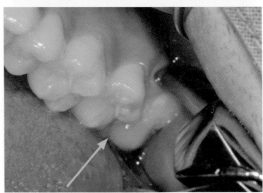

When the wisdom tooth is located this way, be careful because the distopalatal side of the second molar can be damaged even with the force you use to grab the tooth. When the wisdom is sloped buccally, you can place an elevator mesial to #8, but first try the forceps extraction of the erupted upper #8 as a rule.

You sometimes need to use forceps and an elevator together. There is no right answer, but see if you can grab the tooth with forceps first.

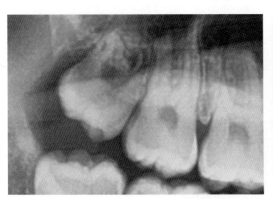

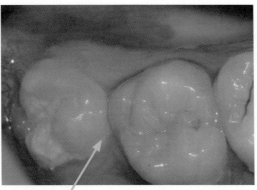

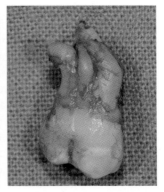

As shown above, the same rule applies to palatally erupted tooth. In this case, be careful not to cause damage to the distobuccal crown of tooth #7. You do not have a good place for an elevator either. Be careful when you grab the tooth with the forceps.

07
Precaution when upper third molars are rotated ★

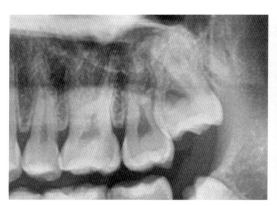 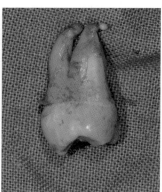

When the thirds are rotated, you first need to consider the anatomical aspect of the teeth and direction of forceps movement in order to avoid the damage to the adjacent teeth or the surrounding tissue before grabbing the teeth with forceps.

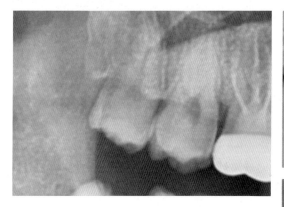

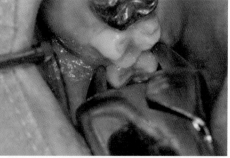

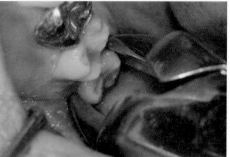

Even when wisdom teeth are not located buccally, most of the time you need to be careful of the distopalatal side of tooth #7. When you grab the tooth with forceps, there is less space between the beak and the adjacent tooth in the palatal side. When you grab the tooth with forceps, check if any part of beak touches the adjacent tooth. It becomes second instinct when you have done many wisdom teeth extractions but beginners can damage the adjacent tooth just by the force you get from grabbing the wisdom tooth with forceps.

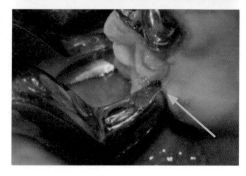

08
Axial view of the cervical area where forceps grab a tooth ★

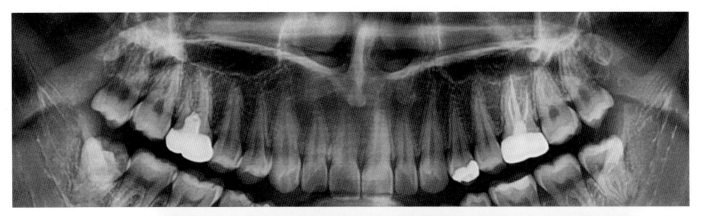

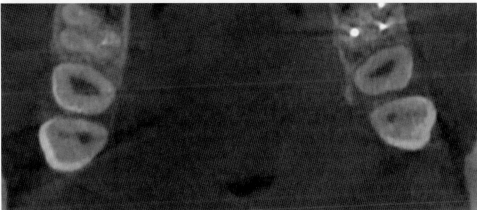

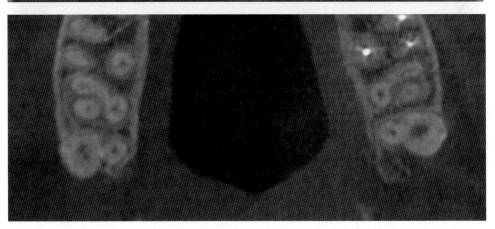

Let us take a look at the axial view of the cervical area where forceps forcefully grab the tooth. It becomes narrower as it goes palatal because there is one palatal root. This explains how beaks do not grab each side of the tooth evenly. When the beaks slip or move, it can damage the cervico-distopalatal area or crown of tooth #7. This is the precise reason why you need to extract as you rotate the tooth distobuccaly.

09
Cases that forceps extraction becomes very useful ★★★

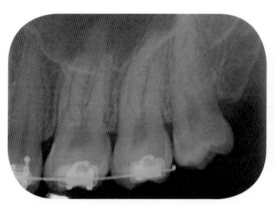 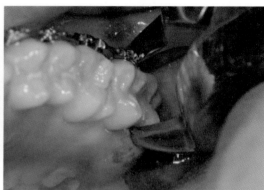

When a patient is undergoing orthodontic treatment, tooth #7 is often luxated and more mobile. Placing an elevator on distal to tooth #7 is not a good idea. When tooth #7 has an ortho wire, you should use forceps to avoid any force acting on #7.

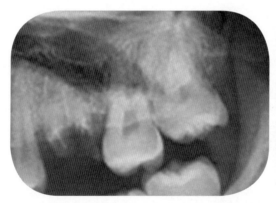 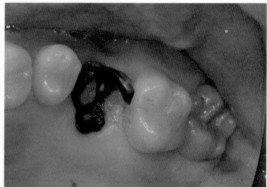

Let us assume there is a dentist who performs a wisdom tooth extraction by placing an elevator between tooth #7 and 8. Will tooth #8 come out? It looks like #8 is bigger and more anchored than #7. Even if tooth #7 is much bigger and more anchored, you want to treat, as #8 was bigger. If you push after placing the elevator and open a space, you are not moving just one tooth, but both teeth. In this case, forceps extraction is a much safer and better option. There are often many careless dentists working without thinking the consequence. Some dentists place an elevator distal to tooth #7 in the similar case where tooth #6 lost the crown due to caries and distal of #8 is blocked by a mandibular ramus.(????)

10
New forceps to avoid adjacent tooth damage

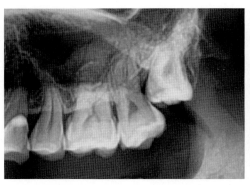
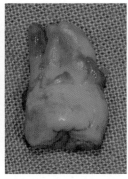
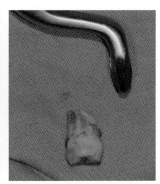

There are new forceps with small beaks from Hu-Friedy as shown in the previous chapter. I own one pair of each for upper and lower and they are useful in some cases. I hesitate to use these in routine surgeries because it looks weaker, but when a wisdom tooth is located deeply in a narrow space, it becomes useful. You could use an elevator, but if it is not easy to place an elevator, these forceps can be used as a supplement. Beaks of 10S forceps are too big to enter and grab the tooth in narrow space. I recommend this kind of forceps in those cases and to get a pair for upper and lower in your office. I will emphasize one more time; a dentist is not different from the general public if you do not have proper instruments.

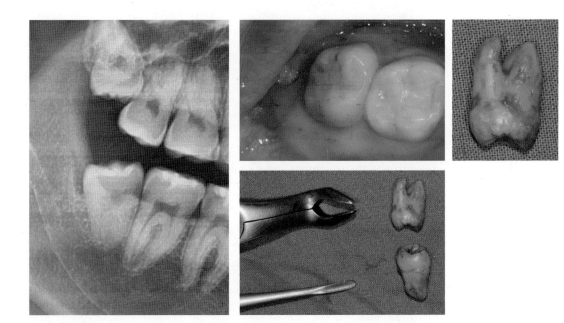

The forceps that were used in this case are shown above. You do not have to worry about damaging the adjacent tooth by the forceps if you follow my forceps movement direction. For both cases, it was hard to place an elevator at a good fulcrum point, therefore I used forceps to extract the wisdom teeth.

11
Useful in small tooth extraction

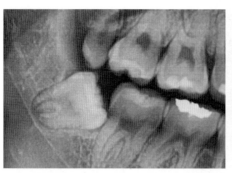
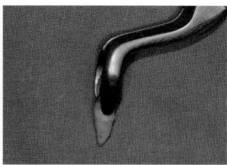

In this small tooth extraction, it is not easy to place an elevator in the mesiobuccal bone, so dentists often place an elevator between #7 and 8, and push away #8. Usually it comes out easily because the wisdom tooth is small and has one root. However, it is not a good habit to place an elevator distal to tooth #7. You can use forceps that have small beaks. You still need to be careful of the distal of tooth #7. You can try using lower small forceps if you do not have the upper forceps. Be careful to avoid damage to the opposing tooth. Always wring the forceps to the side to extract the teeth.

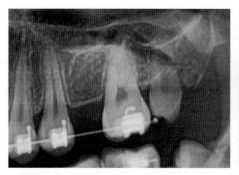
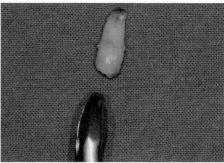

In this case tooth #6 is missing and the wisdom tooth is small. The patient is also undergoing orthodontic treatment and #7 might be luxated. You should never place an elevator between #7, 8 in this case. The forceps with small beaks would be a good choice. It's always better not to touch #7 at all.

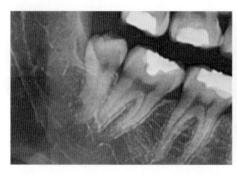
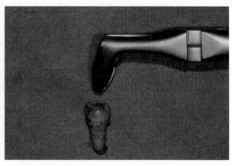

There are new forceps with small beaks for a mandibular tooth. These forceps are useful for a mandibular small tooth. I used the small beak forceps for this tooth shown in the picture.

12
Movie clips for the maxillary wisdom teeth forceps extraction ★★★

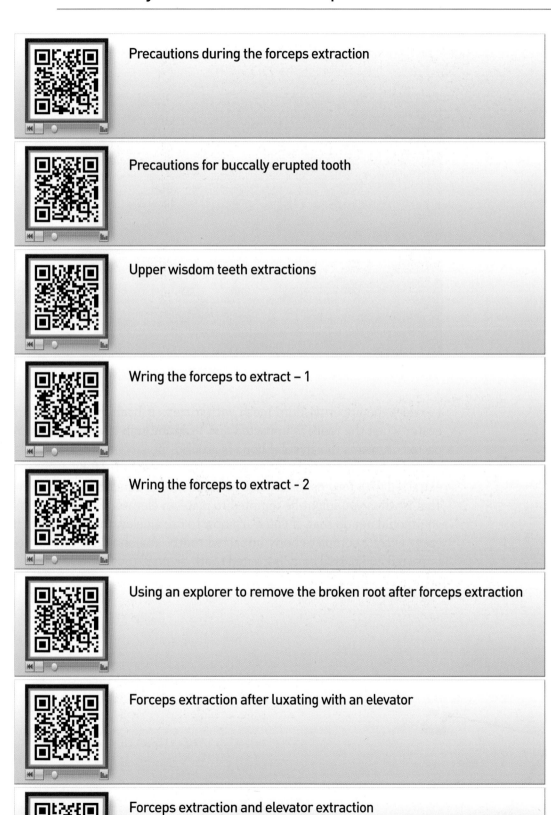

Precautions during the forceps extraction

Precautions for buccally erupted tooth

Upper wisdom teeth extractions

Wring the forceps to extract – 1

Wring the forceps to extract - 2

Using an explorer to remove the broken root after forceps extraction

Forceps extraction after luxating with an elevator

Forceps extraction and elevator extraction

Elevator Extraction ★★

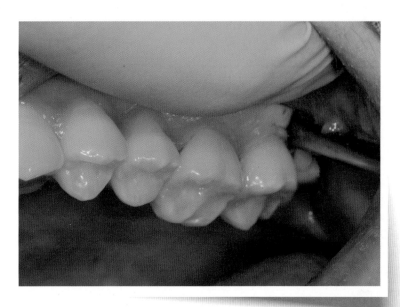

I extract the upper wisdom teeth with forceps if I can grab it with forceps. I use an elevator when the tooth is impacted and I cannot grab it with forceps. When tooth is impacted, it means the alveolar bone is around the crown and the alveolar bone will act as a good fulcrum lever action for the elevator. In case of a fully erupted tooth that can be extracted with forceps, there is no alveolar bone around the crown to engage the elevator. That is when you might be tempted to place an elevator between the tooth #7 and 8, but you should not do that. If you learn how to use an elevator and engage it in bone, you can easily extract complete bony impacted tooth. You should first practice with soft tissue impacted and partial bony impacted tooth or small tooth.

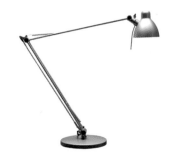

01
My workhorse elevator, Hu-Friedy EL3C ★★

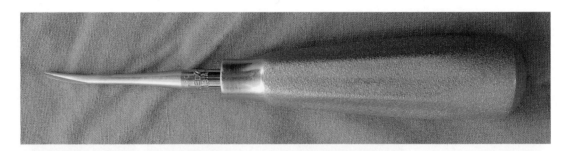

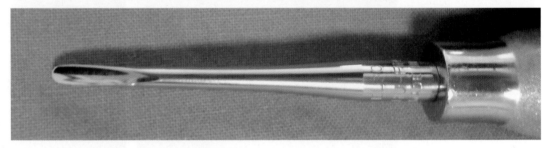

Hu-Friedy EL3C, this luxating elevator is thin and slightly curved. These features allow it engage well between the tooth and the buccal alveolar bone. No more explanation is needed. If you do not have this elevator, you are still a novice in extraction. I taught many wisdom teeth extractions lectures and hands-on courses. Everyone in the course was very satisfied and greatly appreciated to learn about this elevator.

This elevator is very sharp, so you need to be careful of using it. If you are used to create a deep trough on the buccal bone and use a 4S elevator to extract, it might be uncomfortable. If you are new to this elevator or a beginner for wisdom teeth extraction, I recommend getting an EL5C elevator as well. This has a 5 mm wider tip. Even if you have done many extractions before, I highly recommend getting the EL3C elevator this time. You can engage the bone most of the time without doing buccal trough on the lowerand you can use it on upper due to the curvature of the elevator

To improve accuracy, I often used mirror to place the elevator disto-buccally. If you are already used to use mirror to do dentistry, you may try. I even use a mirror during implant placement.

Dr. Jaewook Lee's comment

I want to ask those who think that the upper second molars do not get traumatized at all from the extraction of the upper third molars. In which case do you think would be easier to extract the third molar: when the second molar is present vs. missing?

02
How to use an elevator ★★★

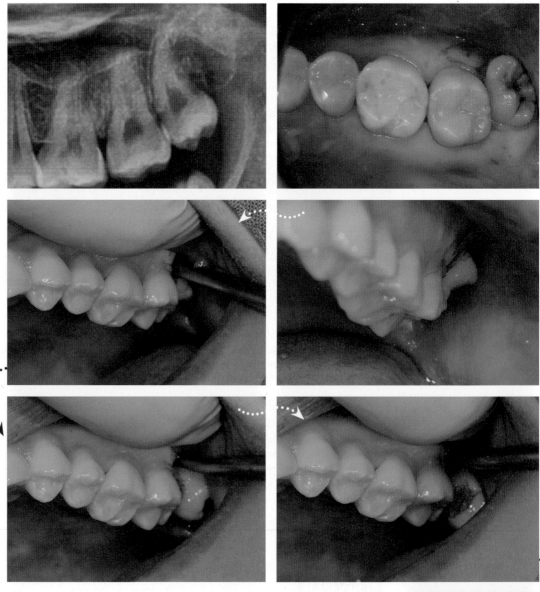

Basically, when you use an elevator to extract an upper wisdom tooth, you need to place an elevator between the alveolar bone and mesio-buccal of the tooth as shown in the pictures above. You need to be cautious to avoid damage to the distobuccal root of tooth #7. If you have extracted an upper second molar, you probably noticed how thin and weak the distobuccal root of the tooth is. Therefore, when wisdom teeth are fully erupted and you can grab the teeth with forceps, I usu-ally do not use an elevator. Alveolar bone and PDL is well established around fully erupted tooth, thus if you use an elevator, it can strain the surrounding tissue. An elevator plays an important role in the deeply impacted wisdom teeth. Forceps extraction is the first choice, but an elevator should supplement it.

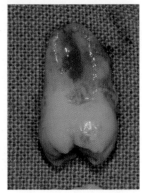

03
Placing an elevator between #7 and #8? ★★★

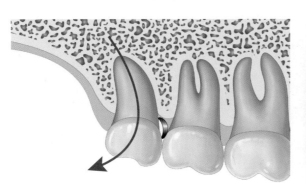
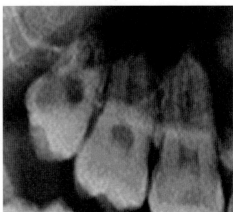

I have drawn a picture that was shown in some textbook. It is very dangerous to use an elevator like this. Of course, it is a bit less dangerous to place an elevator between #7 and #8 in upper than in lower. I used to like this technique when I was a beginner because the tooth comes out easily as I push #8 after placing an elevator between tooth #7 and tooth #8. However, this is not always the case. Less than 50% of cases did not cause any problems with this technique. The picture shows some alveolar bone between #7 and #8, but in most clinical cases, teeth #7 and 8 are in close proximity as shown in the right x-ray. It is because there is usually no space for #8 to erupt. You need to be careful of any damage to tooth #7 when you use an elevator.

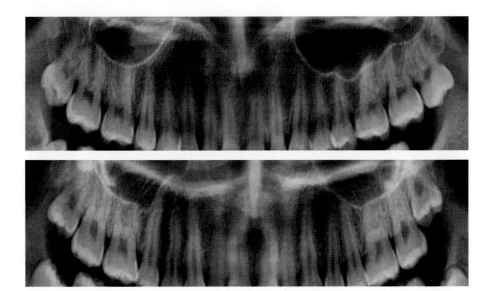

Let us look at these two cases of panoramic x-rays. In most cases, there is thin and weak alveolar bone between #7 and #8. When an elevator is placed between the two teeth, elevator is usually pushed deeply toward the roots and it can potentially cause a damage to the distobuccal root of the tooth #7.

04
When placing an elevator between #7 and #8 ★★

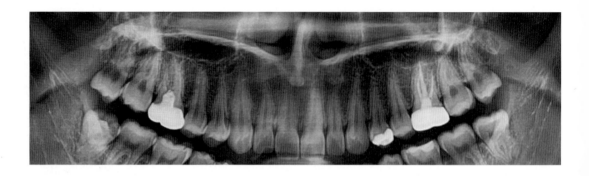

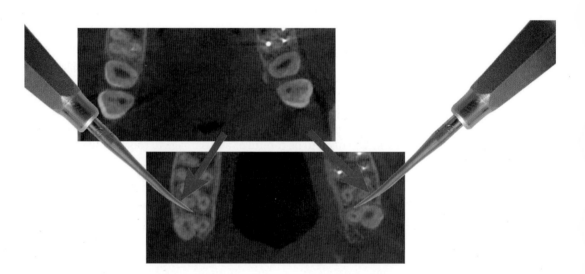

This is a CT scan that we saw earlier. This is a very common upper third molar case. It is slightly hyper-erupted and the crowns are located low. When we see the CT scan, the crown of the most wisdom teeth are located very close to the distobuccal root of tooth #7. The two last pictures demonstrate placing an elevator in between two teeth. The distobuccal roots become a fulcrum of the lever.

05
Elevator extraction on these wisdom teeth? ★★

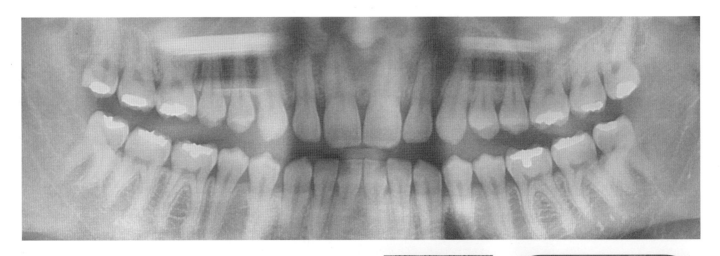

If you try to extract these wisdom teeth with an elevator, will this work? Before you extract the wisdom teeth, tooth #7 and #8 will break or crack. Elevators should only be used when you need light force to extract so you do not cause damage to the surrounding tissue. In this case, it will not be easy with forceps, either.

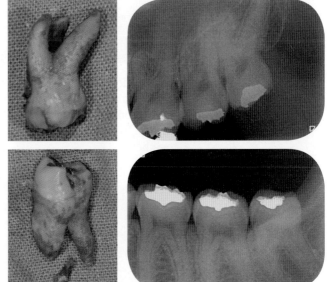

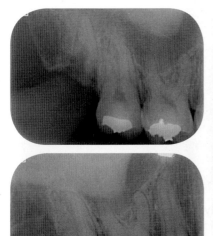

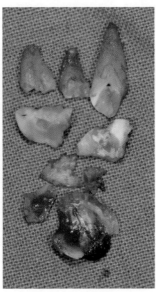

Let's take a look at this tooth #18 (US#1). In this case, I could not extract with forceps, so I cut the crown off and sectioned the roots to extract. Keep in mind; if you try to extract this tooth with an elevator, you will need to prepare #7 to be extracted as well. Some dentists give up the wisdom teeth extraction due to the post op sensitivity from the adjacent tooth.

06
Simple extraction that can be done w/ an elevator ★

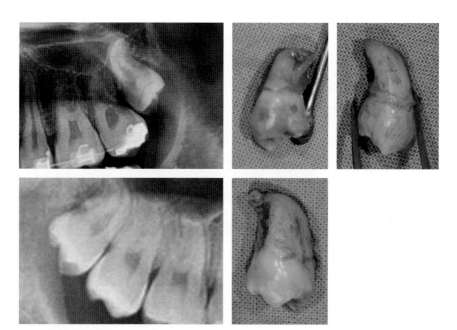

Cases which doesn't involve sectioning of a tooth, usually no photos are taken. There is no information regarding the extraction except the comparison between clinical and radiographic extracted tooth. When a tooth is below the plane of the occlusion, it is hard to grab the tooth with forceps. In this case, I tried to extract with an elevator, but I usually use an elevator and forceps together.

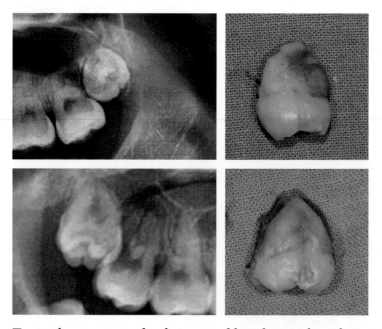

The teeth may appear deeply impacted but they are buccaly erupted. Buccaly erupted wisdom teeth are generally easier. In most cases, I give a slight incision distal to #7 with a No.12 scalpel. When a tooth is buccally erupted, it is possible the tooth can tear the gingiva as it comes out. I sometimes have to make a vertical incision and raise a mucoperiosteal flap. I rarely remove crestal bone and section the tooth.

Full Bony Impacted Third Molar Extraction

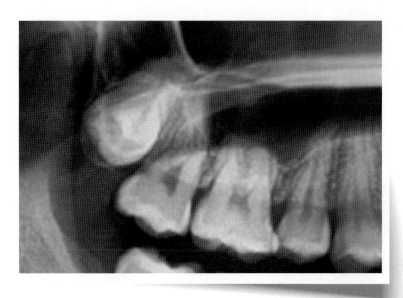

When a tooth is partially soft tissue impacted, I usually extract without any incision or give a small incision in the direction the tooth will come out. When the tooth is not shown in the oral cavity at all, incision is needed for extraction. For maxillary, the wisdom tooth is usually twisted and erupted buccally because of the dense palatal bone. For the same reason, the impacted tooth is generally located on the buccal side. Therefore, the incision is made on the buccal side and an elevator is to be placed mesio-buccal side of the wisdom tooth. Since the impacted wisdom tooth is pushed out distobuccally, you need consider the direction of the force and where to place an incision. If you are not confident in wisdom tooth extraction, I do not recommend trying extraction of a wisdom tooth located on the palatal side. However, once you start enjoying doing more challenging wisdom extraction cases, it's hard not to do these type of cases. Even for me, who has performed many extractions, I still have a little curiosity and little fear when I extract an upper impacted wisdom tooth. It might be because I cannot directly visualize and need to extract with my senses due to my spine problem. However, I still do many wisdom tooth extractions because I cannot forget the pleasure when my elevator gets in the right spot and tooth comes out.

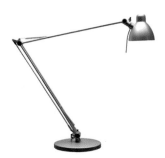

01
Flap design for the impacted maxillary wisdom teeth ★★★

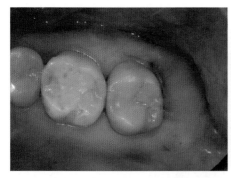
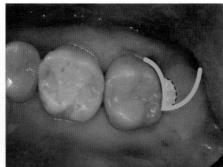

When the tooth is fully soft tissue impacted, it is important to make an incision. If a part of the wisdom tooth is throughout the gingiva, we can logically guess its location, therefore, this is an important parameter when deciding difficulty of wisdom tooth extractions. When I am busy, I sometimes do not make an incision, but the soft tissue around the maxillary wisdom teeth are weak and easily torn, so it is better to give an incision in the direction you want.

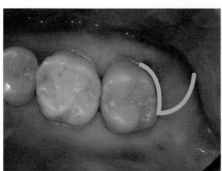
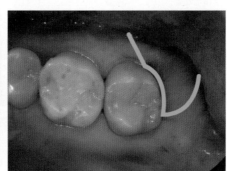

This shows general flap designs for the impacted maxillary wisdom teeth. My first rule is to make a small incision, so I give a small incision to the distal surface. When the tooth is located buccally or if the crown is large, I give a vertical incision on the buccal side. Otherwise, the gingiva on this area can be torn frequently.

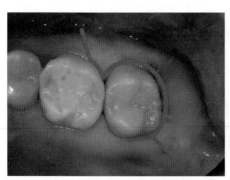
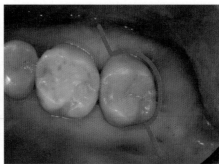

When the tooth is palatally located or the crown is large, incisions needs to be made on the palatal side. Additionally, when the patient has thick gingiva, you will need to make a larger incision. Sometimes you need to make an incision on the palatal side as shown in the picture. When I do not make an incision on the palatal side, I often see soft tissue torn, just like the drawing. Remember, it is better to make an incision than the tissue getting torn unintentionally.

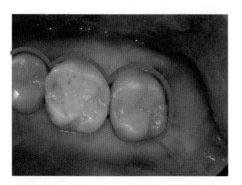

I do not prefer this design but I often see some dentists extend the incision mesially instead of vertically. Many dentists seem to be more familiar to vertical incisions during implant surgeries. Even when an incision is not on the palatal side, if you separate the gingiva from the bone on the palatal side, it helps for the extraction. When I am busy, I sometimes use the sharp and thin EL3C elevator to separate the gingiva from the tooth or bone. However, surgical curette or periosteal elevator is generally used to raise a flap by utilizing class II lever motion.

02
Complete bony impacted wisdom extraction <1> ★★

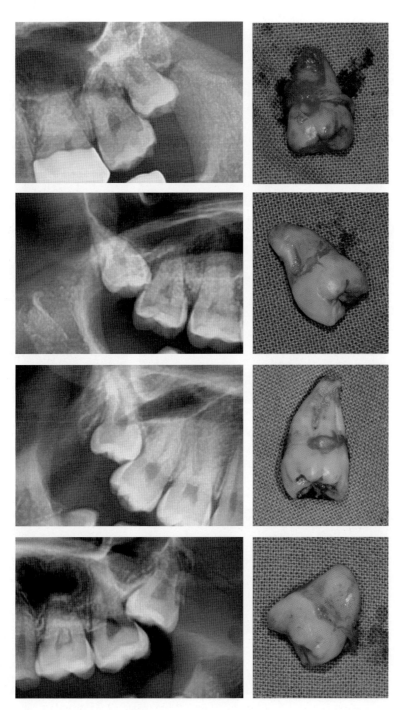

There are not many differences between soft tissue impacted tooth extraction and this. It seems to be correct to say that it comes out as it breaks the alveolar bone on the disto buccal side. Most of time, there is not much resistance and it can be extracted with little effort. However, sometimes it has more resistance, but it is important not to use excessive force. You should not use excessive force to place the elevator into the space between the tooth and bone. It is not good to use excessive force after placing it either. If there is more resistance, first consider making a larger incision and flap.

Complete bony impacted wisdom extraction <2> ★

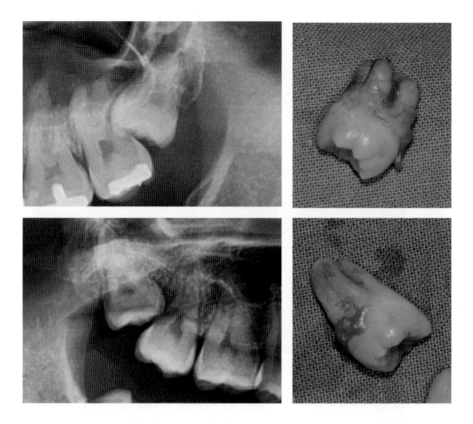

In fact, there are too many cases like these. There are not many pictures of these cases, as the teeth were not sectioned.

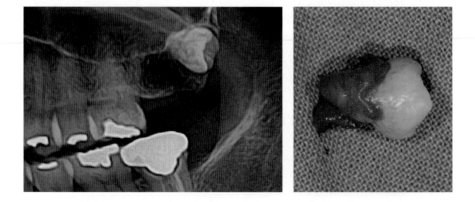

The above case was referred to me for #28(US#16) extraction. Tooth was located bucally. Flap was raised and an elevator was used to remove the bone around the tooth and the extraction was completed.

Complete bony impacted wisdom extraction <3> ★★

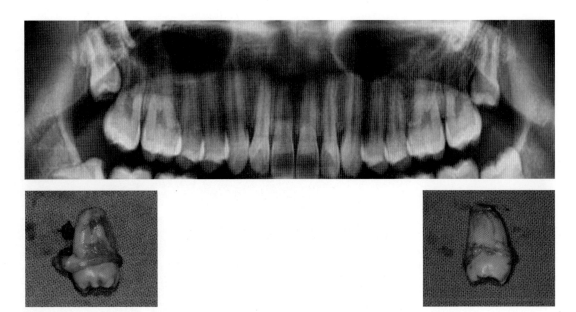

Upper wisdom teeth extraction was referred for non-surgical orthodontic treatment. To tell you in advance, this is my favorite type of extractions. Immature wisdom tooth has incomplete roots, so you can extract simply with an elevator after a small incision. Elevator needs to be placed in mesiobuccal of the tooth. In any case, the elevator should not engage the tooth #7. You also need to check if #7 moves as the wisdom tooth comes out. Occurrence is rare.

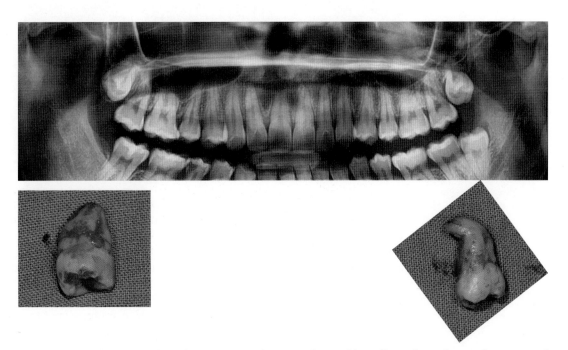

You do not need any bone removal in this case. Tooth #28 is located bucally and can be easily extracted after distal incision on #27 and small vertical incision. The alveolar bone on the occlusal and distal surface of the tooth is thin and weak, so it can break easily and the tooth can be extracted easily. Of course, some mucoperiosteal flap is needed on the buccal side.

03
Three complete bony impacted wisdom teeth extraction in a day

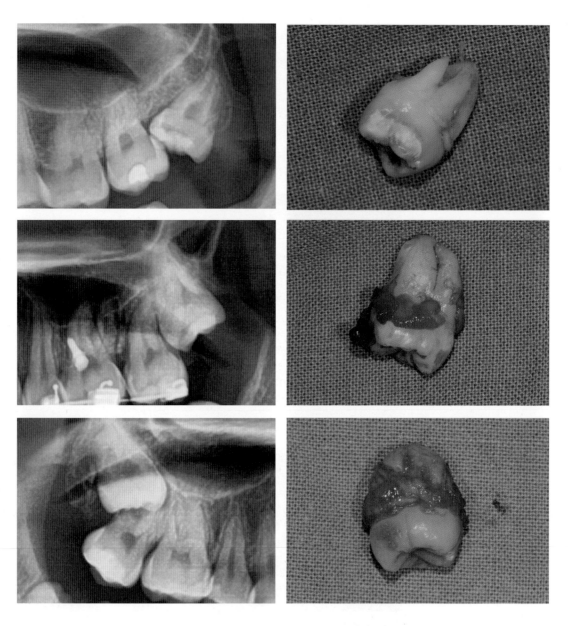

There were three complete bony impacted wisdom teeth extraction in a row. Upper complete bony impaction is not very frequent but when they come, they all come to the clinic on the same day. All these cases were straightforward. It seems like some dentists do not prefer the upper impacted tooth extraction because they are not familiar with it, but once you get used to this, they are very straightforward and easy. In fact, you need to cut the impacted mandibular third molars in certain ways to extract but you can extract the impacted maxillary third molars with an elevator easily for most cases. There are rarely hard cases. When they are located on buccal side, access to the tooth is good and removal of the buccal alveolar bone is not too bad, either.

04
Different elevator I occasionally use ★★

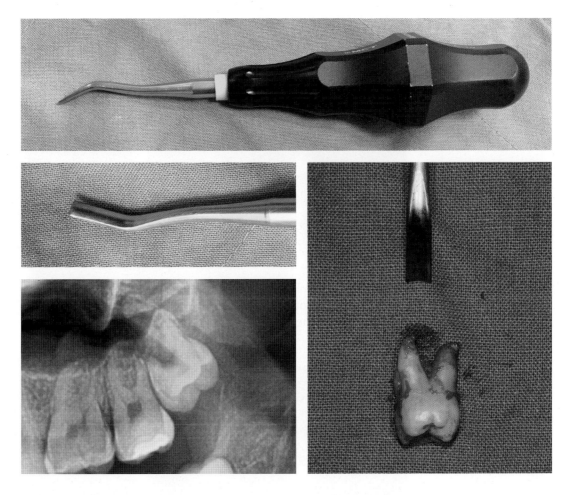

This is an elevator I occasionally use. I use this one when it is hard to grab the tooth with forceps and the angle is not good with the EL3C elevator. I usually get inexpensive elevators for this purpose. I do not use it often, therefore, durability is not an issue. I would rather get different kinds of this elevator and use it when access to the area is different than usual. I can just throw away these inexpensive elevators when they bend or break. You should understand why I included the elevator next to the tooth in the picture.

I bought this on the internet shopping mall "www.2875mart.co.kr". They have a wide variety of elevators. I buy instruments that do not need a lot of strength and high performance (such as scalpel holder, periosteal elevator, unusual elevators or forceps that I don't use often) from the shopping mall.

05
Useful in the carious tooth extraction ★★

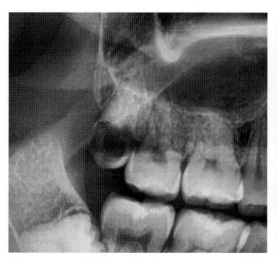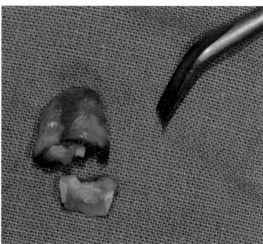

Case of a 31-year-old male patient: I could not use forceps due to the large caries lesion of the crown. EL3C did not engage well on the mesio-buccal side of the tooth. I used a highly curved elevator to extract the tooth.

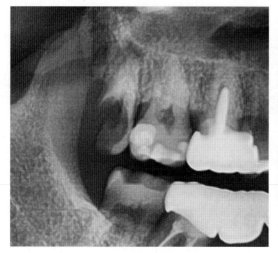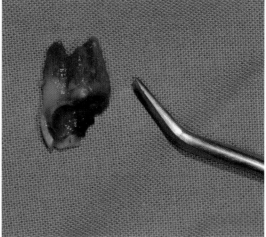

Case of a 35-year-old male patient: I could not use forceps due to the caries lesion. I thought EL3C can fracture the crown so I used the curved elevator to place it deeply to the root and pushed the tooth to buccal side. You can see no damage to the thin and carious enamel of the crown because the elevator did not engage on the crown.

Dr. Jaewook Lee's comment

I recommend using a thick root picker when a general elevator does not engage like in this case.

06
Alveolar bone removal during the upper third molar extraction ★★

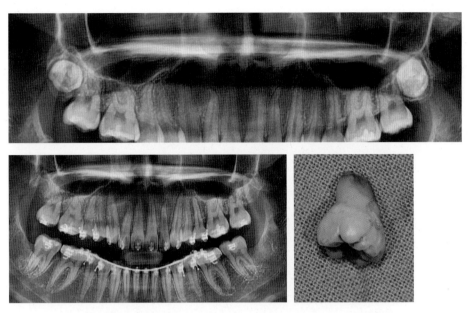

This is a case that I removed the alveolar bone to extract #18(US#1). I do not have a picture for #28. Most of the time, the staff will only take a picture of the teeth that I section. They probably forgot to take this one.

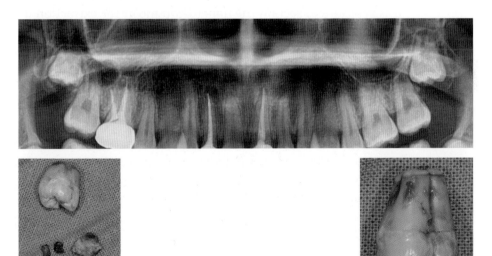

I usually use a bone rongeur to remove upper alveolar bone. I used to have a bad mindset that using a slow-speed handpiece makes you look like a beginner, so I used to use a high-speed handpiece for upper alveolar bone removal. Even if I raise a minimal flap, emphysema is a concern. I use high-speed handpieces less often now. I try to use a wide variety of good instruments. I am considering to start using chisels.

Upper Third Molar Section ★

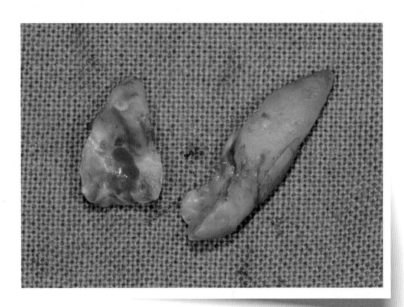

It is very rare to section the upper third molar for extraction. Most of the time, you can extract the tooth with minor removal of buccal and distal alveolar bone. I used to think extracting wisdom teeth by sectioning them was more skillful, so I used to extract them by always sectioning them. Since my back pain got worse due to the spinal problem, I try not to do a procedure that takes too long. It is even challenging to maintain posture for the upper third molar extractions, so I extract the tooth with alveolar bone removal nowadays. I even start to use a bone rongeur and chisel or even an elevator to remove the alveolar bone more often than handpiece. Especially, the technique of maxillary wisdom teeth extraction is very different depending on the surgeon. However, when you try to extract the wisdom teeth and if you feel #7 is moving, it is not a bad idea to cut the crown of the wisdom teeth. These cases are old — when I used to like to section the crown. It is just for reference. I hope you never follow this and use a high-speed handpiece to section the crown.

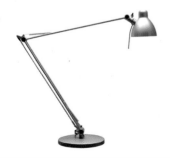

01
Slow-speed straight handpiece in maxillary third molar extraction ★★

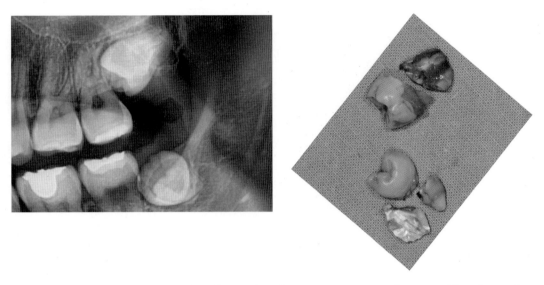

When a lower wisdom tooth is distally angulated, I sometimes use a slow-speed handpiece from the mesial buccal side and cut the crown. In this case, I try to set up simply so I use the same slow hanpiece to extract the upper wisdom tooth as well.

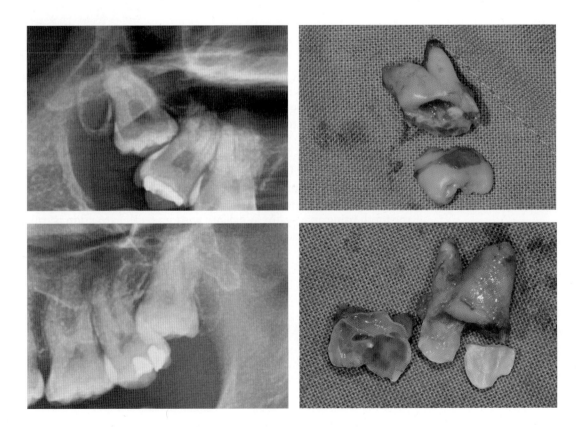

When using a slow-speed, you cut the crown from the side unlike doing vertical cuts with a high-speed, so you will see the cross section like the picture above.

02
Case I extracted by removing the alveolar bone near the occlusal plane

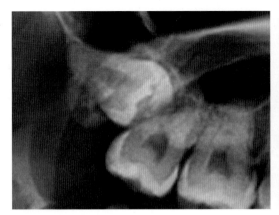

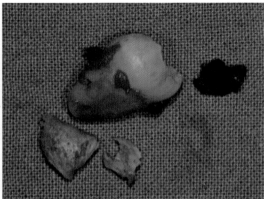

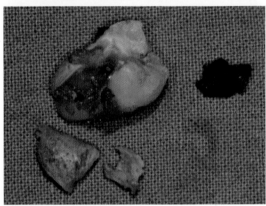

I told the patient it is not necessary to extract this one, but the patient really insisted on extracting it before returning to the US. If this type of tooth is located on the buccal side, it will be easier but the crown of the tooth was located on the palatal side. It is hard, especially for people like me who cannot lean due to a spinal problem. The surgery lasted 35 minutes. It probably took the longest time in the last 500 wisdom teeth extractions. I was deciding whether I should remove the buccal bone and lift or if I should section the tooth in half. In the end, I did neither. The handpiece was not accessible at all. Moreover, the bone underneath the sinus was thin, I was afraid to push the tooth into the sinus. I made an indentation on the tooth with a handpiece and pulled the tooth using an elevator. Maxillary wisdom teeth extraction is usually easier than mandibular wisdom teeth extraction, but you still need to slow down and extract gently.

03
High-speed handpiece in maxillary third molar extraction ★

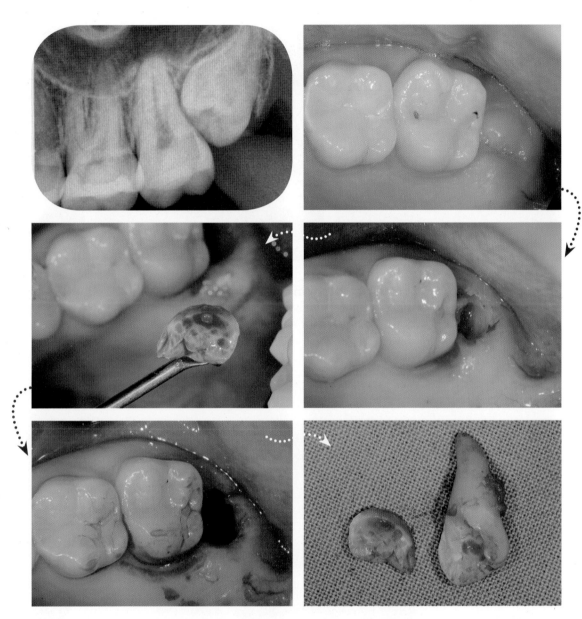

In this case I extracted the mesially angulated maxillary wisdom teeth with a similar technique I used for the mandibular wisdom tooth. In fact, the alveolar bone around the upper third molar is softer than the lower and can be pushed distally. However, since I am good at handling a high-speed handpiece, I just used a high-speed hand piece to extract without raising a flap. Also, I extract the upper wisdom tooth after lower, so I cut the mesial crown to extract with the high-speed handpiece that I used for lower. I use a high-speed handpiece less often for upper wisdom teeth nowadays and I am trying to use different instruments. I do not recommend using a high-speed handpiece for the beginners. If you need to use this method, you can try with the 1:5 contra angle slow-speed handpiece I showed earlier. As I mentioned earlier, flapless surgery needs to be done by a surgeon, who has performed many dento-alveolar surgeries that does not need to raise a flap.

04
Same high-speed handpiece after lower impacted wisdom tooth extraction

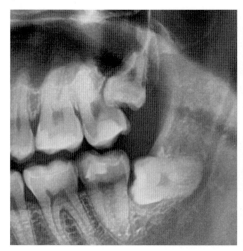 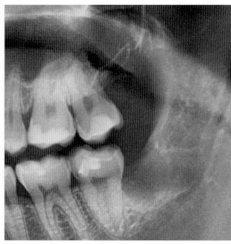 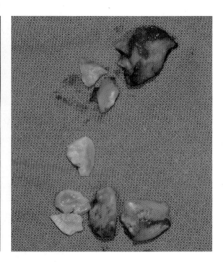

I cut the mesial crown of the upper wisdom tooth to extract with a high-speed, which I used for the lower horizontally impacted tooth. When I am only extracting upper wisdom teeth extraction, I do not ask for a high-speed handpiece. As I said earlier, I am too busy to spend time like that.

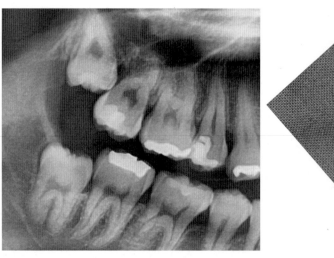 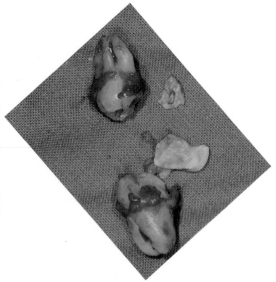

After the distal crown of the lower tooth was sectioned to extract, I used the same handpiece to cut the mesial crown of the upper tooth to extract. The direction of the lower wisdom tooth in the picture is not correct. If our staff took better pictures, we will have more cases. If you are not the dentist who extracted the tooth, it is difficult to visualize how the tooth was extracted by only looking at the picture.

05
Similar technique I use for lower wisdom teeth extraction ★

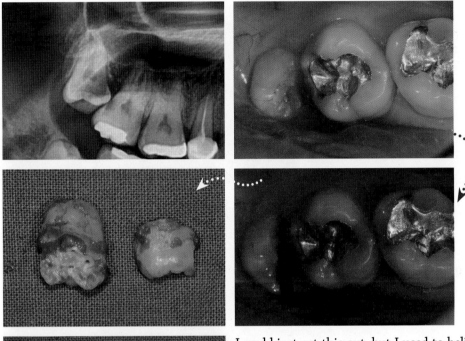

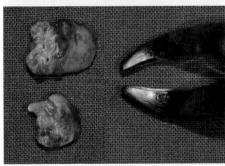

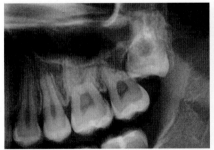

I could just get this out, but I used to believe only using a high-speed handpeice is the only right way to extract. Forceps are in the picture, which means I removed the mesial crown with a high-speed handpiece and extracted the rest of the tooth with forceps.

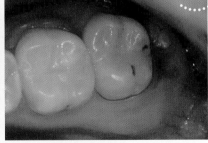

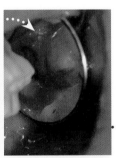

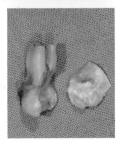

When sectioning the mesial crown, I check the cutting surface as I proceed. In fact, I could have just extracted this tooth with an elevator.

06
High-speed handpiece for mesial angulated wisdom teeth extraction

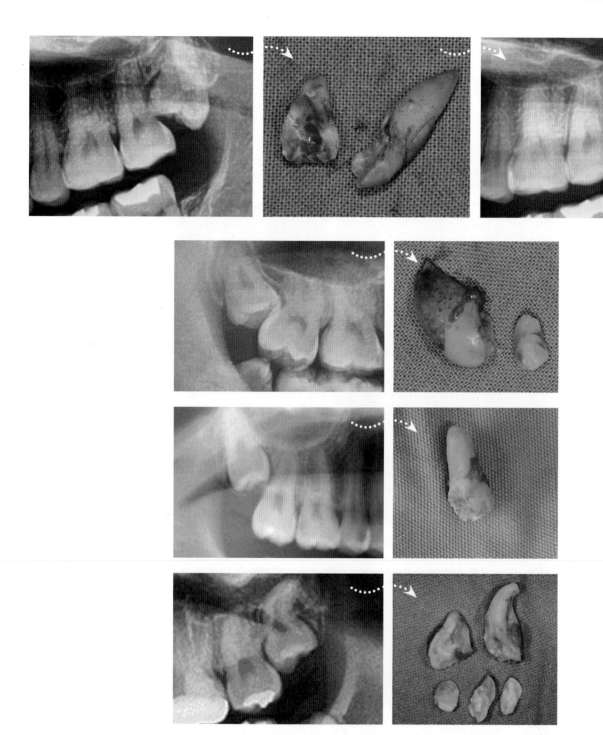

I do not use this technique often anymore, but if contra-angle slow-speed is used frequently for extraction like in Japan, this technique can be handy.

07
When it's clearly caught under the distal of the tooth #7 ★

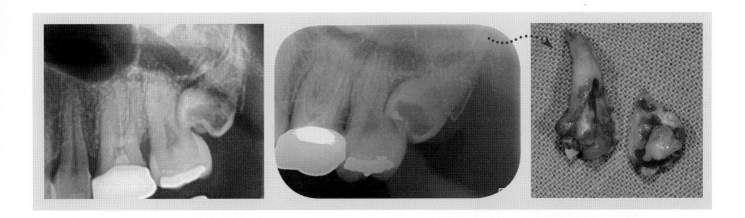

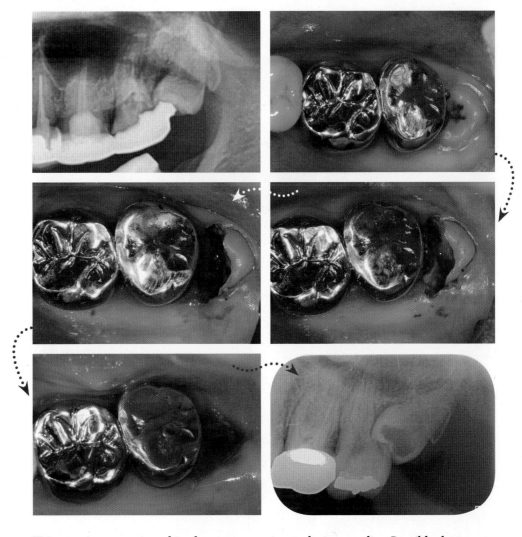

This case was mentioned in the crown cutting technique earlier. Possible damage to the tooth can be expected during extraction using an elevator due to the large overhang of the restoration on #7. I extracted after removing the mesial crown of the wisdom tooth.

08
Travelling extraction

I had lectured a seminar in different area in the past. I have met a e dentist who was interested in the lecture and stopped by my clinic several times. He seemed to be comfortable with implants, prosthetics and surgical extractions. However, he had some fear of the impacted maxillary wisdom teeth extraction. So I decided to stop by his clinic, helped extraction and went to the seminar together when I traveled to that area.

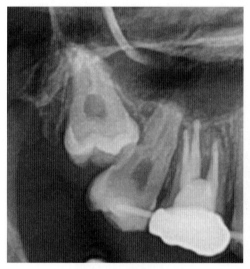
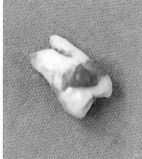

This patient was a staff member of his office. The dentist decided to extract the tooth before proceeding with other treatments. I extracted the tooth while the owner dentist was standing next to me. Even if it was not deeply impacted, it had a large undercut and there was a large amount of alveolar bone distal to the tooth. If this was located buccally, it would have been an easier procedure, but it was located on the palatal side. I believe this was the reason why the owner dentist had asked for my help. I elevated carefully and gently from mesio-buccal side. You need to go slow and gentle in these cases

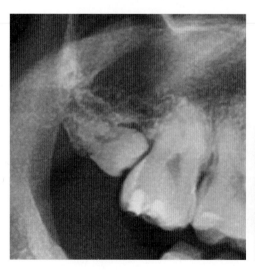
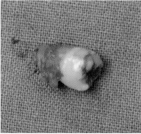

his case was his regular patient. I saw some calculus on the extracted tooth and possibly there was some inflammation. There is not a large undercut and bone distal to the tooth, but it was located on the palatal side. It looks like there is some thick bone under the sinus floor in the panoramic x-ray, but the sinus floor was as thin as 1mm in CBCT. It was not only thin near the roots but all over the tooth. Since I did not want to cause a problem in his clinic, I tried not to push the tooth in the sinus or break the sinus floor. Again, I elevated the tooth out carefully and gently from mesio-buccal side.

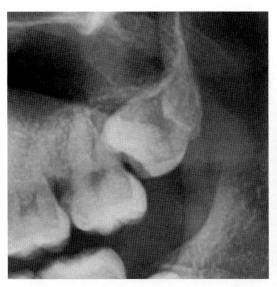 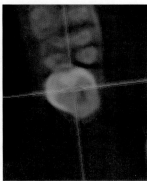

This last case was completed by the doctor after shadowing two previous cases. When you see the CT, you can see the crown is located on the palatal side. I was in his office in case he would need my help.. He soon came back and told me he was done. He told me he used a high-speed handpiece to cut crown as he does in lower wisdom teeth. I told him to be really careful when using a high-speed handpiece on upper wisdom teeth and recommended to use 1:5 contra-angle slowspeed if he was not comfortable with straight slow-speed handpiece. He treated me with a dinner after closing the office and went to my lecture together. I used to travel to other offices for implant placements and extractions when I first opened my practice, but I stopped after the implant procedure became really cheap. It reminded the pleasure of helping fellow dentists again.

Extractions of Maxillary Supernumerary Teeth

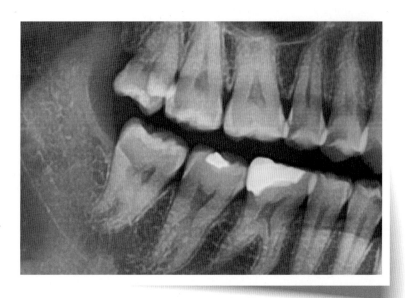

There can be a supernumerary tooth in any area including the area near wisdom teeth. If you have extracted many wisdom teeth, you will know that wisdom teeth have many anatomical variations in shape and size, also has supernumerary tooth around it. You will especially see a cuspid size supernumerary teeth around the maxillary wisdom teeth frequently. I am not sure if designating a tooth ID for this supernumerary is necessary, but I will call it as a 4th molar. It usually needs an additional explanation when billing insurance. It is not difficult to extract this, but since this was not covered in other places, I will discuss it briefly here.

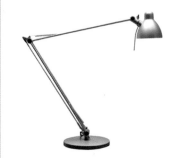

01
4th molar? ★

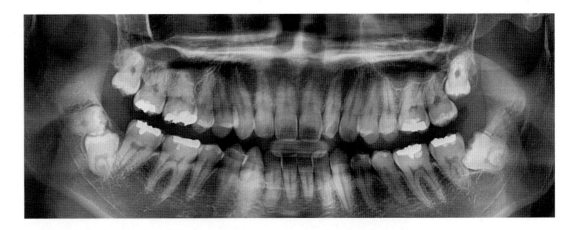

There can be a supernumerary tooth in any area including the area near wisdom teeth. I am not sure if designating a tooth ID for this supernumerary is necessary, but I will call it as a 4th molar or Tooth #9. It is seen more often in maxillary than mandibular but it can certainly appear in mandible just like the panoramic x-ray shown above. I see them frequently, perhaps because I do so many wisdom teeth extraction.

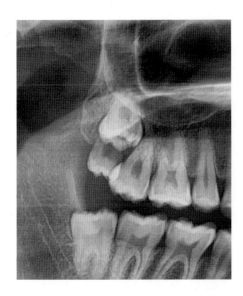

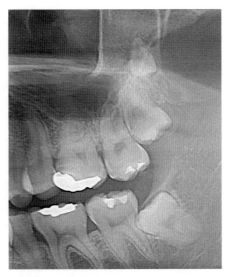

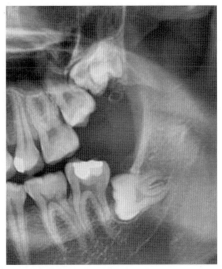

From my experience, I see supernumerary teeth more often in the maxillary than in the mandible. This might be related to the occurrence of more anatomical variations of maxillary wisdom teeth.

Since we see the 4th molar arising from the 3rd molar tooth bud, the 4th molar is usually small. Even if I do not have many pictures of these teeth because my staff only takes pictures when I section the teeth, the 4th molar teeth are quite common. Most of them are located buccal or distal to the third molar. When it is superimposed to the 3rd molar on the buccal side, it is not easily seen in a panoramic x-ray.

It is little hard to call this a 4th molar, but it certainly shows two crowns in the picture. For maxillary wisdom teeth, it is common to have an extra cusp or germination. It often makes extraction difficult.

02
4th molar extraction cases <1> ★

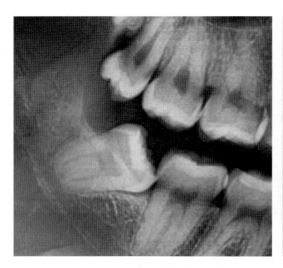 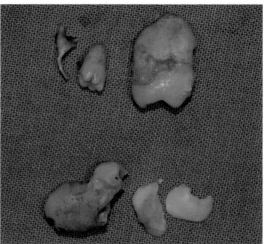

This case is regarding a 26-year-old female patient. It is common to see the 4th molar in the maxilla. It is usually small, so extraction is completed together with the 3rd molar.

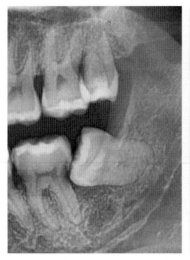 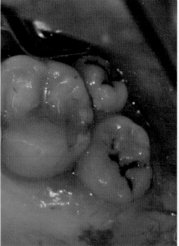 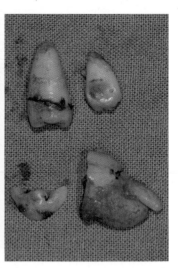

This case is regarding a 41-year-old male patient. It was completed together with the lower third molar. As you can see, it appears buccal and distal to third molar. I elevated the supernumerary tooth and extracted the third molar on the palatal side with the small forceps.

4th molar extraction cases <2> ★

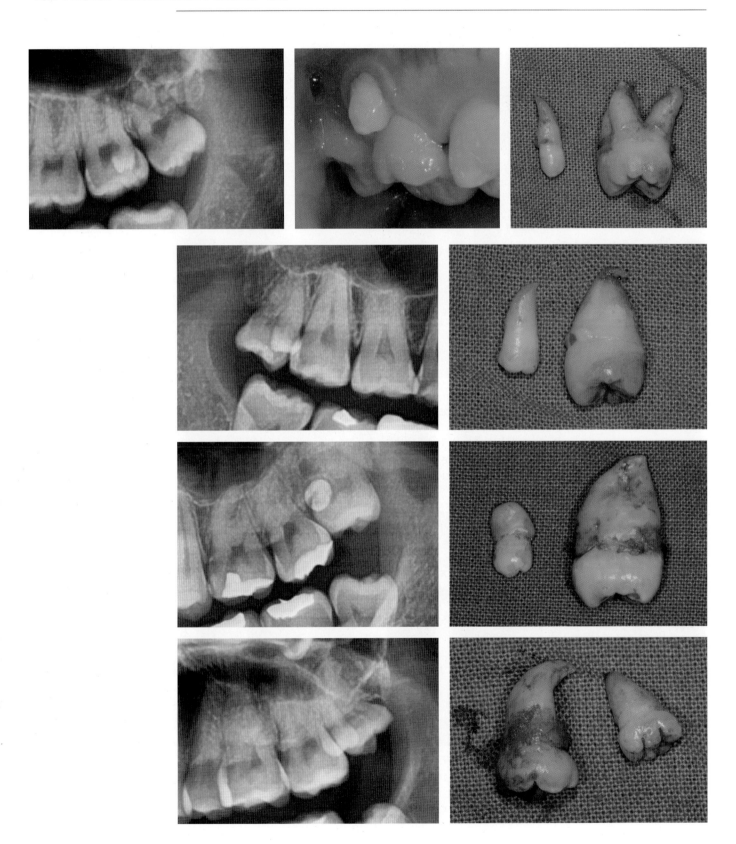

03
Case that I intentionally left the 4th molar ★

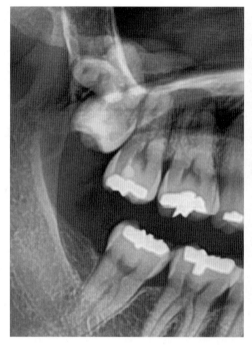 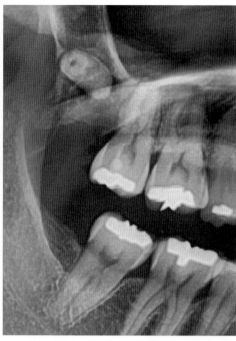 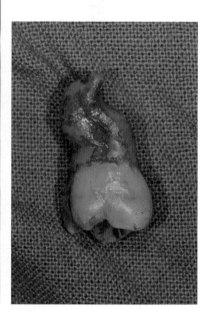

This patient is a 31-year-old female who came to the clinic for the upper right wisdom tooth extraction. When the panoramic x-ray was reviewed, I noticed the 4th molar supernumerary tooth. Patient did not want the tooth to be extracted if it would not become problematic in the future, so we decided to leave it. I was also busy that day and the tooth was located right underneath the sinus floor, so extraction was not recommended either.

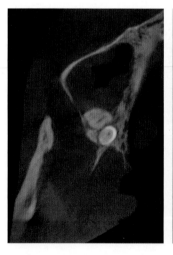 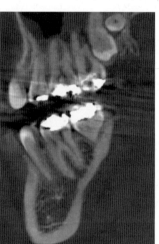 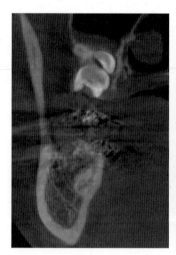 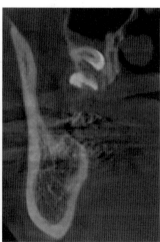

CBCT scan shows that the tooth is horizontally impacted right underneath the sinus floor and the crown is toward the palatal side. Even if she really wished for the extraction, I would hesitate to perform the procedure.

04
The fifth molar ★

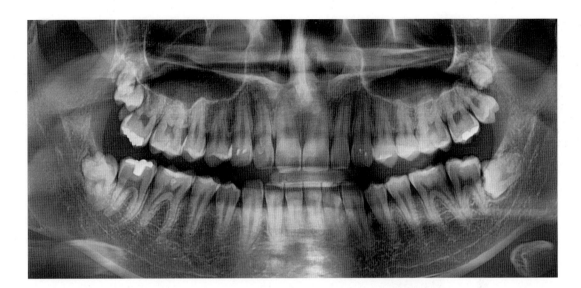

A 23-year-old male patient came to the clinic for all wisdom teeth extraction. He had 7 wisdom teeth. There were 3rd molar, 4th molar and 5th molar on the upper right, and 3rd molar and 4th molar on the left. Patient wanted to extract xxthe right wisdom teeth first, so we extracted the #18, #19 and #20 after #48. The fifth molar is pretty rare even for me who extracts a lot of wisdom teeth.

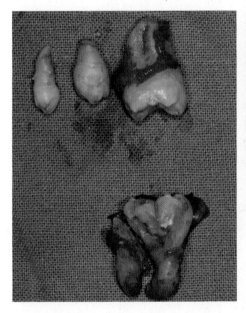

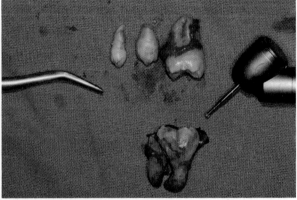

A 23-year-old male patient came to the clinic for all wisdom teeth extraction. He had 7 wisdom teeth. There were 3rd molar, 4th molar and 5th molar on the upper right, and 3rd molar and 4th molar on the left. Patient wanted to extract the right wisdom teeth first, so we extracted the #18, #19 and #20 after #48. The fifth molar is pretty rare even for me who extracts a lot of wisdom teeth.

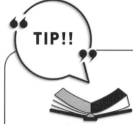

TIP!!

Anatomical variation in upper molars

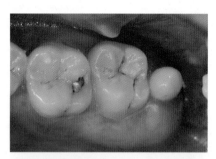

It looks like they are two completely separate teeth in this picture. Anatomical variation is common in upper molars and they show up in different shapes and sizes. It is sometimes hard to tell if it is a separate tooth or an extra cusp.

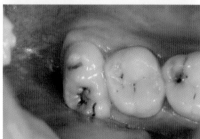

This is a developed cusp on the upper molar. The first picture shows two separate teeth and this one is clearly a cusp on the upper molar. However, it is sometimes hard to distinguish between a separate tooth or an extra cusp.

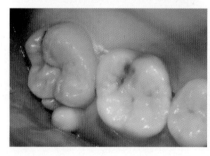 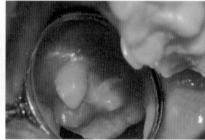

This is a clinical photo from my old lecture material. I could not find the x-ray. I first thought this was a supernumerary tooth and tried to extract. I actually numbed the patient and tried to extract the tooth. During the procedure, I realized that it was actually an extra cusp. Fortunately, we figured this out before it was extracted.

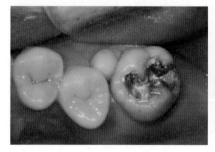 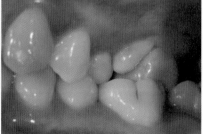

It is hard to distinguish if it is a supernumerary tooth clinically or radiographically. You can try to place floss through the area to confirm. It was an extra cusp in this case.

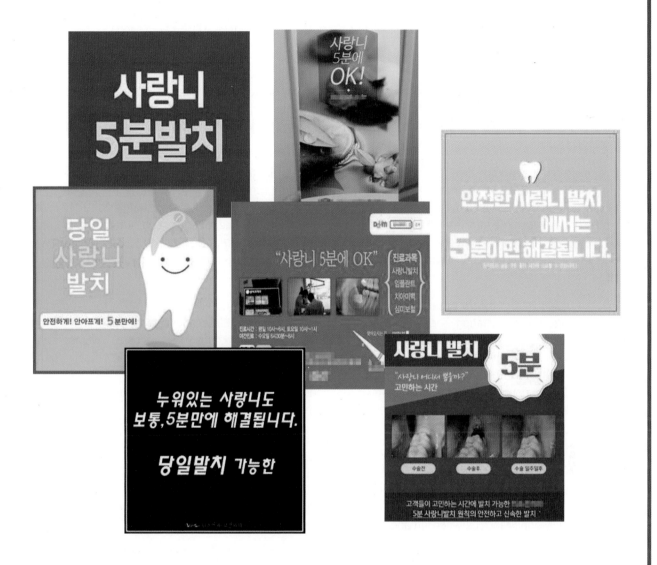

These are some advertisements from the South Korea Dental office offering third molar extractions. Some dentists may think these are false advertising. I do not advertise as this but they can certainly advertise in this way. Even if there are different ways to measure the time spent on the wisdom tooth extraction, it does not take more than 5 minutes for me. Though I do not advertise in this way or speak to patient in this manner.

Of course extraction is the only procedure that patients will truly appreciate when completed quickly. I still think this is not appropriate to just focus on the time and appeal to the patients with this.

However, these advertisements show the dentists who hesitate to offer third molar extraction that third molar extraction is no longer a time-consuming or headache inducing procedure.

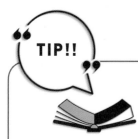

TIP!!

Average time spent on the wisdom tooth extraction?

How long would it take for a wisdom tooth extraction? I have seen some advertisements saying <5 minutes wisdom tooth extraction> on the Internet or on SNS. They seem to compete with each other and I recently saw another advertisement saying <3 minutes extraction>. Perhaps patients or other dentists think that is a false advertisement, but I think this is completely feasible.

I have measured the average time for wisdom tooth extraction several times. I thought it does not help the procedure or seem ethical to patients, so I do not do it often. However, I became curious how other dentists measure their time spent on extraction after seeing the advertisements. When I was finishing up with this book in summer of 2017, I decided to measure the average time for the wisdom tooth extraction (excluding the time for anesthesia, suture) again. I recommend you to try once. However, you need to set a rule. If you are trying to measure, I recommend you try with the way I used. When you try to measure, you will encounter with the similar issues I had, so it might be a good idea to follow the way I used.

The recent result is from the 75 patients (male 30, female 45), (Maxillary 44, and Mandibular 75) for 10 days in a manner of the complete enumeration. The average time for the extraction was 109 seconds (Standard Deviation 136 seconds, minimum to maximum: 10 seconds ~ 690 seconds, confidence interval: 85 seconds ~ 134 seconds). Average for upper extraction was 27 seconds (SD 103 seconds), lower extraction was 157 seconds (SD 137 seconds). To simplify this, I took average of 1 minute 49 seconds for 119 wisdom teeth extraction. The longest one was 11 minutes 30 seconds, average was 27 seconds for the upper extraction and 2 minutes 37 seconds for the lower extraction. The standard deviation is large because difference in time depends on the wisdom teeth. In confidence level, I can take 95% of wisdom teeth in 2 minutes 14 seconds.

In statistical writing, the average time for the upper third molar extraction was 27.27 +/- 102.55 seconds and the average time for the lower third molar extraction was 157.33 +/- 129.99 seconds. There was a statically significant increase in time for the lower third molar extraction. ($P<.01$). The average for the upper third molar extraction on male patients was 10.28 +/- 1.18 seconds, on female patients was 39.04 +/- 133.18 seconds, but it was not statically significant ($P=.367$). There was no statically significance between left and right third molar extraction in different gender ($P=.804$).

Most dentists might think this is not possible. However, if the dentist has performed many third molar extractions, he or she might think they can get a better result. In fact, there are many dentists who can extract as fast as this or even faster. I have not had many extractions recently and sometime when there are more extraction cases, I become faster. I think I had the best result as I was preparing the book and reviewing all the techniques, but I am sure there are many dentists in my country whom can extract faster; they just do not speak up like me. I guarantee there will be readers of this book who can extract faster in near future.

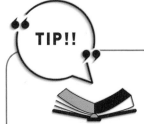

The rules for measuring extraction time for Dr. Youngsam Kim

▬▬ Exclude the time used for anesthesia and suture

It is less painful when giving the injection slowly. If it includes suture time, you might be tempted to finish the case without suturing when it was indicated. This would not be good for patient.

▬▬ Sample size should at least be 100 patients.

Otherwise, the sample can be only simple cases. 100 cases are large enough to include hard cases as well. Do not reject any case.

▬▬ Include every case on the day you start and end.

I wanted to exclude a case in the morning if it took long and start including a simple case or do not want to extract the difficult one on the last day. I might need to adjust the start and end day but all the cases on the day need to be included.

▬▬ Minimum time is 10 sec

It sometimes takes less than 10 seconds, but if you do not set a minimum time, you might rush placing instruments to mouth. You do not want to make the 1% case that makes you sad while trying to measure your average time.

▬▬ Once the tooth is out of the socket, consider this as extracted.

When I see other dentists measuring their extraction time and when the tooth is attached to the little tissue or near the tongue or throat, they can rush the assistants to suction or recklessly use the cotton pliers to take out. It does not take long, but it can rush you, so I decided to exclude this.

▬▬ Do not ask for experienced assistants or new instruments.

It takes less when assisted by an experienced assistant or when using new burs or instruments. However, if I keep asking this, it might interfere with other procedures and other doctors. In fact, I was with a new assistant who recently graduated most of time when we were measuring.

▬▬ Do not include the time the assistant went to back to get another instrument.

If not, I can rush the assistant to run and grab fast. That is not good either.

▬▬ Do not include the time that we had to spend to repair a handpiece during the procedure.

It is rare, but it happens. Handpieces sometimes stops working, the dental chair might not move, the headlight can suddenly go off, or the suction stops working. In this case, you do not want to blame each other, so I decided to exclude this time. I have had couple times the handpiece stopped spinning during the measurement of the extraction time.

▬▬ Include the time if I have to anesthetize the patient more during the procedure.

If I have to anesthetize the patient more, I include the time. Giving profound anesthesia is an important skill set you need to be competent, so I included it.t.

05
Dr. Jeff Lim's visit from Australia ★★

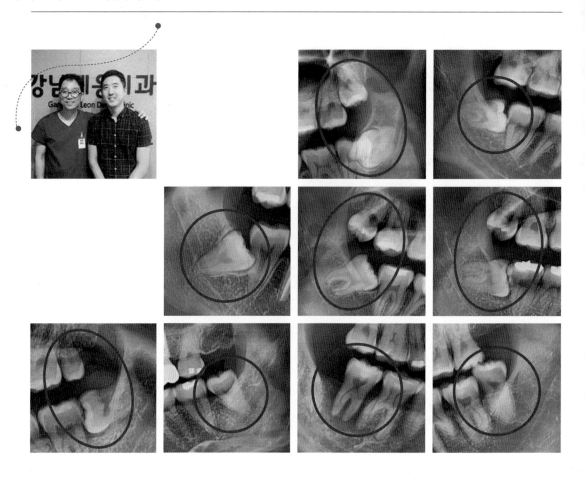

Since Spring 2018, I have been in Los Angles planning to be in USA for couple years. I still had to go back to South Korea once or twice a month to take care of some patients. During the time, a Korean-Australian dentist wanted to visit my office. I welcome any dentist to visit our office, so we often had many dentists not just from other cities, but from other countries as well. I usually see many implant patients when I go back to Korea because the fee schedule for wisdom teeth extraction is terribly low. Since the dentist was visiting us, I decided to take all wisdom teeth cases for the new patients of the day. We had lunch together and he spent morning and afternoon in the office. I took 13 wisdom teeth from 8 patients while seeing other patients. This was a typical day for me and I asked what he thinks about the visit. He answered that he has not measured the time spent on wisdom teeth extraction, but it seems like I take less on extraction than giving anesthesia and suturing. I usually ask Korean dentists to give anesthesia so they can look at the wisdom teeth. I think he was just answering this way because I was jokingly whining about that he did not have a Korean dental license to help me giving anesthesia.

Common Problems related to Extractions of Third Molars

10
CHAPTER

Chapter 10 translated by

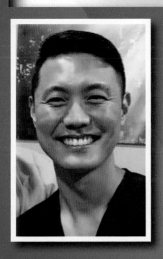

Dr. Joung Lee DMD

Dr. Joung Lee was originally born in South Korea and came to the U.S. at the age of 23. Dr. Lee earned his Bachelor's of Science degree in Chemistry from Georgia Tech with highest honors. He completed his Doctorate of Dental Medicine at the Nova Southeastern University School of Dental Medicine in Florida. He graduated with oral surgery honor and won the award from Academy of General Dentistry. Following his move to San Antonio, Texas, he has worked in private practices as a general dentist. He also teaches dentists at Dr. Kim's live surgery course in Tijuana, Mexico as one of the instructors.

Dr. Joung Lee earned his Bachelor's of Science degree in biochemistry from Georgia Tech with the highest honor. He completed his Doctor of Dental Medicine at Nova Southeastern University School of Dental Medicine in Florida with oral surgery honor and won the Academy of General Dentistry Award. Following his move to San Antonio, Texas, he has worked in private practices as a general dentist and teaches a live surgery course in Tijuana, Mexico with Dr. Kim.

01
Fracture of surgical round burs ★★★

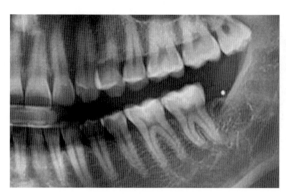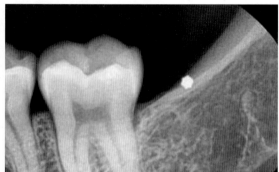

A fractured surgical round bur was noticed from this preoperative panoramic radiograph when the patient presented for maxillary third molar extractions. The patient reported that the previous extraction that resulted in this incident was performed about a year ago. The retained fragment was removed uneventfully, but I don't have a clinical photo of it since it was suctioned when being removed.

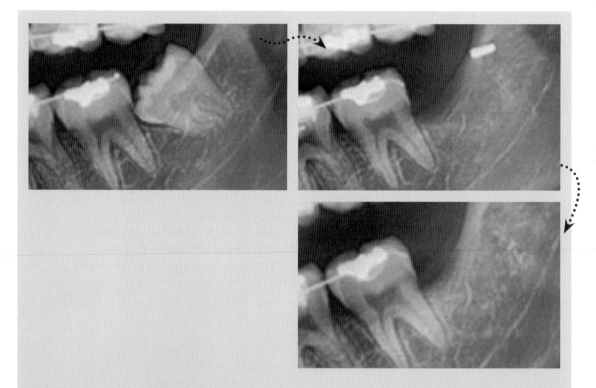

This is a case that a slow speed surgical fissure bur was fractured and retained. This patient was originally referred from my associate orthodontist, and the extraction was done by one of my associate dentists. The orthodontist noticed this fragment a month later and referred the patient back for its removal. The retained fragment was removed uneventfully by the same associate dentist. If I were to extract that third molar, I would have just sectioned the mesial portion of the crown without raising a flap and then extracted the tooth atraumatically. It is totally unnecessary to remove bone all the way to the point where the bur fractured.

02
Fracture of surgical fissure burs ★★★

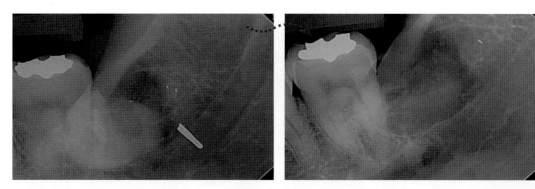

Surgical fissure burs, especially those 28 mm extra long ones, show a significantly higher incidence of fracture. For reference, the length of regular and surgical burs are 21 and 25 mm long respectively. When I visited Pusan National University School of Dentistry in Korea, the 28 mm extra long surgical fissure burs were being discarded after single usage due to the high incidence of fracture. The case above was referred from a resident at a teaching hospital. He said all the burs at the hospital were dull because the residents over there had to re-use them multiple times due to insufficient funds to purchase supplies including burs. Dull burs require more pressure to cut, and that might have caused even more bur fracture incidences he said. When using fissure burs, care must be taken as they fracture very easily. Fortunately, retrieval is not too difficult as fractured fragments are relatively large. In case of surgical round burs, fractured fragments tend to be much smaller and often get suctioned without noticing during the retrieval, so a confirmatory postoperative radiograph is advised.

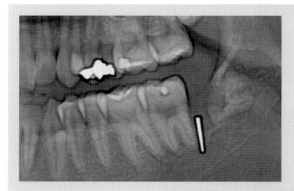

This patient was referred from an oral surgery professor at another teaching hospital. Again, fractured fragments of fissure burs are relatively large, so their removal can be confirmed visually. And that's why we don't see many postoperative radiographs after their removal. However, with fractured surgical round burs, postoperative radiographs are recommended as the retrieved pieces often get lost in the suction and are hard to be confirmed visually.

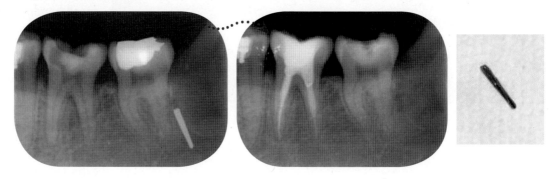

This is a case posted by my Facebook friend. His surgical style is quite different from mine, so I do not understand why the fissure bur got fractured there in the first place. Fortunately, it seems like the fractured fragment was removed uneventfully.

03
Recent cases of surgical round bur fracture (1) ★★

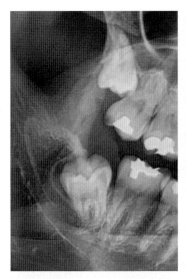
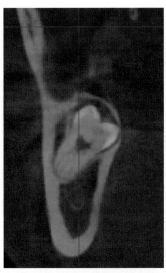
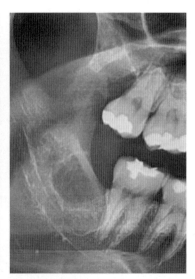

This 28-year-old female patient presented with a disto-lingually impacted #48.

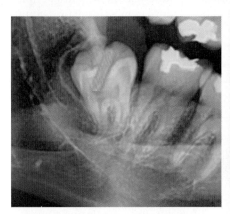
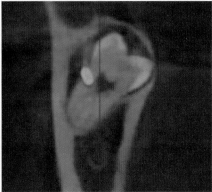

The distal portion of the crown was sectioned by "Distal crown cutting" first. And then, elevation from the buccal side was attempted, but it was not effective due to the lingual inclination of the tooth. So, buccal trough (osteotomy) was made to engage the elevator better. Small diameter burs such as #4 round burs are recommended for this purpose.

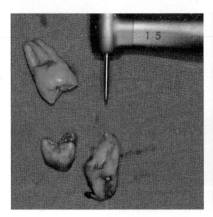
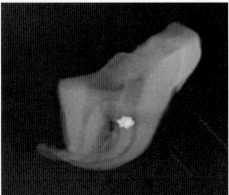

While taking photographs of the extracted teeth along with the instruments used, my assistant noticed that a head of the round bur was missing. I assumed that the black mark on the buccal side of the root was a friction burn as it was common for 5x slow speed handpieces to leave burn marks as such. That's because 5x slow speed handpieces do not spray water like high speed handpieces. However, a radiograph of the extracted tooth confirmed that the black mark was actually the broken bur head embedded in the root. If you notice that your surgical round bur is fractured but cannot locate the broken piece, I strongly recommend taking radiographs of extraction sockets and even extracted teeth. In general, it is quite rare for surgical round burs to be fractured though. I suspect that the vibration and strong torque created by the 5x slow speed handpiece increased the risk in this case.

Recent cases of surgical round bur fracture (2) ★

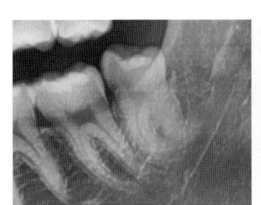
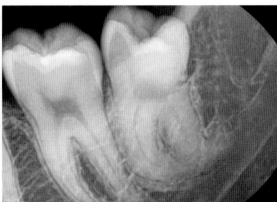

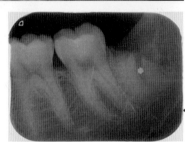

A 26-year-old male patient presented with pain from his third molar and requested the extraction to be done on the same day despite the possible long wait. Due to the severe curvature of the roots, he was informed about the possibility of having to finish the case with coronectomy prior to the procedure.

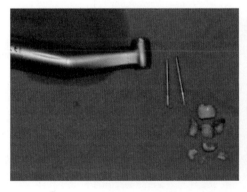
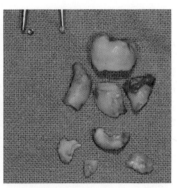

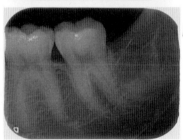

Elevators were tried first instead of a forcep as they generate much greater force than forceps. It was hard to get good leverage with an EL3C elevator, so an EL5C was used, which ended up fracturing the crown. I could have finished the case as coronectomy then, but I refused to stop there. I started sectioning the two roots using a 5x slow speed handpiece, but a #4 round bur was fractured. The fragment was removed using another bur, but the roots kept on breaking afterwards. Whenever some pressure was applied to the remaining roots, the patient felt severe pain, which might have suggested that the roots were in close proximity to the inferior alveolar nerve. Finally, I decided to finish the case as coronectomy by leaving residual roots in the bone. Even though round burs do not fracture nearly as much as fissure burs, they could if their diameter is small and used with slow speed handpieces. I recall only a few fractures out of thousands of those I have used in the last few years even though I use them much more frequently than fissure burs.

04
Retention of foreign objects ★

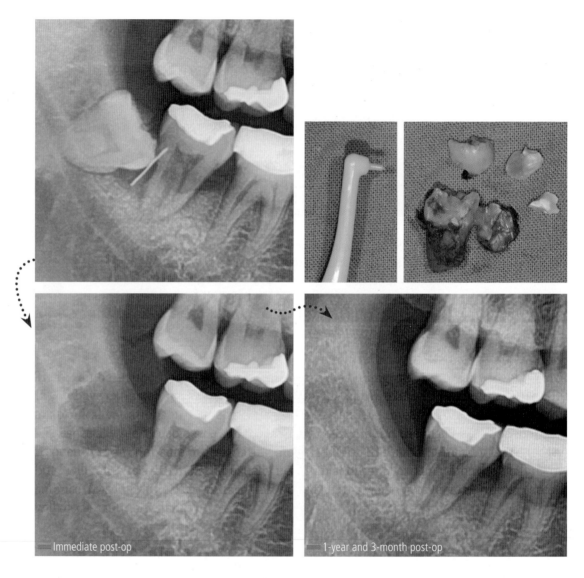

Immediate post-op

1-year and 3-month post-op

A male patient in his late 40s presented with a retained part of an interproximal brush head. The broken piece was removed along with the third molar. A postoperative radiograph was taken to confirm its retrieval as the broken piece went missing in the suction.

05
Chilblain (Ice burn) ★

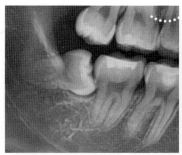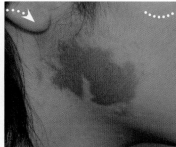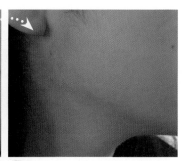

The clinical photograph in the middle was taken a day after #48 extraction. She saw her dermatologist and was told that the skin change was suspectedly due to ice burn. She denied any prolonged application of cold packs, however. Eight days later, the skin reverted back to normal (photo on the right). Generally, ice burn is caused by a prolonged application of cold packs directly on the skin. Cold packs should be applied with adequate breaks after each application. It is more common in females and when patients sleep on cold packs. This is a very rare postoperative complication, so please don't worry too much about it.

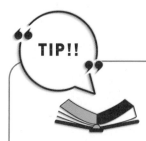

TIP!!

What is Ice Burn?

Dermatologically, it's a type of cold injury, but there is no official diagnostic terminology for that. The term "Ice burn" is often used to help patients understand their conditions better. I have asked my dermatologist friend to explain more about the ice burn for dentists.

Explanation about the case above from Dr. Sung Hyun Park, dermatologist.

Name of the condition: Chilblain.

It is caused by prolonged contact with very cold objects (-2~10°C) which freezes soft tissue and causes localized ischemia as a consequence. The affected area becomes white and waxy in appearance, and initially most patients do not have any symptoms such as pain. However, after warming up the affected area, they usually start having symptoms or lesions based on the severity of tissue damage, which depends on the temperature and the length of exposure to cold. In mild cases, there might be some erythema and discomfort, but the skin will be recovered within hours. In severe cases, tissue necrosis and blisters may develop, and even gangrene in the worst case scenario. Even if there is no tissue damage, symptoms such as paresthesia, hyperhidrosis and cryesthesia may develop and last for months due to the associated adverse effects to blood vessels or the sympathetic nervous system. Therefore, prolonged, greater than 20 minutes, use of cold packs should be avoided, and barriers such as paper towels should be used.

06
Inflammation of extraction sockets (1) ★★★

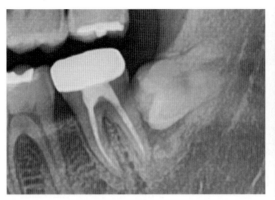 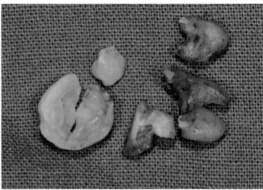

This patient developed pain and swelling 50 days after the extraction. Drainage was performed, and the inflammation eventually resolved within 20 days. Inflammation like this can occur any time after extractions. In most cases, food impaction in the extraction sockets is the underlying cause of suppuration, and it is common to see food particles during drainage.

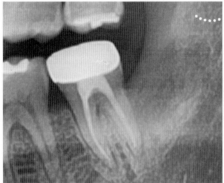 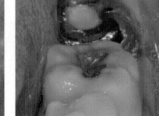 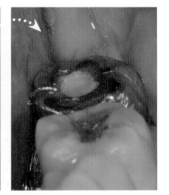

▬Radiograph and clinical photograph taken when the patient presented with pain and swelling. ▬The area was fully healed 20 days after drainage.

Inflammation of extraction sockets (2) ★★

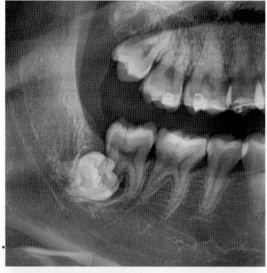

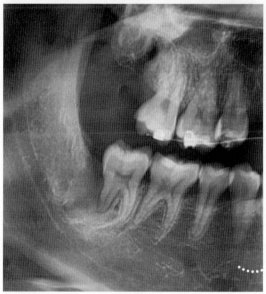

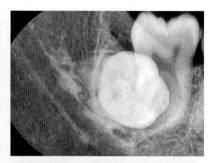

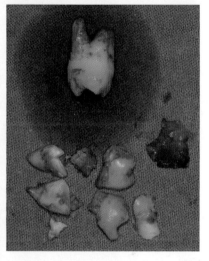

A 23-year-old male patient presented for #48 extraction. It was a difficult extraction, and he developed pain and swelling 2 months later.

This might have been due to the patient's poor oral hygiene with his orthodontic treatment. Much more purulent discharge was drained than what is shown in the photograph.

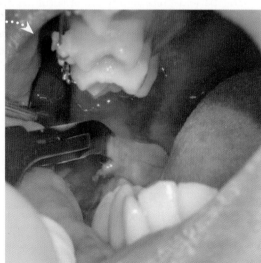

07
Using drains for prolonged drainage ★

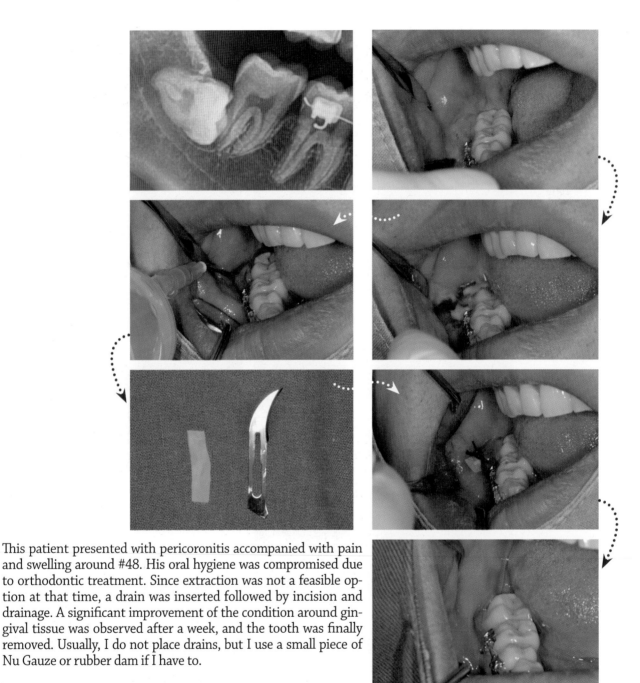

This patient presented with pericoronitis accompanied with pain and swelling around #48. His oral hygiene was compromised due to orthodontic treatment. Since extraction was not a feasible option at that time, a drain was inserted followed by incision and drainage. A significant improvement of the condition around gingival tissue was observed after a week, and the tooth was finally removed. Usually, I do not place drains, but I use a small piece of Nu Gauze or rubber dam if I have to.

Dr. Dae Yong Kim's comment

Do not use a piece of regular gauze as a drain! The gauze fibers can be left within the soft tissues. If you do not have a rubber dam, a small piece of a sterile glove can be used instead. You can place a suture or two in order to stabilize the drain.

08
Causes of suppuration ★★

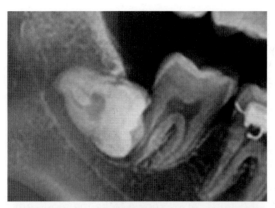

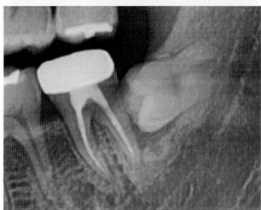

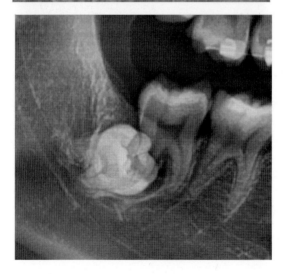

The three cases mentioned previously had narrow socket openings in common. Suppuration is very rare after extractions of fully erupted third molars which result in wide socket openings. When suppuration happens, it usually occurs with narrow socket openings. That is because the epithelium around the socket opening heals faster than other parts, and thus it captures food particles as a consequence. When my patients come back with purulent discharge, I show these radiographs and tell them the analogy that it is easier to clean inside of a bucket than a beer bottle. Based on my experience, this complication is rare and heals uneventfully with drainage and antibiotics.

Wait!

Alveolar Osteitis (Dry socket)

Alveolar Osteitis (AO) is also known as Dry Socket. This typically presents in three to five days after extractions and lasts about five to ten days. Even though the exact underlying pathogenesis of AO is unknown, it is believed to be related to local fibrinolysis leading to premature disintegration of the blood clot in the socket. Hence, it is also known as fibrinolytic alveolitis. To be brief, in AO, plasminogen in the blood clot gets converted to plasmin to induce the fibrinolysis of the blood clot, which in turn causes the release of kinin from kininogen, resulting in the severe pain.

According to several researches, AO happens in 0.5 to 5% of all extractions. Some literatures suggest it to be 1 to 3%. In cases of impacted mandibular third molars, the percentage can be as high as 25 to 30%.

High incidences of AO are mostly reported in teaching hospitals, where extractions are done by residents in training. Contrarily, it is less common among more experienced dentists. AO is known to be the most common with the mandibular premolars. The next commonly involved teeth are the maxillary premolars, followed by the molars, canines, and incisors. Here is some anecdotal evidence about AO even though its exact pathogenesis is not well understood.

- It accompanies halitosis, bad taste, and severe pain with a dull ache radiating to the ear.

- The pain is usually the worst at the onset.

- Vital signs are normal and afebrile.

- There is no suppuration as it is not an infection.

- It is localized within the lamina dura.

- Lab test is unnecessary.

- It does not cause cervical lymphadenopathy.

- Oral bacterial flora might play a role in pathogenesis, but the exact mechanism is not known.

- The risk factors of AO include smoking, pericoronitis, old age, inappropriate irrigation during the procedure. I once believed that AO was associated with the use of tap water as I observed more incidences back in my dental school days where tap water rather than distilled water was used as handpiece coolant. However, this assumption was inaccurate as AO still occurs even though most clinics nowadays use distilled water. In the end, the execution of the procedure itself is what really matters. Quick and atraumatic extraction is the key to prevent AO in my opinion, which depends on the surgeon's skill, finesse, and experience.

- Oral contraceptives might increase the risk of AO. Estrogen in oral contraceptives can activate the fibrinolytic activity of plasminogen, which in turn increases the lysis of blood clot in the socket. However, such increased risk can be considered insignificant.

- Contrary to popular belief, the use of vasoconstrictors such as epinephrine, seasonal factors, amount of bacteria in the socket, flap design and negative pressure caused by straws or spitting have not been found to increase the prevalence of AO.

- The localized use of intra-alveolar antibiotics either before or after AO is still controversial, but many researches show no benefits of doing it. Even prophylactic IV antibiotics have been reported to have no efficacy to prevent AO.

- From many researches, copious irrigation of extraction wounds with chlorhexidine and saline has been found to decrease the incidence of AO by as much as 50%.

Dr. Dae Yong Kim's comment

Excessive mouth rinsing after extraction can also cause AO

Treatment for AO

- Re-curettage of the affected socket was often practiced in the past as iatrogenic bleeding in the socket was believed to expedite the healing, but it is no longer recommended.

- The most common treatment these days is the placement of a gauze with eugenol into the affected socket mainly for pain relief. This has to be repeated every day or every other day for three to six days. Once the pain subsides, the gauze should be removed to prevent foreign body reaction.

Dr. Dae Yong Kim's comment

Instead of eugenol, I recommend applying some topical anesthetics into the socket with cotton applicators.

- Eugenol is known to be neurotoxic, and thus there is a risk of nerve damage if it is placed too close to the inferior alveolar nerve.

- I recommend placing a collagen plug to treat AO or pain from the extraction sockets. Eugenol has a strong smell, and many young dentists don't even have it in their offices. As we will see later in this chapter, AO patients from other dentists healed quickly after placing collagen plugs.

- We need to think if re-curettage before placing collagen plugs is mandatory. I personally try to keep the extraction sockets as clean as possible before placing collagen plugs by performing minimal re-curettage.

- In most cases, the pain subsides rapidly without any local anesthesia. The need for antibiotics is controversial. Generally, I do not routinely prescribe oral antibiotics post procedure, but I would prescribe it for patient management reasons if patients want it.

- The prognosis of AO with proper management is good, and no further treatment is usually needed.

- However, more proactive management and follow-ups are needed for those patients at an increased risk of osteonecrosis (ie, diabetes, chronic steroid use, radiation therapy).

- If a patient does not respond to the treatments explained above, a specialist referral is recommended to evaluate pathological processes from other unknown underlying conditions.

09
Severe pain after extraction from another dentist ★★

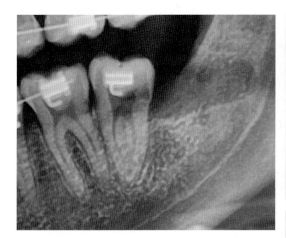

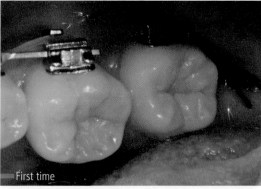

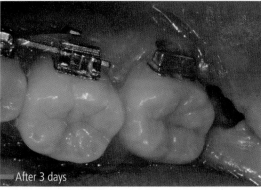

The clinical photograph on top was taken during the initial examination. As AO was suspected, the sutures were removed, the socket was lightly re-curetted under local anesthesia, and a collagen plug was placed. He returned asymptomatic three days later. According to Professor Seung-O Goh, pain control and irrigation are all you need to do when treating AO. If eugenol is to be used, it can be applied for 30 minutes to an hour followed by removal and irrigation. As with the intra-alveolar dressing, he also recommends using only those that are clinically proven to be safe.

10
Severe pain and halitosis after extraction from another dentist ★★★

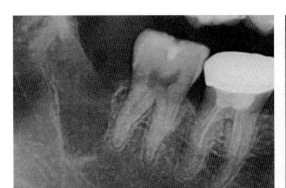

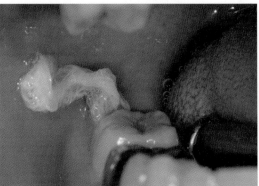

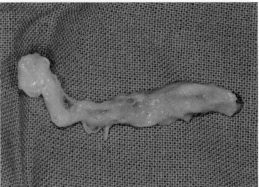

According to the patient, the dentist who performed the surgery suspected AO and placed a gauze with Vaseline in the socket. However, it smelled like eugenol when I examined it. As usual, under local anesthesia, the gauze was removed, and a collagen plug was placed after gentle curettage.

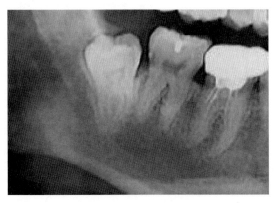

The patient reported instant pain relief. Thankfully, he provided us with the preoperative radiograph from his previous dentist to be used for this book and left a great review on our website.

Dr. Dae Yong kim's comment

Use of Vaseline gauze is not recommended. Like bone wax, it is known to delay tissue healing by inhibiting blood flow to the socket.

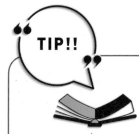

In Korea, local anesthesia and sutures were billed separately, however, in total, it is still ~$25

발치와재소파술

대한민국 건강보험 규정에서 발치와재소파술을 보면 아래와 같다.

(김영삼 원장의 [치과건강보험 달인되기] 2017년도 9판에서 발췌)

■ 발치와재소파 (Recurettage of extracted socket)

진료비 : 8,080원 (2017년 기준)

– 발치 후, 발치와에 염증이 생긴 경우로 발치와 내부를 소파하여 염증의 원인이 될만한 요인들을 제거하는 술식이다.

– 건조성 치조염(건성 발치와)의 소파도 해당된다.

– 발치 후 1회만 산정 가능하며, 발치 당일은 인정되지 않는다.

– 타 기관에서 발치한 환자의 경우도 산정 가능하다.

– 유치는 인정되지 않는다.

위의 설명은 발치 후에 치조골을 조금 삭제하거나 틀니 등을 만들기 위해서 광범위하게 치조골을 삭제하는 행위 모두를 포함하고 있다. 여기서는 발치 후에 뽀족하게 잇몸을 뚫고 나온 치조골에 대한 이야기를 해본다.

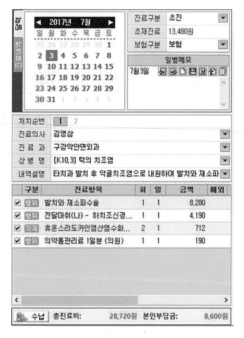

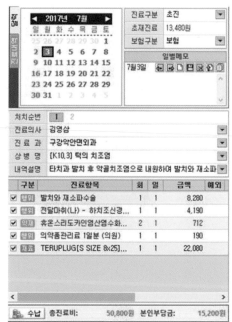

■ 다른 치료 없이 마취와 발치와재소파술만 시행하면 위와 같은 청구화면이 나온다. 비용은 매우 저렴하다.

■ 실제로 발치와재소파술은 거의 의미가 없기 때문에 발치와를 깨끗하게 하는 정도로만 시행하고 콜라겐(Teruplug)을 넣는다. 그 청구화면이다.

In Korea, even if you insert collagen plugs into extractions sockets as an extra procedure, you may only bill the collagen plug material fee.

콜라겐플러그(Teruplug 인정기준)

Teruplug 관련 고시가 최근에 변경되어 올려본다. 관련 내용은 아래와 같다.

■ TERUPLUG 등의 급여기준

1. 창상 보호 및 육아 형성을 촉진하는 마개(Plug) 형태의 치료재료(Teruplug, Ateloplug, Rapiderm Plug)는 다음과 같은 발치의 경우에 요양급여를 인정함.

– 다 음 –

가. 혈액질환 등으로 인한 환자의 발치 후 치유부전이 예상되는 경우

나. 발치 후 출혈이 계속될 경우

다. 구강 상악동 누공

2. 상기 1항의 급여대상 이외 사용한 치료재료비용은 「요양급여비용의 100분의 100 미만의 범위에서 본인부담률을 달리 적용하는 항목 및 부담률의 결정 등에 관한 기준」에 따라 본인부담률을 80%로 적용함.

관련근거 – 보건복지부 고시 제2016–147호

그렇게 되어서 위 인정기준에 맞지 않으면, 발치 직후나 재소파술 시행 시에 환자는 본인부담금 80%를 부담해야 한다. 필자의 경우는 지속적인 출혈이나 건조성 치조염, 상악동 천공의 경우는 본래 급여 기준(30% 본인 부담)으로 하고 있으며, 그 외 기준으로는 최근 변경기준 본인부담금 80%로 시행하고 있다.

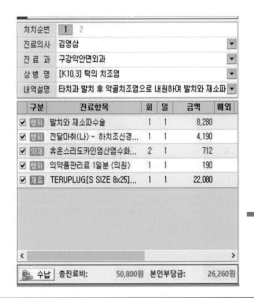

■ 본인부담금 80%로 적용하여 청구한 경우로 치과는 아무런 금전적 이익은 없이, 구매한 비용을 전액 청구하는 것이므로 손해가 아닌 것만으로 만족해야 할 듯하다.

11
Various hemostatic and collagen materials ★

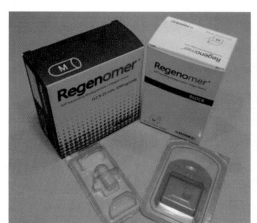
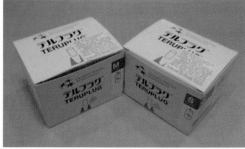
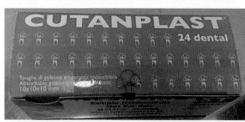
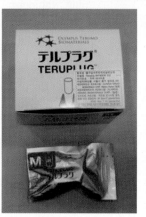
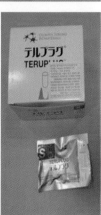
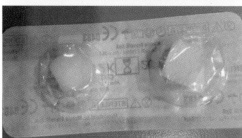
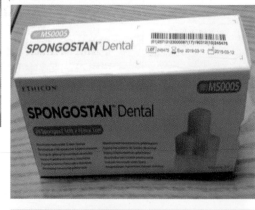
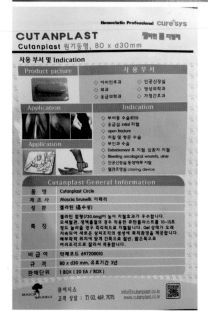
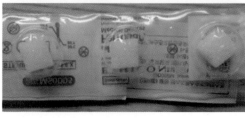

There are many different types of gelatin foams and collagen plugs.

12
Teruplug seems to be the most effective collagen plug to me

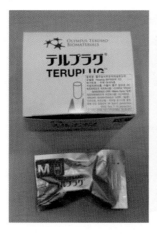
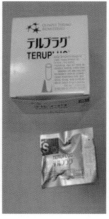
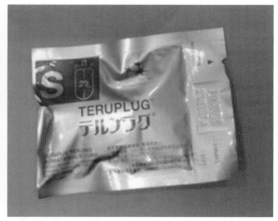

The small size Teruplugs are used most of the time. Even though I rarely perforate sinus membranes, the medium size ones are in stock just in case to manage sinus perforation.

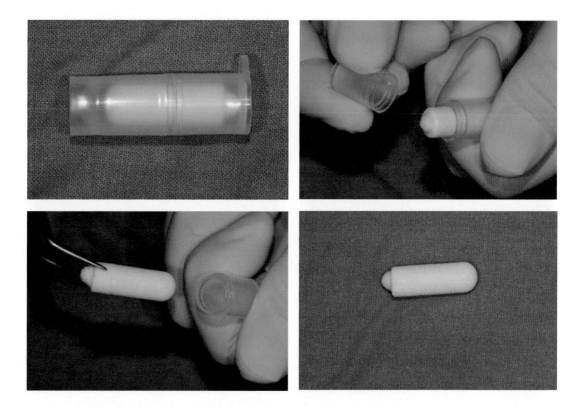

It can be applied directly into the socket, or you can soak it in saline first, but it becomes very soft as soon as it gets wet. I do not think it is a good idea to use it by itself for perforated sinuses. If you have no other option, the medium size one is recommended with primary closure. Also, postoperative instructions equivalent to those for sinus lift surgeries should be given.

13
Maxillary sinus perforation ★★

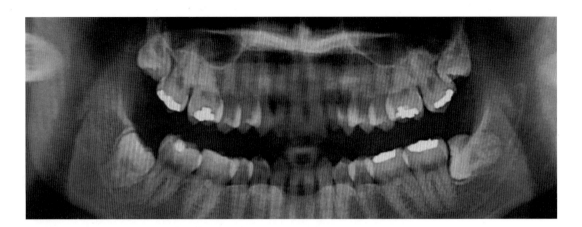

As mentioned previously, sinus perforations rarely happened to me. This panoramic radiograph is from a patient who presented for a second opinion after being told that his maxillary sinus was perforated during the extraction of #28. As in this case and also based on my experience, sinus perforations usually occur when a tooth is abutting the sinus floor sideways, all the way from the crown to the root tip. In this case, the force generated by elevators from the mesiobuccal aspect likely caused the fracture of the sinus floor which led to sinus perforation as a consequence.

Dr. Jong Hwan Lim's comment

Test for sinus perforation (The Valsalva maneuver)

Ask the patient to blow air out through his/her nose while you hold it. While he/she's doing it, monitor the socket closely. If you see air bubbles, that means the Schneiderian membrane is perforated. Generally, over 90% of the cases heal uneventfully with placement of collagen plugs.

Many clinicians do this Valsalva maneuver to check for the sinus perforation and have learned many different ways to deal with sinus perforations during implant surgeries. In my opinion, it is more important to ensure that the patient adheres to the postoperative instructions and precautions (e.g., do not blow your nose, do not drink with a straw, do not sneeze through your nose, etc.) to allow the perforation to close spontaneously. If placing a collagen membrane does not resolve the issue, physical closure should be achieved with a flap or a small piece of bone block in the socket, hence oro-antral communication can be closed physically.

Dr. Dae Yong Kim's comment

It is possible to cause sinus perforation during the Valsalva maneuver, so to be safe, I irrigate the socket with saline to see if there is any oro-antral communication.

Dr. Jae Wook Lee's comment

Keeping a stable blood clot in the socket is very important. This can be achieved by placing a figure eight (Criss-cross) suture.

14
Lingual nerve injury ★

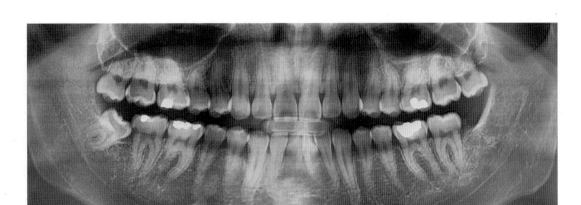

This is a panoramic radiograph of a patient presented for #18 and #48 extractions. She reported having suffered from lingual nerve damage following #38 extraction five years ago, which lasted more than six months before resolving spontaneously. The anatomy of the lingual nerve varies greatly, and therefore clinicians must take the utmost caution with it. The patient's radiograph demonstrates that the lingual nerve injury can occur to anybody with typical anatomy.

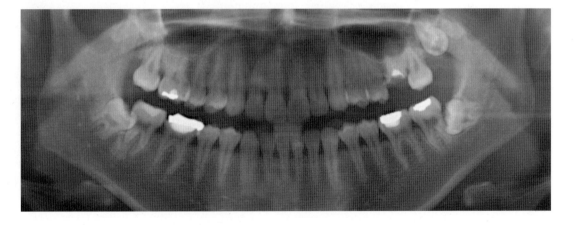

This patient is my friend's wife. She has been suffering from lingual nerve paresthesia ever since her #48 was extracted by another dentist five years ago. From this radiograph, other than the roots being in close proximity to the inferior alveolar nerve, I was not able to identify any anatomical risk factors for possible lingual nerve damage. The nerve was likely damaged while making incisions or raising a flap. Because one can never be sure about the exact location of the lingual nerve, never touch the lingual side of the mandibular third molars when extracting them.

15
Inferior alveolar nerve (IAN) injury ★

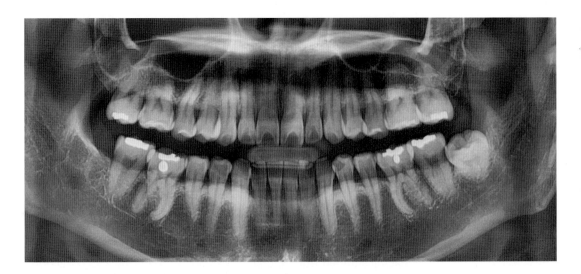

A 50-year-old female patient presented for the extraction of #38. She reported that #48 was extracted by another dentist 20 years ago and the IAN was damaged during the procedure. She has been having discomfort since then.

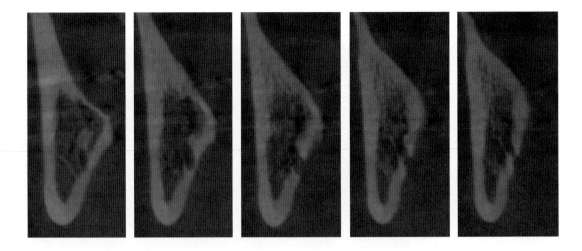

The patient requested a preoperative CBCT for #38 to reduce such a risk this time. Along with #38, the extraction site of #48 was also scanned. As shown above, a residual root tip and perforation of the lingual plate by the IAN were observed. Without a preoperative image, I can only suspect that the IAN might have been either compressed or transported by the abutting root during the extraction.

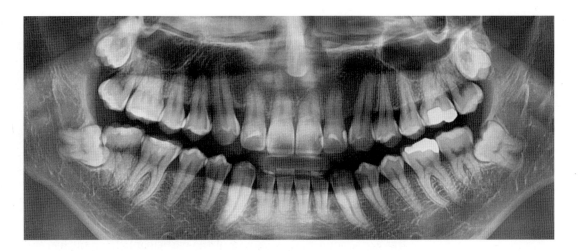

One of my associate oral surgeons extracted #48. Right after the local anesthetics wore off, the patient started complaining of symptoms of paresthesia for a month, suggestive of the IAN injury. In the panoramic radiograph, Youngsam's sign and a dark band are observed around the roots. This indicates that the roots were abutting the IAN and in close proximity to the lingual plate. The surgeon only used a slow speed handpiece for the procedure, and I suspect that the IAN might have been damaged while he was sectioning the roots along the furcation.

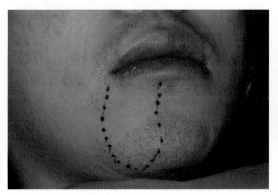

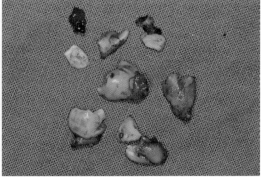

Nerve mapping of the IAN injury. Patients typically present altered sensation in the area shown.

16
Recent cases of IAN injury ★★

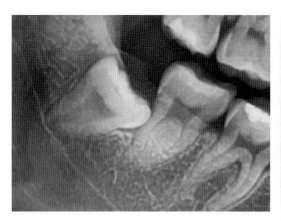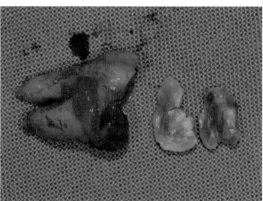

This extraction was done by one of the participants from my live surgery course. The tooth was extracted using 'Mesial crown cutting' followed by 'Lingual crown cutting' or 'Oblique cutting'. The whole procedure took about 30 minutes. The next day, the patient complained of numbness around his lower lip. You can see Youngsam's sign and a dark band around the roots of #38.

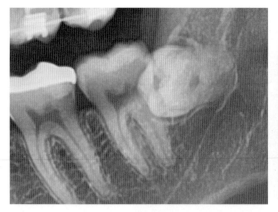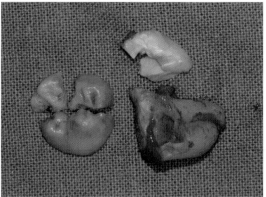

This is my own case. From the panoramic radiograph, the roots of #38 appear to be overlapping with the IAN canal, but no dark band could be seen as the tooth is rotated and tipped. The patient was informed of the difficult nature of the procedure and the possibility of having to finish the case with coronectomy. The crown was sectioned and removed first. When the roots were being elevated, the patient complained of discomfort and tingly sensations on her lower left lip. As the luxated roots were against the distal surface of #37, they were again 'Lifted then sectioned' to allow passage. From the photograph above, it seems as if 'Oblique cutting' was done since the tooth was rotated 90 degrees lingually with its mesial surface facing the buccal and the buccal surface facing the occlusal. Even after the extraction, the patient complained of some altered sensation on her lip, but fortunately it resolved spontaneously the next day. This could have been my very first case resulting in iatrogenic nerve damage ever.

17
IAN injury induced by apical periodontitis

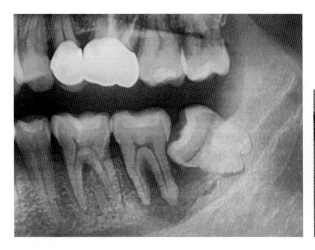
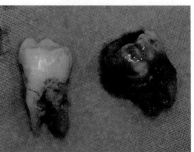

This patient complained of pain from his third molar, but it was actually coming from the second molar. As the radiograph shows, the periapical infection was spread to the vicinity of the IAN. After extractions, the sockets were not curetted due to the risk of nerve injury. The patient reported some altered sensation after the extractions, so follow-ups are being done.

Prescription for suspected nerve injury

I have never caused any iatrogenic nerve injury and believe that spontaneous resolution eventually occurs without any intervention in most cases. However, for liability purposes, I recommend prescribing medications as soon as possible if any kind of nerve injury is suspected. Steroids, vitamins, and Neurontin (Gabapentin) are typically prescribed even though their therapeutic effects are still questionable. Also, referral to a specialist in a timely manner for further evaluation and treatment should also be considered.

18
Clinical note of a patient with IAN injury – Dr. Min Kyo Seo's case ★★

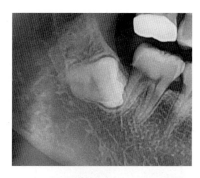

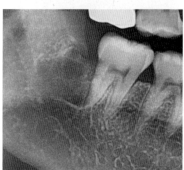

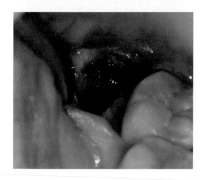

Steroid – Prednisolone: reduces neuritis in paraesthesia quickly and effectively.

Eg: after wisdom extraction, numbness / tingly sensation : 12 ts #3 tid sig Po for 5 days (for a healthy adult)
5 mg/Tab 5~60 mg/day, many brands available

01/27/2016
44yo female
C.C: "The right side lower gum in the back was swollen and painful."
Exposed IAN.
Soaking Dexamethasone 1 ample in the socket (5 min), Dexamethasone 1 ample IM injection given.
Solondo (prednisolone).
Day 1 and 2: Take two tablets three times a day.
Day 3: Take one tablet three times a day.
Cefaclor (2nd gen Cephalosporin ABX), Almagest (Almagate) tid for 3 days.

01/28/2016
S: "I still feel slight numbness."
Hypoesthesia – right lower lip & chin
Not significant compared to the contralateral
Dexamethasone 1 ample IM injection given
Sellalux laser Tx 15 min
Instructed to use hot pack from tomorrow

01/30/2016
Diagnosis: hypoesthesia on the right lower lip & chin due to IAN exposure
- ~70% sensory depression on the right lower lip compared to the contralateral
- Delayed response to painful stimuli
- Ginexin-F 40 mg (ginkgo biloba ex), take 1 tab bid for 14 days
- Beecom-C Tab (multi vitamins), take 1 tab bid for 14 days
- Tyrenol ER, take 1 tab bid for 14 days
- Warm massage

03/08/2016 (6 weeks post operative)
S: "It is better now."
O & P
Sensation came back more than 90%
No sensation of tightening of anterior teeth
Ginexin-F 40 mg, 1tab bid for 14 days
Will do a follow up in 3 weeks

03/29/2016
S: "It seems to be back to normal."
O: Right lip and chin sensory recovery 100% comparable the contralateral side #48 extraction socket causes food impaction but is self-cleansable by the patient.

Dr. Min Kyo Seo's comment

Prednisolone quickly and effectively reduces neuritis in the early stage of nerve injury. I did not prescribe Neurontin (gabapentin) as I did not feel comfortable prescribing it myself without consulting oral medicine specialists.

19
Fracture of alveolar bone from maxillary third molar extractions ★★★

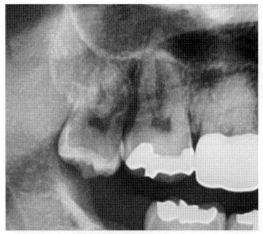

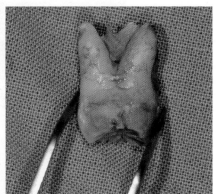

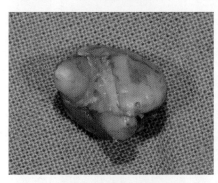

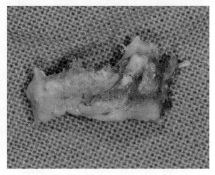

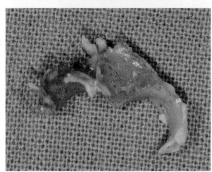

Bone fractures can occur during the extractions of both maxillary and mandibular third molars. Maxillary tuberosity fractures occur more commonly when elevators rather than forceps are used. Also, in my experience, they can be observed more from middle-aged males and also females with osteoporosis. It seems like bone fractures do not affect the healing, and they do not accompany excessive hemorrhage, either. Fractures even larger than the cases shown here are frequently observed, but they usually all heal without any complications. This also means that we do not need to concern too much about removing the buccal bone using a slow speed handpiece while extracting impacted maxillary third molars.

20
Alveolar bone attached to extracted maxillary third molars ★★

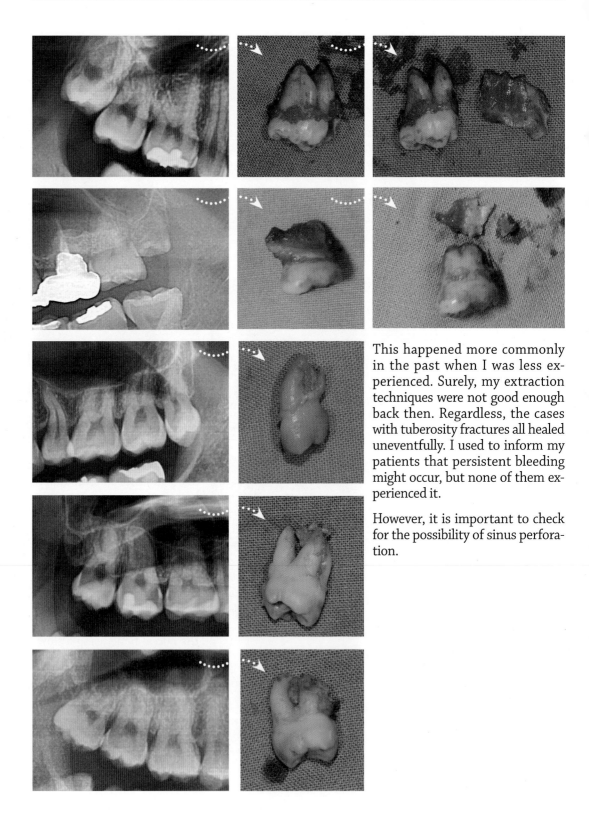

This happened more commonly in the past when I was less experienced. Surely, my extraction techniques were not good enough back then. Regardless, the cases with tuberosity fractures all healed uneventfully. I used to inform my patients that persistent bleeding might occur, but none of them experienced it.

However, it is important to check for the possibility of sinus perforation.

21
Fracture of interradicular bone from mandibular third molar extractions ★★★

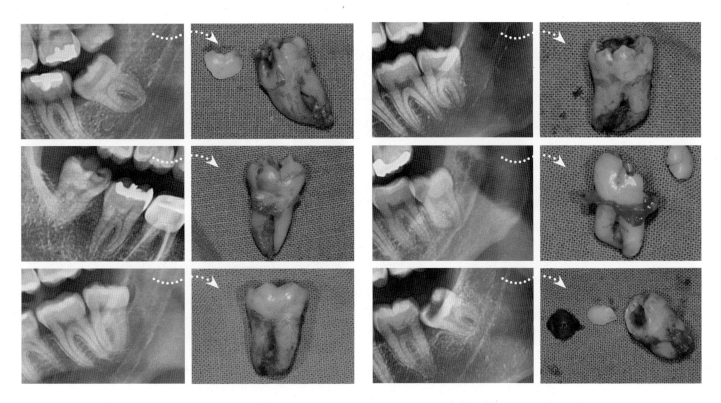

Alveolar bone fractures during extractions occur commonly. Most of them are unnoticed as greenstick fractures, but often you can see interradicular bone fractured off with extracted teeth if their roots are severely dilacerated or converging apically. There is no concern of impaired healing or excessive bleeding with such fractures.

Dr. Jong hwan Lim's comment

If the fractured fragment is too big, we need to place it back to its original position and place tight sutures. Also, we need to inform patients about the possibility of difficulty of swallowing and other potential issues.

Dr. Dae yong Kim's comment

Sectioning the converging roots during the extraction can prevent this from happening if lamina dura can be clearly seen between the roots on the preoperative radiograph.

22
Lingual bone fragment attached to extracted mandibular third molars (1) ★★★

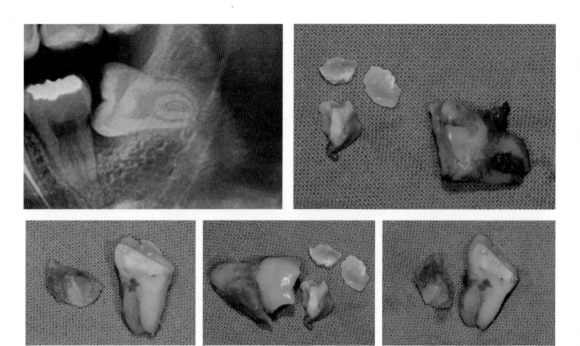

Accidental fractures of the lingual plates are quite common during mandibular third molar extractions. In most cases, the lingual plates are much thinner than the buccal plates. Thus, the elevating force applied from the buccal plate can easily cause those thin lingual plates to break. Occasionally, ankylosis or the lack of periodontal ligament around teeth to be extracted may increase the chances of fracture. Also, there is a higher risk of the lingual plate fracture if Youngsam's sign is observed on preoperative radiographs. Regardless, all such cases showed uneventful recoveries at the follow-ups. If a fragment is large and thus difficult to be removed along with a tooth, it can be separated from the tooth and left in the socket. And then, you should do your best to stabilize the fragment and the soft tissue by placing sutures.

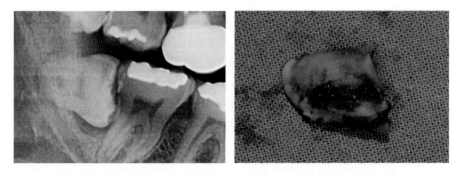

Due to Youngsam's sign along the roots and the presence of interradicular bone, lingual plate fracture was expected.

Lingual bone fragment attached to extracted mandibular third molars (2) ★

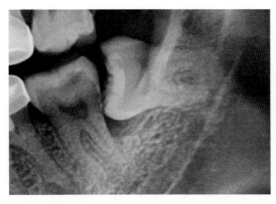

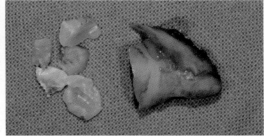

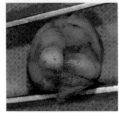
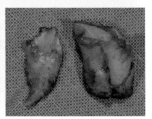

Lingual plate fractures occur much less in my cases since I do "Oblique cutting" before extracting third molars. However, inexperienced clinicians often apply unnecessarily strong and prolonged force from the buccal side of the tooth towards the lingual plate, and this leads to the higher rate of fracture incidence.

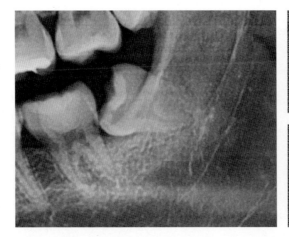

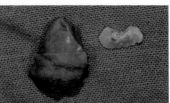

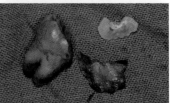

At times, mylohyoid muscle can be seen along with the lingual plate fragment. I was very nervous when this happened to me for the first time, but I carefully dissected it from the fractured lingual plate with a scalpel and placed it back in. Mylohyoid muscles attach to the whole length of the mylohyoid ridge of the mandible, so even if a small portion of it is severed, it does not cause any major problems, at most some discomfort upon swallowing for a few days.

Dr. Dae yong Kim's comment

Mylohyoid muscles can cause trouble to denture patients as well. Sometimes, smoothing the sharp edges of the mylohyoid ridge makes dentures feel much more comfortable to wear.

23
Exposure of mylohyoid muscle ★★

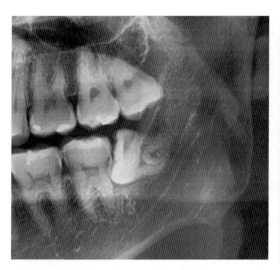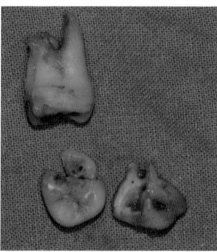

This is a 33-year-old male's horizontally impacted #38. Its roots were curved and converging, but there were no other significant radiological findings. As usual, the crown was sectioned and removed. And then the elevator was applied from the buccal aspect, but the tooth was not extracted easily. Because the tooth was small and I only had a #6 round bur, 'Disto-Cervical Cutting' instead of 'Oblique Cutting' was performed to luxate the tooth more.

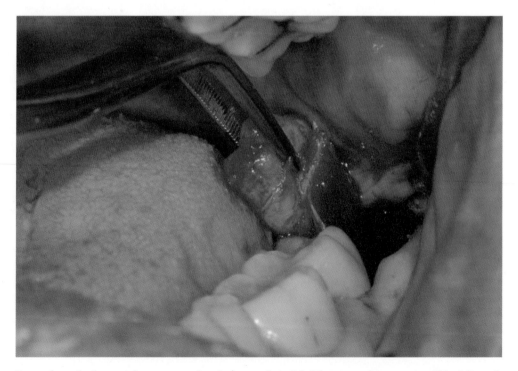

Even though the tooth was completely luxated, it felt like something was still holding the tooth. When I picked up the tooth with a cotton plier, it was found to be attached to the mylohyoid muscle through the fractured lingual plate. In this photograph, the tooth is rotated so that it can be positioned lingually to show the mylohyoid muscle. Usually, exposed muscles are smaller and thinner than the one shown in this case.

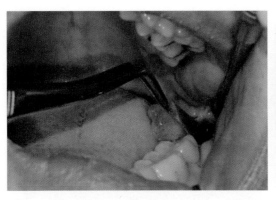 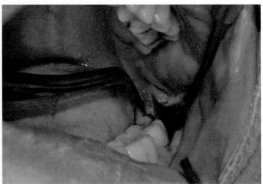

If the exposed muscle is small, it can be cut with scissors or a scalpel close to its attachment, and the fractured lingual plate can be removed together with the tooth. However, because the exposed muscle was quite large in this case, the fractured lingual plate was separated from the tooth first. The photograph on the right shows the separated lingual bone fragment with the muscle attached.

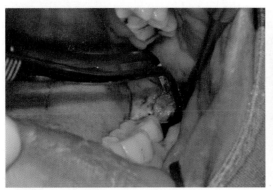 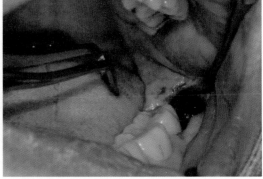

The lingual bone fragment and the attached muscle were then repositioned to their original position. In order to stabilize the fragment and the soft tissue, interrupted sutures were placed after. The patient did not experience any postoperative discomfort. The size of exposed muscle and bone fragment and the level of difficulty to separate the bone fragments from extracted teeth are the factors that you need to consider when managing this kind of problem. All of my exposed mylohyoid muscle cases recovered uneventfully regardless of the treatment methods I used.

Dr. Jae wook Lee's comment

The mylohyoid muscle should be separated from the bone fragment by dissecting, not cutting.

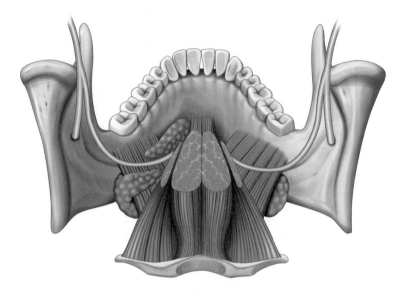

However, the mylohyoid muscle should not be pulled excessively any more than shown in the previous photograph since the lingual nerve lies superior to the mylohyoid muscle. The attached muscle should be separated within the socket without being pulled out. One of my oral surgeon colleagues even recommends doing blunt dissections using the back of a scalpel to prevent any potential damage to the lingual nerve.

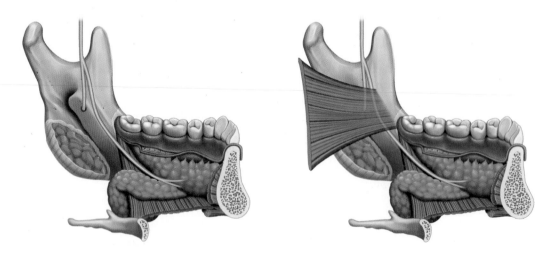

These illustrations show the anatomical relationship between the lingual nerve and the mylohyoid muscle. Extra care should be taken when dissecting this muscle.

24
Pictures posted online ★★★

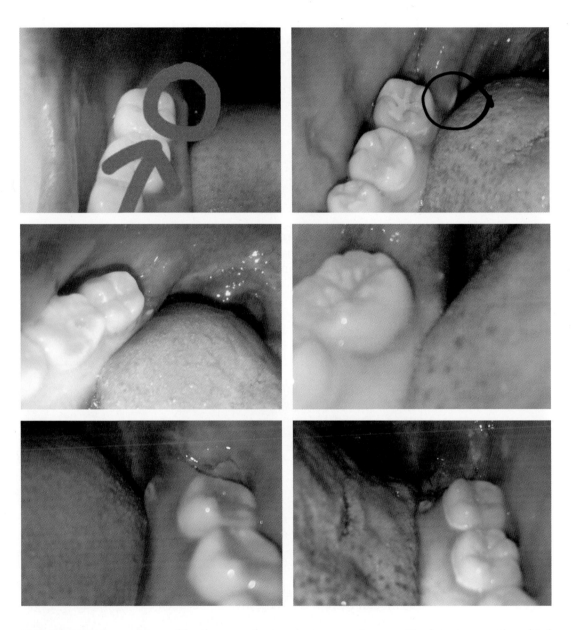

Patients often post pictures like these on the internet suspecting a residual root or another third molar erupting. In most cases, the mandibular third molars have been extracted within a few months. This occurs commonly, but what could be causing this condition?

25
Formation of lingual bone spicule after third molar extractions

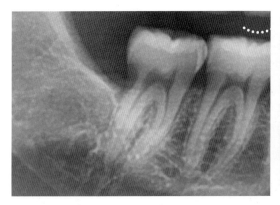 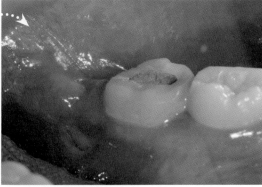

This patient was referred by a dentist who noticed an unusual bony lesion close to the disto- lingual side of #47 during an endodontic treatment. When asked, the patient reported that #48 was extracted a year ago and the bony lesion appeared soon after.

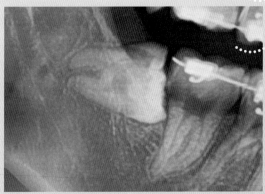 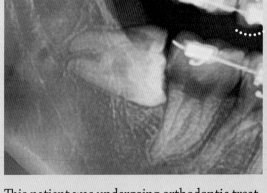 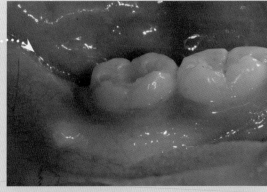

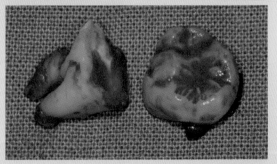

This patient was undergoing orthodontic treatment, and there was a space created between #47 and #48, which allowed the crown of #48 to be removed easily. But, there was inadequate disto-buccal purchase point for the elevator, so 'Disto-Cervical Cutting' was done followed by 'L-Extraction'. It is likely that the lingual plate was fractured from the strong force during the elevation and luxation. One month later, the patient returned to the office wondering if an extra third molar was erupting. There are many different ways to manage this, but I usually just reduce and smooth the exposed bone with a high speed round bur under local anesthesia.

26
The cause of lingual bone spicule after third molar extractions ★

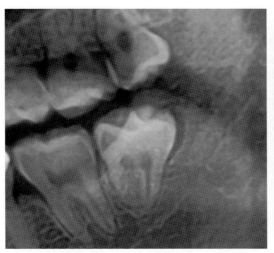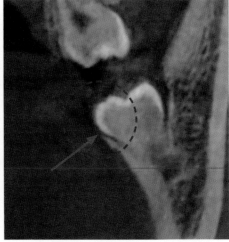

These are the panoramic radiograph and the coronal view of CBCT of an impacted third molar. I show these images to patients who complain of post-extraction lingual bone spicules. The sharp tip of the lingual plate is evident in this CBCT. With the third molar present, the bone is flush with the tooth and therefore is not palpated clinically. However, it gets exposed after the tooth is extracted and consequently causes discomfort. Lingually directed force during extractions may displace the lingual plate more lingually or even fracture it, which can result in fragments left in the lingual gingiva.

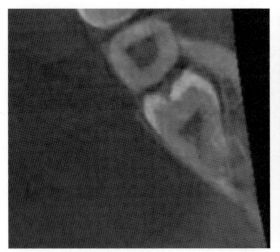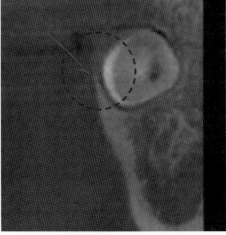

These are the axial and coronal views of CBCT of a horizontally impacted third molar. The sharp edge of the lingual plate is commonly seen, but not every case with it develops the lingual bone spicules. So, please do not be afraid if you observe the sharp edge of the lingual plate from CBCT images. Instead, you can utilize them to explain to your patients when the lingual bone spicules occur. As described later in this chapter, they can be treated easily.

27
Lingual bone is easily fractured ★★★

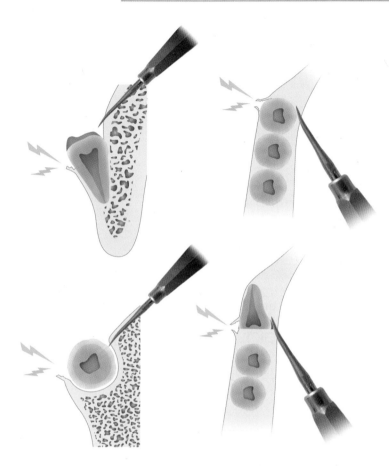

Regardless of the angle of impaction, we approach mandibular third molars from the buccal aspect. For this reason, the thin lingual bone is easily fractured.

Dr. Jong hwan Lim's comment

This happens to 3~4% of patients. I tend to tell my patients "this is due to the hypertrophy of the bone" (Similar to the development of torus, but in this case the bone comes through the soft tissue).

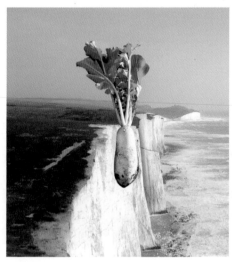
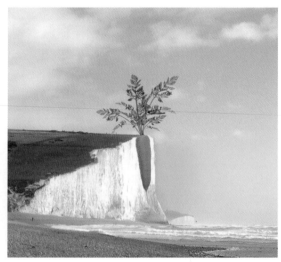

Extracting a third molar can be compared to harvesting a radish or a carrot from the edge of a cliff. We should keep in mind that the lingual bone adjacent to the tooth may be paper-thin and not exert too much force against it.

28
Management of lingual bone spicule ★★

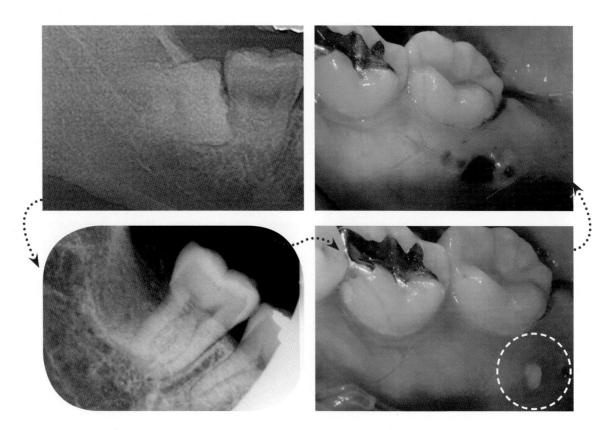

This is a patient of mine. He thought there was either a new tooth erupting or a part of the third molar was still remaining. In such cases, I simply reduce and smooth the exposed bone with a high speed surgical round bur without any further management. All of them have recovered uneventfully. One thing you should remember is that a proper retraction of the posterior soft tissue should be done during the procedure to prevent soft tissue injuries.

29
Formation of lingual bone spicule after second and third molar extractions ★

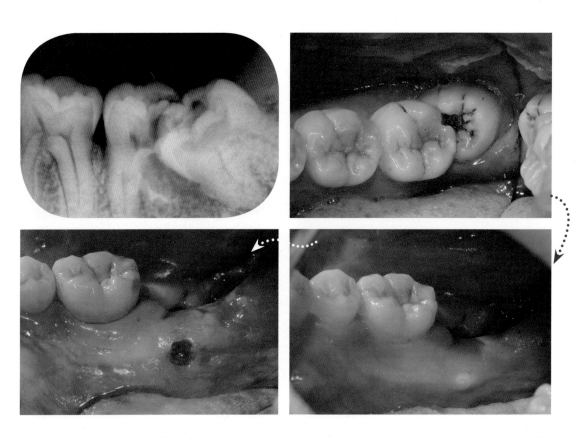

This is a case after #37 and #38 extractions. The management was the same. While retracting the soft tissue and the tongue with a mirror, the exposed bone was reduced and smoothed with a high speed surgical round bur without raising a flap.

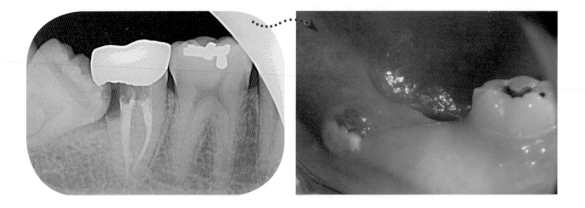

This is a similar case after #47 and #48 extractions. The bone spicule was treated the same way.

30
It is more common in cases with lingually impacted third molars ★

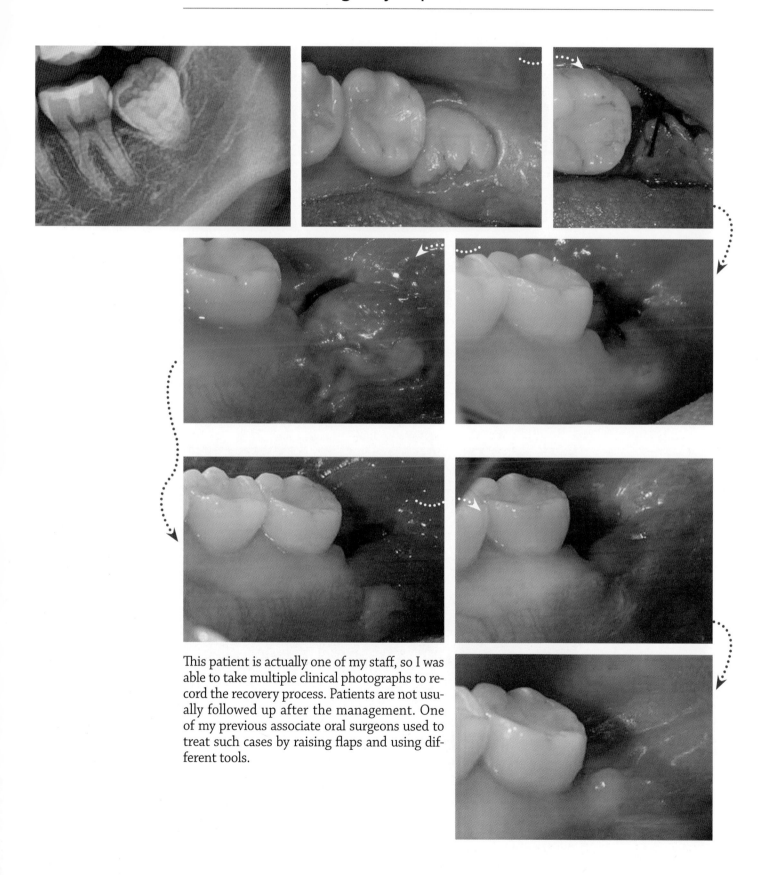

This patient is actually one of my staff, so I was able to take multiple clinical photographs to record the recovery process. Patients are not usually followed up after the management. One of my previous associate oral surgeons used to treat such cases by raising flaps and using different tools.

31
Removal of lingual bone fragments (1) ★

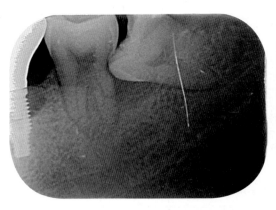

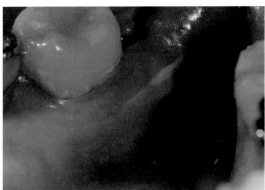

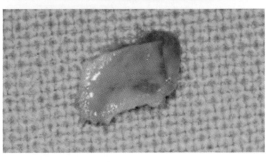

The lingual cortical bone was exposed post extraction. A rongeur was used to fracture and remove the exposed portion without raising a flap. I prefer flapless management even though some oral surgeons prefer to raise a large flap for better access.

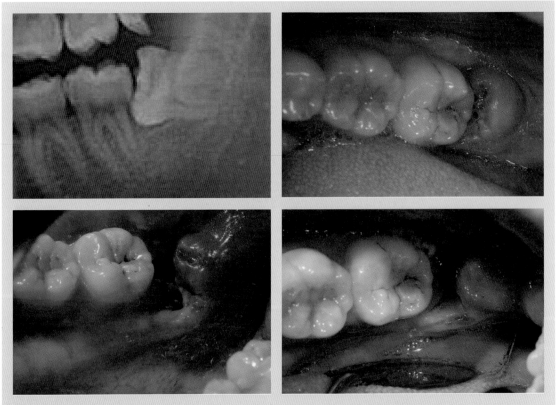

This is a similar case, where the sharp lingual bone fragment was removed.

32
Removal of lingual bone fragments (2) ★

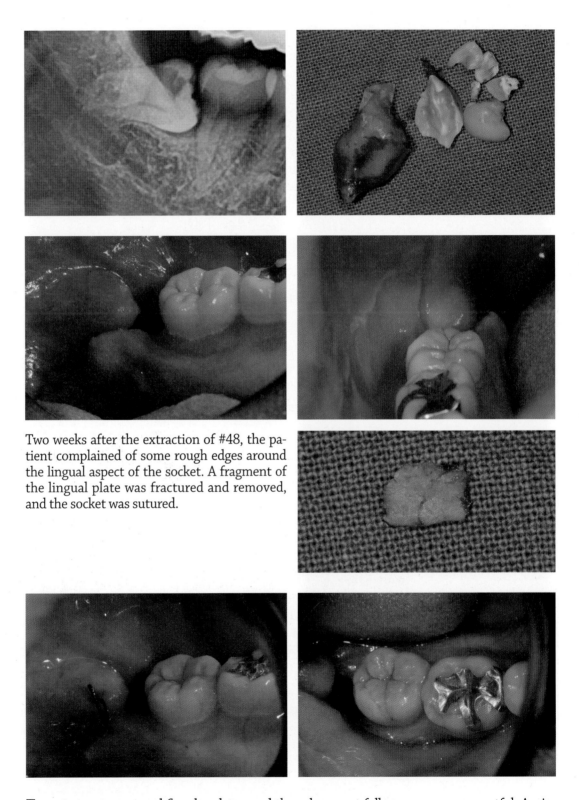

Two weeks after the extraction of #48, the patient complained of some rough edges around the lingual aspect of the socket. A fragment of the lingual plate was fractured and removed, and the socket was sutured.

The suture was removed five days later, and the subsequent follow-ups were uneventful. Again, we must be mindful of the lingual nerve in these cases.

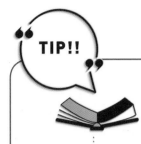

TIP!!

In Korea, if further alveolaplasty is required after extractions in cases of bony spicules, extra $35 will be billed including local anesthesia and a x-ray.

치조골성형술 ★

대한민국 건강보험 규정에서 발치와재소파술을 보면 아래와 같다.

(김영삼 원장의 [치과건강보험 달인되기] 2017년도 9판에서 발췌)

> ■ 치조골성형수술 (Alveoloplasty)
>
> 진료비 : 8,720원
>
> 발치 후 발치와는 잔존 치조골에 의해 둘러싸여 지는데, 잔존 치조골이 너무 뾰족하게 형성되거나 하여 수술 후 불편을 야기할 수 있다. 발치와 동시에 시행하거나 발치 후 환자가 불편감을 호소하는 경우에 시행한다.
>
> 임플란트의 발달 등으로 일반적인 구치부의 경우 개념이 약간 바뀐 듯하다.
>
> – 발치와 동시에 시행 시 낮은 수가는 50%만 산정한다.
>
> – 치주판막술과 동시에 시행했을 경우는 산정할 수 없다.
>
> 위의 설명은 발치 후에 치조골을 조금 삭제하거나 틀니 등을 만들기 위해서 광범위하게 치조골을 삭제하는 행위 모두를 포함하고 있다. 여기서는 발치 후에 뾰족하게 잇몸을 뚫고 나온 치조골에 대한 이야기를 해본다.

처치순번	**1** 2			
진료의사	김영삼			▼
진 료 과	구강악안면외과			▼
상 병 명	[K08,81] 불규칙한 치조돌기			▼
내역설명				▼

구분	진료항목	회	일	금액	예외
☑ 행위	치조골성형수술	1	1	9,100	
☑ 행위	전달마취(나) - 하치조신경...	1	1	4,210	
☑ 의재	휴온스리도카인염산염수화...	1	1	356	
☑ 행위	의약품관리료 1일분 (의원)	1	1	190	
☑ 재료	100:100 발치, 치근, 치조골...	1	1	6,980	
☑ 재료	SILK	1	1	1,910	
☑ 행위	치근단 촬영판독	1	1	3,250	

수납 총진료비: 37,420원 본인부담금: 11,200원

처치순번	**1** 2			
진료의사	김영삼			▼
진 료 과	구강악안면외과			▼
상 병 명	[K10,3] 턱의 치조염			▼
내역설명				▼

구분	진료항목	회	일	금액	예외
☑ 행위	치조골성형수술	1	1	9,100	
☑ 행위	전달마취(나) - 하치조신경...	1	1	4,210	
☑ 의재	휴온스리도카인염산염수화...	1	1	356	
☑ 행위	의약품관리료 1일분 (의원)	1	1	190	
☑ 재료	100:100 발치, 치근, 치조골...	1	1	6,980	
☑ 재료	SILK	1	1	1,910	
☑ 행위	치근단 촬영판독	1	1	3,250	
☑ 행위	발치와 재소파수술	1	1	8,280	

수납 총진료비: 46,940원 본인부담금: 14,000원

〈치과의원 수가 기준〉

33
Mucocele formation after extraction

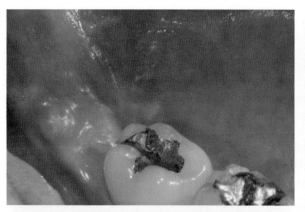

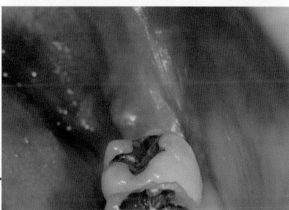

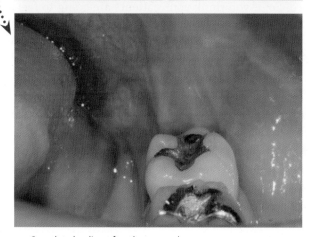

Complete healing after the removal.

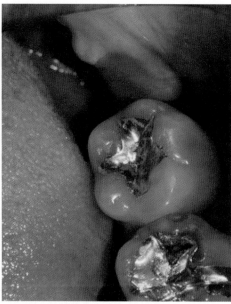

A 26-year-old male complained of a soft tissue swelling at the extraction site two months after his #38 was extracted. He reported that it was constantly bothersome and became bigger during meal times. Mucocele was diagnosed based on the history and the appearance of the lesion, and it was removed subsequently by electrocautery under local anesthesia. The biopsy result confirmed the initial diagnosis of mucocele. I suspect that this might have been caused during the infiltration injection or while raising the flap. Even though I have heard that some dentists had one or two cases like this, this was the first case that I have come across. Unlike mucoceles around the lips, the ones on the posterior gingiva do not tend to recur due to the decreased number of minor salivary glands.

34
The best management of wisdom teeth extractions

The best treatment you could provide for your patients would be for them to experience the least pain during and after the procedure. No matter how well you explain the procedure or how good your technique is, if the patient feels severe pain postoperatively, I would consider it as a failure. My maxillary third molars were congenitally missing, and I only had mandibular ones, one vertically erupted and the other horizontally impacted. Both were extracted by my senior colleagues when I was a dental student. The erupted one was extracted first, and I suffered so much pain throughout the procedure. It took several students taking turns and struggling, and it was the worst experience of my life. However, after the local anesthetics wore off, there was no postoperative pain. A few years later, one of my senior colleagues removed the other horizontally impacted third molar. It was a painless procedure, but once the anesthetics wore off, I had to suffer excruciating pain. It was a very different experience from the first one.

Having done many third molar extractions myself, now I understand why the two experiences were so different. It is difficult to achieve an adequate local anesthesia with vertically erupted third molars due to the thick cortical bone around their apices, and of course, a functional, fully erupted mandibular third molar, especially in a young healthy male patient, is probably the most difficult case for a training student to practice on.

It is relatively easier to adequately anesthetize horizontally impacted third molars as the cortical bone is thin around their apices. However, done by an inexperienced student, the procedure perhaps involved a large flap and extensive buccal bone reduction, which in turn resulted in the worst pain I have ever experienced in my life. I could not sleep that night and just wished the time would pass quickly.

I cannot emphasize enough the importance of painless third molar extractions because having gone through some difficult and painful experiences, patients are not likely to return to you for other treatment needs. On the other hand, the opposite holds true if the pain is much less than what they expected. So, if you think your patients are going to feel so much pain after procedures, It would probably be better for you to refer them out than to make bad impressions. If you want to do third molar extractions, you must learn the minimally invasive extraction technique that will cause the least pain and discomfort.

Tips on the Painless Extractions

- Minimize the size of incision and flap.
- Section the tooth to minimize bone reduction.
- Minimize the use of distilled water on the exposed bone.
- Saline irrigation before the roots were removed.
- Ensure adequate local anesthesia, especially infiltration around the tooth.
- Prescribe prophylactic antibiotics and analgesics.
- Manage pain actively with medications. Especially, prescribe Ultracet along with ibuprofen when severe pain is expected.
- IM injection of antibiotics with severe infection (also if severe pain and swelling are expected).
- If possible, place collagen plugs.
- Last but not least, upskill yourself and extract efficiently, not forcefully.

35
Post-operative instructions are given and also sent via text/email ★

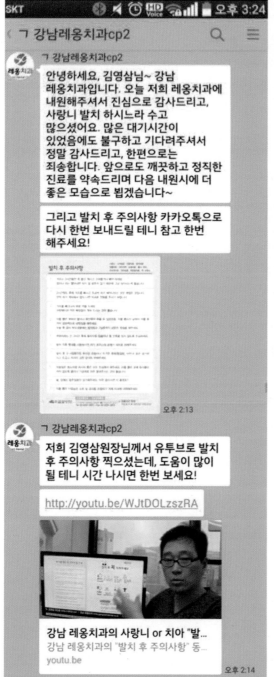

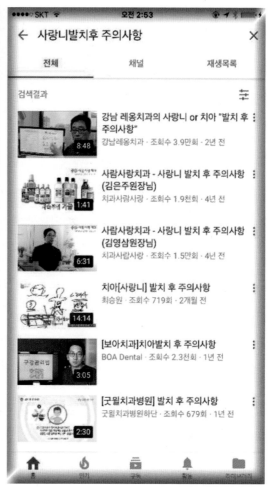

If you Google YouTube: "Postoperative instructions after a wisdom extraction", you can see numerous clips uploaded by dentists. It is not a bad idea to make your own version.

Post-operative instructions for the wisdom tooth extraction
(Recorded in Gangnam Leon Dental Clinic)

36
Post-operative instructions for patients

발치 후 주의사항

사랑니 | 스케일링 | 잇몸치료 | 충치치료
임플란트 | 치아미백 | 보철치료 | 틀니·의치
라미네이트 | 치아성형 | 턱관절치료 | 턱·보톡스

1. The gauze pad placed over the sockets should be kept in place for two hours. Please do not remove or reposition it. Spitting saliva and blood can cause prolonged bleeding, so it is better to swallow them.

2. Please discard the gauze pad after two hours. Slight oozing of blood from the surgical site is normal. Please call us for further instructions if excessive or persistent bleeding occurs.

3. Take the prescribed pain medication straight after the gauze pad is removed. Please follow directions and finish them as scheduled for the maximum effect.

4. For the first 48 hours after the extractions, place cold packs on the affected side of your face to minimize the swelling of the face/neck/surgical site. You should switch to warm packs after the 48 hours.

5. The numbness from local anesthetics will wear off within two to three hours after the surgery. Please be careful not to chew on your lips and cheeks during this period.

6. Avoid using straws as it can dislodge blood clots and cause more bleeding.

7. Avoid heavy exercises, hot spa and sauna for the next three to four days. Also avoid hot or spicy food.

8. Continue with normal brushing, but be careful around the surgical area. It is recommended to rinse gently with water or mouth rinse after meals to avoid food impaction in the socket.

9. No alcohol or smoking for a week. It is even better if you can quit for good.

10. Please come back tomorrow for disinfection and follow-up.

건강보험진료 | 진료상담환영

강남 레옹치과
Gangnam Leon Dental Clinic

H.P 010-4569-1848 ☎ (카카오톡 가능)
H.P 010-2804-1848 ☎ (보존,보철전용)
서울시 서초구 강남대로 415 대동빌딩 8층
Tel 02-535-2119 Fax 02-591-2119

▸ 진료시간 안내
평   일 AM 10:00~PM 7:00
토 요 일 AM 10:00~PM 5:00
점심시간 PM 1:00~PM 2:00
＊월,화,수,목 야간진료 ~PM 9:00

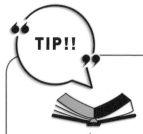

TIP!!

Commonly prescribed medications ★

1. Antibiotics
- I usually prescribe Augmentin 625 mg (amoxicillin 500 mg + clavulanic acid 125 mg) tid for the first 24 hours after extractions. For the next two days, patients are recommended to take the medication twice a day. I don't ask patients to take antibiotics more than three days if there are no odontogenic infections accompanying swelling or fascial space infections. That is because antibiotic therapy should be focused on preventing infections during the surgery and the first 24 hours after it.
- In the U.S., Augmentin 1 g (Amoxicillin 875 mg + Clavulanic Acid 125mg) bid for 5 to 7 days is recommended as of March 2020.
- In cases with severe infection or penicillin allergy: Rodogyl (Metronidazole 125 mg, Spiramycin 234.375 mg)
- In the U.S., metronidazole 500 mg tid for 8 days is recommended for dental infection. 250 mg tid with amoxicillin for 7 to 10 days can be used for severe periodontitis.

2. Analgesics
- Ibuprofen 400 mg tid (I usually tell patients to take up to 5 to 6 times on the day of the surgery. Maximum daily dosage is 3200 mg)
- If you expect severe pain, you can prescribe Ultracet (tramadol/acetaminophen) in addition to ibuprofen 400 mg.

3. Antacid
- Almagel (aluminium hydroxide)

4. Steroids
- Solondo (prednisolone)

5. Mouthwash
- Hexamedine (chlorhexidine gluconate)

1. Antibiotics

Amoxicillin 500 mg tid used to be my first-line antibiotic because it is the most commonly prescribed antibiotic amongst dentists around the world. It is effective against Streptococcus mutans, the main bacteria in the oral flora, and is also the first-line prophylactic antibiotic for patients at risk of infective endocarditis.

The second-line antibiotics would be Augmentin, clindamycin, or cephalosporins. In South Korea, Augmentin seems to be the primary antibiotic used in pediatric medicine because of its wider antimicrobial coverage. This is why I started to prescribe Augmentin as my first-line antibiotic. To me, it does not make sense to prescribe amoxicillin when patients had taken mostly Augmentin in their childhood. American Dental Association

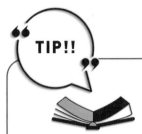

TIP!!

also recommends the use of Augmentin instead of increasing dosage of amoxicillin.

The first generation cephalosporins are not better antibiotics than amoxicillin in dentistry because they are not effective against anaerobes. Patients allergic to penicillin are also likely to be allergic to cephalosporin, making it even less useful as a second-line option. The reason why clindamycin is not used as a first-line antibiotic is that it can cause pseudomembranous colitis and needs to be used in case the first-line ones do not work. Rodogyl is a combination of two antibiotics, metronidazole and spiramycin. Metronida- zole is extremely effective against the obligate anaerobes and together with spiramycin, they are great for dental infections accompanying swelling or fascial space infections. Also, patients allergic to penicillin are not likely to be allergic to metronidazole and spiramycin, which makes Rodogyl as my most prescribed antibiotics along with Augmentin.

2. Analgesics

Analgesics have more side effects than antibiotics. I prefer ibuprofen due to its rapid onset of action. The effect of ibuprofen would kick in within half an hour, reaching its maximum effect within 1~2 hours with the duration of effect up to 4~6 hours. In view of this property, I generally prescribe ibuprofen half an hour before any surgical extractions. Ibuprofen being a non-steroidal anti-inflammatory drug (NSAID) is more effective in reducing inflammation and fever than Tylenol (acetaminophen). It is recommended not to exceed the recommended dosage of NSAIDs as supratherapeutic dose will not provide additional analgesic effect. Instead, Tylenol can be co-prescribed for a synergetic effect.

If the patient complains of side effects with NSAIDS or is pregnant or breastfeeding, Tylenol may be prescribed. Unlike NSAIDS, acetaminophen will not cause gastric side effects, hence it can be taken with an empty stomach. However, it does not have anti-inflammatory effect, and one should be mindful of its known liver toxicity when taken excessively or with alcohol.

Lastly for severe pain relief, I prescribe Ultracet, a combination drug consists of acetaminophen and tramadol, along with ibuprofen. Drowsiness and dizziness are common side effects, so it is advisable to inform the patient ahead of time.

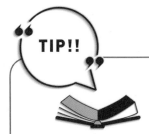

TIP!!

3. Mouthwash

I do not think that this plays a big role in recovery, but I prescribe chlorhexidine gluconate oral rinse along with antibiotics and analgesics if patients want something to rinse their mouths. Please make sure that you are not supposed to prescribe mouthwash alone.

Please consider this as a guideline. Final decisions should be made based on the health care policies in your countries. Key point is, pain after third molar extraction is not a common incident like cold, hence, please prescribe medications more proactively.

APPENDIX

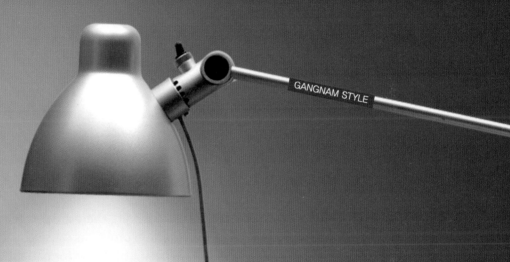

Issues with Third Molars

Issues with Third Molars

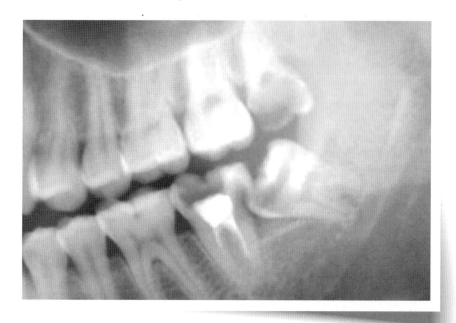

As we can see from this radiograph, there are severe carious lesions on both #37 and 38. This is one of the most common problems caused by third molars. This radiograph means a lot to me because I have been utilizing it for patient consultation since 2002. And that's why I elected to use this as the first radiograph of this chapter to illustrate the problems with third molars.

You must be wondering why I have included so many case studies here to just talk about the problems caused by third molars. I am hoping this book can be used as a reference for clinicians as well as a graphical tool to show patients potential issues related to their third molars. I myself will use this chapter to explain patients why it is important to extract third molars. Let's have a look at the problems caused by third molars.

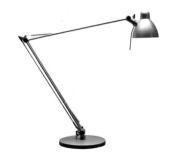

Wait!

Do we really need to extract third molars?

Do we really need to extract third molars? Why do we need to extract intact third molars? We, as dentists, receive questions like these many times. Let's read the next paragraph with an evidence based approach in order to answer those questions.

In England, third molar extractions have been provided at no charge to the public by the National Health Service. Presumably because of that, from the middle of 1990s, dentists in England had negative views toward third molar extractions based on the results from national researches reporting the complications of third molar extractions and the needlessness of prophylactic removal. Finally, on May 27, 2000 in England, National Institute for Health and Care Excellence (NICE) published the guidance on the extraction of wisdom teeth. According to that, the extraction should be limited to the third molars with non-restorable conditions such as severe carious lesions, periapical lesions, cysts or tumors. This guideline appeared promising at first, but numerous problems arose after five years. In May 2012, one article was published in British Dental Journal to evaluate the 10-year results of the NICE guideline, and many other articles were published to report the negative impacts of the guideline. According to them, the average age for third molar extraction was increased from 25 to 32, and there was more than 200% increase in the occurrence of carious lesions in third molars. Furthermore, they reported an increased number of cases of endodontic treatments and extractions of the adjacent teeth since third molars were not extracted in a timely manner. There is a greater chance of postoperative complications after the age of 38. In the beginning, the guideline resulted in 30% reduction in the number of third molar extractions. However, the number of difficult extractions (e.g. performed by specialists) has increased by 97% from the third year onwards. There was initial saving on the national budget, but currently it is causing much greater expense than before. Many researches indicated that it will be medically and economically beneficial if third molars with potential pathology are removed prophylactically. Since these researches did not take potential damage on the adjacent teeth into account, there are even more benefits from the prophylactic removal of third molars. Recent researches show that pathologic conditions from third molars are rarely resolved without extractions and more than 70% asymptomatic third molars develop pathology which requires extractions.

Wait!

Do we really need to extract third molars?

Some people say that we are not supposed to extract intact third molars since they develop and erupt as an important part of normal dentition. However, we need to discuss this statement in more detail. Around six years of age, permanent teeth start erupting and replacing deciduous dentition. By around 12 to 13 years of age, all of the permanent teeth are erupted except third molars. On average, the eruption of third molars occurs in the later teenage years which is about six years after the eruption of permanent second molars. This also means it takes about 12 years for the third molars to erupt after the appearance of the first permanent dentition. In the past, due to poor oral hygiene, it was common to see patients with missing permanent molars before the eruption of third molars. This can lead to shifting of dentition, which creates enough space for third molars to erupt. However, in the 21st century, studies have shown most people have better oral hygiene, which helps the modern people retain their permanent dentition for much longer years than the past. As a consequence, cases with inadequate space for the eruption of third molars have been increased more and more, and many researches have proven that.

In the past, many clinicians and patients believed that third molars should not be extracted prophylactically since they could be used as abutments for prostheses. However, dental treatments such as dental implants have evolved and progressed along with the advancement in technology. Nowadays, it is very rare to plan a third molar to be a functional part of dental prosthesis, and this kind of plan will make the dentist look old school. Another argument can be made for preserving third molars in order to use as an autogenous bone graft material in future implant surgery. In my opinion, preserving third molars can cause more damage to the surrounding dentition which could lead to more dental implants. There is a wide range of excellent bone graft materials available, and it is very important not to sacrifice other teeth in order to save the third molars as a source of bone grafting.

Now, you can confidently and professionally answer your patients'questions regarding their third molars, so they can make informed decisions. In my opinion, if you as a dental care provider observes symptoms from third molars or believes that they will cause problems in the future, it is better to remove them early rather than deal with the consequences at a later stage.

Written by Dr Ki Yong Kim from Gangnam Midas Dental Clinic

01
Carious lesions on third molars

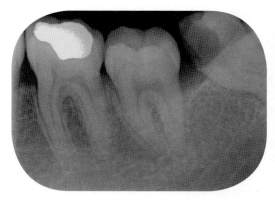 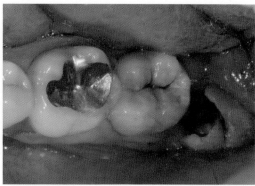 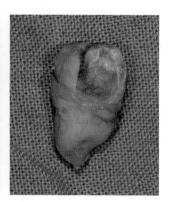

Due to a severe carious lesion, the mesial half of the third molar was fractured off causing food impaction. This could lead to halitosis, but many patients are not aware of it.

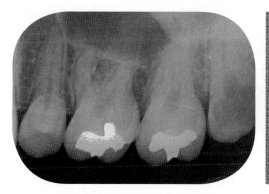 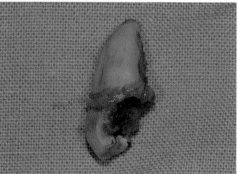

This maxillary third molar shows a severe carious lesion, which left only a thin layer of enamel. Halitosis could develop even one hour after oral hygiene.

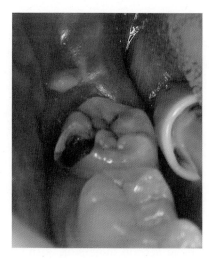 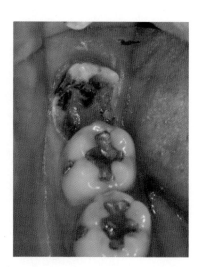

As shown above, only the third molar presented with a severe carious lesion while other teeth are intact. This kind of case is frequently observed.

Pulp polyp suggests that the carious lesion was progressing gradually over a long period of time.

02
Carious lesions on adjacent teeth due to third molars

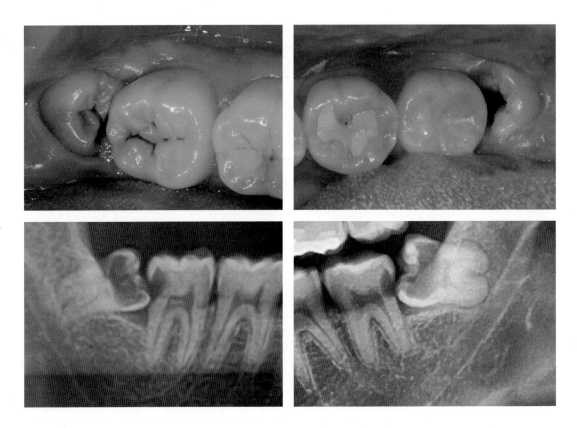

It is common to observe carious lesions not only on third molars but also on second molars. As shown above, mesially impacted third molars can cause carious lesions on the adjacent second molars, and thus it is best to extract these impacted ones as early as possible to prevent any possible damages. Carious lesions on the adjacent teeth due to third molars are also common on the maxilla. When examining radiographs, we need to pay close attention since sometimes distinct radiolucent patterns of carious lesions may not appear on them.

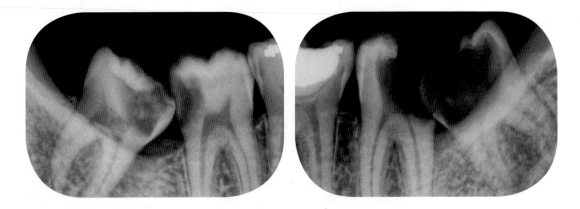

Unfortunately, this patient's mandibular second molars on both sides have developed severe carious lesions due to the impacted third molars. It is very important to evaluate and extract the third molars in a timely manner in order to save the second molars.

03
Carious lesions between maxillary second and third molars

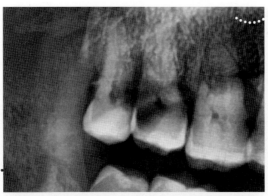
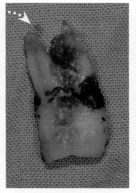
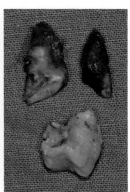

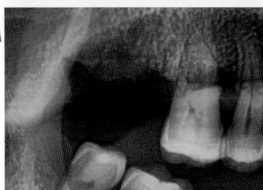

A 59-year-old male had severe carious lesions between his second and third molar. This is common due to food impaction. When this happens, most patients complain of cold sensitivity. Most of the time, the third molars are extracted first, and then the second molars are endodontically or restoratively treated. But unfortunately, there are cases when both teeth are unsalvageable. Therefore, it is important to consider prophylactic third molar extractions before the second molars are damaged.

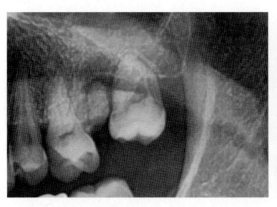
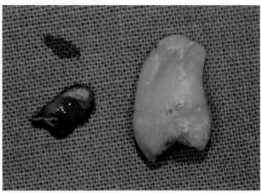

This is a case of a 55-year-old male who only has one root of #27 remaining due to the mesially impacted #28. When he was young, he was advised to have #28 removed, but he never followed the advice due to dental anxiety. He is currently undergoing implant treatments for #27.

04
Various types of carious lesions on third molars

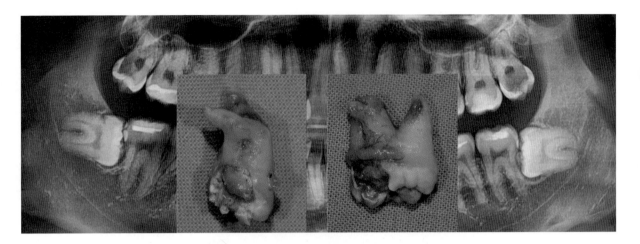

Both maxillary third molars were extracted due to severe carious lesions.

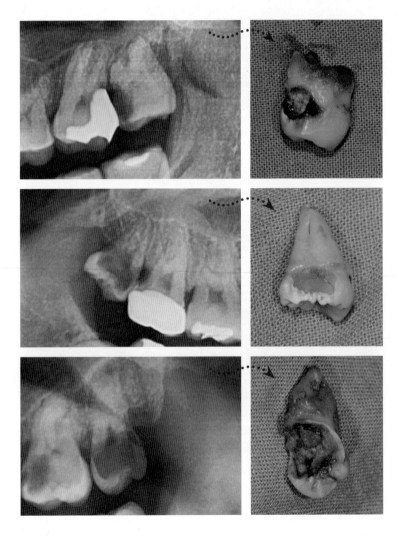

Carious lesions on maxillary third molars can occur on any surfaces.

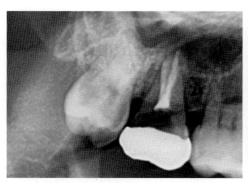 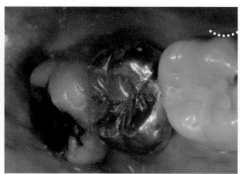 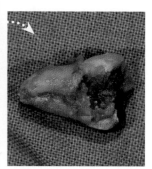

Severe carious lesions between the second and third molar are shown. This is common due to food impaction.

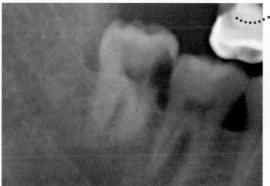 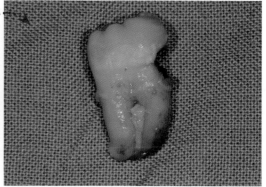

The mesial surface of this third molar has severe carious lesion which could affect the distal surface of the second molar. Halitosis from the region is frequent also due to food impaction.

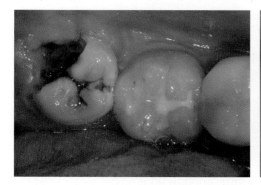 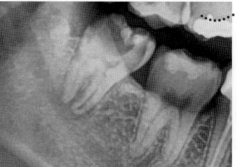 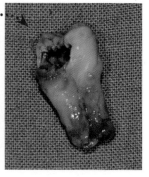

Severe carious lesion on the distal side of this third molar is most likely due to the difficulty in brushing. In addition, heavily occluding with the opposing third molar can also cause this problem. Chronic halitosis can occur from the carious lesion.

05
Carious lesions caused by food impaction

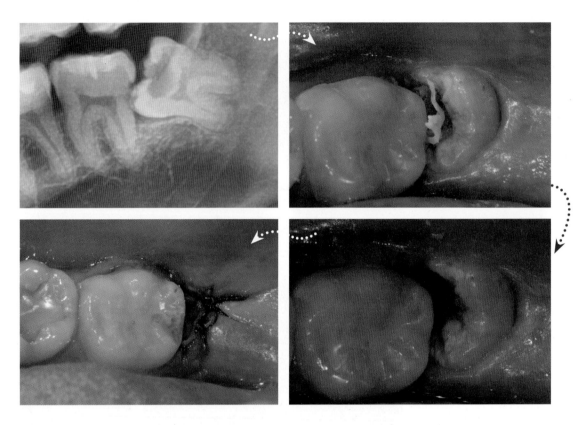

The chief complaint of this patient was food impaction between his second and third molar. Due to the restricted spacing and angulation, patients may find it hard to clean the area adequately. This may cause carious lesions but also periodontal diseases and inflammation.

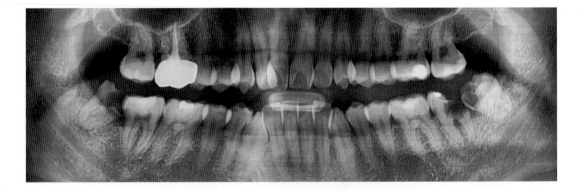

A patient who was in her early 20s presented with carious lesions on her second and third molars on both sides due to food impaction. Even though she was still very young, the carious lesions were severe enough to lead to the extraction of one of the second molars. We can assume that those third molars should have been extracted many years ago, probably during her early teenage years. Thus, this case highlights the fact that there is no early age for third molar extractions.

06
Endodontic treatments of adjacent teeth

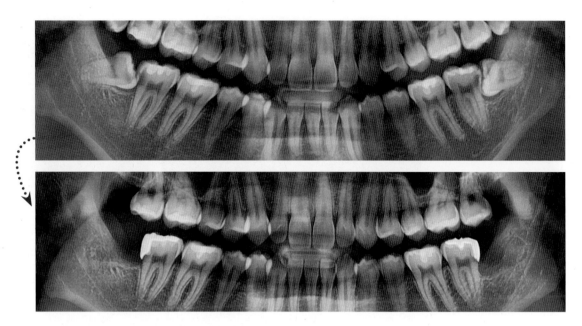

If the mandibular third molars were not there, or extracted earlier, such caries on the mandibular second molars would not have occurred.

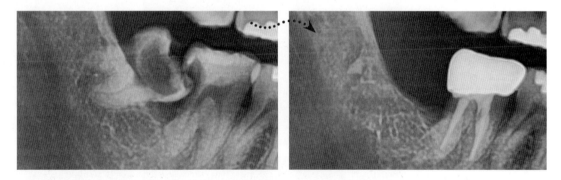

A crown was placed followed by endodontic treatment due to a carious lesion caused by the third molar. This would not have occurred if there was no third molar.

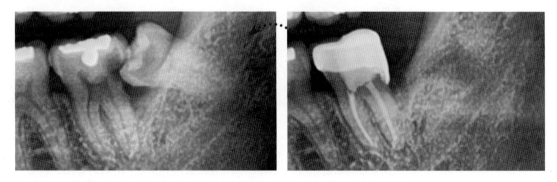

Again, #37 had endodontic treatment, and a crown was placed. Restorability of the tooth is determined by the extent of caries to the roots rather than the size of them.

07
Extraction of adjacent teeth

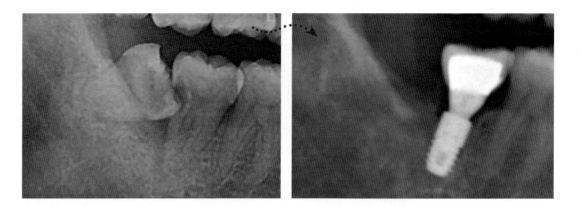

This is a case of my 40-year-old cousin. Caries on the distal of #47 extended to the roots, and periapical inflammation was along the distal side of the tooth. Endodontic treatment was attempted after removing #48, but it failed. Hence, #47 was extracted, and an implant was placed. This case has been over 10 years, and there is no problem with the implant so far.

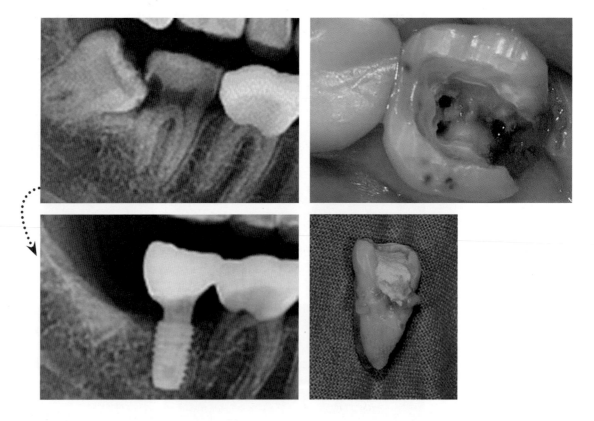

This is a case of a 28-year-old female who complained of pain around the third molar. Upon examination, pain was found to be coming from irreversible pulpitis of #47. Again, after #48 was extracted, endodontic treatment was attempted. However, the tooth was found to be nonrestorable due to the extent of the root caries, so extraction was performed. An implant was placed after the extraction.

08
Spread of infection into local tissue spaces

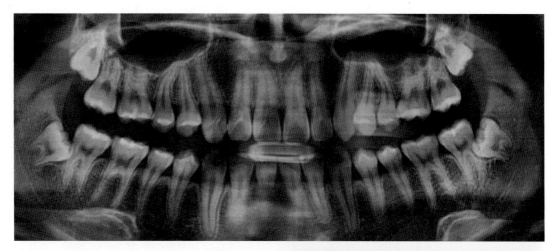

This patient presented with pain and extra and intra-oral swelling around #38. Drainage was provided as the first-line of treatment. After several rounds of drainage, purulent discharge finally stopped. I have even seen patients who came back from overseas in the middle of their business trips because of the acutely spreading infection. I have also seen that it caused a lot of problems for pregnant women and students who need to take important exams the very next day.

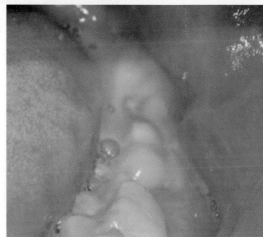

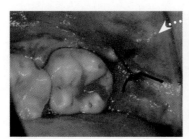

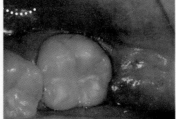

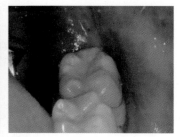

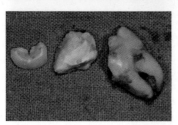

The affected tooth was removed with "Mesial crown cutting" and "Lingual crown cutting" methods once the infection was under control.

09
Calculus and periodontitis

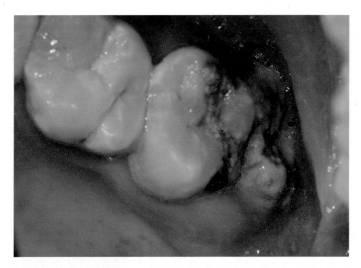

This is a clinical photograph of #28. Third molars are difficult to clean by brushing due to their position and location. In addition to that, even though most teeth can self-cleanse during mastication, non-functional third molars cannot. Therefore, plaque and calculus can easily build up around third molars, which can lead to periodontitis and halitosis.

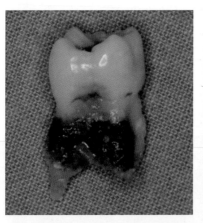

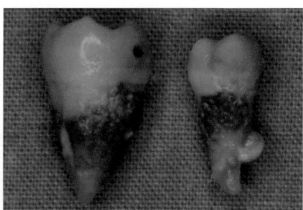

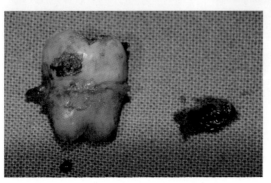

You can see the subgingival calculus almost all the way down to the apex of the root, and it means the adjacent tooth is already periodontally affected as well. From the bottom photograph, you can also see calculus around the crown. This usually causes chronic periodontitis with severe gingival edema and halitosis.

10
What do you think this is?

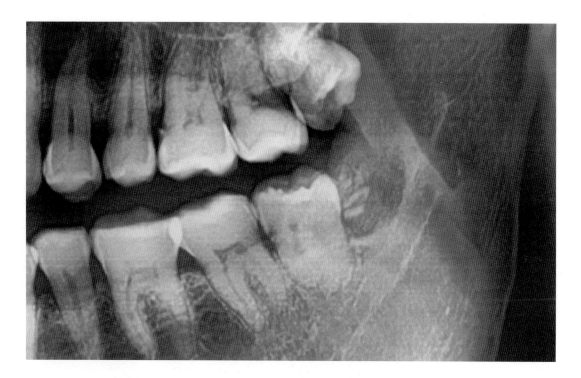

This is a panoramic radiograph of a 47-year-old radiologist at a university hospital. What is that radiolucency on the distal side of #38? And what is that radiopaque object? Even this radiologist patient was not sure about them. My differential diagnosis was OKC (odontogenic Keratocyst), calcified cyst, or tumor.

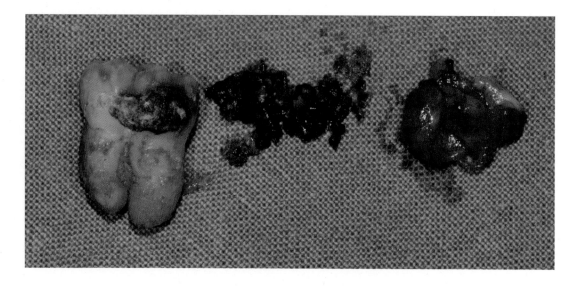

The biopsy results were chronic inflammation and calculus. Chronic inflammation can cause bone resorption and displacement of the tooth.

11
Periodontitis on second molars caused by third molars

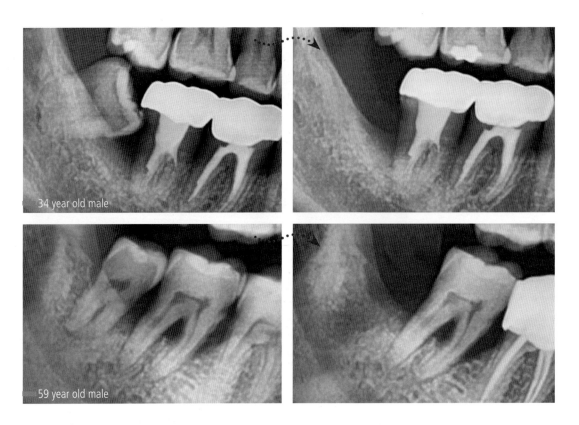

These radiographs of 34-year-old and 59-year-old male patients respectively show chronic periodontitis around the second and third molars. Continued periodontal maintenance has been performed after the third molar extractions.

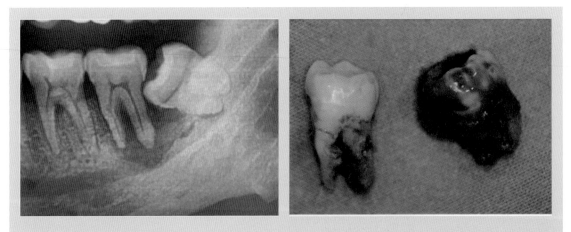

A 50-year-old male patient presented with a chief complaint of severe pain from his third molar. However, upon examination, the pain was actually coming from #37. Both #37 and #38 were removed.

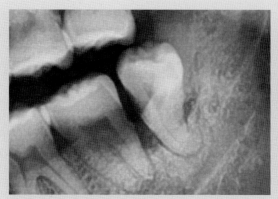 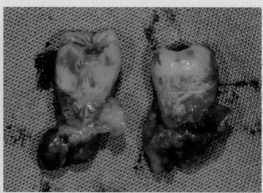

A 41-year-old female patient had discomfort around #38. Since clinical examination showed both #37 and #38 had severe inflammation and mobility, both molars were extracted with a forcep. We can see the granulation tissue from the extracted teeth.

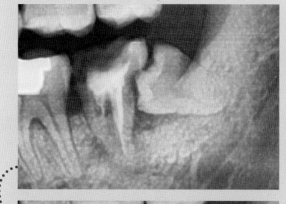 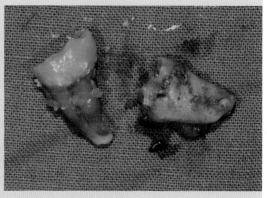

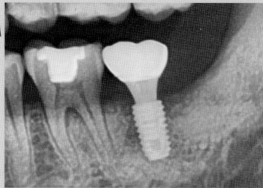

A 35-year-old male patient had #37 and #38 extracted, and an implant was placed. As you can see from the first radiograph, #37 had caries, root resorption and periodontitis. It is common to see the combination of pathologies like this around the third molars and their adjacent teeth.

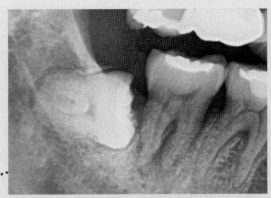
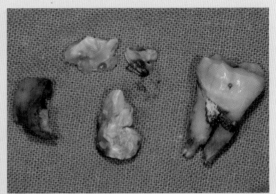
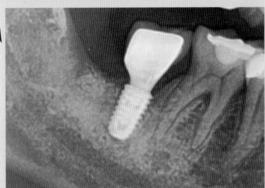

A 50-year-old male patient presented with a chief complaint of severe pain from his third molar. However, the actual etiology of inflammation was the second molar. There were food impaction, calculus and granulation tissue in between #47 and 48. After cleaning them, both teeth were extracted.

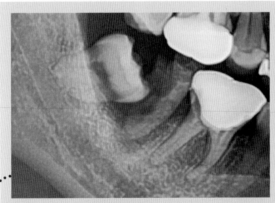
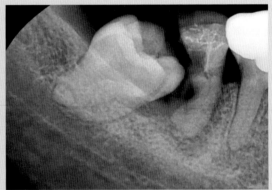
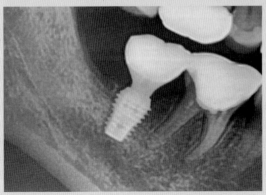

Due to a severe carious lesion and periodontitis on #47 caused by #48, a female patient in her 30s had #47 and #48 removed, and an implant was placed. We would all agree that the state of #47 would have been different if #48 was absent.

12
Mandibular gingival trauma caused by maxillary third molars

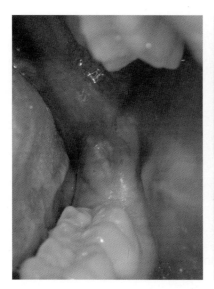
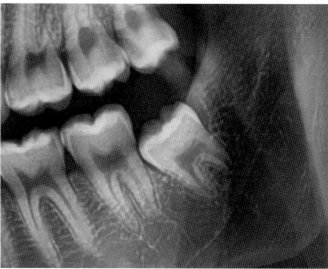

This case shows mandibular gingival trauma caused by the maxillary third molar. Initially, this kind of trauma starts as an oral ulcer and transitions to pericoronitis and then back to oral ulcer again. Oftentimes, this cycle keeps repeating. Many dentists recommend extracting mandibular third molars as a solution to interrupt this cycle of inflammation. However, since extraction of maxillary third molars is easier, it is actually a good idea to extract maxillary ones only in order to reduce this type of acute inflammation.

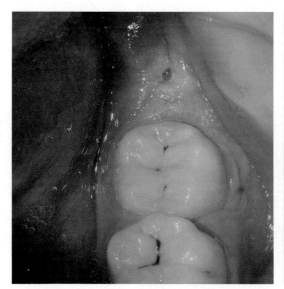
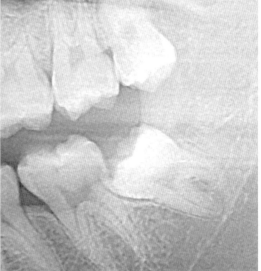

The upper third molar has made a 'hole' on mandibular gingiva. This could cause periodic gingival ulceration and pericoronitis. If mandibular third molars do not need to be extracted immediately, extracting maxillary third molars only can solve the problem.

13
Inflammation from cheek biting caused by maxillary third molars

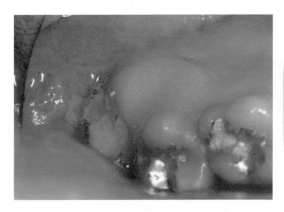 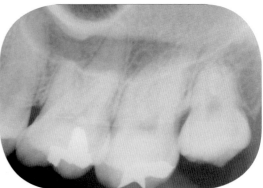

Upper third molars tend to erupt buccally and be out of the normal alignment of dentition. It causes ulceration on buccal mucosa with moderate to severe pain. Ulcers caused by the third molars are usually accompanied by more pain compared to other ones because the third molars keep irritating the ulcerated areas.

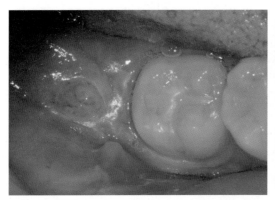 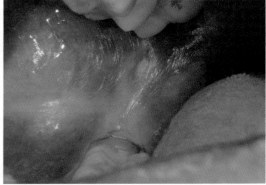

Traumatic ulcers are common around third molars.

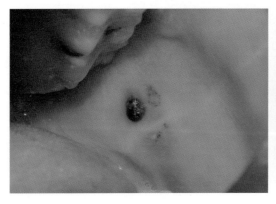 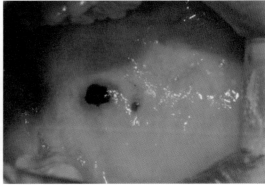

Chronic cheek biting has caused hematoma. This occurs more frequently around third molars. I have seen hematoma greater than 1 cm in diameter quite often.

Can we remove the lower third molars only?

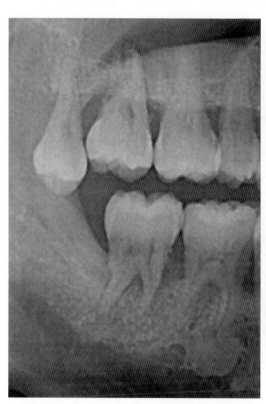
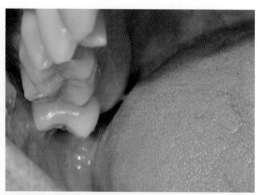
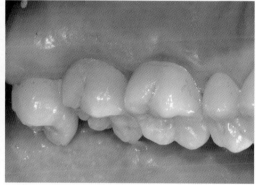

There are some patients who want to extract mandibular third molars only as the maxillary ones are not causing any problems at the time. However, without the opposing mandibular third molars, the maxillary third molars can be supraerupted excessively and cause cheek biting or occlusal interference, which in turn might create problems on other teeth.

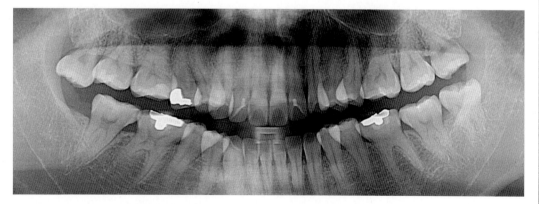

After extracting #48, #18 has supraerupted and is at a different occlusal plane from #28.

Wait!

Can we remove the lower third molars only? -Continued

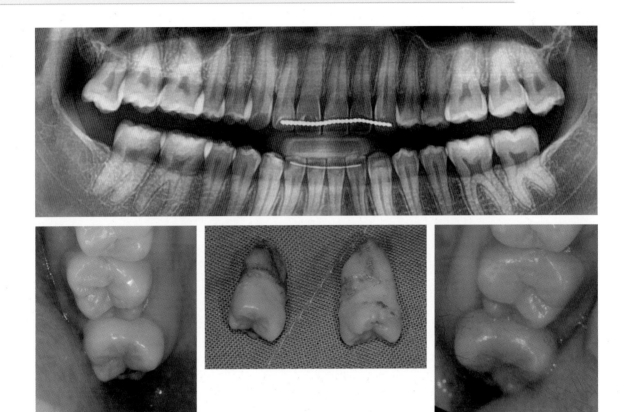

This is a case of a 25-year-old female patient. Despite her relatively young age, both #18 and #28 have been supraerupted. In order to prevent this kind of problem, the non-functional maxillary third molars need to be extracted with the mandibular third molars at the same time. That's also because the remaining third molars may develop caries and cause damage to their adjacent teeth anyways even if supraeruption does not happen.

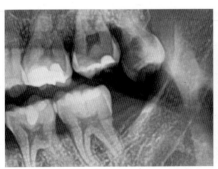
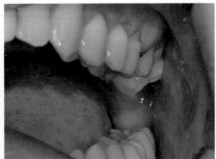
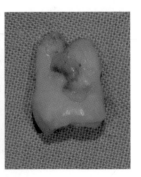

A 27-year-old male patient wanted to extract #28 which was supraerupted shortly after #38 was removed. Maxillary third molars tend to be supraerupted more often than mandibular third molars, probably because of the gravity. When I heard about this "gravity theory" for the first time, I did not believe it. But, as I was gaining more experience with third molars, that theory was making more sense because it is a fact that maxillary third molars become supraerupted more than mandibular third molars.

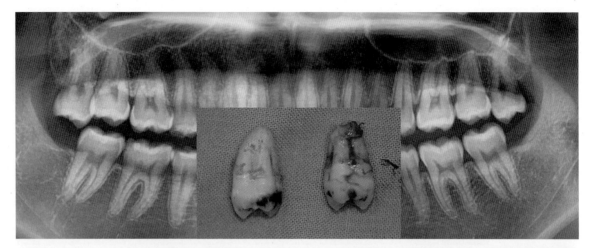

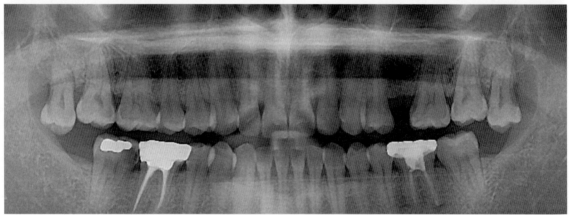

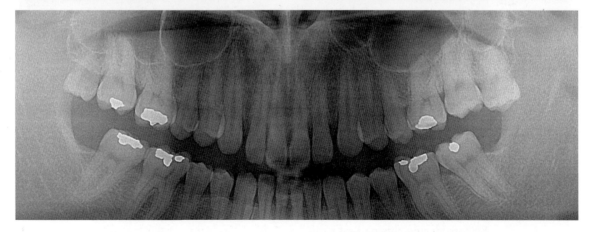

To avoid supraeruption of maxillary third molars, it is recommended to extract both maxillary and mandibular third molars at the same time. However if a patient is already undergoing or planning to start orthodontic treatment, it is best to discuss with an orthodontist. I usually extract the mandibular third molars first and then the maxillary third molars because the mandibular ones take more time than the maxillary ones.

14
Supra-erupted mandibular third molars

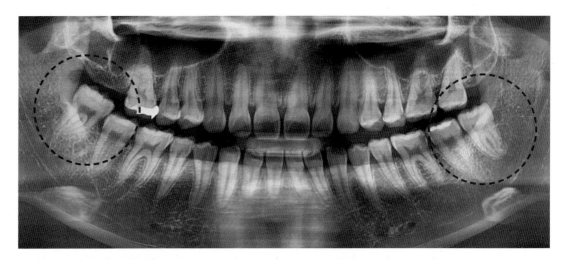

A 21-year-old female patient presented and mentioned that her #17 and #18 were removed not too long ago due to severe carious lesions. The patient was told that #48 needs to be extracted due to the supraeruption and recommended to have the #38 extracted later.

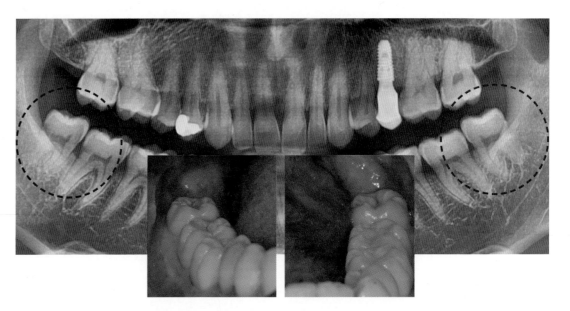

A 38-year-old male patient said he had maxillary third molars removed a few years ago but not the mandibular ones. Even though this panoramic radiograph shows mild supraeruption of the mandibular third molars, moderate supraeruption of both third molars was observed clinically. By considering this patient's mild class II malocclusion and forwarded mandible position while taking the panoramic radiograph, we can assume that the third molars merely occlude with the maxillary second molars.

15
Mandibular fracture

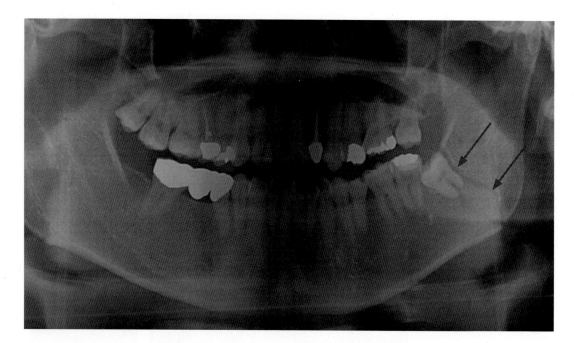

In this panoramic radiograph, you can see an angle fracture around an impacted third molar. Even though condylar fractures are more common in the absence of third molars, there is not enough evidence to say that the angle fractures are caused by the presence of third molars which presumably weaken the bone around them. Actually, regardless of the presence or absence of the third molars, mandibular fractures can happen with any force that is strong enough to fracture the weakest point of the mandible. Therefore, it's not convincing that we need to remove third molars in order to prevent the mandibular fractures, but I just want you to know for future reference that there are some theories like this.

16
Root resorption of second molars

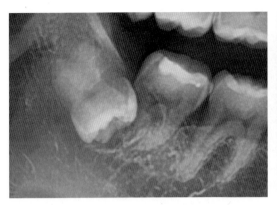
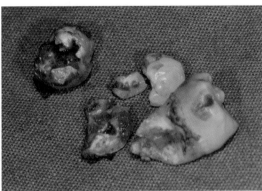

Even though it does not happen all the time, third molars often cause resorption on second molars. It usually involves roots when it happens, so a lot of times both second and third molars end up being extracted unfortunately.

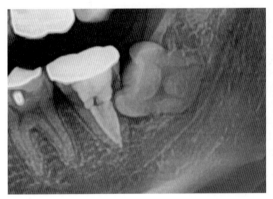
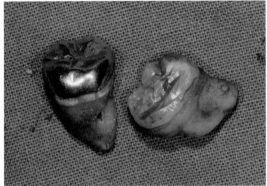

#37 has undergone an endodontic treatment followed by a crown placement. However, the root resorption caused by the third molar could not be prevented.

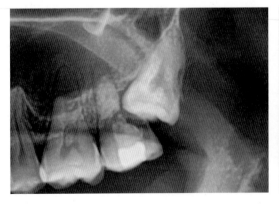
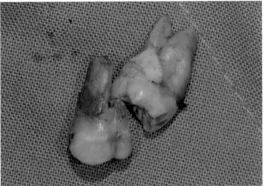

This shows the resorption of a maxillary second molar. Carious lesions caused by third molars on the adjacent teeth are more common on the mandible, but the root resorption caused by third molars on the adjacent teeth happens on the maxilla as frequently as on the mandible. In this case, it is possible to extract #27 and orthodontically reposition #28 to the second molar site. However, many factors including the location and anatomy of the tooth, patient's age and other treatment options such as dental implants need to be considered.

17
Cysts and tumours around third molar crowns

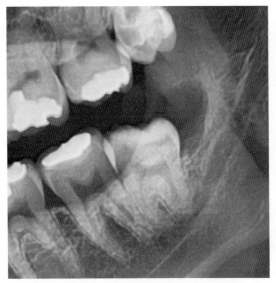

A biopsy was ordered after the extraction due to a radiolucency around the distal aspect of #38, and it was confirmed to be just inflammation instead of a dentigerous cyst.

It can be assumed that #38 has been displaced vertically due to the pericoronal cyst.

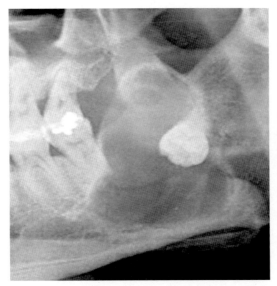

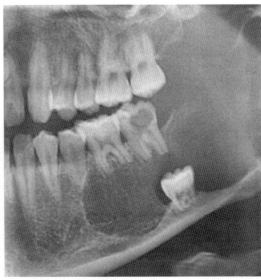

Since I extract so many third molars, I see some serious cysts and tumours like these from time to time.

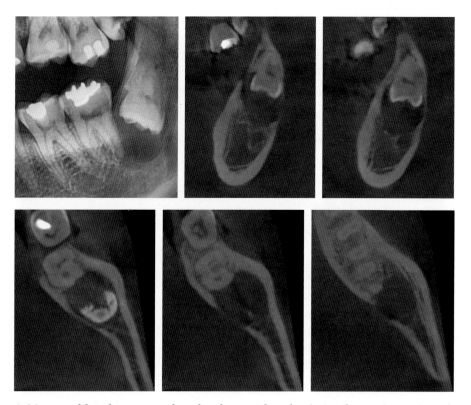

A 30-year-old male presented to the clinic with a chief complaint of pain from his third molar. A large pericoronal radiolucency was observed from a panoramic radiograph, so CBCT was taken. Due to the cyst, #38 was found to be displaced, and there was almost no cortical bone left because the alveolar bone around the height of contour of the crown was resorbed too much. It is important to order a biopsy as dentigerous cysts can sometimes but not often become malignant.

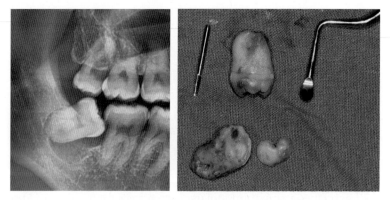

This 39-year-old male originally presented to another clinic with chief complaints of severe pain, edema and halitosis. The dentist referred him to a university hospital, but he came to my clinic instead. I was a little afraid of the cyst because it was developed around the crown, but it was found to be a paradental cyst after biopsy. The extracted third molar shows root surface calculus and remnants of granulation tissue. Due to the close proximity to the inferior alveolar nerve, curettage of the socket from the bottom was not performed. Instead, a serrated surgical curette was carefully used to pull the cyst up from the middle of the socket.

18
It was thought to be another typical third molar case, but...

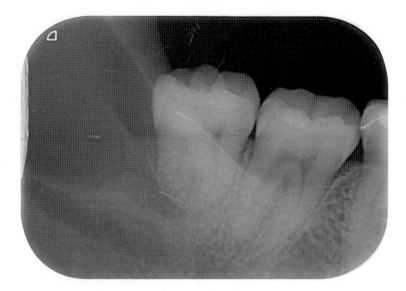

A female patient in her mid 20s wanted to have her #48 removed. Because Korean Health Insurance Review and Assessment Service suggested that dentists should reduce the number of panoramic radiographs during new patient examinations at that time, a periapical radiograph was taken initially. As shown above, the distal of #48 looked suspicious, so a panoramic radiograph was taken to evaluate the area better.

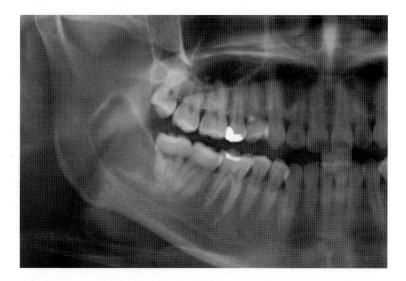

The patient was referred to a university hospital as the radiolucency did not appear as a typical dentigerous cyst. She was diagnosed with ameloblastoma, and I felt sorry for her. It would have been better if she had gotten her dental examination done earlier since early detection is important for a better prognosis. Please google ameloblastoma if you want to know more about it.

DR. YOUNGSAM KIM'S CLINICAL NOTES;
EXTRACTION OF THIRD MOLARS

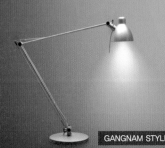

GANGNAM STYLE　Easy Simple Safe Efficient Minimally Invasive & atraumatic **Extraction of Third Molars**